Surgical Research

Basic Principles and Clinical Practice

Third Edition

Edited by

H. Troidl   M.F. McKneally   D.S. Mulder
A.S. Wechsler   B. McPeek   W.O. Spitzer

With Foreword by Sir James Black

With 99 Illustrations

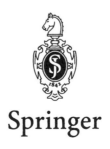

Springer

Hans Troidl, Department of Surgery, University of Cologne, Ostmerheimer Strasse 200, D-51109 Cologne, Germany

Martin F. McKneally, University of Toronto, Joint Centre for Bioethics, and The Toronto Hospital, 200 Elizabeth Street, EN 10-230, Toronto, Ontario M5G 2C4, Canada

David S. Mulder, Department of Surgery, McGill University, Montreal General Hospital, Montreal, Quebec, Canada H3G 1A4

Andrew S. Wechsler, Department of Surgery, Medical College of Virginia, Virginia Commonwealth University, Richmond, VA 23298-0645, USA

Bucknam McPeek, Department of Anaesthesia, Harvard University, Massachusetts General Hospital, Boston, MA 02114-2696, USA

Walter O. Spitzer, Genentech, Inc., 460 Point San Bruno Boulevard, South San Francisco, California 94080-4990, USA

Library of Congress Cataloging-in-Publication Data
Surgical research : basic principles and clinical practice / [edited
 by] H. Troidl . . . [et al.]. — 3rd ed.
    p. cm.
  Rev. ed. of: Principles and practice of research. 2nd ed. c1991.
  Includes bibliographical references and index.
  ISBN 0-387-94699-3 (hardcover : alk. paper)
  1. Surgery—Research—Methodology. I. Troidl, Hans, 1938– .
 II. Principles and practice of research.
  [DNLM: 1. Surgery. 2. Research. 3. Research Support. WO 20
 S961 1997]
 RD29.S87 1997
 617′.0072—dc21   97-13782

Printed on acid-free paper.

RD
29
.S87
1998

Previously published under the title: *Principles and Practice of Research: Strategies for Surgical Investigators.*

Production coordinated by Impressions Book and Journals Services, Inc., and managed by Lesley Poliner; manufacturing supervised by Joe Quatela.
Typeset by Impressions Book and Journal Services, Inc., Madison, WI.
Printed and bound by Edwards Brothers, Inc., Ann Arbor, MI.
Printed in the United States of America.

9 8 7 6 5 4 3 2 1

ISBN 0-387-94699-3 Springer-Verlag New York Berlin Heidelberg   SPIN 10015879

This book is dedicated to
our students and to our teachers.

Foreword to Third Edition

Sir James Black

Fifty years ago, I was learning the elementary principles of surgery as a medical student. That was still the era when surgery was about pus and blood; medicine was about prayers and poultices! The surgical imagination was circumscribed by what could be seen. The bedrock of surgery, in those days, was gross anatomy. *Gray's Anatomy* was every medical student's incubus. I have to say that I had no interest in a career in surgery. My school motto was "Lux in tenebris" (light in darkness) and to me it was physiology, not anatomy, that I thought would shine light in to the dark places of medicine. Fifty years ago, I had no idea that illumination would come from a new kind of anatomy, a chemical anatomy. The molecular and genetic revolution was an unimagined future.

Today, the excitement in surgery is about espousing the new molecular anatomy. Surgeons still see the blood and gross anatomical structures as the operation progresses, but their mind's eye is now focused on invisible structures—the growth factors, interleukins, adhesion molecules, second messengers, and transcription factors—that may be disturbed by the disease and by the knife. Today's surgeon is an implicit molecular biologist. The laboratory is becoming as important as the operating theater. Concerns about measurement, evaluation, concepts, and theories have led to the development *theoretical surgery*, a wholly new academic discipline. The name may sound like an oxymoron, but it aptly sums up the nature of the revolution. In addition to excursions to the laboratory, the database of academic surgery has been expanded by development of controlled clinical trials and clinical audit. Surgical judgment is constantly being sharpened by evaluation.

Fifty years from now, what will surgery be like? Trauma will always be with us. So, so will surgery! Perhaps it will have a new millennial name, like "tissue engineering," but we can be sure that surgeons as we know them today will still be around, and we can be sure that they will have adapted to changes in both understanding and patterns of disease. The speed with which surgeons responded to the loss of their bread and butter with the arrival of the histamine H_2-receptor antagonists was truly remarkable. So what will they be up to? Before the middle of the next century there will be deep insight into how the physiological processes of cell division, chemotaxis, and apoptosis are controlled and regulated. The kinetics and rate-limiting steps of control sequences of commands will be common knowledge. The parallel-coupled interactions between simultaneously operating linear pathways, both within and between cells, will be well understood. Many control arrangements will probably be recognized to have neural-net complexity, with built-in redundancy, operating at the edge of chaos. We can speak and write only in narrative form, one event following another in a linear pathway. Comprehension of nonlinear, parallel-coupled, hierarchically organized biological systems can probably be achieved only by mathematical models that will probably have become accepted by surgeons as indispensable working tools. Why do I imagine that surgeons will ever be bothered to master all this stuff? Because I think that then as now, surgeons will be where the action is. Organ transplantation, one of the major successes of surgery in this century, was built on the back of advances in immunology. I imagine that, in the next century, surgeons will be busy with programmed cell transplantation that will exploit advances in cell biology. Cells from a patient's sick sinoatrial node, incompetent sphincter, or diseased brain might be removed, cultured with specific growth factors, and transfected with genes for specific chemotactic factors to create a command center that will attract appropriate nerve endings when it is sur-

gically grafted back into the sinoatrial node or sphincter or brain. Surgical cell and tissue engineering could add another revolution to medical science. Fantasy? Probably. We can be sure, however, that there will be surgeons, busy as always, and closely in touch with the biomedical science of the day.

This book, written by an outstanding group of thoughtful surgical scientists, clearly indicates that their eyes are cocked to the surgical science of the future. Their energy and scholarship make me feel confident about the future of surgical research.

68 Half Moon Lane
Dulwich, London, England SE24 9JE

Foreword to Second Edition

R.L. Cruess

This book addresses problems that are fundamental to the future of surgical practice. Although the enormous impact of technology on the practice of medicine has broadened the types of therapy that are possible, it has tended to reemphasize the age-old pressures to make surgeons into technicians rather than compassionate physicians or scientists. Nevertheless, without an ongoing and regularly updated scientific basis for surgical practice, surgeons do indeed become mere technicians.

John Hunter became a surgeon in the late 18th century when surgery was a craft rather than a science. By the time he died, he had incorporated science as an essential part of surgery and had founded a tradition of investigation that has remained unbroken ever since. The pride of surgeons in their skills and knowledge, and the intellectual satisfaction they gain from the surgical act are derived from this tradition.

It is surgeons who must pose the questions about the surgical aspects of the diseases they treat. The nutritional problems and requirements of surgical patients were not defined until they were investigated by surgeons, and the therapeutic intravenous solutions we now use were developed in surgical research laboratories.

Modern joint replacements are the result of surgeons' investigations of the problems posed by arthritic patients, and surgeons have participated actively in identifying the causes of arthritis. Much of our present understanding of epilepsy developed in response to questions posed by neurosurgeons, and a host of other examples demonstrate how patients have benefitted from the questions surgeons ask.

Shifts in the academic centers of surgery during the last 150 years have been uniformly based on surgeons' perceptions of the state of the surgical sciences throughout the world. Surgeons have traveled for their training and intellectual enrichment to the centers at the forefront at any given time. The European centers that had such great influence in the late 19th and early 20th centuries, the renowned teaching hospitals in the United Kingdom, and the great academic centers in North America have all been built around research laboratories and inquiring surgical minds.

No operating surgeon or anaesthetist is satisfied with all aspects of contemporary surgical and clinical management. Accordingly, research is not just desirable, it is a necessity imposed upon us. The authors of this book are attempting to lay down a proper framework for the organization of surgical research. The benefits will not be for surgeons but for mankind.

McGill University
Montreal, Canada

Foreword to First Edition

J.C. Goligher

For some readers, the title of this book will immediately raise the question, what exactly is meant by surgical research? In the very broadest sense, the term can be taken to include all endeavors, however elementary or limited in scope, to advance surgical knowledge. Ideally, it refers to well-organized attempts to establish on a proper scientific basis (i.e., to place beyond reasonable doubt) the truth or otherwise of any concepts, old or new, within the ambit of surgery and, of course, anaesthesia.

The methods used to achieve that end vary enormously, depending on the issue being investigated. They comprise a wide range of activities in the wards, outpatient clinics, operating rooms, or laboratories, such as simple clinical or operative observations and clinical or laboratory investigations involving biophysics, biochemistry, pathology, bacteriology, and other disciplines. Well-planned animal experimentation is exceedingly important, and it is well to remember the old truism that every surgical operation is a biological experiment whose results, unfortunately, are not always as carefully documented and analyzed as they should be. When the findings of any clinical, operative, or laboratory study are being considered, stringent statistical methods must be applied to ensure that any conclusions rest on a statistically sound basis.

Surgery provides an almost unlimited range of topics for research. Much of what is practiced and taught in surgery consists of traditional concepts passed from surgical teacher to surgical trainee by example, by word of mouth, or by standard texts, without ever having been submitted to really objective assessment. Every year we see scores of promising new ideas emerging on the surgical scene to challenge orthodoxy. Although these innovations are often greeted with great optimism, a factual basis for that enthusiasm is sometimes far from secure, and much further work is frequently required to discover whether we are dealing with genuine advances.

The most exciting and attractive scenario for surgical research is unquestionably one that depicts a successful attempt by a researcher to establish the accuracy of some bold innovation for which he himself is responsible. Joseph Lister, demonstrating by clinical trial that wound suppuration could be combated by antiseptic measures, comes to mind, along with Lester Dragstedt showing by experimental and clinical studies that vagotomy could play a valuable role in the treatment of peptic ulcer disease.

In all well-developed countries, and most notably in the United States, there is now strong pressure on surgeons in training to engage in a period of research in order to foster a critical attitude toward the appraisal of the results of surgical treatment, and to stimulate a continuing interest in combining investigative work with clinical practice.

Hitherto, acquainting the tyro researcher with the methods appropriate to his or her particular project has usually depended on the guidance of more experienced colleagues working in the same field, and on the acquisition of a gradually increasing understanding of how to conduct research as the result of being in a research environment. It is very surprising that there has been no textbook to which the young researcher could turn to secure a more systematic presentation of the various matters of importance in undertaking surgical research. Hans Troidl, David Mulder, Martin McKneally, Walter Spitzer, and Bucknam McPeek are to be congratulated most warmly on their great perspicacity in recognizing the claimant need for a work providing this sort of information and, even more, on the supremely effective way in which they have met that need by the production of their new book.

Principles and Practice of Research covers its subject in an unusually comprehensive way that includes not only the conduct of research in general, but also the special facilities and problems encountered in several personal attributes that are conducive to success in research, such as a certain amount of open-mindedness combined with the enthusiasm and determination needed to carry a project through to its ultimate conclusion despite the various obstacles that may be encountered en route. Not to be forgotten in this connection is the decisive role played by sheer good luck in achieving a successful outcome in research—as is true of many other activities in life. An important subsidiary matter in the prosecution of investigative work is how to present an account of that work and its results most effectively, at subsequent meetings or discussion groups and in publications; this book offers very helpful advice on all these points. Very appropriately, a concluding section affords an inspiring appraisal of future prospects in surgical research by that great surgeon-researcher, Francis Moore of Boston, whose contributions to surgical knowledge are legion.

I have no doubts that *Principles and Practice of Research* will be very widely read and greatly appreciated, not only by surgical trainees starting on research work, but also by experienced researchers and established surgeons who will welcome the wealth of information it provides on every facet of surgical research. Since research follows essentially the same principles in anaesthesia, medicine, obstetrics, gynecology, and other fields of clinical activity, this book should prove equally helpful to beginning or established investigators in other branches of health care. It cannot, in my judgment, fail to secure an assured place in the libraries of all medical schools, departments of surgery, and clinical departments the world over, as well as in the studies of many individual purchasers.

University of Leeds
Leeds, England

Acknowledgments

The editors acknowledge indebtedness to the authors of this textbook, who have generously given their time to share knowledge and experience in diverse fields with us, and with you, the reader. Like all truly able people, they are heavily committed, with active lives of scientific inquiry. We encourage them to take pride in their creative ownership of this third edition.

Dr. Troidl thanks all of his friends who worked so hard to finish their chapters, and his devoted office staff, Heidrun Mindhoff, Regina Langen, and Hedi Vier. He acknowledges in particular Martin McKneally, "He is the editor of the third edition," and his wife Deborah McKneally, "She was the heart of the book personally and professionally."

Dr. Mulder acknowledges the sacrifices his wife and family have made to give him the time to work on this and other academic tasks, and the surgical colleagues who provided clinical care in his absence. They recognized and supported this activity as part of the academic mission of their division, and share responsibility for its completion. He thanks Deborah and Martin McKneally for managing the organizational and editorial work, and all of the editors for their positive impact on his academic life, the international camaraderie and the resulting broader perspectives in thought, exchange of surgical residents, readings, and friendship.

Dr. McPeek thanks the other editors' families for their hard work, grace, and kindness during the preparation of this book, and the editors jointly and severally for their thoughtful ideas, comment, and advice, along with many friends at Harvard, Massachusetts General Hospital, Cologne, Montreal, Toronto, Richmond, and Marburg. He thanks Alexandra McPeek, his daughter, for her constant support that made his work on the third edition possible, the residents and students from Harvard, Cologne, McGill, and Toronto, and Mrs. Jeanette Cohan for her help with the manuscripts.

Dr. Wechsler acknowledges the warm friendship among the editors, and the strong efforts of Deborah and Martin McKneally, enabling the completion of the book. He thanks his wife Donna and daughters Jennifer and Hollis for their uncompromising support and tolerance of absences and distractions from their lives together, his colleagues and students for intellectual stimulation, and his secretarial associates Susan Clarke and Debbie Crenshaw.

Dr. McKneally thanks his wife Deborah for managing manuscripts, reading and correcting all page proofs, and keeping the book on a realistic production schedule; his son Gregory for editorial help and for the design on the chapter headings and cover; and the surgical residents in the Thoracic Surgical Laboratory at the University of Toronto, Dr. Stephen Cassivi and Dr. Andrew Pierre, and student Tim Jancelewicz for technical help with the intensive review and production phase; the production team at Springer-Verlag; the Surgical Directorate at The Toronto Hospital; and the University of Toronto Department of Surgery for support during the writing of this book.

Contents

Contributors

John Alexander-Williams, MD, ChM, FRCS, FACS
Consultant Surgeon, Birmingham, Nuffield, & Priory Hospitals, 5 Farquhar Road East, Birmingham B15 3RD, United Kingdom

Dmitri J. Anastakis, MD, MEd
Assistant Professor, University of Toronto, Divisions of Plastic and Orthopaedic Surgery, The Toronto Hospital Western Division, 399 Bathurst Street, West Wing 5-832, Toronto, Ontario M5T 2S8 Canada

Charles M Balch, MD
President and CEO, City of Hope, 1500 East Duarte Road, Duarte, California 91010-3000, U.S.A.

J.K. Banerjee, MD
Rural Medicare Centre, Department of Surgery, Ward No. 6, Peelkhana Mehrauli, New Delhi 110030, India

D. Bartsch, MD
Department of General Surgery, Philipps-University, Baldingerstrasse, D-35043 Marburg, Germany

J. Benbassat, MD
JDC Brookdale Institute of Gerontology and Human Development, P.O. Box 13087, Jerusalem 91130, Israel

James Bennett, PhD
Associate Professor, Division of Cardiothoracic Surgery and Department of Pharmacology, Albany Medical College, ME-514/A-62, Albany, New York 12208, U.S.A.

Sir James Black
J. Black Foundation, 68 Halfmoon Lane, Dulwich, London SE24 9JE, United Kingdom

Peter McL. Black, MD
Professor of Surgery, Harvard Medical School, Chief of Neurosurgery, Brigham and Women's Hospital, Boston, Massachusetts 02115, U.S.A.

Bertil Bouillon, MD
II. Department of Surgery, University of Cologne, Ostmerheimer Strasse 200, D-51109 Cologne, Germany

Stephen D. Cassivi, MD
Research Fellow, Thoracic Surgery Research Laboratory, The Toronto Hospital, CCRW 1-810, 101 College Street, Toronto, Ontario M5G 1L7 Canada

Mary E. Charlson, MD
Associate Professor of Medicine, Cornell University Medical Center, Attending Physician and Director, The Clinical Epidemiology Unit, New York Hospital, New York, New York 10021, U.S.A.

Chu-Jeng (Ray) Chiu, MD, PhD
Professor of Surgery, McGill University,
Montreal General Hospital, 1650 Cedar
Avenue, #947, Montreal, Quebec H3G 1A4,
Canada

W. Randolph Chitwood, Jr., MD
Professor and Chairman, Department of
Surgery, Division of Cardiothoracic Surgery, E.
Carolina University School of Medicine, Moye
Boulevard, Greenville, North Carolina 27858,
U.S.A.

R.P. (Pat) Cochran, MD
Associate Professor, Division of Cardiothoracic
Surgery, University of Washington School of
Medicine, Seattle, Washington 98195-6310,
U.S.A.

Robert Cohen, PhD
Surgical Education Office, University of
Toronto, The Banting Institute, 100 College
Street, Toronto, Ontario M5G 1L5, Canada

George T. Christakis, MD
Cardiovascular Surgery, Sunnybrook Health
Science Center, Toronto, Ontario M4N 3M5,
Canada

Deborah J. Cook, MD
Department of Medicine, McMaster University,
St. Joseph's Hospital, Fontbonne Building,
Room 505-2, Hamilton, Ontario L8N 4A6,
Canada

H. Brendan Devlin, CBE, MD
Fir Tree House, Hilton, Yarm, Cleveland
TS15 9JY, United Kingdom

Chadli Dziri, MD
General Surgery, Hôpital Charles Nicolle,
1006 Tunis, Tunisia

Stanley Dziuban, MD
Chief of Thoracic Surgery, St. Peter's Hospital,
319 South Manning Blvd., Suite 301, Albany,
New York 12208, U.S.A.

Mary E. Evans
Freelance Technical Editor, Scarborough
Hospital, Scarborough, North Yorkshire
YO12 6QL, United Kingdom

Ernst Eypasch, MD
II. Department of Surgery, University of
Cologne, Ostmerheimer Strasse 200, D-51109
Cologne, Germany

P.-L. Fagniez, MD
Service de Chirurgie Générale, Hôpital Henri-
Mondor, 51, av. De Lattre de Tassigny, F-94010
Creteil, France

John R. Farndon, MD
Professor of Surgery, University of Bristol, Level
7, Bristol Royal Infirmary, Bristol BS2 8HW,
United Kingdom

Abe Fingerhut, MD
Centre Hospitalier Intercommunal, 10, rue de
Champ Gaillard, Poissy 78303, France

Josef E. Fischer, MD
Chairman, Department of Surgery, University of
Cincinnati College of Medicine, 231 Bethesda
Avenue, Cincinnati, Ohio 45267-0558, U.S.A.

David M. Fleiszer, MD
Department of Surgery, Montreal General
Hospital, Room L9-313, Montreal, Quebec
H3G 1A4, Canada

Steven Gallinger, MD, MSc
Associate Professor of Surgery, University of
Toronto, Mt. Sinai Hospital, 600 University
Avenue, Suite 1225, Toronto, Ontario
M5G 1Z5, Canada

Dietrich Götze, MD
Springer-Verlag, D-6900 Heidelberg, Germany

David J. Hackam, MD
Department of Surgery, The Toronto Hospital,
200 Elizabeth Street, Toronto, Ontario
M5G 2C4, Canada

Paul C. Hébert, MD
Associate Professor of Medicine and
Epidemiology, University of Ottawa, Ottawa
General Hospital, Toom LM-11, 501 Smyth
Road, Mailbox 205, Ottawa, Ontario K1H 8L6,
Canada

Kathryn J. Hoffman, MSLS
Executive Director, Research Medical Library,
M.D. Anderson Cancer Center, Houston, Texas
77030-4095, U.S.A.

Jürgen Höher, MD
II. Department of Surgery, University of
Cologne, Ostmerheimer Strasse 200, D-51109
Cologne, Germany

E. Carmack Holmes, MD
William P. Longmire Jr. Chair in Surgery,
UCLA School of Medicine, 72-131 Center for
the Health Sciences, Box 951749, Los Angeles,
California 90024, U.S.A.

Sarah M. Horwitz, MD
Department of Epidemiology and Public
Health, Yale University School of Medicine,
New Haven, Connecticut 06510, U.S.A.

Wolf H. Isselhard, MD
Professor of Experimental Surgery, Director,
Institute of Experimental Medicine, University
of Cologne, Robert Koch-Strasse 10, D-50931
Cologne, Germany

Christopher Jamieson, MBBS
Office of Surgical Education, University of
Toronto, The Banting Institute, 100 College
Street, Toronto, Ontario M5G 1L5, Canada

Norman A. Johanson, MD
Professor of Orthopaedic Surgery, Cornell
University Medical College, Chief of
Orthopaedics, Bronx Veterans Administration
Medical Center, New York, New York 10021,
U.S.A.

Shaf Keshavjee, MD, MSc
Assistant Professor of Surgery, University of
Toronto, Division of Thoracic Surgery, The
Toronto Hospital, 200 Elizabeth Street,
EN10–224, Toronto, Ontario M5G 2C4,
Canada

Job Kievit, MD
Medical Decision Making Unit, Leiden
University Medical School, Building 1 K6-R,
P.O. Box 9600, 2300 RC Leiden, The
Netherlands

L. Köhler, MD
II. Department of Surgery, University of
Cologne, Ostmerheimer Strasse 200, D-51109
Cologne, Germany

Irving Kron, MD, FACS
Department of Surgery, University of Virginia
Health Science Center, Box 181, Charlottesville,
Virginia 22908, U.S.A.

Cheng-kiong Kum, MD
Senior Lecturer in Surgery, The National
University of Singapore, 5 Lower Kent Ridge
Road, Singapore 0511

Karyn S. Kunzelman, PhD
Research Associate Professor, Division of
Cardiothoracic Surgery, University of
Washington Medical Center, Mailstop: Box
356310, 1959 NE Pacific Street, Seattle,
Washington 98195, U.S.A.

Jürgen Kusche
Professor, Madaus GmbH, D-5000 Cologne-
Merheim, Germany

Karl W. Lauterbach, MD, ScD
Institut für Gesundheitsökonomik, Gleuler
Strasse 176, 50931 Cologne, Germany

Valerie A. Lawrence, MD
Department of Medicine, University of Texas
Health Science Center, San Antonio, Texas
78284-7879, U.S.A.

Francis E. LeBlanc, MD
Professor and Chairman, Division of
Neurosurgery, Foothills Hospital, Calgary,
Alberta T2N 2T9, Canada

Rolf Lefering, MD
Biochemical & Experimental Division, II.
Department of Surgery, University of Cologne,
Ostmerheimer Strasse 200, D-51109 Cologne,
Germany

Bernard Lewerich
Springer-Verlag, D-6900 Heidelberg, Germany

J.M. Little, MD
Emeritus Professor, Centre for Values, Ethics,
and the Law in Medicine, University of Sydney,
Department of Surgery, Black Burn Building,
DO6, Sydney N.S.W. 2006, Australia

Stephen Lock, CBE, MD
110 Seddon House, The Barbican, London
EC2Y 8BX, United Kingdom

Prof. Dr. Wilfried Lorenz
Head, Institute of Theoretical Surgery, Centre
of Operative Medicine, Philipps-University of
Marburg, Baldingerstrasse, 35033 Marburg,
Germany

Thomas A. Louis, PhD
Division of Biostatistics, School of Public
Health, University of Minnesota, Minneapolis,
Minnesota, U.S.A.

Helen M. MacRae, MA, MD
Mt. Sinai Hospital, Room 1525, 600 University
Avenue, Toronto, Ontario M5G 1X5, Canada

Stephen A. Marion, MD
Department of Health Care and Epidemiology,
University of British Columbia, Vancouver,
British Columbia V6T 1W5, Canada

John C. Marshall, MD, FRCSC, FACS
General and Critical Care Surgery, The Toronto
Hospital, EN 9-234, 200 Elizabeth Street,
Toronto, Ontario M5G 2C4, Canada

Douglas Martin, PhD
University of Toronto Joint Centre for Bioethics,
88 College Street, Toronto, Ontario M5G 1L4,
Canada

Arthur D. Mason, Jr., MD
Chief of Laboratory Division, U.S. Army
Institute of Surgical Research, 2322 Harney
Road, Fort Sam Houston, Texas 78234-6315,
U.S.A.

Kevin McGovern
Ciné-Med, 127 Main Street North, Woodbury,
Connecticut 06798, U.S.A.

Leo McGovern
Ciné-Med, 127 Main Street North, Woodbury,
Connecticut 06798, U.S.A.

Robert J. McKenna, Jr., MD
Medical Director, Chapman Lung Center,
Chapman Medical Center, East Chapman
Avenue, Orange, California 92669-3296, U.S.A.

Martin F. McKneally, MD, PhD
Professor of Surgery, University of Toronto,
Joint Centre for Bioethics, and The Toronto
Hospital, 200 Elizabeth Street, EN 10-230,
Toronto, Ontario M5G 2C4, Canada

Bucknam McPeek, MD
Department of Anesthesia, Massachusetts
General Hospital, 15 Parkman Street, Wang
Building, Suite 333, Boston, Massachusetts
02114, U.S.A.

Marc Miserez, MD
Chirurgie, U.Z. Gasthuisberg, Herestraat 49,
B–300 Leuven, Belgium

Francis D. Moore, MD
Moseley Professor of Surgery, Emeritus,
Harvard Medical School, 10 Shattuck Street,
Countway, Boston, Massachusetts 02115,
U.S.A.

Lincoln Moses, PhD
Stanford University School of Medicine,
Department of Statistics, Room G-100,
Stanford, California 94305, U.S.A.

Frederick Mosteller, PhD
Roger I. Lee Professor of Mathematical
Statistics, Harvard University, Science Center,
One Oxford Street, Cambridge, Massachusetts
02138, U.S.A.

David S. Mulder, MD
Chairman, Department of Surgery, McGill
University, Montreal General Hospital, 1650
Cedar Avenue, Suite 633, Montreal, Quebec
H3G 1A4, Canada

E.A.M. Neugebauer, PhD
Biochemical & Experimental Division, II.
Department of Surgery, University of Cologne,
Ostmerheimer Strasse 200, D-51109 Cologne,
Germany

Jemi Olak, MD
Department of Surgery, University of Chicago,
Box 255, 5841 South Maryland Avenue,
Chicago, Illinois 60637, U.S.A.

John E. Niederhuber, MD
Professor of Surgery, Johns Hopkins University
School of Medicine, Baltimore, Maryland
21205, U.S.A.

Andreas Paul, MD
II. Department of Surgery, University of
Cologne, Ostmerheimer Strasse 200, D-51109
Cologne, Germany

Jacques Perisat, MD
Centre Hospitalier Universitaire de Bordeaux,
Centre de Chirurgie Laparoscopique, Maison du
Haut-Lévêque, Avenue de Magellan, 33604
Pessac Cedex, France

Andrew F. Pierre, MD
Research Fellow, Thoracic Surgery Research
Laboratory, The Toronto Hospital,
CCRW–1–810, 101 College Street, Toronto,
Ontario M5G 1L7, Canada

Peter W.T. Pisters, MD
Assistant Professor, Department of Surgical
Oncology, M.D. Anderson Cancer Center, 1515
Holcombe Boulevard, Houston, Texas
77030–4095, U.S.A.

Alan V. Pollock, MB, ChB, BSc, FRCS
Honorary Consultant Surgeon, Scarborough
Hospital, Scarborough, North Yorkshire,
Y012 6QL, United Kingdom

Raphael E. Pollock, MD
Chairman, Department of Surgical Oncology,
M.D.. Anderson Cancer Center, 1515
Holcombe Boulevard, Houston, Texas 77030,
U.S.A.

Basil A. Pruitt, Jr., MD
Commander and Director, U.S. Army Institute
of Surgical Research, 2322 Harney Road, Fort
Sam Houston, Texas 78234-6315, U.S.A.

Vivek Rao, MD
Division of Cardiovascular Surgery, The
Toronto Hospital, EN 14-215, 200 Elizabeth
Street, Toronto, Ontario M5G 2C4, Canada

Richard Reznick, MEd, MD
Department of Surgery, The Toronto Hospital,
200 Elizabeth Street, Toronto, Ontario
M5G 2C4, Canada

Povl Riis, MD
Physician-in-Chief, Medical Gastroenterological
Department C, Herlev University Hospital,
DK-2730 Herlev, Denmark

Dicter Rixen, MD
II. Department of Surgery, University of
Cologne, Ostmerheimer Strasse 200, D-51109
Cologne, Germany

Lawrence Rosenberg, MD, PhD
Professor of Surgery, McGill University,
Director, Pancreatic Disease Center, Montreal
General Hospital, Room L9-424, 1650 Cedar
Avenue, Montreal, Quebec H3G 1A4, Canada

Bernard Rosner, PhD
Professor, Department of Statistics, Harvard
University, Channing Laboratory, 181
Longwood Avenue, Boston, Massachusetts
02115, U.S.A.

Jack A. Roth, MD
Chairman, Department of Thoracic Surgery,
M.S. Anderson Cancer Center, 1515 Holcombe
Boulevard, Box 109, Houston, Texas 77030,
U.S.A.

Mathias Rothmund, MD
Professor and Chairman, Department of
General Surgery, Philipps-University,
Baldingerstrasse, 35043 Marburg, Germany

Ori Rotstein, MD
Department of Surgery, The Toronto Hospital, EN 9-236, 200 Elizabeth Street, Toronto, Ontario M5G 2C4, Canada

David J. Roy, PhD
Director, Center for Bioethics, Clinical Research Institute of Montreal, 110 Pine Avenue West, Montreal, Quebec H2W 1R7, Canada

Stefano Saad, MD
II. Department of Surgery, University of Cologne, Ostmerheimer Strasse 200, D-51109 Cologne, Germany

David C. Sabiston, Jr., MD
James B. Duke Professor of Surgery, Duke University Medical Center, MSRB DUMC-2600, Durham, North Carolina 27710

Martin T. Schechter, MD, PhD, FRCP
Chairman, Division of Epidemiology and Biostatistics, University of British Columbia, Vancouver, British Columbia V6T 1W5, Canada

Walter O. Spitzer, MD
Professor Emeritus, McGill University, Director of Epidemiology, Genentech, Inc., 460 Point San Bruno Boulevard, South San Francisco, California 94080-4990, U.S.A.

B. Stinner, MD
Department of General Surgery, Philipps-University, Baldingerstrasse, 35043 Marburg, Germany

Hans Troidl, MD
Professor and Chairman, II. Department of Surgery, University of Cologne, Ostmerheimer Strasse 200, D-51109 Cologne, Germany

Paul M. Walker, MD, PhD
Vice President, Surgical Directorate, Surgeon-in-Chief, The Toronto Hospital, Bell Wing 1-635, 585 University Avenue, Toronto, Ontario M5G 2C4, Canada

Andrew S. Wechsler, MD
Professor and Chairman, Department of Surgery, Medical College of Virginia, MCV Station, Box 645, Richmond, Virginia 23298-0645, U.S.A.

Richard D. Weisel, MD
Division of Cardiovascular Surgery, The Toronto Hospital, EN 14-215, 200 Elizabeth Street, Toronto, Ontario M5G 2C4, Canada

J.I. Williams, PhD
Institute for Clinical Evaluative Sciences, Sunnybrook Health Science Centre, 2075 Bayview Avenue, G-260, North York, Ontario M4N 3M5, Canada

Pamela G. Williams, MD
Clinical Epidemiology Unit, Cornell University Medical Center—New York Hospital, Assistant Attending Physician, New York Hospital and the Hospital for Special Surgery, New York, New York 10021, U.S.A.

John Wong, MD
Department of Surgery, The University of Hong Kong, Queen Mary Hospital, Hong Kong

Sharon Wood-Dauphinee, PhD
Director, School of Physical and Occupational Therapy, McGill University, 3654 Drummond Street, Montreal, Quebec H3G 1Y5, Canada

H.R. Wulff, MD
Department of Medical Philosophy and Clinical Theory, University of Copenhagen, Panum Institute, Blegdamsvej 3, DK-2200 Copenhagen N, Denmark

John Yee, MD
Research Fellow, Department of Surgery, McGill University, 602 Stanstead, Town of Mount Royal, Quebec H3R 1Z7, Canada

Thomas Yeh, Jr., MD
Cardiovascular Surgery Fellow, Department of Cardiac Surgery, Hospital for Sick Children, 555 University Avenue, Suite 1525, Toronto, Ontario M5G 1X8, Canada

Introduction to Third Edition

Hans Troidl

Six years have passed since the publication of the second edition of our textbook on *Surgical Research*, and it is now 11 years since the introduction of the first edition. The editors and publishers felt compelled to present a third edition for several reasons. As always, there was the need to improve upon our work. Our friends, colleagues, and reviewers have given us good ideas. We have attempted to respond by condensing discussion, reducing overlap, and filling in missing components. We have added topics that have recently come into prominence, and strengthened areas needing improvement. We are motivated not just as a reaction to deficiencies; we are writing for the fun of working together. We favor fun as a motivating force in scholarship, balanced carefully with the work of learning, thinking, and writing.

We have continued to use the format of brief chapters, permitting them to be comfortably read between dinner and bedtime. After 11 years of emphasis on the academic surgeon as our target audience, we realize today that every surgeon needs these same methodological tools, because every surgeon is a scientist. We have changed the name of the book to reflect this realization. In the current era, the collection of data, the derivation of inferences, and the communication of results is mandated by strong societal and economic forces. Every surgeon needs information management,

communication, understanding of the analytic process, comparison of individual experience with the experience of others for quality control, audit, budget justification, and management of a clinical service. Surgeons will be more successful in their practice and their negotiations if they have the necessary methods and tools for these tasks, which are no longer limited in their application to laboratory experiments or clinical trials.

The third edition has more than 40 new topics treated in new chapters, including "Developing New Information in Community Practice," "Computer-Based Literature Searches," "Research in Surgical Education," and expanded sections on technology assessment, outcomes analysis, and ethics. Sir James Black, who was awarded the Nobel Prize for Physiology and Medicine in 1989, has contributed the foreword to the third edition.

In this edition we try again to define surgical research, recognizing the limitation of definitions. We discuss research as a search for certainty, going from ideas through proofs, using the best available methods of validation. Our book is fundamentally about methods and processes. We attempt to familiarize our readers with the best methods currently available, as we understand them. We are fortunate to have over 60 international experts representing 10 countries and 15 disciplines to help us toward this goal.[1]

Our concepts and our thinking are derived from our teachers, including reading works of the great philosopher of science Sir Karl Popper, from the questions of our students, and objections and discourse with our friends and our opponents. Discourse, particularly among the editors, has been the most enjoyable and fruitful part of writing this book. "First of all, it should be fun!" has been the first principle of the methodology of "how to write a book about surgical research."

The current pressures and grinding problems undermining academic life as we knew it just a few years ago forced a change in our modus operandi. The organization and communication formerly achieved by meeting together regularly was replaced in this edition by smaller, serial meetings. The McKneallys provided newsletters, personal visits and encouragement to the editors to insure continuity, communication, and timely completion of manuscripts. I am grateful for their contribution.

Though we continue to try to be broadly international, we realize that our book is driven largely by Western, predominantly Anglosaxon, scientific thinking. Other important countries and cultures, may be underrepresented, but they are not excluded intentionally. The ethical dilemmas created by modern technology are addressed briefly. Perhaps this topic will be covered better by our students in the next edition. This book is written for them, and we look to them to do a better job. Preparing them for this responsibility is our life's work.

Cologne, Germany

---

[1]Though others define science more broadly, we will attempt in chapter 1 to develop the position espoused by Descartes and Nietzsche, viz., that methodology is the defining essential element of science.

Introduction to Second Edition

Hans Troidl

My colleagues and I have been most pleased at the reception given to the first edition of this book. We conceived the idea for *Principles and Practice of Research* because we could not find in one volume a clear exposition of research methods for clinical disciplines. We saw a need to cover the principles of experimental design, biostatistics, epidemiology, strategies for beginning and finishing research, and finally the diffusion of results. We sought a book in which a clinician-scholar could find an introduction to specific research methods, an introduction that would start at square one and give a complete overview of each issue, ending with suggestions for further readings on special topics. We deliberately tried to keep our chapters rather brief, to permit them to be comfortably read by a tired clinician between dinner and bedtime. We carefully sought authors who were good at exposition, who shared with us a special concern for helping others develop careers in clinical science.

The first edition was favorably reviewed in journals across the world, and their reviewers made many helpful suggestions. In the preparation of this second edition, we have tried to respond to them.

We have been particularly pleased by the letters received from readers in many countries, some from old friends, many from well-known clinical scholars and teachers. Perhaps the most heartening have been letters from young men and women just starting to build careers of practice and research. Most of our correspondents offered helpful suggestions for future revisions. They kindly pointed out important topics we failed to cover, issues we touched on too briefly, or explanations that seemed unclear. Their comments have been of prime importance in planning, writing, and edition this present edition.

When our publisher, Springer-Verlag, first approached us about preparing a second edition we were eager to do so. After all, we read the book too, and while we were proud of what had been done and pleased that both reviewers and individual readers liked it and found it met their needs, we could see ways to improve it even before our friends helped us by pointing out some of the warts and blemishes.

After a series of planning meetings, Professor David Mulder from Montreal, Professor Martin McKneally from Albany, Professor Jack McPeek from Boston, and I sat down together in Chicago during a meeting of the American College of Surgeons to discuss the best way of approaching a second edition. All of us were busy, none more so than Professor Walter Spitzer, who had just committed himself to a year's sabbatical in the United Kingdom coordinating a major research project in epidemiology. The temptation to do only a quick revision, a cosmetic job, was strong, but our hearts were not in that. We and Springer knew that our readers deserved something more. More meant a larger, more complete volume. To do this, we needed help and turned to two of the most respected and innovative clinical scholars in North America: Professor Andrew Wechsler, chairman of the Department of Surgery at Virginia Commonwealth University in Richmond, and Professor Charles Balch, chairman of the Division of General Surgery at the University of Texas–M.D. Anderson Cancer Institute in Houston. Andy and Charles agreed without hesitation. This edition shows the effect of their outstanding teaching and editorial skills.

Thus began a busy 2-year process, at planning meetings in the United States, Canada, and Europe, research seminars in Boston, Montreal, and Cologne, and correspondence with methodologists and clinical scholars across the world to decide on a choice of emphasis, topics, and authors. We were indeed fortunate in again enlisting the collaboration of the distinguished Canadian editor, clinician, and research administrator, Dr. N.B.J. Wiggin. Authors and editors circulated drafts and redrafts of chapters by telefax, courier, and, occasionally, by mail. Gradually a new book took shape.

Over the last 6 months, as we had been putting the final touches on this second edition, I reread each of the letters sent in by readers. I wanted to make sure that we have responded seriously to readers' suggestions. We have retained the format you liked, revised chapters that needed to be strengthened, and completely rewritten others that required more help. We have added new chapters to cover areas you felt got short shrift before. Especially helpful have been a series of research seminars held for budding academicians at Harvard University, McGill University, and the University of Cologne. These young academicians and their teachers offered many practical suggestions.

We hope that this second edition meets your needs and expectations. I am truly grateful to my friends, both old and new, who have helped in its preparation as critics and reviewers, authors, editors, and now to you as readers.

Cologne, Germany
August 1990

Introduction to First Edition

Hans Troidl

Early in my career as an academic surgeon, Professor H. Hamelmann encouraged me to venture from my home department at the University of Marburg to visit other academic surgical departments in Germany. I was immediately struck by the variety of approaches to similar clinical challenges and surgical research problems. When my good fortune took me to other university centers in Europe, I was particularly impressed by Professor John Goligher's philosophy and approach to surgical scholarship in Leeds. During the several months I subsequently spent working with him in 1973, I learned as much as I could about his way of doing clinical research and found his and other British perspectives especially valuable because my previous experience in Germany had been largely confined to basic laboratory research. The following year, Professor Wilfried Lorenz of Marburg accompanied me to North America to visit basic research laboratories, clinical departments of surgery and anesthesia, and clinical research centers. We consulted researchers at the National Institutes of Health, Cornell University, and the University of California at Los Angeles, and clinicians at Albany, Chicago, and the Mayo Clinic.

When I left Marburg to become first assistant to Professor Hamelmann in the Department of Surgery at Kiel, I continued my laboratory research activities while I acquired further experience as a clinical surgeon. During this period, the necessity for an academic surgeon to be an exemplary clinician, a skilled and uncompromising technician in the operating theater, an inspiring teacher, and a competent researcher, *simultaneously*, was brought home to me.

Once again, I was struck by the similarity of the unanswered questions in surgery and anesthesia, no matter where they arose in the world. The problems had common themes, but the solutions proposed were very different in different cities and countries, whether they were related to the organization of medical care, levels and sources of funding, or the design of research studies. Even the organization of research facilities varies not only between countries, but within countries; differences among the individual units of a single university or hospital are the rule, not the exception.

As I traveled and corresponded with friends in other centers, I realized that some of the ideas and solutions developed in Sweden had relevance to the problems we faced in Marburg and Kiel. Some of the ideas I discovered in North America, the United Kingdom, or Japan could be profitably brought home to Germany. My colleagues at home showed me that only a little modification was sometimes required to make them applicable and useful in Marburg. I was delighted to find that colleagues around the world were curious to know how we cope with problems in Germany, and that new friends in Boston and Montreal were not only open to sharing their problems but very receptive to ideas and potential solutions that my colleagues and I had worked out in Germany.

When I became Professor of Surgery at Cologne, I instituted an open-door policy. I invited senior scholars to visit us in Cologne and arranged for my younger colleagues to be exposed to leaders and new ideas elsewhere. A number were able to present the results of their own work and to learn, firsthand, the techniques that I had discovered for myself, earlier.

My most trusted colleagues and I gradually recognized that while research problems had much in common around the world and many scientists had developed fruitful strategies and tactics for dealing with the problems associated with surgical research, there was no readily accessible source of information about much of the methodology that was evolving so rapidly. The idea of a book on feasible technology for research in surgery and other clinical disciplines became compelling. It would cover the principles of experimental design, biostatistics, epidemiology, starting and finishing research, and the diffusion of results.

Many a scholarly undertaking, whether it is a book or a research project, starts with an idea. Taking the idea from conception to fruition is often aided by interactions with friends—with whom I am still blessed!

The first step toward converting my idea of a book into a reality took place on October 14, 1984, in a chalet nestled in the hills near St. Adolphe, north of Montreal. My friend and host, Professor Walter Spitzer, spent half the night arguing with me about a possible table of contents. Early in the morning, we reached a consensus and quickly wrote down the headings and subheadings. When we called our mutual friend, Professor Jack McPeek in Boston, he immediately pronounced a benediction on our plan and agreed to work on it with us without hesitation. Professor Martin McKneally was the next to hear from us at four in the morning—it's hard to contact busy surgeons at any other time of the day. He was already up preparing slides for a paper and enthusiastically joined our growing team as soon as he had heard the details. Within a few hours, Walter and I succeeded in reaching Professor David Mulder in Montreal and found that he needed no

persuasion before volunteering to contribute his considerable effort and resources.

Over a period of years, most clinical scholars develop an appreciation of the elements of experimental design and the recruitment and management of research resources. The acquisition of this knowledge is unpredictable in different academic settings and all too often is a matter of trial and error learning under the supervision of senior colleagues who have also learned by the trial and error method. It need not be so, because a much better understanding and consensus about scientifically acceptable methodology has been developing around the world.

The editors of this book share my concern about this state of affairs and my commitment to doing something about it. Each is a scholar with a special responsibility for advancing research. Three of us are clinical surgeons charged with the care of patients, the supervision of research laboratories, and the development of younger surgical research colleagues in Albany, Cologne, and Montreal. One is a professor with a long track record of clinical epidemiologic research and teaching who now directs the affairs of the major Department of Epidemiology and Biostatistics at McGill University. One is an anesthetist, clinician-teacher, and research administrator at the Massachusetts General Hospital and Harvard University. Each is single-minded about helping colleagues with research problems and establishing an atmosphere and facilities to advance applied science. The underlying motive of all is to improve the care of patients through better understanding of relevant biological phenomena. We all give priority to the task of nurturing the academic growth of younger associates. A significant number of individuals who are world experts in their fields have joined our undertaking. Investigators in clinical disciplines, epidemiology, biostatistics, and the basic medical sciences have created a complementary ensemble of chapters giving advice on how to make research the creative, exciting, stimulating, intellectual endeavor it should be.

We offer practical suggestions and describe approaches and methods that have a proven record of success. The treatments prescribed for some of the most common ailments that afflict many well-intended clinical research endeavors are straightforward, but not simplistic or superficial. Most chapters are the product of collaborative efforts among clinicians and methodologists. Although the exposition of each topic is by no means exhaustive, sources of additional information are provided.

I sincerely hope that this book will help many of my colleagues, especially those who are newer in the field of clinical investigation, to avoid the errors and frustrations I have encountered in my search for a deeper understanding of clinical surgical research. The rewards and excitement of seeking and finding new knowledge can only be accelerated and enhanced by having a roadmap in hand when you start on your journey of discovery.

Cologne, Germany
August 1986

The Surgeon as Investigator

CHAPTER 1

Toward a Definition of Surgical Research

H. Troidl and M.F. McKneally

The most important quality of a scientist is intellectual humility.

Die Einsicht mahnt zur intellektuellen Bescheidenheit.

—Popper, 1984[1]

Writing a book about research requires some definitions and formulation of the relationship between research, science, and knowledge. We discuss these relationships here with humility, recognizing that we are not experts in the philosophy of science.

Historical Background

Hippocrates's careful observations of patients' symptoms, the natural history of disease, and the outcome of treatment provide an early example of the scientific study of patients, leading to induction of some generalizable principles about empyema, wound healing, and other surgical subjects. Hippocrates recorded no systematic method, but left a rich legacy of medical knowledge, passed on by "apprentice learning," with a generous dose of authoritarian dogmatism. The written record of formal western science may be said to begin with the systematic and logical approach to nature documented in the essays of Ar-

istotle, who emphasized systematic catalogs and methodical development of knowledge through observation, inference, and deduction. Descartes helped to open the period of enlightenment by rejecting blind acceptance of authoritarian dogma. "Unable to find anyone whose opinions struck me as preferable to those of all others, I found myself as it were forced to become my own guide. . . . Like a man who walks alone in the dark, I resolved to proceed so slowly, and to use such circumspection in all things, that even if I made but little progress I should at least be sure not to fall."[2] In his landmark "*Discours de la Méthode*" for rightly conducting one's reason and seeking the truth in the sciences, Descartes presented four basic rules in 1637 (see box) that illuminate the modern era of western science. Many other scholars of the period of enlightenment fought off the darkness of authoritarian dogmatism at their peril (e.g., Galileo). It persists in other forms and carries other perils to the present day.

The expansion of rationalism led to two major streams of scientific thinking:

Reason and methodology. The principle-based, deductive, and less empirical approach to scientific knowledge is exemplified in the writings of Kant, who believed that scientific truth could be attained by the process of careful, logical thought. Nietzsche emphatically advocated the paramount importance of developing knowledge, in contrast to the acceptance of dogma ("know or die"), and

---

Descartes' Four Basic Rules

1. Never accept anything as true without evidence of its truth; avoid precipitate conclusions and preconceptions.
2. Divide problems into as many parts as possible and as may be required to resolve them.
3. Begin with the simplest, and ascend in an orderly manner, step by step, to the most complex.
4. Make reviews so comprehensive, and enumerations so complete that you can be sure of leaving nothing out.

Discours de la Méthode, 1637
René Descartes

---

vividly described how resistant we are to knowledge that challenges our beliefs "unless it cuts through our flesh like a scalpel." Jaspers identified science with the perfection of methodology; if knowledge evolved using well-developed and generally accepted methods, its truth became an inescapable conclusion. The reliance on methodology and deductive reasoning in the philosophy of these thinkers is still evident in contemporary research approaches of many scientists, especially in France and Germany.

Empiricism. Bacon, Locke, and Hume took a different approach. While they followed Descartes' lead in questioning dogma from established authority as the primary source for the derivation of knowledge, they were inspired by the discoveries in the New World to look for new and unexpected sources of knowledge and to emphasize the empiric and observational. The recognition and pursuit of entirely new phenomena outside the accustomed sphere of knowledge and experience provided a pathway to new understanding. Multiple consistent and reproducible observations of perceptible phenomena allowed inductive inference of generalizable principles. This major stream of thought in the history of ideas, the empirical, inductive approach, is preserved in the English and American traditions of surgical research, with their reliance on chance or unexpected observations, clinical trials involving multiple patients, and multiple replications in laboratory experiments to strengthen inference.

In this century Popper pointed out how neither approach, nor both of them together, suffice. He persuasively defended the position that positive hypotheses cannot be proven, using the simple and memorable example of the swans: "no matter how many instances of white swans we may have observed, this does not justify the conclusion that *all* swans are white; you have not yet seen the black swan."[3] In contrast, negative or null hypotheses can be constructed and refuted to achieve objective knowledge. His synthesis of the inductive and deductive approaches, combined with analytic testing of hypotheses formulated as "null" or negative statements, comprise the scientific method as we practice it in surgery today in the Western world.

Discovery

The experience of scientific discovery begins with an inspiration derived from initiators, such as innovative ideas, observations, accidents, or problems. Discovery or inspiration precedes the application of methods discussed more formally elsewhere in this textbook. These are psychologically complex experiences that seem to come more easily to open-minded risk takers such as Einstein or Beethoven, who were often regarded by their more rigid and traditional colleagues as exotic or eccentric in their thinking.* Initiators are extremely important to the progress of science. What preparation of the mind enables chance observations to lead to discovery? Why did Semmelweiss uniquely discover the value of handwashing, despite the knowledge and beliefs of science at the time? This rich and complex subject is an area of study beyond the scope of this book.

Science

From the inspiration derived from initiators, science brings us to an approximation of certainty through careful application of reliable methods.

---

*DeBono has characterized this quality as "lateral thinking."[4] In his celebrated example of a crowded elevator at rush hour, many "vertical" engineering solutions are offered for rebuilding the transport system. The problem of waiting for the elevators was solved by distracting the workers with mirrors added in the waiting area. This example is fun to discuss since the elevator is truly vertical, and it has become a reference standard example for lateral thinking.

Our book will focus on methods presented in an introductory form for working surgeons who care for real patients. We refer the readers to more extensive sources for more complete treatment of the methods we discuss, and for the knowledge developed from their application.

We recognize that there are limits to science; it does not lead to an understanding of being, even if it does clarify our understanding of the universe. Science does not always include common sense. The obvious, the intuitive, and the personal relationship to the patient are not learned through science. The overarching considerations of impact, relevance, and common sense are not necessarily derivable through scientific methodology, but they are essential for its productive application. These aspects are more intuitive than rational.

The dark side of an emphasis on methods is the potential suppression of thinking through excessive application of methods. "When you have only a hammer, every problem seems like a nail."[5] Examples in surgery are the use of the PET scanner for every disease, the endoscopic approach applied to every surgical problem, or hammering with the same surgical laboratory model or mediator assay on a mindless assortment of research questions. Nietzsche characterized this excess as "the victory of scientific methodology over science."[6]

Research

Vollmer defines research as a process or activity within science: "Research is scientific activity intended to collect new results."[7] Science is a particular domain of knowledge that includes research; surgical research is a smaller domain of science.[8] Some components of science extend outside research, such as texts, tables, and organizations. Similarly, some aspects of surgery extend outside science and research, such as the art of surgery.

The *Oxford English Reference Dictionary* defines research as "systematic investigation into and study of materials, sources, etc. in order to establish facts and reach new conclusions." The *American Heritage Dictionary* introduces the possibility of employing the scientific method: "Research is scientific investigation or inquiry." It also includes the colloquial usage "to study thoroughly," as in "go to the library and do a little research on that subject." The Council for International Organizations of Medical Sciences proposes this definition: "The term 'research' refers to a class of activities designed to develop or contribute to generalizable knowledge. Generalizable knowledge consists of theories, principles or relationships, or the accumulation of information on which they are based, that can be corroborated by accepted scientific methods of observation and inference."

Defining Surgical Research

When the editors met as a group to plan the third edition of our textbook, we tried once again to develop a definition of the term *surgical research*. We agreed that a definition of research, such as those described above, could be further narrowed by a qualifier limiting the systematic investigation to subjects related to surgery, the work of our hands (from *chirurg*, meaning hand, and *ergon*, meaning work). We were troubled, however, by the narrowness of the definition.

During the evolution of this book Hans Troidl had many conversations with Sir Karl Popper about this problem. We hoped Sir Karl could write a chapter for this edition, but failing health leading to his death in 1994 prevented him from developing a formal essay for our book. He was keenly interested in surgical research and held strong views on the necessity for surgeons to emphasize *hypothesis testing* in their thinking, and *failure analysis* in their assessment of technology and outcomes. We will try first to explain Popper's thinking about definitions, and then develop our expanded definition of surgical research using his method.

Popper on Definitions

Narrow definitions tend to create exclusionary boundaries. They are useful in argument to help advance the definer's proposition, but they are limiting, somewhat artificial, and require defense against exceptions and variations. Popper felt that definitions become more durable and more easily defensible if they are developed not from exclusionary characteristics (as in "man is a featherless, spined biped"), but from inclusive, commonsense lists of many defining characteristics and components. The aggregate picture developed from the list then serves as a tentative definition and is presented as a hypothetical summation (such as, "all this might be called surgical research"). The list for surgical research might include, inter alia, the treatment of war wounds and Listerian antisepsis in an earlier era, cost-benefit analysis, robotic surgery, and the molecular genetics of wound healing in the current era. This approach provides flexibility and leads to discussion of the underlying thoughts, rather than defense of a narrowly constructed label. Erroneous components can be modified by progressive refinement in the way that hypotheses are extended, refuted, or confirmed in the evolution of scientific knowledge.

Our Definition of Surgical Research

Hours of thoughtful discussion, reflection, revision, and critical review have led us to believe that *the application of the scientific method to surgery comes closest to providing an accurate definition of surgical research*. Surgical research examines and evaluates innovative and conventional ideas related to surgery through scholarly analysis of data and the generation and investigation of hypotheses. The subject of surgical research includes anything that a thoughtful surgeon or serious scholar thinks will benefit the science and practice of surgery, including new ideas, observations, accidents, and problems.

Surgical research includes laboratory experiments and clinical experiments. Clinical research may include, for example, the development of algorithms, decision theory, the development and study of endpoints, clinical trials, multicenter trials, meta-analysis, research in the operating room, research in the surgical intensive care unit, health services research, and the analysis of clinical outcomes. Laboratory research may include hypothesis-driven studies of patients' tissues, cells, and subcellular particles including genes and gene products.

The goal of our book is to provide access to useful methods for testing hypotheses within these domains of surgery.

Hypothesis testing is the essence of the daily life of a surgeon. We do it every time we hypothesize the presence of acute appendicitis or a perforated ulcer, then methodically validate our hypothesis using the time-proven methodology of surgical exploration followed by gross and microscopic examination of the surgical specimen. "Too often we test only for differences, like the differences in outcome, cost, or benefit between open versus laparoscopic cholecystectomy, and undervalue the importance of hypotheses."[9]

Returning to our task of developing a definition, *surgical research* "might be defined" as a searching for certainty through hypothesis testing in a long, commonsense list of subjects related to surgery, using a broad variety of methods. In the expanding age of technology, our list of subjects and methods could include a nearly infinite number of problems and methods. Examples might include the cost and effectiveness of prehospital care for the trauma patient, using the techniques of modern economics; the optimal timing of operative interventions, using logistic regression; the immunosuppressive effects of trauma, transfusion, or drugs, using cellular and molecular markers; the complex interaction of mediators in the systemic inflammatory response syndrome, using the tools of contemporary molecular biology; the molecular genetics of wound-healing deficiencies; or assessments of the outcome of surgery, using measuring instruments developed in surgical patients for the evaluation of pain or disability. When all of these and many hundreds of other components are summed up, we have a 1997 hypothesis for the definition of surgical research. It is not surprising that we had trouble developing a definition for earlier editions.[10] We are more comfortable with Popper's broader, inclusive approach.

References

1. Popper KR. Logic der Forschung. Tübingen: JCB Mohr, 1984, p. xxv.
2. Cottingham J, Stoothoff R, Murdoch D, eds. and trans. Descartes Selected Philosophical Writings.

Cambridge, England: Cambridge University, 1988, p. 28.

3. Popper KR. The Logic of Scientific Discovery. London: Routledge, 1992, p. 27.

4. DeBono E. Die positive Revolution. Düsseldorf: ECON Verlag, 1992.

5. Maslow AH. Die Psychologie der Wissenschaft. München: Goldmann-Sachbücher, 1977.

6. Nietzsche F, cited in Bretschneider HJ. Physiologic und Patho-Physiologie, Grundlagen-Forschung und Therapie-Forschung, Göttinger Universitätsreden. Göttingen: Vandenhoeck & Ruprecht, 1979.

7. Vollmer G. Evolutionäre Erkenntnistheorie, 6th edn. Stuttgart: Hirzel, 1994.

8. Böcher W. Natur, Wissenschaft und Ganzheit. Opladen: Westdeutscher Verlag, 1992.

9. Jennett B. High Technology Medicine: Benefits and Burdens. London: Oxford University, 1986.

10. Troidl H, Spitzer WO, McPeek B, Mulder DS, McKneally MF, Wechsler AS, Balch CM, eds. Principles and Practice of Research: Strategies for Surgical Investigators, 2nd edn. New York: Springer-Verlag, 1991.

Commentary

This chapter sets the tone for our textbook. It is a distillate of many discussions among the editors about what constitutes surgical research. It begins with a historical background and documents the development of the two major streams of scientific thinking, the principle-based deductive method and the empirical method which champions the development of scientific truth from observation. The elusive concepts of "discovery," the development of the "prepared mind" emphasized by Pasteur, and the recommendations to surgeons from Sir Karl Popper are discussed. For further discussion of the concept of science and the pitfalls of sole reliance on the scientific method, the reader is referred to *What Is This Thing Called Science?* by A.F. Chalmers (Hackett, Indianapolis, 1982). This chapter finally provides the reader with the editors' best approximation of a definition of surgical research, "the application of the scientific method to surgery." From this chapter forward, the mission of the textbook will be to provide the reader with access to useful methods for testing hypotheses within the scientific domain of surgery.

D.S.M.

CHAPTER 2

The Ideal of Surgical Research: From the Bedside to the Laboratory and Back

R.C.-J. Chiu and D.S. Mulder

A number of strategies for planning a research project and organizing a competent team of clinician-scientists to execute it are discussed in this book. The "horizontal interaction" approach, illustrated by the Marburg experiment,[1] joins a team of basic scientists with clinicians to attack a problem. "Vertical interaction," another effective approach, draws collaborators with differing areas of expertise into a study as it progresses.

The vertical approach may be more cost-effective for a complex project, because collaborators are recruited as and when the need for their particular areas of expertise arises. Success with this approach depends on the availability of a wide variety of experts and the establishment of an extensive communication network within the research community. An attempt to develop a new "biomechanically activated cardiac assist device," undertaken in our laboratory at McGill University, illustrates the vertical approach to a research project in the North American context.

The Clinical Problems to Be Addressed

The problem addressed by our study is chronic heart failure, which afflicts approximately 2.3 million patients in the United States alone; 400,000 new cases occur each year, and the five-year sur-

vival rate is about 50%. The patients who fall into the New York Heart Association class IV functional category have a one-year survival rate of only 50%, and half their deaths are sudden. Long-term cardiac assist devices might benefit between 35,000 (NIH study) and 160,000 (Heart Failure study) patients per year. For many of these patients, cardiac transplantation is the most established and acceptable mode of therapy now available; but even the most optimistic estimate of cardiac donors is only about 2,000 per year in the United States for the foreseeable future.

Despite considerable relaxation in donor criteria in recent years, the waiting period for donor organs has increased eightfold in some cardiac transplantation centers in North America. The epidemiologic impact of this mode of therapy is obviously very limited, without even considering that cyclosporin has not solved all the allograft rejection problems, and that continued monitoring with endomyocardial biopsies is required for all the transplant recipients. The alternative is to use mechanical artificial hearts or cardiac assist devices; but existing long-term devices are plagued by thromboembolic and external power source problems. The tethers connecting the patient to the external power source limit the patient's mobility and are a constant potential source of infection. Another approach to cardiac assist would be valuable, if feasible.

The Conceptualization of a Hypothesis

We postulated that powering a cardiac assist device from an intrinsic energy source, such as the patient's skeletal muscle, would offer many advantages. Accordingly, the research question of our project was, Can the energy generated by skeletal muscle be harvested and modified, if necessary, to activate a totally implantable cardiac assist device capable of producing significant hemodynamic improvement?

The Rationale

Using the patient's skeletal muscle as the power source would eliminate the need for donors, immunosuppression, and external power sources; it also would restore patients' mobility and avoid the risk of infection by eradicating tethers. Careful selection of the assist mode could also exclude such thrombogenic components as artificial valves that now exist in cardiac assist devices. Obviously, an effective skeletal-muscle-powered device would be a useful addition to the spectrum of cardiac assist devices currently under development.

Review of the Literature and Identification of Specific Problems to Be Solved

An extensive literature review revealed that the idea of utilizing skeletal muscle to assist circulation was expressed several decades ago. Two types of approach were described. One uses a skeletal muscle flap to replace damaged myocardium, or to enlarge a hypoplastic right or left ventricle, and is called today "dynamic cardiomyoplasty." The second approach uses skeletal muscle to activate a pump device, in series or in parallel with the heart, to improve the circulation. Critical appraisal of previous experiments identified two major problems that must be addressed before either technique can become clinically applicable. The first problem is skeletal muscle fatigue; the second is that skeletal muscle's response to stimulation by a single electrical impulse is a contraction of much shorter duration and smaller amplitude than a cardiac muscle contraction. Nevertheless, we felt that recent advances in muscle physiology and electronics could make these problems resolvable.

Physiologists have discovered that electrical stimulation at 10 Hz for 4 to 6 weeks can transform type II, fast-twitch skeletal muscle fibers, into type I, slow, fatigue-resistant muscle fibers. This conferred fatigue resistance may solve the first problem; microchip and computer technology now make it feasible to construct miniaturized, implantable, programmable electronic stimulators to solve the second problem.

Our research plans were developed and pursued in the light shed by the work on transforming skeletal muscle to confer resistance performed by John Macoviak and Larry Stephenson and associates at the University of Pennsylvania, in collaboration with Stanley Salmons, a muscle biologist and pioneer in muscle transformation at the University of Birmingham. We learned the technique of muscle transformation from these investigators and adopted it for the purpose of cardiac assists, particularly the augmentation of left ventricular function.

Simultaneously, we pushed the idea that a new stimulator that sensed the R-wave of the heart, processed the signal with appropriate delay, and added a burst of electrical "pulse train" stimuli, could produce summation of the skeletal muscle contraction and modulate it to match the duration and amplitude of a myocardial contraction. This would compensate for the fact that skeletal muscle, even after transformation, consists of individual muscle fibers and "motor units," whereas cardiac muscle is a syncitium in which all the myocytes are connected by the intercalated discs. To be hemodynamically effective, the pulse train stimuli would have to be injected precisely into the selected segment of the cardiac cycle.

Preliminary Studies and the Animal Model

To evaluate the feasibility of the foregoing ideas, we consulted an electrical engineer to work out the specifications for a pulse train stimulator capable of being synchronized with the R-waves of the electrocardiogram. We then connected an available generator, the bulky model 5837 of Medtronics, Inc., to an Interstate Electronics Corporation stimulator, purchased with a modest grant from the Quebec Heart Foundation, to obtain the desired capabilities.

A canine model was chosen, primarily on the grounds of size and availability. The new stimulator was tested using a rectus muscle pouch; it produced the expected effects and was then used for a cardiomyoplasty approach to augmenting left ventricular function. The isometric left ventricular function was assessed by intraventricular balloon measurement during cardiopulmonary bypass, with the pulse train stimulator turned on, and turned off. This on-off "paired design" was advantageous, because it reduced the sample size required for the study.

A preliminary report on the concept of pulse train stimulation timed to the cardiac cycle was published in 1980.[2] The efficacy of synchronously stimulated skeletal muscle graft for myocardial repair was reported in 1984.[3] In 1985 the feasibility of transforming a skeletal muscle to make it fatigue resistant for myocardial assist and for powering an accessory ventricle was described.[4]

To obtain maximum muscle stretch prior to contraction, and thereby derive a powerful contractile force (Frank Starling's law), we selected the extra-aortic balloon pump as the most feasible design for our skeletal-muscle-powered assist device. Hemodynamically significant diastolic augmentation was achieved with it in a canine study reported in 1985,[5] and further improvements were made in subsequent years.[6,7]

Progress and Interaction with Other Disciplines

Throughout this project we interacted with various experts in muscle physiology and electronic technology. In 1985 a symposium sponsored by the Neuroelectric Society brought together for the first time international groups of investigators in this field and facilitated their interaction.[8]

To continue the elucidation of the muscle transformation phenomenon, we collaborated with—

David Ianuzzo, an expert in muscle biochemistry at York University in Toronto, Canada, in an investigation of changes in phenotype expression of genes during transformation, species differences, and the effects of various stimulation parameters.[9] Our concept of "working transformation"—achieving muscle transformation while extracting a measure of hemodynamic work—has gained acceptance in both laboratory and clinical settings.

During the foregoing we also interacted with electronic and device engineers at Medtronics, Inc., in Minneapolis and in Maastricht, Holland. The engineers of this leading pacemaker company improved and miniaturized our prototype stimulator; an implantable, synchronized burst stimulator (Medtronics model SPI005)—the first of its kind—is currently undergoing clinical trial.[10]

To expand the capability of our stimulator to muscle-powered counterpulsation systems, we acted as consultants to Medtronics in their project to develop a new generation of pacemakers; "Prometheus" is currently being tested in our laboratory.[11] Thus, as the project progresses, it obtains necessary expertise from both academic and industrial sources.

From the Bedside to the Lab and Back Again

The clinical problem we chose for investigation was taken to the laboratory, where the feasibility of muscle-powered cardiac assist was demonstrated; we are now trying to bring the results back to the patient.

Clinically, we perform "dynamic cardiomyoplasty" by wrapping the latissimus dorsi muscle around the patient's failing heart and stimulating it to contract during systole. Bruce Williams, a plastic surgeon with experience in the muscle flap procedure, and John Burgess, a senior cardiologist who coordinates case selection and pre- and postoperative studies, joined us for this phase of our continuing "vertical interaction" in this project.

By 1995, worldwide, more than 500 patients had undergone dynamic cardiomyoplasty. While a rigorous, prospective randomized study under a Food and Drug Administration protocol is under way in North America, the cardiomyostimulator for this procedure is now approved for clinical use in Europe. With the inclusion of the cardiomyoplasty procedure in a forthcoming textbook on adult cardiac surgery, this approach is now being accepted into the mainstream of surgical therapy. With an increasing number of investigators and companies with expertise in mechanical cardiac assist and artificial hearts turning to the transformed skeletal muscle as the possible power source, further research and possible clinical application can be expected in the coming decade.[12]

The Roles of Surgeon-Scientists

> **"A surgical investigator is a bridge tender."**
> Francis D. Moore, 1958

In projects such as this, surgeon-scientists can play a unique and important role in coordinating a multidisciplinary team, and bringing the information from the bedside to the laboratory and back. Nevertheless, the difficulties faced by surgeon-scientists have been felt for a long time. As far back as 1958 Francis D. Moore had been quoted to state that

> A surgical investigator is a bridge tender, channelling knowledge from biological science to the patient's bedside and back again. He traces his origin from both ends of the bridge. He is thus a bastard and is called this by everybody. Those at one end of the bridge say he is not a very good scientist, and those at the other say that he does not spend enough time in the operating room. If only he is willing to live with the abuse, he can continue to do his job effectively.[13]

By the last decade of this century, this dilemma faced by surgeon-scientists has become so overwhelming that they are now an endangered species facing possible extinction. This situation is due to developments on a number of fronts at both sides of the bridge. Health care cost crises in many countries are forcing surgeons to do more clinical work with less financial income, depriving them of time for research, and depleting the clinical earnings of surgical departments which used

to be available to support surgical investigators. Limited research funding increases the fierce competition for research grants, and rapid advances in science demand greater sophistication in research. The share of national research funding received by surgeon-scientists is decreasing, and many surgeon-scientists are being forced to turn to revenue-generating clinical practice.

In order to combat this worrisome trend, efforts are being made to train young surgeons for research, and to improve their ability to compete for research funds. In Canada, the Royal College of Physicians and Surgeons approved a Clinician Scientist program in which surgical residents can be trained simultaneously as future clinical scientists. Seminars to upgrade grantsmanship have been sponsored by many surgical organizations, with good attendance. However, although important, these efforts are analogous to breeding an endangered species in zoo nurseries, which by itself does not guarantee the survival of this species. Once these newly bred neophytes are returned to the wild, their survival depends on the availability of a viable habitat, as well as their ability to adapt to changing environments. The viable habitat for surgeon-scientists has to be provided by surgical departments and divisions. Because of the great time demands, it is increasingly difficult for a busy clinical surgeon without protected time to pursue strong research and remain competitive for peer-reviewed funding. The divisional and departmental strategy could be to spread the goals of an academic service, namely, patient care, teaching, and research, among the members of the faculty, rather than to expect each faculty member to accomplish all three goals. A talented and well-trained surgeon should be selected, and both his research time and income protected, the latter by various means such as grants, block funding, or a clinical-academic practice plan. Periodic review of faculty members so protected may assure their continued productivity in research. Some departments attempt to quantify the productivity by point systems, but the arbitrary weight of points as well as quantity versus quality of published papers are issues that may mitigate against the validity of such a system. A peer-review system of productivity analogous to that employed by granting agencies and promotions committees may be more appropriate. The surgeon-scientist, on the other hand, would have to focus both his clinical and his research activities in order to maintain clinical competence and achieve depth in research. Clearly, the life of an academic surgeon can be challenging, but it is also very exciting. One may ask, In what other job can you have the humanitarian satisfaction of treating patients, the artistic satisfaction of surgery, the scientific satisfaction of research, and the professional satisfaction of training a lot of people?[14]

Conclusion

A surgical research project can be initiated, guided, and coordinated by a principal investigator. He or she freely consults needed experts and interacts with collaborators to achieve success for the project. Such a collaboration can be done by "horizontal interaction" within a research team composed of a variety of multidisciplinary experts from the outset, or by "vertical interaction" with experts who are consulted and recruited as the project progresses. Horizontal and vertical interaction may occur simultaneously in a large project. Given the increasing sophistication of science and technology, the ability to communicate and the willingness to collaborate are becoming important attributes in a surgical investigator. A surgeon-scientist is uniquely suited to provide the bridge between the patient and the bench, between the clinicians and the basic scientists.

References

1. Lorenz W, Troidl H, Rothmund M. The Marburg experiment: developing the new specialty of theoretical surgery. In: Troidl H, Spitzer WO, McPeek B, et al, eds. Principles and Practice of Research: Strategies for Surgical Investigators, 2nd edn. New York: Springer-Verlag, 1991.
2. Drinkwater DC, Chiu RC-J, Modry D, Wittnich C, Brown PR. Cardiac assist and myocardial repair with synchronously stimulated skeletal muscle. Surg Forum 1980;31:271–274.
3. Dewar ML, Drinkwater DC, Wittnich C, Chiu RC-J. Synchronously stimulated skeletal muscle graft for myocardial repair: an experimental study. J Thorac Cardiovasc Surg 1984;87:325–331.
4. Brister S, Fradet G, Dewar M, Wittnich C, Lough J, Chiu RC-J. Transforming skeletal muscle for myocardial assist: a feasibility study. Can J Surg 1985;28:341–344.
5. Neilson IR, Brister SJ, Khalafalla AS, Chiu RC-J. Left ventricular assist using a skeletal muscle powered device for diastolic augmentation: a canine study. J Heart Transplant 1985;4:343–347.
6. Chiu RC-J, Walsh GL, Dewar ML, De Simon JH, Khalafalla A, Ianuzzo D. Implantable extra-aortic balloon assist powered by transformed fatigue resistant skeletal muscle. J Thorac Cardiovasc Surg 1987;94:694–701.
7. Kochamba G, Dexrosiers C, Dewar ML, Chiu RC-J. The muscle powered dual-chamber counterpulsator: rheologically superior implantable cardiac assist device. Ann Thorac Surg 1988;45:620–625.
8. Chiu RC-J, ed. Biomechanical Cardiac Assist—Cardiomyoplasty and Muscle Powered Devices. Mount Kisco, NY: Futura, 1986.
9. Ianuzzo CD, Hamilton N, O'Brien PJ, Desrosiers C, Chiu R. Biochemical transformation of canine skeletal muscle for use in cardiac assist devices. J Appl Physiol 1990;68:1481–1485.
10. Hill A, Chiu RC-J. Dynamic cardiomyoplasty for treatment of heart failure. Clin Cardiol 1989; 12:681–688.
11. Li CM, Hill A, Desrosiers C, Grandjean P, Chiu RC-J. A new implantable burst generator for skeletal muscle powered aortic counterpulsation. Proc Am Soc Artif Intern Organs 1989;35:405–407.
12. Chiu RC-J, Bourgeois I, eds. Transformed Muscle for Cardiac Assist and Repair. Mount Kisco, NY: Futura, 1990.
13. Moore FD. The university in American surgery. Surgery 1958;44:1–10.
14. McHarg N. Beating as one. McGill News 1990;Fall:12–13.

Commentary

This chapter describes an example of a systematic program of surgical research, driven by a common clinical problem. Ray Chiu is an established cardiovascular surgical scientist. He describes an approach to the problem of heart failure based on the hypothesis that an intrinsic energy source, skeletal muscle, can be adapted to become an effective cardiac assist device. The concept required the recruitment of basic scientists with expertise in the transformation of skeletal muscle, as well as a cohort of engineers who were able to develop pacing technology to train the muscle for continuous work. A senior cardiologist and a plastic surgeon were added as the program proceeded to clinical application. The cooperation of industry and several basic scientists was required in order to bring the project to fruition.

The project is now in the phase of clinical trials, and currently more than 500 patients have un-dergone dynamic cardioplasty. As the technique is moving toward general clinical application, several new problems have evolved that required a return to the laboratory and the recruitment of new investigators. This chapter provides an example of the vertical approach to a research project in the area of cardiovascular disease and is an excellent illustration of the concept of the surgeon-scientist as a "bridge-tender," which was first enunciated by Francis D. Moore.

D.S.M.
M.F.M.

CHAPTER 3

Developing New Knowledge in Community Practice

R.J. McKenna Jr.

Introduction

The continuous development and testing of new ideas and treatments is essential for progress in medicine. Surgeons can participate in this process via the creation of new technology, its early development and testing, or the initial application of new technology into clinical practice after it has been proven to be safe and efficacious. Evaluation of outcome by clinical trials or other analyses should become an inherent part of every surgeon's practice. This chapter discusses the opportunities and reasons for involvement of the community surgeon in clinical research.

Case Study

In 1994, surgery for diffuse emphysema was being performed by ablation with the laser (Wakabayashi method) and by stapled resection (Cooper method). There were several unresolved questions regarding patient selection, optimal operative technique, mechanism of improvement following the operation, and the duration of benefit. We established a lung-volume reduction surgery program at Chapman Medical Center in 1994 to study these questions.

Wakabayashi had been performing laser bullectomy as a form of treatment for emphysema at Chapman Medical Center for four years. When

he moved elsewhere, the hospital wanted to continue the program. The hospital had an experienced team of anesthesiologists, a thoracic surgeon who had assisted on most of the prior cases, nurses, and a rehabilitation team, but there was no organized research program. The results of the procedure had not been presented at major medical meetings and had not been reported in major medical journals.

The hospital administrator asked me if I was interested in developing the program, so I began making inquiries. The experienced thoracic surgeon, anesthesiologists, nurses, and the rehabilitation team all agreed to remain. The nurse coordinator for the program agreed to stay and help expand the program in new directions. Although I had clinical experience with the surgical treatment of emphysema, a research team needed to be developed. I invited Dr. Matt Brenner, a university-based pulmonologist with expertise in clinical research on emphysema, and Dr. Arthur Gelb, a pulmonologist who studied elastic recoil and exercise physiology in patients with severe emphysema to join the program.

The hospital administrator understood the importance of the program and agreed to fund the development of a lung center designed to support both clinical and research activities. The lung center required examination rooms and physician offices that would allow severely debilitated patients to be seen by the surgeon, anesthesiologist, pulmonologist, internist, and psychologist in one location. The new center was equipped with the necessary office equipment, telephones, copiers, and fax machines, as well as a computer system and support staff to collect research data. The team developed protocols to study the unanswered questions regarding lung-volume reduction surgery. With the help of the hospital institutional review board (IRB),we began a randomized, prospective trial of laser lung reduction versus a stapled lung reduction. A weekly conference was established to screen patients for the procedure; the conference also served as a forum to discuss morbidity and mortality, patient care issues, ideas for directions for clinical research, and data from current research studies.

This program was developed at a 125-bed hospital, based primarily on the commitment of the hospital and the physicians. Financial support has been provided by the hospital and a $10,000 research grant from the Heart and Lung Surgery Foundation.

The research from the program has generated considerable interest; our data have been presented at several national and international meetings. To date, we have published 13 papers[1] in major medical journals regarding operative technique, postoperative care, the mechanism of improvement, and the results of the procedure. The hospital is happy with the development of the program, and all members of the team are proud of the contribution that we are making to the understanding of lung-volume reduction surgery.

This case study demonstrates the need for as well as the kinds of benefits that can result from contributions by community physicians toward research and clinical study. The vast majority of private-practice surgeons participate in the process of advancing medicine only by their involvement in the integration of new treatments into patient care. The development and testing of new treatments occurs primarily in the university setting, but surgeons in private practice in the community have made and will continue to make significant contributions to the advancement of our field; indeed, important changes in medicine, such as the development of the laparoscopic cholecystectomy, have come from the private sector. Community surgeons have much to offer to the development and initial testing of new treatments.

For the surgeon who is interested in clinical research, there is a wide range of involvement available, depending on the desired level of participation. With only a small time commitment, physicians can offer new treatments to patients at their local hospitals through clinical trials groups. This level of involvement requires that the physician be aware of the available studies and request the assistance of the hospital research staff in entering patients into trials. For greater involvement in research, one can attend the meetings of the clinical trials groups, join a committee in the clinical trials group, or even participate in the development of new trials.

What Are the Benefits of Involvement?

Clinical research offers many rewards for the surgeon, the patient, and hospitals. Intellectually, it keeps the clinical practice of surgery new and interesting. It helps to keep the surgeon's medical knowledge current and may even provide an edge in today's very competitive health care market. Patients and their family doctors know that physician participation in surgical and other research is critical to progress in medical care.

Increased Patient Accrual for Trials

The National Institutes of Health (NIH) encourages community outreach by clinical trials groups because patient accrual to National Cancer Institute (NCI)–supported cancer clinical trials is currently low. There is a substantial untapped pool of patients in the community that can provide good candidates for enrollment in clinical trials.[2] Only 3% of the more than 150,000 patients with newly diagnosed breast cancers, and fewer than 2% of the 160,000 patients with newly diagnosed colon cancers participated in clinical trials in 1991.[3] Overall, less than 3% of the 1.17 million patients with newly diagnosed cancers at all sites are entered into clinical trials.[4] In medicine, the proper testing of ideas frequently requires large-scale, reliable clinical trials; the advancement of medicine is slowed by low accrual. It is estimated that over 90% of all cancer patients are now treated in the community setting without ever being seen at a teaching institution.[3] The inclusion of these community patients into clinical research studies would substantially help the progress of medicine and would allow a much better reflection of the "real world."

Dr. Bernard Fischer has clearly proven that it is certainly possible to enter large numbers of patients into trials. The National Surgical Adjuvant Breast Project (NSABP) has completed multicenter trials involving over 16,000 patients. In 1992, the NIH initiated a breast cancer prevention trial that involved 250 health care organizations, 40 Community Clinical Oncology Programs (CCOPs), and 16,000 patients.[5] In 1992, the Johns Hopkins Hospital entered 2,880 of 3,508 (82%) patients with newly diagnosed cancers into clinical trials.[6] Large-sized trials and high accrual to clinical trials are possible, but they depend on the commitment of the institution and its physicians.

While overall clinical trial accrual is low, accrual to surgical studies is even lower, and very few of the NIH-funded studies are surgical studies. There are very few examples of surgical groups, such as the Lung Cancer Study Group, established to run surgical studies. There have not been enough surgeons who have taken a leadership role in clinical research. Studies to compare the survival of melanoma patients with and without a regional lymph dissection, or after mastectomy versus lumpectomy for breast cancer have been performed, but there have been relatively few trials that compared the efficacy of different operative procedures. More surgeons are needed in leadership roles in clinical research to address these issues and to clarify the role of various perioperative adjuvant procedures.

New Challenges

After a surgeon has performed the same operation hundreds of times, the thrill is gone. Participation in the development of new treatments keeps the practice of medicine new and exciting.

Keeping Current

Medical care is constantly evolving, so, at the very least, practitioners need to stay up-to-date with these changes. Participation in clinical research can help keep a physician abreast of the latest changes in medicine. Attendance at clinical trial group meetings keeps the physicians' medical knowledge current by exposure to multiple protocols in addition to the particular protocols on which they have personally entered patients.

When video-assisted thoracic surgery (VATS) was first introduced, thoracic surgeons desiring to learn about the technique attended courses sponsored by the American Association of Thoracic Surgery (AATS) and the Society of Thoracic Surgeons (STS). The faculty for the courses came from all over the United States and Canada; they were often in private practice in the community. The opportunity to interact with faculty members on the frontiers in the development of these procedures and share ideas about new VATS techniques and instruments was beneficial and educational to both students and faculty. Collegiality and critical discussions of evolving techniques strengthen the initiation and diffusion process and provide a broader base for assessment of this new technology in a standardized fashion.

Improvement of Quality of Patient Care

Participation in clinical trials improves patient care in community hospitals through earlier introduction of state-of-the-art treatments. The physician-patient relationship is strengthened by the patients' realization that the physician is at the leading edge of medical knowledge.

Benefits for the Hospital

Although the hospital may be reluctant to invest resources in clinical research, in many cases it can be very beneficial to the hospital and accomplished at a minimal cost. Many patients seek state-of-the-art care or may feel more comfortable at a hospital where it is provided. The community's impression of the facility is enhanced when it offers state-of-the-art treatment. This can be emphasized in the hospital's marketing efforts.

Involvement in clinical trials is generally not a significant financial burden for the community hospital. Clinical trials groups pay the institution for each patient entered into a trial. In my experience, this reimbursement can essentially cover the costs of the research. Patient recruitment can be increased at a nominal expense. For example, Methodist hospital in Indiana sent letters to approximately 3,000 dentists and oral surgeons in an attempt to accrue patients for an oral leukoplakia chemoprevention study. The mailing list was obtained from the Health Professional Bureau at a cost of $35. An initial request for patients, a reminder about the ongoing study, and a thank you note for referrals were put in envelopes by hospital volunteers. The total cost of this marketing was only $822. This inexpensive effort presented the hospital as a positive resource to the community; 30 new patients were entered in the clinical trial, and 40 additional patients were screened.[7]

What Are the Difficulties with Involvement?

Time and Effort

The required paperwork for the studies and the effort required to obtain appropriate follow-up at the appropriate times can be time-consuming and frustrating. For those in private practice, there is no significant monetary reimbursement for the time, effort, and office resources spent obtaining institutional approval of the research project, obtaining proper follow-up, and attending administrative meetings about the research.

In addition, clinical research involves a team effort by both physicians and the hospital. The hospital's role includes a serious philosophical commitment to clinical research, help with data management, and an active IRB, all of which can enormously reduce workload. These elements are often present in today's hospitals. If you have to create them, you may be considering the wrong hospital. If your hospital does not have these in place, it may not be positioned to survive the current revolution in health care with its emphasis on emerging technology and outcome assessment. Community hospitals actually have access to a wide variety of clinical research and support services to go along with the trials. To learn how

hospitals have become effective contributors and leaders, talk to colleagues who are engaged in research and have taken advantage of these opportunities.

Hospital data managers greatly facilitate effective participation in clinical research. They provide details about existing protocols that are available at the hospital and have access to information about additional protocols. They can help remind the physician of the data needed for the studies and can collect the follow-up data by reviewing charts in the physician's office. These efforts save the physician a great deal of paperwork and time. With the help of hospital data managers, minimal physician time, effort, and expense are needed for this level of participation in clinical research.

Another helpful addition to a community research program is a research nurse. The nurse can identify patients who are candidates for the trials, confirm eligibility requirements, explain treatment to the patient, and help with data collection schedules.[8] Research nurses may serve as full-time data managers, or may work part-time on the research protocols while holding a clinical position in the hospital or office. The latter role often increases their access to potential study patients and enhances accrual to research protocols.

Obstacles to Accrual

Obstacles to accrual of patients for clinical trials are related to organizational issues, health care system factors, patients, and physicians.[2] One study showed that the major obstacles to patient accrual, in descending order, were as follows:[9]

OBSTACLES TO ACCRUAL
Time demands on physician and staff
Explanation of trial to patients
Completion of flow sheets
Perception of increased costs
Protocol breaks

Aids identified as potentially helpful for increasing accrual are as follows:[3]

> **AIDS TO ACCRUAL**
>
> Pocket-size lists of available protocols
>
> Computer-generated prompts
>
> Clinical trial specialist to explain protocol to patient and obtain informed consent
>
> Video to explain protocol to patient

No obstacle to accrual is greater than the issue of cost. Some payers point to escalating costs and deny patient access to clinical trials by refusing to pay for any "experimental" treatment.[10] We are facing the daunting prospect that health care reform may curtail or bias future clinical trials.[11,12] Consumers, providers, and politicians must be educated to protect and expand the clinical research structure so that we can continue to evaluate and improve patient care.

Another cause of low accrual may be that patients are concerned about the physician's primary allegiance being toward the trial, rather than the specific health needs of the patient, time or travel constraints, the quality of research care versus clinical care, consent; and a primitive fear of "being a guinea pig."[11]

Developing Research Protocols

Development of new research protocols can be very rewarding, but it is often impractical in the community hospital because the process involves creation and development of the concept, possible laboratory work to develop the treatment, drafting a protocol, presenting the protocol to the hospital IRB, conducting the trial, collecting and analyzing all the data, and reporting the results to the IRB and possibly at a medical meeting. This process can be undertaken in private practice, but it is very time-consuming and can be difficult in a community hospital with limited support for research.

Increased Responsibility

Participation in clinical research brings additional responsibilities regarding patient safety. After informed consent has been obtained, both patients and families frequently do not know the stage of disease and correct details of the proposed treatment.[13,14] Patients who are desperately ill will agree to almost any treatment if there is a possibility that it might help them. Patients with severe emphysema who are potential candidates for lung-volume reduction surgery are vivid examples. Generally, their quality of life is so bad that they become severely dyspneic with eating, walking short distances, or attempting minimal activities of daily living. Be careful about offering a treatment that desperate patients are likely to accept regardless of the risk. The physician has an extra burden of responsibility to protect patients from recklessness born of desperation.

All institutions participating in NIH research are required to have a current assurance that guarantees the protection of human research subjects. A copy of this is kept on file at the NIH. Compliance with this assurance includes annual review of all protocols performed at the hospital.

Involvement in clinical research carries the extra burden of carefully watching for any associated morbidity and mortality. For example, when laparoscopic cholecystectomy was rapidly incorporated into clinical practice, early experience showed a significantly increased risk of biliary tract injury when compared to the conventional open procedure. Recent reports show that the current risk of biliary tract injury is the same for both techniques. This emphasizes the need for physicians to carefully monitor the clinical outcomes of new treatments that they use and to stay current with any new measures to minimize side effects and complications.

Some new treatments require little change in existing patterns of care, while others require extensive education and the involvement of a multidisciplinary team. For example, because of the promising initial results of lung-volume reduction surgery, it was attempted in many hospitals with a very high morbidity and mortality in some cases. This in part led to the Health Care Finance Administration's decision to stop payment for the procedure, and the creation of a national randomized trial in centers of excellence to evaluate the safety and efficacy of the procedure.

How to Get Involved

What Is the Easiest Way to Participate in Clinical Research?

The easiest way is to become involved with an established program at your hospital. Many community hospitals already have programs in place that provide access to research protocols. The hospital data manager or research nurse in the program can provide a list of all clinical trials available through the hospital. The data manager or research nurse can also help you to audit your practice to determine what types of protocols would fit your patient mix. If there are additional protocols that are not currently available at the institution to which you would like to enter patients, the hospital data manager can obtain copies of the protocols from the clinical trials group and submit them to the IRB for institutional approval. You should attend the IRB meeting at which the protocol is presented and discussed.

What Clinical Groups Are There to Join?

Community-based physicians can participate in many cooperative clinical trials groups sponsored by grants through the NCI and the NIH. Most of the clinical trials groups are regionally based, but they may also depend on hospital association (e.g., the M. D. Anderson Cancer Center system). Other cooperative groups are organized by disease type or treatment. Examples of cancer cooperative groups sponsored by the NCI are seen in Table 3-1.

These groups have made a big difference during

Table 3-1. List of NCI sponsored cancer cooperative clinical trials groups.

Southwest Oncology Group (SWOG)

Eastern Cooperative Oncology Group (ECOG)

North Central Cancer Treatment Group (NCCTG)

Brain Therapy Cancer Group (BTCG)

Cancer and Leukemia Group B (CALGB)

Gynecological Oncology Group (GOG)

Radiation Therapy Oncology Group (RTOG)

MD Anderson Cancer Center (MDACC)

the past two decades. Clinical cancer research in the United States has grown; this growth has been enhanced by participation of community hospitals, practicing oncologists, and the creation of community cancer clinical trials organizations. More than 102,000 patients have been enrolled by community-based groups.[12] This is progress, but most community patients are still not offered clinical trials.

In terms of hospitals, the NIH has established programs for community hospitals to participate in cancer clinical trials as a Cooperative Group Outreach Program (CGOP) hospital or as a Community Clinical Oncology Program (CCOP) hospital. The former functions under the direction of a university hospital cancer program. In contrast, CCOPs are more autonomous; they have access to a wider variety of clinical trials than are available to a CGOP. For a hospital to become a member of CCOP requires greater oncologic expertise, clinical trials experience, and a higher patient accrual. There are only 52 CCOPs throughout the United States.

As either a CCOP or a CGOP, a hospital cancer program becomes aligned with one of the clinical trials groups (Table 3-1) which encourage hospitals to recruit patients. The clinical trials group is responsible for data management, quality control, and registration of all patients. Hospital participation in these programs requires attainment of baseline accrual of patients and attendance by hospital physicians at clinical trials group meetings. The groups monitor the hospitals for quality and quantity of contributions and performance.

What If You Want to Actually Conduct Research?

If you want to go a step further than joining a clinical trials group, the NIH has devised a new curriculum for teaching doctors how to conduct and report quality clinical research. Currently, the program is conducted at the Clinical Center at the NIH in Bethesda, Md. The curriculum includes modules on methods in epidemiology, study design, ethical issues related to patients and the researcher's potential conflicts of interest, monitoring research, data management and analysis, methods of meta-analysis, and preparation of grant proposals for funding for clinical research. In 1996 approximately 150 physicians took the program for credit. In order to expand availability of the program to more physicians, it may soon be on the Internet. More information regarding the program may be obtained from Dr. John Gallin at the NIH Clinical Center (telephone 301-496-4114).

What Else Needs to Be Done?

The surgical societies should play a greater role in encouraging surgeons to participate and help establish surgical protocols. The general public and its political leaders need to be educated about the importance of funding and performing clinical trials. Finally, surgeons need to assume a more active role in clinical trials. I believe this should start during surgical training, with greater exposure to the development and performance of clinical trials.

References

1. McKenna RJ Jr, Brenner M, Fischel RJ, Gelb AF. Should lung volume reduction for emphysema be unilateral or bilateral? J Thorac Cardiovasc Surg 1996;112:1331–1339.
2. Winn RJ. Obstacles to the accrual of patients to clinical trials in the community setting. Semin Oncol 1994;21:112–117.
3. Fisher WB, Cohen SJ, Hammond MK, Turner S, Loehrer PJ. Clinical trials in cancer therapy: efforts to improve patient enrollment by community oncologists. Med Pediatr Oncol 1991;19:165–168.
4. Mansour EG. Barriers to clinical trials. Part III. Knowledge and attitudes of health care providers. Cancer 1994;74:2672–2675.
5. Klabunde CN, Kaluzny AD. Accrual to the breast cancer prevention trial by participating Community Clinical Oncology Programs: a panel data analysis. Breast Cancer Res Treat 1995;35:43–50.
6. Lenhard RE Jr. A large private university hospital system: the Johns Hopkins Oncology Center. Cancer 1993;72:2820–2823.
7. Battiato LA. Recruitment strategies for a chemoprevention trial. Oncol Issues 1992;7:17.
8. Cassidy J, MacFarlane DK. The role of the nurse in clinical cancer research. Cancer Nurs 1991;14:124–131.
9. Stoller RG, Earle MF, Jacobs SA. Protocol participation in a private practice setting: a successful model. Proc Annu Meet Am Soc Clin Oncol 1991;10:A229.
10. Mortenson LE. Health care policies affecting the treatment of patients with cancer and cancer research. Cancer 1994;74:2204–2207.
11. Schain WS. Barriers to clinical trials. Part II. Knowledge and attitudes of potential participants. Cancer 1994;74:2666–2671.
12. Avent RA, Dillman RO. Cancer clinical trials in the community setting: a 20 year retrospective. Cancer Biother 1995;10:95–113.
13. Eguchi K, Hyodou K, Kobayashi T, et al. Informed consent in cancer clinical trials: simultaneous questionnaires for patients, families, and physicians. Proc Annu Meet Am Soc Clin Oncol 1995; 14: A1776.
14. Olver IN, Buchanan L, Laidlaw C, Poulton G. Are consent forms for anticancer clinical trials adequate for informing patients? Ann Oncol 1994;5:216.

Commentary

McKenna's chapter exemplifies the revised mission and scope of this textbook on surgical research. He illustrates how a surgeon in private practice can contribute effectively to technology assessment as it applies to video-assisted thoracic surgery. Through his leadership, a private hospital group established a highly credible clinical research team approach to the assessment of lung reduction surgery. He clearly defines how research methodology interacts with surgical practice.

In attempting to change the mission of this textbook, the editors had consulted Alexander Walt during his tenure as president of the American College of Surgeons in 1993–1994. He was an enthusiastic supporter of the concept that every surgeon is a scientist. In his challenging presidential address delivered during the 78th convocation of the American College of Surgeons on October 13th, 1994, he praised the uniqueness of American surgical education. Most important was his message that since World War II there has been tremendous energy directed toward health sciences. He said that "basic science investigators returned to their laboratories and there was soon an unprecedented flow of new scientific breakthroughs and technical advances. These successes were typified in the early 1950s by the advent of cardiopulmonary bypass and open heart surgery, carotid and other vascular endarterectomies and substitutions, the development of highly sophisticated intensive care units, and the wonders of successful organ transplantation. It is ironic that these university-acclaimed technical triumphs and acknowledged marvels of American enterprise, designed to improve the health of patients, are now significant contributors to the cost of health care and the clamor for the attenuation of specialty training. Some cynics, or perhaps realists, may argue that we have succeeded too well. I would argue that it is not possible to train surgeons too well."[1] In his recommendations for the maintenance and growth of surgical education in North America, Walt emphasized the importance of teaching the history of surgery, particularly the history of surgical research and its accomplishments, and the importance of strengthening training and research methodology early in the surgical residency program. It is not a coincidence that in McKenna's closing words to this chapter he makes a plea for further clinical research training in all our residency programs as the solution to improving the interface between surgical research and patient care.

D.S.M.

1. Walt AJ. Presidential address: the uniqueness of American surgical education, and its preservation. Bull Am Coll Surg 1994;79:8–20.

CHAPTER 4

Selected Historical Perspectives on the Evolution of Surgical Science

W.R. Chitwood Jr. and D.C. Sabiston Jr.

But when I tried the experiment, the result was different.

—John Hunter

Over the years, advances in surgery have been made through observation, experimentation, innovation, application, and . . . *serendipity*. The continual development of new information in surgery has maintained the vibrancy of our science and specialty. Although the history of surgery is lengthy, the evolution of the scientific approach is relatively brief, spanning just over 250 years. Surgeons have always been on the leading edge of science and have served as a wellspring for new ideas.

Our heritage is rich with successes; however, the evolution of surgical science is fertilized equally by failures. Many operations that sprouted with great promise and fanfare were discarded without even a footnote of remembrance. This chapter will focus on the accomplishments of several springboard surgeons who typify this surgical evolution. However, others have influenced surgical science just as much through their skepticism, negative observations, failed experiments, or discarded operations. Benjamin A. Barnes reviewed the *Transactions of the American Surgical Association* between 1880 and 1942 for potentially promising operations that had been discarded.[1] Subsequently abandoned operations for ptosis included suturing abdominal organs into improved positions and the Lane operation (excision of the right and transverse colon with anastomosis of the ileum to the left colon). Constipation was treated by excision of a redundant sigmoid colon, ileosigmoidostomy, appendectomy, and duodenojejunostomy. Peripheral nerves were stretched to improve circulation, and sympathectomies were performed as treatment for epilepsy and various other disorders. All of these operations were considered meritorious but were cast aside, often with far too much delay. Discarded operations and failed experiments serve as reliable compasses, just as do the scientific successes.

The Darkness before the Dawn

Early surgery had little scientific basis, and empirical application of unproved treatments was routine. As the darkness of the Middle Ages descended, medical care in Europe was delivered by monks, barbers, and poorly apprenticed surgeons. In Britain monks were free to practice medical therapy without training or supervision. Surgical therapy consisted mainly of amputations, scarifications, leechings, lithotomies, and drainage of abscesses. Antisepsis and anesthesia were not considered until the nineteenth century.

To protect society against charlatans and inept practitioners, an organized guild of surgeons was formed in 1423 by the surgeon to Henry V.[2] In 1540 the Company of Barber Surgeons was formed by Henry VIII. With the development of Harveian physiology and anatomy during the first quarter of the seventeenth century, surgeons demanded a broader education. The schism between barbers and surgeons was prompted by William Cheselden, the mentor of John Hunter. Through his efforts, the Company of Surgeons was formed, and the Royal College of Surgeons was to become its lineal descendant. During this pre-Hunterian era, observation was the only semblance of scientific procedure, and surgery improved very little either in England or on the Continent.

The discipline of surgery has been fortunate in having had a number of investigators who have made significant, basic scientific contributions with practical clinical application. The great medical historian, Garrison, considered Ambroise Paré, John Hunter, and Joseph Lister to be the three greatest surgeons of all time.

Ambroise Paré: An Early Clinical Trial

Paré (Figure 4-1) reintroduced and popularized the ancient use of the ligature to control hemorrhage and placed its use on a firm basis. He also introduced the concept of the controlled experiment, when treating two soldiers with similar wounds lying side by side in a tent near the battlefield. The first soldier's wound was managed by the standard method of cauterization with boiling oil. The second was managed by debridement, cleansing, and the application of a clean dressing. Paré wrote that he spent a restless night, worrying that the second patient would do very poorly since

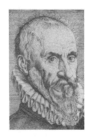

Figure 4-1.   Ambroise Paré.

his treatment defied the standard therapy of that time. The following morning, however, he found the second patient to be essentially without systemic symptoms, whereas the other had high fever, tachycardia, and disorientation. When he was congratulated on the outcome of this new approach, Paré very humbly replied, "Je le pansay, Dieu le guarit" [I treated him, God cured him], a quotation subsequently inscribed on his statue.

John Hunter: The Founder of Scientific Surgery

John Hunter illuminated the darkness by providing important experiments and clinical contributions to surgery, while similarly enlightening the fields of comparative anatomy and natural history (Figure 4-2). Osler said of Hunter, "He made all thinking physicians naturalists. He lent dignity to the study of organic life, and re-established a close union between medicine and the natural sciences." Hunter's impact was realized in his time, and in his shadow new scientific information began to change the course of surgery. Questions

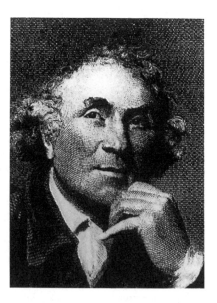

Figure 4-2.   John Hunter. In this Sharp engraving of Sir Joshua Reynolds's painting, Hunter is shown during his most productive clinical and investigative period.

became experiments and experiments became operations. For the first time, students came to learn the method rather than rote material. For perspective, this was the eighteenth century, the era of the writers Samuel Johnson and Richard Sheridan, the artists Thomas Gainsborough and William Hogarth, and the scientists Joseph Priestley, Henry Cavendish, Sir Humphry Davy, and John Dalton. The Royal Society was just 100 years old, and science was in the cradle. It was the age of discovery; experimentation was replacing speculation. The world of science was fertile for a John Hunter.

Born in 1728 near Glasgow, Hunter was interested in everything, even as a youth . . . except a formal education.[3,4] He had a penchant for natural history and once said, "When I was a boy I wanted to know all about the clouds and grasses. I watched the ants, bees, birds, tadpoles, and caddis worms. I pestered people with questions about what nobody knew . . . or cared anything about." He apprenticed in London with his university-educated brother, William, who was well known for his expertise in anatomic dissection. At the Surgeons' Hall, Cheselden and Pott taught John the basics of clinical surgery. He had an insatiable scientific curiosity and thirst for new knowledge, as well as a fanatical enthusiasm for the experimental approach. Many of Hunter's detailed dissections and experiments remain as a time capsule at the Royal College of Surgeons. The Hunters educated the most venerated English surgeons of the day including Jenner, Abernethy, Cline, Bell, and Cooper. In America the Hunterian spirit was spread through his surgical students Post, Morgan, Shippen, and Physick, who was to become the father of American surgery.

John Hunter's contributions to new knowledge in natural science surgery were voluminous. His studies in transplantation and vascular collateralization typify the Hunterian method for scientific analysis. He once moved the spur of one cock to the comb on the head of another. He also performed perhaps what was the first xenograft transplant by placing a human tooth in the comb of a cock. The relatively inert tooth and the highly vascular comb allowed the transplant to succeed without rejection, and subsequent blood vessel injections indicated revascularization. Later, he attempted to transplant teeth from one patient to another. Hunter described these collective findings by saying, "It is equally possible to unite different parts of the same, or different bodies, by bringing them into contact under certain circumstances."

By examining seasonal deer antler changes, Hunter became interested in collateral blood vessel development. Using arterial injections, he observed that new growth enlisted neovascularity, and he proceeded by experiment to determine the "stimulus." After ligating the external carotid of a deer in Richmond Park, the antler velvet lost warmth and arterial pulsations (1785). A week later, warmth returned with restored blood flow. Hunter established that with "the stimulus of necessity, the smaller channels quickly increased to do the work of the larger." Based on these studies, he operated on a 45-year-old coachman with a popliteal aneurysm (1785).[4,5] Hunter ligated the superficial femoral artery in the proximal thigh at a distance from the aneurysm, to diminish the risk of hemorrhage (Figure 4-3). This provided arterial occlusion over a sound portion of the vessel, with collateral protection of the distal extremity.

To John Hunter is due the primary credit for introducing the *experimental method* by using animals to develop surgical techniques prior to their application to humans. His philosophy and practice are appropriately summarized in his often-quoted response to a question from Edward Jenner, the developer of smallpox vaccination. When Jenner was speculating about hibernation in the hedgehog, Hunter responded tersely, "I think your solution is just; but why *think?* Why not *try* the experiment?"[6]

Hunter's observations are preserved in four books: *The Natural History of Teeth* (1771), *A Treatise on the Venereal Disease* (1786), *Observations on Certain Parts of the Animal Oeconomy* (1786), and *A Treatise On Blood, Inflammation and Gunshot Wounds* (1794).[7–10] William Clift's transcriptions from his casebooks represent many of the best examples of Hunter's skilled deductive reasoning.[11] Hunter's admonition reveals his scientific philosophy:

In pursuing any subject most things come to light . . . , by accident, . . . that is, many things arise out of investigation[s] that were not at first conceived, . . . even misfortunes in experiments have brought things to our knowledge that were not . . . and probably could not have been . . . previously conceived. . . . On the other hand, I have often devised experiments by the fire-side, or in my carriage, and have also conceived the result . . . , but when I tried the experiment, the result was different . . . or I found that the experiment could not be attended with all the circumstances that were suggested.[12]

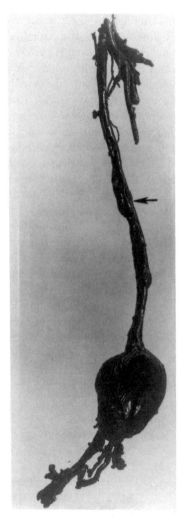

Figure 4-3. Hunterian operation. First operation done by Hunter for popliteal aneurysm. Four ligatures were used to occlude the femoral artery in the thigh at a distance from the aneurysm. This specimen resides in the Hunterian Museum at the Royal College of Surgeons of England. Courtesy of Elizabeth Allen, Curator of the Royal College of Surgeons of England.

Hunter died in 1793, and later the Royal College of Surgeons placed the following inscription on his Westminster Abbey tomb: ". . . to record their admiration of his genius as a gifted teacher and interpreter of the divine power and wisdom at work in the Laws of Organic Life, and their grateful veneration for his services to mankind as the Founder of Scientific Surgery.[4]

Lord Lister: The Discovery of Antisepsis

In the 1927 Hunterian Lecture, Sir Berkeley Moynihan compared the contributions of Hunter, Lister, and Pasteur to a rugby match: "If I may borrow a simile from the football field to express the relation of these three great men . . . I would say that it was Pasteur who made the final pass to Lister possible. . . . [However] it was Hunter's captaincy in the scrum that placed Lister in the scoring position." Joseph Lister was born in 1827 (Figure 4-4).[13] By this time, surgical training had evolved considerably. Lister obtained a university education and was influenced by the physiologist Sharpey. His first clinical post was as a house surgeon to the master surgeon James Syme, in Edinburgh. At the age of 33, he was appointed Professor at the University of Glasgow. Two years later he became surgeon to the Royal Infirmary, where he made many of his lasting contributions. During this period his publications reflected experimental and clinical observations on tissue viability, involuntary muscle fibers, inflammation, gangrene, and coagulation. On the wards he observed many surgical infections that stimulated him to experiment. From the combination of examining infected surgical wounds, performing ex-

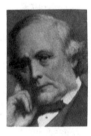

Figure 4-4. Joseph Lister.

periments, and applying the results clinically, he developed and popularized his theories on surgical antisepsis.

Before application of Lister's discoveries, nearly every wound became infected and suppurated.[14] Union by first intention was rare, and closed wounds usually became reddened, painful, and opened spontaneously. Patients either healed secondarily or developed major complications including hemorrhage, sepsis, erysipelas, tetanus, or septic gangrene. In the two years before introduction of Lister's antiseptic techniques, the surgical mortality at the Royal Infirmary was 45%, and operations were limited to those considered lifesaving. For practical purposes, abdominal and thoracic surgery did not exist.

In 1865 a Glasgow chemist alerted Lister to the experiments of Pasteur. Lister became convinced that infections were caused by minute organisms suspended in particulate airborne material. He selected carbolic acid for sterilization during surgery, rather than dry heat, as proposed by Pasteur. In his first publication on the subject, he stated, "In the year of 1864, I was much struck with an account of the remarkable effects produced by carbolic acid upon the sewage of the town of Carlisle."[14] In March of 1865 he began his first clinical studies using carbolic acid–soaked dressings. By 1867 he had published his seminal work on surgical antisepsis, describing compound fracture patients that were treated successfully with carbolic acid–soaked dressings. The transcript of his exhaustive 1868 address to the Medico-Chirurgical Society of Glasgow provided the best descriptions of his experiments. His classic work on arterial ligations suggested that infections and hemorrhage should decrease markedly if absorbable catgut was substituted for silk ligatures. Lister eventually expanded his antiseptic methods to include vaporized carbolic acid, which became standard in his operating theater. He boldly applied his antiseptic principles to even the most difficult cases, and by 1879 the surgical mortality at the Royal Infirmary had fallen to 1.8% from 45% 15 years earlier.

His successive posts in Edinburgh and London were achieved through persistence and dedication to his theory and application of surgical antisepsis. Despite successes in London and the United States, Listerism was not embraced. When he re-turned to London in 1877, operating room conditions were similar to those of his student days 20 years earlier. At the third meeting of the American Surgical Association in 1883, over half of the speakers and discussants opposed Lister's methods.[15] Although principles of antisepsis evolved slowly, in some European clinics Listerism was adopted early. On his 1875 tour through Germany, he was welcomed by Volkman, Nussbaum, Thiersch, and Mikulicz. Lister merits a place near the summit of scientific surgery for paving the way to the surgical asepsis practiced today. As Osler said, "Only those who have lived in the pre-Listerian days can appreciate the revolution which has taken place in surgery."

The Development of Formal Training Programs

The original patterns of surgical training were established in Europe during the latter half of the nineteenth century, particularly in the university clinics of Germany, Austria, and Switzerland. The surgical masters, who were all-powerful in their respective hospitals, established the principle of stepwise assumption of responsibility in residency training programs, culminating in the concept of full completion of the training during the chief residency. Bernhard von Langenbeck, professor of surgery at the University of Berlin, is regarded as the father of modern training programs (Figure 4-5). An extraordinary teacher, clinical investigator, and master surgeon, he is credited with devising 33 original operative procedures.[16] At the famed Charité Hospital in Berlin, he attracted a remarkable group of trainees, including Billroth, Kocher, Trendelenburg, and many others (Figure 4-6). Each became a leader of his own school and a great contributor in his own right. Langenbeck was also the first to initiate a journal devoted solely to surgery, *Archiv für klinische Chirurgie*, also known as *Langenbeck's Archiv* (Figure 4-7). After completing Langenbeck's program, Billroth became professor of surgery at Zurich, and later at the University of Vienna, where he was chief surgeon to Allegemeines Krankenhaus. Theodor Kocher was appointed professor at the University of Berne at the amaz-

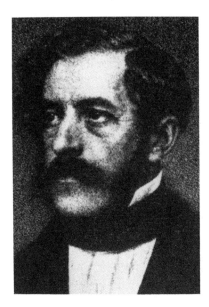

Figure 4-5. Bernhard von Langenbeck, professor of surgery at the University of Berlin.

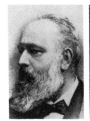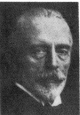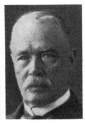

Figure 4-6. Billroth, Kocher, and Trendelenburg: students of Professor Bernhard von Langenbeck.

ing age of 31; Trendelenburg was appointed to the chair in Leipzig.

William Stewart Halsted: The Father of the Modern Surgical Residency in the United States

The intellectual life of Halsted parallels closely that of Lister. In the 45 years between Halsted's graduation from the College of Physicians and Surgeons in New York and his death in 1922, surgery advanced remarkably.[17,18] This transformation was due largely to his intellect, original laboratory studies, and clinical application. Harvey Cushing's description of Halsted (Figure 4-8) provides an accurate insight into his character:

> He was a man of unique personality, shy, something of a recluse, fastidious in his tastes and in his friendships, an aristocrat in breeding, scholarly in his habits, the victim for many years of indifferent health. He nevertheless may be considered to have established in America a school of surgery comparable to that of Billroth in Vienna. . . . He had that rare form of imagination which sees problems, and the technical ability,

combined with persistence, which enabled him to attack them with the promise of a successful issue. Many of his contributions to his craft and medicine in general were fundamental and of enduring importance.

At Bellevue Hospital, Halsted was first exposed to the appalling sight of suppurating surgical wounds. Despite overall skepticism, several surgeons at Bellvue used some antiseptic methods. Through their practices, Halsted compared the surgical results. Thereafter, his interest in eradicating surgical infections developed, and these investigations became a lifelong pursuit. William Welch, the pathologist at Bellvue, became a major influence on Halsted's professional training, scientific curiosity, and personal life. At Welch's suggestion he traveled to the clinics of Billroth, von Bergmann, and Volkmann. On his return he developed the beginnings of aseptic surgery by establishing the importance of minimal tissue damage and hemorrhage.[19]

In 1886 Halsted accepted a faculty position with Welch at the newly established Johns Hopkins Medical School and worked solely in the research laboratory until the hospital opened (1889). Then Halsted was made surgeon pro tempore and in 1892 was elevated to Professor and Surgeon-in-Chief. He and Welch showed that bacteria were still present on the skin even after vigorous cleansing with antiseptics. His detailed wound microscopic studies lead him to realize that careful tissue handling was as important in preventing infections as avoidance of bacteria.

Halsted's life at Johns Hopkins was replete with multiple, independent advancements in scientific surgery.[20] He first established experimentally that

ARCHIV

FÜR

KLINISCHE CHIRURGIE

HERAUSGEGEBEN

VON

Dr. B. LANGENBECK,

Geh. Medicinal-Rath und Professor der Chirurgie, Director des chirurgisch-
ophthalmologischen Klinikums der Universität etc. etc.

REDIGIRT

von

Dr. BILLROTH,   und   Dr. GURLT,
Prof. der Chirurgie in Zürich.   Docent der Chirurgie in Berlin.

ERSTER BAND.

Mit 6 Tafeln Abbildungen und 22 Holzschnitten.

7448

BERLIN, 1861.
VERLAG VON AUGUST HIRSCHWALD,
Unter den Linden, Ecke der Schadowstrasse.

Figure 4-7. Title page of the first issue of Langenbeck's *Archiv für klinische chirurgie.*

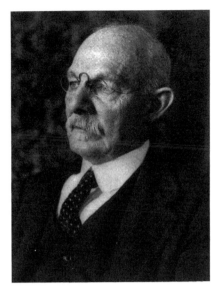

Figure 4-8. William Stewart Halsted. This photograph shows Halsted in 1922, the year of his
death. During his most productive investigative
years, few portraits were made of him.

strength of the intestinal wall is delivered primarily by the submucosa, which led to the development of improved, safer intestinal anastomoses.
His laboratory coworker, Councilman, said of
Halsted:

> It is difficult to think of surgery more carefully
> conducted than was this experimental surgery by
> Halsted. . . . The dog was treated as a human
> patient. . . . The surgery of Halsted was differ-
> ent, it was scientific in that he tested by the ex-
> periment all theoretical conceptions of the art.
> Not since the time of John Hunter had the ex-
> periment been so fully useful in the development
> of surgery.[21]

From his early experiments Halsted developed an
appreciation for specific "rules" of technique in

operative surgery. For the first time, he closed
clean wounds without drainage. His 1913 publication on the use of fine silk in preference to
catgut, the introduction of gloves, gutta-percha
tissue, and silver foil, and the advantages of transfixing tissues and vessels in controlling hemorrhage remains a classic in surgery.[22] Halsted's new
or improved operations resulted from his scientific
approach and included the radical mastectomy,
the radical cure for hernia, ligations of aneurysms,
and the operation for goiter.

   In the United States, the development of surgical residency training programs followed the
Langenbeck-Billroth schools, as introduced by
William Stewart Halsted. Generally regarded as
the most outstanding surgeon in North America,
Halsted regularly visited the major surgical clinics
in Europe from 1878 until the end of his life. He
was impressed by the progressive system of surgical training and completely devoted to the concept that highly selected, bright young trainees
should begin as interns and gradually progress
through the residency with increasing responsibility. He believed that, upon completion of the
chief residency, the trainee should have essentially
the same abilities as the teachers in the university

clinic. Consequently, many trainees were appointed to prestigious academic chairs immediately following their completion of Halsted's training program at the Johns Hopkins Hospital[23] (Figure 4-9). His astonishing success in the training of surgeons was later duplicated by such other notable figures as Blalock,[24] Wangensteen[25] (Figure 4-10), Ravdin (Figure 4-11), and Rhoads (Figure 4-12).

Halsted said, "It was our intention originally to adopt as closely as feasible the German plan, which, in the main, is the same for all the principal clinics." He emphasized further, "Every facility and the greatest encouragement is [sic] given each member of the staff to do work in *research*." Halsted was deeply impressed by the contributions of those who involved themselves in original research, and he specifically cited the discoveries of Hunter, Pasteur, and Lister as being the foundation of modern surgical practice.

In his classic address, "The Training of a Surgeon," delivered at Yale in 1904, Halsted said:

> The assistants are expected in addition to their ward and operating duties to prosecute original investigations and to keep in close touch with the work in surgical pathology, bacteriology, and so far as possible physiology. . . . Young men contemplating the study of surgery should early in life seek to acquire knowledge of the subjects fundamental to the study of their profession.[23]

"Halsted's men" were subsequently appointed to the most prestigious academic posts, and his con-

cepts of surgical training with emphasis on clinical excellence, combined with research, spread rapidly and became widely adopted.[26] Emile Holman, his last chief resident, alluded to Halsted's future impact by saying, "In the world of science, the rewards go to the thinkers. . . . In the history of surgery, Halsted clearly and uniquely embodied the role of an original and productive thinker, to whom all surgeons the world over are deeply indebted . . . now and in the limitless future."[27]

Responsibility for the training of surgical investigators is an obligation of surgical faculty members everywhere. More than two centuries ago, Samuel Johnson said:

> Every science has been advanced to a perfection by the diligence of *contemporary* students and the gradual discovery of one age improving on another, either truths, hitherto unknown, must be enforced by stronger evidence, facilitated by a clearer method, or more ably elucidated by brighter illustrations.

The distinguished Nobel laureate, Arthur Kornberg, in an essay entitled "Research—The Lifeline of Medicine," stated:

> Advances in medicine spring from discoveries in physics, chemistry, and biology. Among key contributions to the diagnosis, treatment and pre-

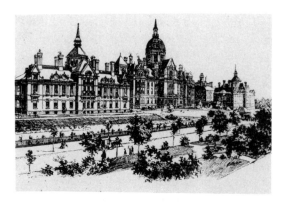

Figure 4-9.   Johns Hopkins Hospital as it appeared when built in 1889 (from an original etching).

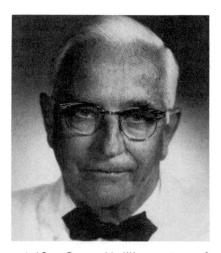

Figure 4-10.   Owen H. Wangensteen, famed academic surgeon who trained many of the current leaders in surgery.

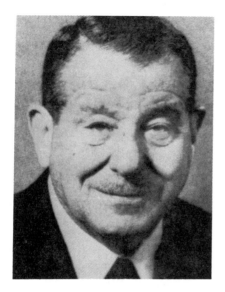

Figure 4-11.   Isador S. Ravdin.

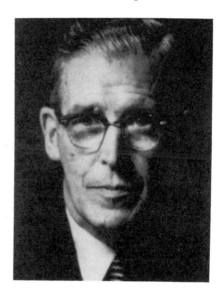

Figure 4-12.   Jonathan E. Rhoads.

vention of disease, an analysis has shown that two-thirds of these discoveries have originated with basic observations, rather than applied research. Without a firm foundation in basic scientific knowledge, innovations perceived as advances frequently prove hollow and collapse.

Surgical teachers are well advised to bear persistently in mind a comment of one of our greatest physiologists, Julius Comroe:

> I have always believed that a main responsibility of a faculty member is to be a talent source—to determine the special abilities of medical students in clinical care, in teaching, or in research and then to encourage them to do the very best they can in their field of unusual competence. One field, of course, is research. I see no way for faculty to determine this special talent of their students unless students have contact with research while they are still in medical school.

Quite clearly, it is highly desirable that students begin investigative work as soon as practicable.

Alfred Blalock: Discoveries in Shock and Heart Surgery

Isadore Ravdin related Dr. Alfred Blalock's importance in this chain by saying, "Alfred Blalock represents the finest of the physiologically minded surgeons who followed after the death of Dr. Halsted."[24] Blalock was born in 1899 and graduated from the University of Georgia. As a second year student at the Johns Hopkins Medical School, he was influenced by Dr. Halsted. He completed his residency at Vanderbilt and remained on the staff for 16 years. There and at Johns Hopkins he developed studies leading to monumental advances in the treatment of shock and congenital heart disease.[28,29]

The story of shock is fascinating. In 1925, Alfred Blalock and Tinsley Harrison began their early investigations which showed the inverse relationship between serum pH and cardiac output. After contracting tuberculosis, Blalock withdrew from clinical work and during 1928 worked with Anrep and Barcroft at Cambridge where he learned techniques needed to complete his shock studies. These studies were reborn at Vanderbilt, and in 1930 he published his classic paper, "Experimental Shock: The Cause of the Low Blood Pressure Produced by Muscle Injury." His twelve seminal papers showed that multiple conditions can result in shock and intravascular fluid imbalances. He showed that with massive soft tissue injury, intravascular fluids extravasate and deplete up to 66% of circulating blood volume. Blalock first determined that vasoactive toxin release was not the cause of shock, and that intravenous fluid infusions were beneficial.

The investigative spirit in surgery at Johns Hopkins had dissipated after Halsted's death. Everyone there considered the return of the 41-year-old Blalock to be the renaissance of scientific surgery (Figure 4-13).[24] Dr. Helen Taussig was following a large number of children with irreparable cyanotic heart disease. To approach this problem, Blalock relied on results of an earlier "failed" Vanderbilt experiment. He and Vivian Thomas had attempted to create the histologic changes of pulmonary hypertension in dogs by performing a subclavian to pulmonary artery shunt. In Blalock's words, "The left lung was pinker than the right on gross examination during life. Microscopic examination revealed no noteworthy alterations in either the left pulmonary artery or lung." Although pulmonary blood flow was augmented, he had not achieved his goal.[28] The negative results of that study were to launch a serendipitous treatment for Taussig's "blue babies." On November 29, 1944, Drs. Blalock and Longmire performed the first successful shunt operation for the tetralogy of Fallot. Later Drs. Blalock and Taussig reported 610 patients treated successfully by this operation. This operation,

more than any other, became the stimulus for a new age in cardiac surgery.

Will Camp Sealy: The Father of Arrhythmia Surgery

A North Carolina fisherman with multiple episodes of medically refractory supraventricular tachycardia was diagnosed at Duke University as having Wolff-Parkinson-White syndrome (WPWS). On May 2, 1968, Drs. Will C. Sealy and his team mapped the epicardial surface before instituting cardiopulmonary bypass. Boineau, a colleague, later wrote, "We found the site of pre-excitation [Kent Bundle] in the right ventricle during sinus rhythm and in the right atrium during PSVT." Cardiopulmonary perfusion was established, and through the mapped site Sealy wrote, "A 5 to 6 cm incision, extending from the base of the right atrial appendage to the right boarder of the right atrium and completely transecting the communication between the atrium and ventricle, was made." Remapping showed the earliest activation area arising from the normal right ventricular location, and the point of earliest activation now the latest. The fisherman returned home with a normal pulse, and Dr. Sealy had provided clear evidence that WPWS resulted from an anomalous pathway. Twenty-seven years later, the fisherman remained cured.[30]

The cardiac conduction system interested and bewildered physiologists, cardiologists, and surgeons for many years. Dr. Sealy played a pivotal role in the development of clinical electrophysiology (Figure 4-14).[30] He determined experimentally that abnormal conduction could be altered surgically. In this milieu, by meeting "the fisherman with a fast pulse," he and his colleagues at Duke University affected the first direct surgical cure for arrhythmias generated over an abnormal conduction pathway. Over the next 25 years, Sealy either trained or influenced a school of arrhythmia surgeons who perfected the surgical treatment for these patients worldwide. These accomplishments clearly established Dr. Sealy as the father of arrhythmia surgery.

Prior to this success, he had contributed much to surgery through his experimental and clinical

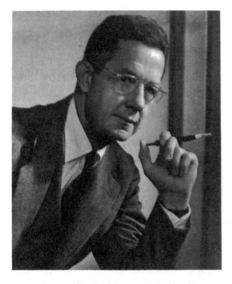

Figure 4-13. Alfred Blalock. This Karsh portrait of Blalock was made in 1950 to celebrate his 1,000th "blue baby" operation.

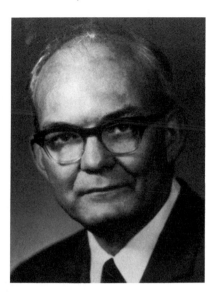

Figure 4-14. Will Camp Sealy. This portrait was made during the peak era of the Sealy operation for cardiac preexcitation due to the Wolff-Parkinson-White syndrome.

work on hypothermia, aortic coarctation, and thoracic surgery. As early as 1957, he and his colleagues wrote extensively on both experimental and clinical hypothermia. Sealy's interest in cardiac arrhythmias developed from this latter work. He said:

> The biggest problem [during deep hypothermia] related to patients developing ventricular fibrillation when their body temperature fell below 28°C. To get them out of fibrillation, we hooked the 120 volt AC power from the wall directly to the heart and this usually converted them to a normal rhythm. At that time we became interested in arrhythmias associated with deep hypothermia.[30]

Sealy, Boineau, and a third colleague, Wallace, played pivotal roles in attempting to understand the electrocardiogram under different pathologic conditions. They asked, Why does the electrocardiogram look different in congenital and acquired conditions? Sealy performed mapping on patients with atrial septal defects, tetralogy of Fallot, and left ventricular hypertrophy, among other cardiac lesions. Experimentally, he excised the sinus node of dogs and attempted to define the location of

the new intrinsic pacemaker. One of these animals developed atrial flutter, and the aberrant electrogram whetted an interest in supraventricular arrhythmias.

The early cases were done by the epicardial approach. The next patient after the fisherman developed an unstable arrhythmia pattern, and the pathway was never located. She died of intractable arrhythmias postoperatively, and her loss cast a pall over the surgical arrhythmia program.[30] Serendipity had played a major role in the first success. In retrospect, it was discovered that the second patient had a more complex paraseptal pathway, and if the simpler WPWS pathology had not been present in the fisherman, neither arrhythmia surgery nor catheter ablation may have been launched. Techniques were modified, and in 1974 Sealy presented the first 20 cases, with one death. The combined Duke series of 200 consecutive WPWS cases operated on by Sealy and Dr. James Cox were detailed in 1984, and right free wall paths were found in only 18% of patients. Worldwide, over 1,000 WPWS operations were reported by 1987, a time when radio frequency ablation was beginning to replace surgery. The WPWS operation and the pioneering efforts of Sealy and his colleagues paved the way for modern catheter-based methods and laid the foundation for future successes.

Research by Students

The major discoveries made by medical students are fascinating. Andreas Vesalius (Figure 4-15) prepared his great anatomical text, *De humani corporis fabrica* (Figure 4-16) while a medical student and had it published four months after his graduation from the University of Padua as a doctor of medicine. The first microscopic observation of the function of the capillary circulation was made in 1665 by a medical student, Jun Swammerdum, who noted erythrocytes flowing through the capillary network. In 1799 Humphry Davy, a 19-year-old medical student, prepared and inhaled quantities of nitrous oxide, discovered its marked analgesic effect, and predicted that it would someday be used to prevent the pain associated with surgical operations. In 1846 another medical stu-

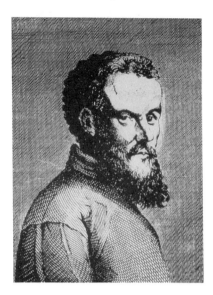

Figure 4-15. Andreas Vesalius, famed scientific anatomist.

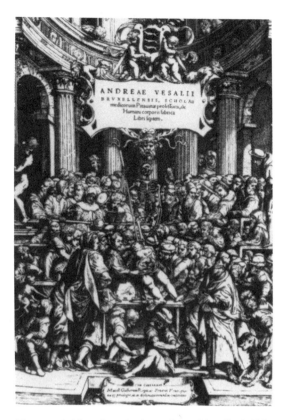

Figure 4-16. Frontispiece from Vesalius' *Fabrica,* published in 1543.

dent, William T.G. Morton, administered ether as an anesthetic at the Massachusetts General Hospital. Paul Langerhans, a medical student working with Virchow in Berlin, first described the islets in the pancreas that now bear his name. Ivar Sandstrom, a medical student at the University of Uppsala in Sweden, discovered the parathyroid glands and wrote a monograph documenting his observations. In the team of Banting, Macleod, and Best, who pioneered the discovery of insulin, Best was a medical student, but only Banting and Macleod received the Nobel prize. Jay MacLeod was a second-year medical student working in the physiology laboratory of William H. Howell when he discovered heparin in 1916.

In 1929 Werner Forssmann became a superb example of a surgical intern, making a major discovery with great courage, by passing a ureteral catheter through a vein in his left arm into his own heart, after failing to convince a volunteer to undergo the experimental procedure. Once the catheter was in his heart, Forssmann pondered whether he would be believed unless he had objective proof of this daring human experiment. Consequently, he arose from the operating table, walked up several flights of stairs, had a chest radiograph taken (Figure 4-17), and returned to re-

move the catheter. His forthright honesty is reflected in the last sentence of his report, in which he apologized to his readers because, when he removed the bandage from his forearm a week later, he had a superficial wound infection. He felt he must have inadvertently broken sterile technique during that historic procedure.[31]

Louis Pasteur made the famous statement, "Chance favors the prepared mind." Modern educational systems now approach complex subjects much earlier in a student's life, and child prodigies are becoming much more frequent. Although such individuals account for a small percentage of those who become scientific investigators, stepwise progression of education remains the usual and most reliable means of nurturing productive investigators. Many medical students now begin original investigation while in college and continue in medical school. Although M.D.-Ph.D. programs have played an influential role in the

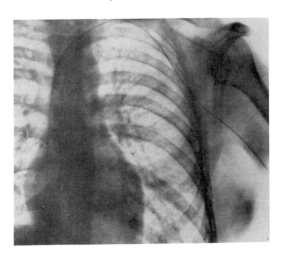

Figure 4-17.   Chest film showing catheter self-inserted in the left antecubital vein and passed into the heart of Werner Forssmann.

training of medical investigators, research fellowships during surgical residency training have been of greater significance. Many residency training programs foster the concept of spending one or more years in research, and in many centers most trainees obtain investigative experience. In the Duke University program nearly all surgical residents elect to spend two full-time years in basic research with a member of the faculty, a group of researchers, or, occasionally, in a laboratory position elsewhere. Such programs have been the source of most recent academic surgical appointees in medical schools and centers. An academic appointment now generally depends on demonstrated competence in research, confirmed by significant publications.

Conclusion: The Past May Predict the Future!

As the late Alexander Walt, a consummate surgical thinker, said in his Presidential Address to the American College of Surgeons, "The history of surgery should be taught as one would do in a graduate school so as to avoid repetition of past errors and to stimulate excitement at the recognition of how past challenges were overcome by serendipity or design."[32] Unfortunately, in most surgical curricula today, historical relevance has been crowded out by the specter of managed care, new technology, and more complex patient care. We must teach ourselves and our residents to review the accomplishments and failures of the past before launching new experiments and operations. We must ask ourselves Has this been done before? Halsted's admonition that "the wards (and operating rooms) are laboratories . . . laboratories of the highest order" should be heeded, since these are the vineyards for observation and application that lead to surgical discovery. For any of us, a careful historical search will often result in a head start on a surgical problem, whether it is clinical or experimental. Hunter's innovative deer studies, Lister's groundbreaking use of carbolic acid, Halsted's meticulous observations, Blalock's failed experiment, and Sealy's operation have each been a step in the evolution of scientific surgery. We will continue to see excellent operations that will be replaced by minimally invasive or less complex technologic advances. However, it is our charge to not become discouraged, but to continuously add new knowledge to the area of scientific surgery. Remember what Sir Berkeley Moynihan said in his Hunterian Oration: "The young surgeon of today can learn almost as much from [John] Hunter's mistakes as from his triumphs."[33]

The young surgeon planning a career in academic surgery is wise to reflect upon the present fabric of the field and recognize that the *biological* basis of modern surgical practice grows increasingly significant. Depth of knowledge is particularly important in the fields of physiology, pathology, biochemistry, immunology, pharmacology, biostatistics, genetics, and other emerging areas of research. It is difficult to make significant surgical advances without such knowledge of one or more of these disciplines, and the ability to perform and utilize the associated laboratory techniques. Close association with a recognized investigator or team, over a significant period of time, merits considerable emphasis and should be thoughtfully planned in advance, in consultation with acknowledged contributors in the field and the director of the surgical residency training program.

A career in academic surgery is demanding but is also the source of much excitement and many pleasures. Alfred Blalock stated this very well:

No satisfaction is quite like that which accompanies productive investigation, particularly if it leads to better treatment of the sick. The important discoveries in medicine are generally simple, and one is apt to wonder why they were not made earlier. I believe that they are made usually by a dedicated person who is willing to work and to cultivate his power of observation rather than by the so-called intellectual genius. Discoveries may be made by the individual worker as opposed to the current practice of a large research team. Simple apparatus may suffice; all the analyses need not be performed by technicians; large sums of money are not always necessary. Important basic ideas will probably continue to come from the individual. Whether by accident, design or hunch, the diligent investigator has a fair chance of making an important discovery. If he is unwilling to take his chance, he should avoid this type of work.[24]

Finally, all those planning to enter investigative surgery should be continuously aware of the words of William Osler (Figure 4-18), generally regarded as the greatest physician, worldwide, in the first half of this century; his astonishing career was characterized by tremendous happiness as well as achievement. While in his thirties, he became professor and chief of the department of medicine at McGill University and the Montreal General Hospital in Montreal. Shortly thereafter, he was offered and accepted what was then the leading post in medicine in the United States, at the University of Pennsylvania. Several years later, in 1889, he was offered the position of physician-in-chief and professor of medicine at the newly formed Johns Hopkins Hospital and Medical School, with a large number of beds and laboratories completely under his control. Since these beds were endowed and could be occupied by patients of any economic group, selected by the physician-in-chief, Osler was able to introduce medical students to the wards and to allow them to perform clinical examinations on patients. He was also a distinguished medical scholar who edited an extraordinary textbook of medicine that remained in publication for half a century; he was a skilled diagnostician, a superb speaker, and a clinical scientist of great renown. In 1905 Osler was offered the most prestigious post in medicine of that day, the Regius Chair at the University of Oxford in England.

When asked why he had been so successful in his career and why he was well known by his friends and colleagues to be an exceedingly happy individual who thoroughly enjoyed all aspects of the medical profession, Osler simply said:

It seems a bounden duty on such an occasion to be honest and frank, so I propose to tell you the secret of life as I have seen the game played, and as I have tried to play it myself. . . . This I propose to give you in the hope, yes, in the full assurance that some of you at least will lay hold upon it to your profit. Though a little one, the master-word looms large in meaning.— WORK—It is the open sesame to every portal, the great equalizer in the world, the true philosopher's stone, which transmutes all the base metal of humanity into gold. The stupid man among you, it will make bright, the bright man brilliant, and the brilliant student steady. With the magic word in your heart all things are possible, and without it all study is vanity and vexation. The miracles of life are with it. . . . To the youth it brings hope, to the middle-aged confidence, and to the aged repose. . . . It is directly responsible for all advances in medicine during the past twenty-five centuries.[34]

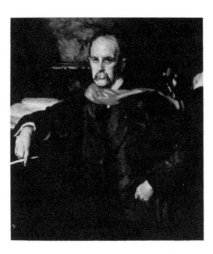

Figure 4-18.   Sir William Osler, 1849–1919, Regius Professor of Medicine at the University of Oxford, England.

References

1. Barnes BA. Discarded operations: surgical innovation by trial and error. In: Bunker JP, Barnes BA, and Mosteller F, eds. Costs, Risks, and Benefits of Surgery. New York: Oxford University, 1977, pp. 109-123.

2. Cope Z. The History of Royal College of Surgeons of England. London: Anthony Blond, 1959.

3. Dobson J. John Hunter. London: E. & S. Livingstone, 1969.

4. Rohrer CWG. John Hunter: his life and labors. Bull Johns Hopkins Hosp 1914;25:10-25.

5. Chitwood WR. John and William Hunter on aneurysms. Arch Surg 1977;112:829-836.

6. Gloyne SR. John Hunter. Edinburgh: E. & S. Livingstone, 1950.

7. Hunter J. The Natural History of the Teeth: Explaining Their Structure, Use, Formation, Growth, and Diseases. London: J. Johnson, 1778.

8. Hunter J. A Treatise on the Venereal Disease. London: John Hunter—Castle Street, 1786.

9. Hunter J. Observations on Certain Parts of the Animal Oeconomy. London: John Hunter—Castle Street, 1786.

10. Hunter J. A Treatise on the Blood, Inflammation, and Gunshot Wounds. London: J. Richardson, 1794.

11. Allen E, Turk JL, Murley R. The Case Books of John Hunter. London: Royal Society of Medicine and Whitstable Litho, 1993.

12. Palmer JF. The Works of John Hunter, vol. 3. London: Longman, Rees, Orme, Brown, Green, and Longman, 1835.

13. Godlee RJ. Lord Lister. London: Macmillan, 1917.

14. Cameron HC, Cheyne WW, Godlee RJ, Martin CJ, Williams D. The Collected Papers of Joseph, Baron Lister. Oxford: Clarendon, 1909.

15. Ravitch MM. A Century of Surgery: The History of the American Surgical Association. Philadelphia: J. B. Lippincott, 1982.

16. Garrison FH. History of Medicine. Philadelphia: W. B. Saunders, 1929.

17. Heuer GW. Dr. Halsted. Bull Johns Hopkins Hosp 1952;90:(Supp) 1-105.

18. MacCallum WG. William Stewart Halsted: Surgeon. Baltimore: Johns Hopkins, 1930.

19. Halsted WS. Surgical Papers of William Stewart Halsted. Baltimore: Johns Hopkins, 1924.

20. Blalock A. William Stewart Halsted and his influence on surgery. Proc R Soc Med 1952;45:555-563.

21. MacCallum WG. William Stewart Halsted: Surgeon. Baltimore: Johns Hopkins, 1930, p. 67.

22. Halsted WS. The employment of fine silk in preference to catgut, and the advantages of transfixing tissues and vessels in controlling hemorrhage; also an account of the introduction of gloves, gutta-percha tissue, and silver foil. JAMA 1913;60:1119-1126.

23. Halsted WS. The training of the surgeon. In: Surgical Papers of William Steward Halsted, vol 2. Baltimore: Johns Hopkins, 1924:512-531.

24. Sabiston DC Jr. Presidential address: Alfred Blalock. Ann Surg 1978;188:255-270.

25. Wangensteen OH. Teacher's oath. J Med Educ 1978;53(6):524.

26. Carter BN. The fruition of Halsted's concept of surgical training. Surgery 1952;32:518.

27. Holman, E. The legacy of William Steward Halsted. Bull Am Coll Surgeons. Apr 1969; 1-5.

28. Thomas V. Pioneering Research in Surgical Shock and Cardiovascular Surgery: Vivien Thomas and His Work with Alfred Blalock. Philadelphia: University of Pennsylvania, 1985.

29. Ravitch MM. The Papers of Alfred Blalock. Baltimore: Johns Hopkins, 1966.

30. Chitwood WR. Will C. Sealy, MD: The father of arrhythmia surgery—the story of the fisherman with a fast pulse. Ann Thorac Surg 1994;58:1228-1239.

31. Forssmann W. Experiments on myself. Klin Wonchenschr 1929;8:2085.

32. Walt AJ. The uniqueness of American surgical education and its preservation. Bull Am Coll Surgeons. Dec 1994;8.

33. Moynihan B. Hunterian Oration: Hunter's ideals and Lister's principles. Lancet 1 (Feb 27, 1927): 372-379.

34. Osler, Sir William. Aequanimitas, with Other Addresses. Philadelphia: P. Blakiston's Son, 1932.

Commentary

This chapter provides selective historical perspectives on how scientific surgery evolved as seen from the vantage point of one of the deans of

American surgery and his former student, now chairman of a surgical department. It is not meant to be a comprehensive history of surgery, since that is available in numerous other sources. Each author of this chapter has written separate and somewhat different accounts of this material. Dr. Sabiston's chapter appeared in our second edition. With the authors' permission we have combined their contributions. The strengths of the chapter should be credited to the writers; the editors take responsibility for any inconsistencies or overlap that may have resulted from the fusion.

The authors emphasize the contributions of Paré, Hunter, and Lister as being pivotal in our emergence from the dark days of the barber surgeons. Halstead's leadership role in establishing residency programs in the United States based on his exposure to the classic training in the German surgical schools provides us with an understanding of the roots of current surgical residency training programs. Exciting examples of the contributions of Alfred Blalock to the pathophysiology of shock, and Will Sealy to dysrhythmia surgery can serve as models for the young investigator facing current surgical challenges.

D.S.M.
M.F.M.

CHAPTER 5

Surgeons Who Have Won the Nobel Prize

J. Yee and D.S. Mulder

Surgery is practiced at the crossroads of clinical intuition and scientific deduction. Although exigency often dictates that irreversible decisions must be made within the context of incomplete or conflicting data, the "imprecise science" of surgery has demonstrated that astute observation of signs and symptoms and constant reappraisal of the results of therapy can lead to profound insights into the nature of illness. The rhythm of observing protean manifestations of disease, progressing to death or disability unless correctly analyzed and treated, forms the core of a surgeon's daily life. The relentlessness of this march could lead to fatalism when effective treatment is unavailable, or inspire determination to understand and influence the biological forces at work. This determination has characterized the surgeons who have been recognized by the Nobel prize in physiology or medicine. It may seem incongruous that surgeons, with their very workmanlike focus on practical solutions to common problems, would draw accolades from the august world of scientists and academics, but the surgical specialties have produced nine Nobel prize winners in medical science. The reasons for this success are derived from the attributes cultivated in every generation of surgeons:

> Care for the Sick;
> Scientific Curiosity;
> Concentrated Activity
> Commitment to Excellence

The bequest of Alfred Nobel stipulated that annual prizes be awarded to those individuals who, through work in their chosen field, had "conferred the greatest benefit on mankind." Since 1901 the Nobel prize in physiology or medicine has identified pivotal contributors to medical knowledge whose impact has been widespread and enduring.[1] Nine surgeons have been recognized: Emil Theodore Kocher, Allvar Gullstrand, Alexis Carrel, Robert Bárány, Frederick G. Banting, Walter R. Hess, Werner O. Forssman, Charles B. Huggins, and Joseph E. Murray. Some of these surgeons remained invisible to their contemporaries, and the importance of their work was recognized only many years later. A few were immediately identified and celebrated. Despite their pursuit of distinctly different interests in separate countries and historical eras, all of these surgeons shared the essential attributes that still define the profession. Their careers were concerned with solving human problems and the puzzles of nature. The Nobel prize would come as a recognition of a career well spent, but was never a goal for these men.[1,2] Their accomplishments are recorded here as reminders of our profession's foundations and to serve as a guide for meeting the challenges of the future. This chapter, necessarily brief and citing sources mainly in the English language, can serve only as an introduction to their lives and work. The interested reader is referred to other published works that similarly celebrate our surgical heritage in more detail. The series of articles by Jain, Swan, and Casey are especially interesting reading.[3–8]

Emil Theodore Kocher

Emil Theodore Kocher was born in Bern, Switzerland, on August 25, 1841, and graduated with honors from the Medical College of the University of Bern in 1865. During the following year, he traveled to expand his surgical and scientific outlook, visiting the clinics of Billroth in Vienna, Lister in Edinburgh, and Pasteur in Paris. He returned to Bern in 1866 to join the university's surgical clinic. Kocher was appointed professor and director in 1872, a post he held until his death 45 years later. Widely respected as a meticulous and skilled technical surgeon, his career was marked by the breadth of his interests. He authored articles on subjects as diverse as orthopedics, gastrointestinal and biliary tract surgery, techniques of asepsis, the management of penetrating trauma, and the repair of inguinal hernia. His textbook of surgery was first published in 1892 and remained in print for four more editions.[9]

Because he lived and worked his entire life in an area of endemic goiter, Kocher obtained extensive experience in surgery of the thyroid gland.[10] He performed more than 9,000 thyroidectomies with less than 1% mortality. As he reviewed his own results on total thyroidectomy, which were widely regarded as unparalleled, Kocher identified a disturbing postoperative condition he termed *cachexia strumipriva*. This complication of hypothyroidism, now called *myxedema*, would later provide an explanation for congenital cretinism and form a rational basis for thyroid replacement therapy.[11] He was awarded the Nobel prize in 1909 for his work on the physiology, pathology, and surgery of diseases of the thyroid.

He continued as an operating surgeon until a few weeks prior to his death at age 75 on July 27, 1917. The eponyms in modern surgery that celebrate his career are the Kocher maneuver, to mobilize the duodenum; the subcostal Kocher incision, for open cholecystectomy; the transverse Kocher incision, for thyroidectomy; and the Kocher reduction of the dislocated shoulder.

Allvar Gullstrand

Allvar Gullstrand was born in Landskrona, a small town near Copenhagen (then a part of Sweden) on June 5, 1862. He followed in the footsteps of his physician father and graduated with a doctorate in medicine from the University of Uppsala in 1888. His dissertation in 1890 at the Royal Caroline Institute on the origins of astigmatism formed the basis for a scientific career in ophthalmology. In 1894 at the age of 32 years, Gullstrand became the professor and chairman of the newly created Department of Ophthalmology at the University of Uppsala and guided the development of objective laboratory tests in the clinical diagnosis of ophthalmologic disorders.[1,2,12]

Largely self-educated in mathematics and physics, Gullstrand theorized that geometric abnormalities in the cornea formed the basis for the distortion of light and the associated disorders of visual perception. He correlated disparities in the horizontal and vertical axes of the cornea to patient symptoms and invented the punctual lens as a corrective measure. He further demonstrated that the process of accommodation involved a gain in the refractile power of the lens that was due to both a change in the convexity of the lens and to previously undescribed changes in the internal structure of the lens itself. Gullstrand understood that the existing laws of optics, based on glass and other homogenous materials, could not be generally applied to the live tissues of the human eye. Gullstrand developed an operation for the treatment of symblepharon and designed both the slit lamp and modern reflex-free ophthalmoscope. The slit lamp, through its ability to inspect the cornea, iris, lens, and vitreous in minute detail, represented a revolutionary improvement in diagnostics.

Gullstrand was awarded the Nobel prize in 1911 for his work on dioptrics and visual accommodation. His remarkable achievements were derived from a focused application of his knowledge of mathematics and physics to the clinical world of ophthalmology.

Alexis Carrel

Alexis Carrel was a pioneer in surgery whose full impact was not truly recognized until many years after his death in 1944. He was born near Lyons, France, on June 28, 1873, and graduated from the University of Lyons in 1900 with a doctorate in medicine. In 1902 and only two years after graduation, Carrel published his first article of a series on the anastomosis of blood vessels. He recognized that the keys to success in vascular surgery resided in delicate and meticulous operative technique: the avoidance of crushing clamps and damage to the endothelial lining, the use of fine nonabsorbable suture, and careful eversion of the vessel edge along suture lines. The anastomosis was constructed using three equidistant retaining sutures placed to unite the ends of the vessels. "By traction on the threads the circumference of the artery can be transformed into a triangle and the perimeter can be dilated at will. Then the edges of each side of the triangle are united by a continuous suture whilst they are under tension." This technique, as described by Carrel nearly a century ago, remains in use today.[13,14]

Most of Carrel's work was carried out in the United States. Frustrated with the academic bureaucracy in France, he emigrated to Canada to raise cattle, and briefly lived in Montreal before eventually assuming a position at the University of Chicago in 1905. His work on vascular anastomoses attracted considerable interest and earned him a fellowship at the Rockefeller Institute in New York. Carrel became a faculty member in 1912 and would remain at the Rockefeller Institute until his retirement in 1939. The freedom and support offered at the Institute allowed Carrel to extend his studies to include interpositional grafting by autogenous veins, vessel patches, aortic surgery, tissue culture, and early animal experiments on the technique of organ transplantation. He was the first to describe the use of shunts during surgery on the thoracic aorta as a means of preventing paraplegia from spinal cord ischemia. His descriptions of valvular cardiac surgery and coronary artery bypass grafting were prophetic. Even more remarkable were his ideas for the transplantation of organs. Carrel's experience with vascular anastomoses led to experiments on limb reimplantation and the autotransplantation of various organs, including the kidney. He described how harvesting a patch of the proximal vessel (e.g., aorta) in continuity with the vascular supply of the organ could technically facilitate

later implantation. Carrel also noted that autografts survived longer than heterografts. He recognized that the feasibility of organ transplantation would depend on a deeper understanding of the biological processes that mediated the phenomenon of host rejection.

The Nobel prize was awarded to Carrel in 1912 for his work on vascular suturing and the transplantation of blood vessels and organs. Further recognition would follow as Carrel, while a volunteer military surgeon stationed in France during World War I, developed a wound-cleansing solution of sodium hypochlorite, with the famed British chemist Henry Drysdale Dakin. Carrel received the United States Distinguished Service Medal but failed to gain the recognition he most wanted from his native France.

His book, *Man, the Unknown*, was published in 1935 and reflected his growing concern with metaphysics and the dehumanizing effects of materialism and industrial technology.[15] Carrel argued that the principles of science, when applied to people and society, would help restore civilization to its intellectual and humanistic roots. Carrel and Charles A. Lindbergh published a book entitled *The Culture of Organs* in 1938. In this work, the surgeon and the famous pilot described their experiments on organ preservation.[16] Carrel and Lindbergh had worked on the concept of an artificial heart and hoped to develop a mechanical pumping device that could perfuse and preserve excised organs.

Conflicts within the Rockefeller Institute would soon force Carrel to leave the United States and ultimately return to France. His efforts as a medical advisor to the French Ministry of Public Health and his association with the Vichy regime after the fall of France in 1940 led to harsh criticism and later accusations of collaboration with the Axis powers. Carrel, the surgeon and scientist whose own sparkling accomplishments lay intertwined with his disillusioned witness of two world wars, died in November 1944.[17]

Robert Bárány

Robert Bárány was born in Vienna, Austria, on April 22, 1876, and graduated with a doctorate in medicine in 1900. He studied neurology under

Kraeplin in Heidelberg before returning to his native Austria to train in surgery at the renowned Vienna General Hospital. His interest in neurology led him to the surgical discipline of otology and the influence of Adam Politzer. Bárány observed that patients developed nystagmus and dizziness on irrigation of the auditory canal, and that the ocular findings varied with the temperature of the irrigating solution. He theorized that temperature changes in the vestibular canal induced movement of the liquid within and resulted in the perception of body movement. Vertigo resulted when other senses, such as sight, perceived no such motion. Bárány further hypothesized that this normal response to caloric stimulation would be lost in patients with disease of the middle ear. Detailed investigations on patients and normal volunteers substantiated his hypotheses and formed the basis for his *Investigations on Rhythmic Nystagmus and its Accompanying Manifestations Arising from the Vestibular Apparatus of the Ear*, published in 1906.

During World War I, Bárány was sent to organize a military surgical unit. His subsequent management of wartime neurosurgical injuries, which included the heretofore unaccepted primary closure of debrided cerebral gunshot wounds, predated the essentially similar practice later promoted by and credited to Harvey Cushing, the famed American neurosurgeon. Bárány was captured by the Russian army in 1915 and interred at a prisoner of war camp in Turkistan. It was here that he received the news that his work on the vestibular apparatus had won the 1914 Nobel prize. He was released in 1916 only to return to Vienna and be accused by his colleagues of plagiarism. Fully exonerated of these accusations, Bárány chose to move to Sweden and accepted the rather modest appointment of assistant professor at the University of Uppsala. He remained in Sweden until his death in 1936.[18]

Frederick Banting

Frederick Banting was born November 14, 1891, in Alliston, a small town near Toronto, Canada. His parents were hardworking farmers who hoped that he would become a Methodist minister. Much to his father's dismay, Banting enrolled in the University of Toronto's medical school in 1912. During World War I, Banting enlisted with the Medical Corps of the Royal Canadian Army and left for England. He saw service in France and was decorated with the Military Cross. Despite sustaining a serious injury to his right arm, Banting returned to Toronto in 1919 and completed training in orthopedic surgery under his mentor, Clarence Starr. He accepted a hospital position in London, Ontario, but soon began to grow restless. Lecturing at the Department of Physiology at the University of Western Ontario was his outlet. He developed a keen interest in diabetes mellitus and physiology of the pancreas. Basing his reasoning on the pathophysiology of gallstone pancreatitis, Banting thought that the endocrine function of the gland could be better studied if its exocrine function was somehow removed. He approached J.J.R. MacLeod, professor of physiology at the University of Toronto, with his research proposal but was rebuffed repeatedly. Banting persisted and MacLeod finally relented, allowing the young surgeon to use his Toronto laboratory during his absence. Charles H. Best, one of MacLeod's students, was assigned to work with Banting for the summer of 1921. MacLeod himself was in Scotland.[19]

Banting and Best proceeded with a classic series of experiments that involved ligation of the pancreatic duct and the induction of exocrine atrophy.[20,21] They found that an extract of the atrophic pancreas could reverse diabetic coma in dogs. In January 1922 a crude preparation was used to treat a young boy with diabetic ketoacidosis at Toronto General Hospital. The Nobel prize was awarded in 1923 to Banting and MacLeod for the discovery of insulin. The committee's decision to recognize MacLeod and to exclude Best deeply wounded Banting's sense of fairness. He shared his half of the money award with Best and evoked a controversy on the anatomy of scientific collaboration, which remains pertinent even now.[22]

The Nobel prize, which Banting won at the age of 32, brought fame to the university and heightened public optimism for research in other diseases. The Banting Research Foundation and the

Banting Institute were formed at the University of Toronto to concentrate medical research at this time of intense expectation. The onset of World War II led Banting to rejoin the military, this time to coordinate war-related research in North America. The Banting Institute had helped develop a pressurized flight suit that would protect pilots during high-*g*-force maneuvers. On his way to England to test this device, Charles Banting lost his life in a Newfoundland airplane crash. Once again, a life devoted to medicine and science was caught up in the social currents of the time and the inexorable rhythm of the drumbeat of war.[23]

Walter Hess

Walter Hess was born in Frauenfeld, Switzerland, on March 17, 1881. He received his degree in medicine from the University of Zurich in 1905 and entered a residency in opthalmology during the subsequent year. After several successful and lucrative years in private practice, Hess returned to the University of Zurich to carry out research on hemodynamics and blood viscosity. The influence of Max Verworn from Bonn University served to sharpen Hess's interest in the autonomic control of circulation and respiration. After serving as a field surgeon in the Imperial German army during World War I, Hess resumed his academic career in Zurich and became, at the age of 36, the chairman of the Department of Physiology.[24] His subsequent work concentrated on the use of animal studies to map the functional organization of the brain. Through selective stimulation or ablation of areas in the midbrain, Hess was able to relate the anatomy of what is now known as the diencephalon to the autonomic control of the body's vegetative functions. Insights were also obtained on the biological control of emotion, since electrical stimulation of the hypothalamus was found to elicit rage in experimental animals. Hess was the first to assign a specific physiologic function to a specific area in the brain, a remarkable accomplishment for one who began his professional life in the private practice of opthalmology.[25] Hess was awarded the Nobel prize in 1949 for his work on "the interbrain as a coordinator of the activities of the internal organs."

Werner Theodor Otto Forssman

Werner Theodor Otto Forssman was born on August 29, 1904, in Berlin, Germany, and graduated in medicine from the Fredrich Wilhelm University in 1928. During his subsequent surgical training in 1929 Forssman, after numerous experiments on cadavers, performed the first transvenous catheterization of the human heart on himself. He cut down upon a vein in his left arm and threaded a "well-oiled ureteral catheter" toward the heart. He then walked through the hospital to the radiology department where, despite the ensuing alarm, an X ray was taken to prove the location of the catheter tip in his right ventricle.[26] Although Forssman had originally intended this technique to be an aid in the intracardiac delivery of drugs, its potential application to hemodynamic and metabolic research was apparent. Some of his colleagues condemned him for pursuing what they then believed was a wild and dangerous avenue.

Forssman went on to complete his training as a urologist and served as an army surgeon during World War II. After his capture and release as an Allied prisoner of war, Forssman returned to clinical practice in Germany.[1] His work on heart catheterization had meanwhile been elaborated on by Andre F. Cournand and Dickinson W. Richards in New York. Forssman's contribution to the development of heart catheterization was recognized by the Nobel committee in 1956, more than 25 years after his original publication. He shared the Nobel prize with Cournand and Richards. The modern practice of cardiology and critical care thus became indebted to a urologist and his daring experiments.

Charles B. Huggins

Charles B. Huggins was also a urologist, born in Halifax, Canada, on September 22, 1901. He received his B.A., along with a graduating class of only 25 students, from the nearby Acadia University in Nova Scotia. Huggins earned a medical degree from Harvard University in 1924. He completed a surgical residency at the University of Michigan before joining the newly formed medical school at the University of Chicago in 1927. Huggins studied the physiology of the canine prostate gland, observing that normal prostatic secretion was hormonally regulated by androgens and estrogens. The implications of this on the treatment of prostatic cancer was subsequently realized when Huggins demonstrated that bilateral orchiectomy or exogenous estrogen could lead to a decrease in the serum level of acid phosphatase, a marker of metastatic prostatic cancer.[27] His clinical report on the results of orchiectomy in patients with metastatic prostate cancer showed that clinical improvement and even long-term survival could be attained after manipulation of the hormonal milieu.[28] Huggins later applied this line of reasoning to his research on the endocrine regulation of breast cancer. Ovariectomy and adrenalectomy, followed by cortisone replacement, were advocated as endocrine therapies for advanced breast cancer.[29] His discoveries concerning the hormonal treatment of prostate cancer won him his share of the 1966 Nobel prize for physiology or medicine.

Joseph E. Murray

Joseph E. Murray is the surgeon most recently honored by a Nobel prize. He shared the 1990 award with E. Donnall Thomas for discoveries in the field of organ and cell transplantation. The first successful human kidney transplant was carried out between identical twins in a daring operation performed by Murray on December 23, 1954. The clarity of vision and courage required for this undertaking were formidable. Even today, more than 40 years later, the prospect of subjecting a healthy individual to a donor nephrectomy is not taken lightly. The reasoning and preparation that were necessary, the unwavering conviction that a procedure of this magnitude would work, and the confidence that his technical skills would measure up to the challenge combine to personify the essence of the surgical ideal.[30]

Murray was born on April 1, 1919, in Milford, Massachusetts, and graduated from the Harvard Medical School in 1943. His surgical internship at the Peter Bent Brigham Hospital in Boston was interrupted by service with the United States Army as a First Lieutenant at Valley Forge Hospital. He developed his skills as a plastic surgeon while attending to the wounded, and often burned, soldiers of World War II. After the war, Murray completed his residency at the Brigham Hospital and continued on to further training in both head and neck surgery and plastic surgery at, respectively, Memorial Sloan Kettering and the New York Hospital.[1] He returned to Boston to assume a clinical post in the Department of Surgery at the Brigham Hospital. This hospital had an active dialysis unit and was very involved in the treatment of end-stage renal disease. Murray began a series of animal experiments that served to develop not only the technique of transplantation, but also some means of inducing host tolerance for the new organ. Recognizing, from the work of his colleague David Hume, that a kidney from a cadaveric donor would inevitably fail, and drawing from his own experience in skin grafting, Murray concluded that transplantation would become feasible if the host's immunologic barriers were eliminated. The ultimate test of this hypothesis occurred in 1954 when a patient named Richard Herrick presented with both end-stage renal failure and an identical twin brother willing to donate a kidney. The operation was a success and the patient went on to live 8 more years, marrying his recovery-room nurse and fathering two children during that time. Murray would later demonstrate the feasibility of cadaveric renal transplantation within the context of drug-induced host immunosuppression.[31] Murray's own discipline of plastic surgery would also benefit from his talent as he combined with Donald Matson, the chief of neurosurgery at the Brigham Hospital, to develop a craniofacial approach for the treatment of children with orbital tumors.[32]

Conclusion

This necessarily brief presentation on the nine surgeon Nobel laureates cannot do justice to the color and richness of their professional lives, nor capture their humanity as husbands, fathers, or friends. One cannot help but notice how their lives, separated as they were by time and distance, all resonated with common themes. Kocher, the master technician and dedicated surgeon, was si-

Table 5-1.   Nobel Prize Winners in Surgery.

		Country of Birth	Area of Interest
1901	Emil Kocher	Switzerland	Physiology, pathology and surgery of the thyroid gland
1911	Alver Gullstrand	Sweden	Dioptrics and visual accommodation
1912	Alexis Carrel	France	Vascular suturing and transplantation
1914	Robert Bárány	Austria	Physiology and pathology of the vestibular apparatus
1923	Frederick Banting	Canada	Discovery of insulin
1949	Walter Hess	Switzerland	Functional organization of the interbrain as coordinator of activities of internal organs
1956	Werner Forssman	Germany	Heart catheterization
1966	Charles Huggins	Canada	Hormonal treatment of prostate cancer
1990	Joseph Murray	United States	Kidney transplantation

multaneously a generalist and a highly focused specialist. His work ranged over many topics in surgery, but his approach was always characterized by the same meticulous attention to detail and a constant reappraisal of how surgery could be better done. Gullstrand, with his research on the refraction of light by the human eye and the development of the slit lamp, brought physics and mathematics to be bedside. The seven surgeons that followed were all variously touched by war and went on to serve their country. Carrel, a technical innovator and a visionary scientist in vascular surgery and transplantation, was an enigmatic figure who, despite many honors, died bitterly disappointed from never having gained the recognition he felt he deserved from his native France. Bárány, the founder of otoneurology, received his Nobel prize while a prisoner of war. He too was criticized by contemporaries within his own country and pursued the rest of his academic career outside of Austria. Banting was an orthopedic surgeon who discovered insulin. Hess was an opthalmologist who mapped the brain and defined the diencephalon. Forssman was a urologist who, alone and upon himself, conducted the world's first catheterization of a living human heart. Huggins, a dedicated laboratory scientist and active surgeon, applied his bench findings at the bedside and established the basis for endocrine therapy in cancer. Murray, the plastic surgeon trained in head and neck oncology, performed the world's first kidney transplantation. (See Table 5-1.)

What can we learn from these nine Nobel laureates? All were active participants in patient care. Their research was meticulous yet to the point. Neither easily distracted nor isolated from their social responsibilities, these surgeons concentrated their skills and efforts to solve a technical problem or a biologic puzzle. Like many surgeons, seven of them served their country during times of war to care for the sick and wounded. Their scientific endeavors were characterized by an intellectual curiosity that respected neither the boundaries imposed by their formal training nor the limits placed around them by their colleagues. An openness to self-education and a childlike disregard of contemporary limits on science allowed a urologist and an orthopedic surgeon to become the pioneers of cardiology and endocrinology. Bridges were built across specialties and between the laboratory and the bedside.

The speed and direction of our future progress in the modern practice of surgery will be linked not only to the efforts of individuals, but also to the retained values of the profession. The concerns and pressures faced by surgeons today are unquestionably severe but are no more extreme than those of the past. Subspecialization, the threat of self-interested fragmentation, and the political and economic forces that conspire to make us limit ourselves, pose real challenges to modern surgery. Careers combining clinical care and academic research seem increasingly rare as responsibilities for one's patients, laboratory, and family compete for time and attention. The future of surgery will depend on how we conduct our lives as decisive agents of change in science and society. Surgeons, who rarely hide from the challenges of the operating theater, often fail to recognize how the tallest obstacles to progress, bias and self-doubt, arise insidiously from within. Possibilities may lay unfulfilled unless sparked by an optimistic determination to learn and act. Impressed with the human face of disease and empowered by a trained mind, the surgeon committed to excellence in daily work will always serve as a public witness for what will continue to be a noble profession.

References

1. Magill FN. The Nobel Prize Winners: Physiology or Medicine. Pasadena: Salem, 1991.
2. Sourkes TL. Nobel Prize Winners in Medicine and Physiology, 1901–1965. London: Abelhard-Schuman, 1967.
3. Jain KM, Swan KG, Casey KG. Nobel Prize Winners in Surgery. Part 1. Am Surg 1981;47:195–200.
4. Jain KM, Swan KG, Casey KG. Nobel Prize Winners in Surgery. Part 2. Am Surg 1982;48:191–196.
5. Jain KM, Swan KG, Casey KG. Nobel Prize Winners in Surgery. Part 3. Am Surg 1982;48:287–292.
6. Jain KM, Swan KG, Casey KG. Nobel Prize Winners in Surgery. Part 4. Am Surg 1982;48:495–500.
7. Swan KG, Jain KM, Casey KG. Nobel Prize Winners in Surgery: Summary. Am Surg 1982;48:555–557.
8. Morris JB, Schirmer WJ. The "right stuff": five Nobel prize–winning surgeons. Surgery 1990; 108:71–80.
9. Kocher ET. Textbook of Operative Surgery, 5th edn. New York: MacMillan, 1911.
10. Halstead WS. The operative story of goitre. Johns Hopkins Hosp Rep 1919;19:71–157.
11. Merke F. History and Iconography of Endemic Goitre and Cretinism. Norwell: Kluwer Academic, 1984.
12. Wasson T. Nobel Prize Winners. New York: H. W. Wilson, 1987.
13. Carrel A. Anastomosis and transplantation of blood vessels. Am Med 1905;10:284.
14. Carrel A. La technique operatoire des anastamoses vasculaires et la transplantation des visceres. Lyon Med 1902;xcVIII:859–864.
15. Carrel A. Man, the Unknown. New York: Harper and Row, 1935.
16. Carrel A, Lindbergh CA. The Culture of Organs. New York: Hoeber, 1938.
17. Malinin, TI. Surgery and Life: The Extraordinary Career of Alexis Carrel. New York: Harcourt Brace Jovanovich, 1979.
18. McHenry LC. Garrison's History of Neurology. Springfield: Charles C. Thomas, 1969.
19. Bliss M. Banting: A Biography. Toronto: McClelland and Stewart, 1984.
20. Banting FG, Best CH, MacLeod JJR. The internal secretion of the pancreas. Am J Physiol 1921; 59:439. Abstract.
21. Banting FG, Best CH. Internal secretion of pancreas. J Lab Clin Med 1922; 7:251–326.
22. Bliss M. The Discovery of Insulin. Chicago: University of Chicago, 1982.
23. Harris H. Banting's Miracle: The Story of the Discoverer of Insulin. Philadelphia: J. B. Lippincott, 1946.
24. Hess WR. From medical practice to theoretical medicine. In: Ingle DJ, ed. A Dozen Doctors. Chicago: University of Chicago, 1963.
25. Hess WR. Causality, consciousness, and cerebral organization. Science 1967;158:1279–1283.
26. Forssman, WO. Experiments on Myself: Memoirs of a Surgeon in Germany. New York: St. Martin's, 1974.
27. Huggins CB, Hodges CV. Studies on prostate cancer. I. The effect of castration, estrogen, and androgen injection on serum phosphatases in metastatic carcinoma of the prostate. Cancer Res 1941;1:293–297.
28. Huggins CB, Stevens RE Jr, Hodges CV. Studies on prostate cancer. II The effects of castration on advanced carcinoma of the prostate gland. Arch Surg 1941;43:209–223.
29. Huggins CB. Induction and extinction of mammary cancer. Science 1962;137:257–262.
30. Murray JE, Merrill JP, Harrison JH, Guild WR. Successful homotransplantation of the human kidney between identical twins. JAMA 1956;160: 277–282.
31. Murray JE, Merrill JP, Harrison JH, Wilson RE.

Prolonged survival of human kidney homografts by immunosuppressive drug therapy. N Engl J Med 1963;268:1315–1323.

32. Jurkiewicz MJ. Nobel laureate: Joseph E. Murray, clinical surgeon, scientist, teacher. Surgery 1990; 125:1423–1424. Editorial.

Commentary

The Nobel prize represents the judgment of a distinguished committee from a single country with its own historical criteria and terms of reference. Many in the world community of surgery have their own heroes in surgical science based on criteria that do not enter the calculus of the Nobel committee, such as exemplary patient care, surgical judgment, and technical proficiency. Perhaps surgery will someday have its own honor roll.

Readers are encouraged to develop their own nominations to the "Nobility of Surgery."

It is remarkable that nine surgeons have been recognized with the Nobel prize. This chapter is a refreshing look at the lives, contributions, and professional careers of the nine Nobel prize winners in surgery. They all demonstrated the common characteristics of a high level of care for the sick, intense scientific curiosity, determination, and a level of concentration that allowed them to complete their work despite problems as large as those presented by two major wars. The unqualified commitment to excellence illustrated by each of their lives serves as an example to young surgical investigators not to be deterred by current concerns, pressures, and obstacles that may seem insurmountable.

H.T.
M.F.M.

CHAPTER 6

The Historical Evolution of Clinical Research

A.V. Pollock

Research! A mere excuse for idleness; it has never achieved and will never achieve any results of the slightest value.

—Benjamin Jowett[1]

Surgical research, whether in the laboratory, the animal house, the wards, or the community, relies first and foremost on accurate and honest observation and description. John Ruskin illustrates the challenge of accuracy in observation in *The Stones of Venice:*

> It is not easy to be accurate in an account of anything, however simple. Zoologists often disagree in their descriptions of the curve of a shell, or the plumage of a bird, though they may lay their specimen on the table and examine it at their leisure: how much greater becomes the likelihood of error in the description of things which must be in many parts observed from a distance, or under unfavorable circumstances . . . I believe few people have an idea of the cost of truth in these things; of the expenditure of time necessary to make sure of the simplest facts, and of the strange way in which separate observations will sometimes falsify each other, incapable of reconcilement, owing to some imperceptible inadvertency.[2]

Observation, alone, can lead to fallacies. We still say the sun rises in the east and sets in the west. What could be more natural to medieval observers than to suppose that the sun travels around a stationary earth? It took the genius of Nicolaus Copernicus to refute this theory. The observation was correct, but the ancient proposition ignored the movements of the planets—a new hypothesis was needed, and Copernicus supplied it.

The essence of a scientific statement is that it can be falsified by further observation and replaced by a new statement. Newton gave the world several propositions that explained nearly all astronomical events. Einstein sought the exceptions and propounded the theory of relativity to explain more observations than those supported by Newton's hypotheses. In Einstein's words:

> The new theory of gravitation diverges widely from that of Newton with respect to its basic principle. But in practical application, the two agree so closely that it has been difficult to find cases in which the actual differences could be subjected to observation.[3]

The Philosophy of Research

Two contemporary philosophers of science stand out—Karl Popper and Thomas Kuhn—and their views conflict to some extent.[4] Popper proposed that the distinction between science and nonscience is that it is possible to falsify a scientific proposition. "God created the universe" is a statement of faith—a proposition that cannot be refuted, but "The world was created 7,000 years ago" is a falsifiable hypothesis and therefore a scientific statement.

Popper sees criticism as a chief function of a scientist and has traced logical argument back to the pre-Socratic philosophers of Greece—Thales, Anaximander, and Anaximenes—who initiated the tradition of subjecting speculation to critical discussion that is the basis of the scientific method. In Popper's view, the scientific method comprises the following steps:

1. Seek a problem.
2. Propose a solution.
3. Formulate a testable hypothesis from that proposal.
4. Attempt to refute the hypothesis by observations and experiments.
5. Establish preference between competing theories.

All this means that a young scientist who hopes to make discoveries is badly advised if his or her teacher says: "Go round and observe," but he or she is well advised if the teacher says: "Try to learn what people are discussing nowadays in science. Find out where difficulties arise and take an interest in disagreements. These are the questions that you should take up." In other words, you should study the problems of the day. This means that you pick up, and try to continue, a line of inquiry that has the whole background of the earlier development of science behind it.[5]

Kuhn, in contrast, wrote that scientific knowledge does not progress steadily by criticism of established hypotheses and claimed that *ordinary* research seeks only to solve puzzles within the framework ("paradigm") of the existing accumulation of scientific knowledge. This steady state of puzzle solving is interrupted from time to time by *revolutions* that arrive suddenly, irrationally, and intuitively to establish a new paradigm within which the new scientists do their ordinary research and attempt to solve new puzzles.

Neither Popper nor Kuhn took much interest in biological or medical research, but we can accept both their philosophies. We can try to solve puzzles, and we can also set up hypotheses and devise observations and experiments to refute them. McIntyre and Popper[6] suggested the following ten rules for medical practice and research:

1. Our present conjectural knowledge far transcends what any person can know, even in his own specialty. It changes quickly and radically, and, in the main, not by accumulation but by the correction of erroneous doctrines and ideas. There can be no authorities; there can be better and worse scientists. More often than not, the better the scientist, the more aware he or she will be of personal limitations.
2. We are all fallible; nobody can avoid even all avoidable mistakes. The old idea that we must avoid them has to be revised. It is mistaken and has led to hypocrisy.
3. Nevertheless, it remains our task to avoid errors. But to do so we must recognize the difficulty. It is a task in which nobody succeeds fully—not even the great creative scientist who is led, but quite often misled, by intuition.
4. Errors may lurk even in our best-tested theories, and it is the responsibility of the professional to search for them. The proposal of new alternative theories can help us greatly; we should be tolerant of ideas that differ from the dominant theories of the day and not wait until those theories are in trouble. The discovery that a well-tested and corroborated theory, or a commonly used procedure is erroneous may be a most important discovery.
5. Our attitude toward mistakes must change because it is here that ethical reform must begin. The old attitude leads us to hide our mistakes and to forget them as quickly as we can.
6. The principle that we must learn from our mistakes, so that we avoid them in future, must take precedence even over the acquisition of new information. Hiding mistakes must be regarded as a deadly sin. Such errors as operating on the wrong patient or removing a healthy limb are inevitably exposed. Although the injury may be irreversible, exposure of the error can lead to the adoption of practices designed to prevent its recurrence. Other errors may be equally regrettable, but not so easily exposed. Those who commit

them may not wish to have them brought to light, but they should not be concealed because discussion and analysis may change practice and prevent their repetition.

7. We must search for our mistakes, investigate them fully, and train ourselves to be self-critical.
8. We must recognize that self-criticism is best, but criticism by others is necessary and especially valuable if the critics approach problems from a different background. We must learn to be graceful and even grateful in accepting criticism from those who draw our attention to our errors.
9. When we draw the attention of others to their mistakes, we should remind ourselves of the similar errors we have made; it is human to err, and even the greatest scientists make mistakes.
10. Rational criticism should be directed to definite, clearly identified mistakes. It should contain reasons and should be expressed in a form that allows its refutation. It should make clear which assumptions are being challenged and why. It should never contain insinuations, mere assertions, or only negative evaluations. It should be inspired by the aim of getting nearer to the truth and, for this reason, should be impersonal.

The surgeon, whether solving puzzles or refuting hypotheses, can seek help from three interdependent disciplines: bench work, animal experiments, and clinical practice. Many problems in clinical practice can be solved only in the biochemical and microbiological laboratories. Some questions can be answered ethically only by animal experiments, but laboratory and animal research is sterile unless it has a potential for affecting clinical practice. The historical development of clinical research is outlined here, that of laboratory research in chapter 2.

The Social Responsibility of Scientists

Prometheus was punished for bringing knowledge into the world, and Faust for wanting it too much. Scientists should be aware that they are held responsible for the outcome of the knowledge they generate and must face up to their special responsibilities.

The word *eugenics* was coined by Francis Galton in 1883, and it generated the idea of producing "a highly gifted race of men by judicious marriages during several consecutive generations."[7] In 1904 Charles Davenport persuaded the Carnegie Foundation to set up the Cold Spring Harbor Laboratories to study human evolution. All these activities were undertaken by worthy scientists, but it was only 30 years later that Hitler took up the idea of eliminating undesirable genes from the human stock.

We can now insert genes into human cells. Inserting them into somatic cells gives little cause for argument about the desirability of such research, but inserting new genes into germ cells raises issues of such importance that the public must participate in the debate on its acceptability.

Wolpert[8] advocated letting the community share the responsibility for developing scientific advances, and quoted Thomas Jefferson:

> I know no safe depository of the ultimate powers of the society but the people themselves, and if we think them not enlightened enough to exercise that control with a wholesome discretion, the remedy is not to take it from them, but to inform their discretion.

The History of Clinical Research

The following statement is unscientific because it cannot be refuted: Our forefathers, at least as far back as the fifth century B.C., were no less intelligent than we are. Why, then, is biological and medical research, with a few exceptions, a product of the last century?

Respect for the Doctor-Patient Relationship

There was a time when a doctor was almost universally regarded as being all seeing and all knowing, and this attitude persists in some parts of the world. As a consequence, physicians could never admit that their diagnosis was conjectural or their treatment ineffective. They could never confess ignorance; but the acknowledgment of ignorance is the first step toward research.

Inaccurate Diagnoses

You cannot do clinical research unless you can make precise diagnoses. Diagnostic accuracy improved following the discovery of the causative role of microorganisms in certain diseases, the introduction of diagnostic radiology, and the more recent advances in biochemistry, immunology, and diagnostic imaging techniques.

Ineffective Remedies

When physicians were powerless to influence the course of most diseases, they did not think of doing research. One placebo was as good as the next, and it was merely discourteous to question the practice of colleagues.

Reverence for Authority

Until the late nineteenth century, the task of scholars was to study and interpret the writings of others; reverence for authority was the outstanding virtue. The approach to learning was conceptual rather than empirical. Sir Dominic John Corritan,[9] writing in the *Lancet*, in 1829, said about Harvey's discovery of the circulation of the blood: "Such, however, is the power of prejudice that no physician past the age of forty believed in Harvey's doctrine, and that his practice declined from the moment he published this ever-memorable discovery."[9] Although a few original thinkers have challenged authority in every age in spite of opposing social pressures, it is only recently that respect for logical thinking has generated skepticism and the pursuit of pragmatism.

Lack of Statistical Tests

In therapeutics, scientific testing of remedies is one of the strongest forces for change. The fundamental requirement of a proper clinical trial is the evaluation of the outcome of a treatment regimen by the application of methods based on the mathematics of probability.

Evolution of Population Statistics

During the eight centuries between the compilation of the *Doomsday Book* (an inventory of King William's newly conquered English kingdom) and the nineteenth century, vital statistics were not systematically collected anywhere in Europe. In 1776 the Société Royale de Médicine made one of the first attempts to record births and deaths throughout France, but a reliable system was not introduced until the early 1800s, and later still in other European countries. By 1880, individual cards had taken the place of highly fallible lists in the compiling of statistics, and the Hollerith punch card sorting machine was first used in a national census in the United States in 1890.

It soon became evident that epidemiological studies were stultified by the inaccuracy of death certificates. Even as late as the beginning of the twentieth century, Sir Josiah Stamp was able to write:

> The government are very keen on amassing statistics. They collect them, add them, raise them to the nth power, take the cube root, and prepare wonderful diagrams. But you must never forget that every one of these figures comes in the first instance from the village watchman, who puts down what he damn well pleases.[10]

In 1853 William Farr, who had been a student of Pierre Charles Alexandre Louis, inventor of the "numerical method," in Paris, cooperated with Marc d'Espine in developing the anatomically based system of classification of diseases that formed the foundation of today's *International Classification of Diseases*.

Louis's numerical method received no acclaim until relatively recently. In 1835 he published a paper translated as "Research on the effect of blood-letting in several inflammatory maladies." His main conclusion was that bloodletting had little therapeutic value.[11] The paper attracted adverse comment in the French Academy of Sciences, and François Double issued a report condemning the use of statistical methods in clinical method, and extolling Morgagni's aphorism: *Non numerandae sed perpendendae* (facts must be weighed, not counted). Nevertheless, in 1837 Simon Denis Poisson wrote that if a medication had been successfully used in a large number of similar cases, and if the number of cases in which it had not succeeded was small compared with the total number of cases, it was probable that the medication would succeed in a new trial.

Mathematics of Probability

Games of chance were the original stimulus to sixteenth-century philosophers, including Galileo, to attempt to give mathematical expression to probabilities.[12,13] In the following century, Blaise Pascal corresponded regularly with a fellow mathematician, Pierre de Fermat, on probabilities in relation to card games. The first inkling of modern methods of statistical analysis appeared in 1713 when Jacob Bernoulli's *Ars conjectandi* was published. He proved that the more often a test is repeated, the greater is the probability that the result will be within certain limits.

In eighteenth-century France, Abraham de Moivre published *Doctrines of Chance,* and "The Petersburg Problem" was widely discussed (i.e., if a coin toss comes up tails several times, is it more likely to come up heads the next time?). In 1785 the Marquis de Condorcet declared in his "Essay on the Application of Mathematics to the Theory of Decision Making" that probability calculus "weighs the grounds for belief and calculates the probable truth of testimony or decisions."

The French mathematical philosopher Pierre Simon, Marquis de Laplace, published his *Analytical Theory of Probabilities* in 1812 and wrote, "The theory of probabilities is fundamentally only good sense reduced to calculation."

By 1870, statistical analysis of whole populations was well advanced, but the problems of sampling had not been tackled. Then, the new science of microbiology temporarily eclipsed interest in the application of statistics in medicine, and the development of statistical methods for analyzing samples shifted to brewing and agriculture. The term *random* was first applied in a statistical sense at the end of the nineteenth century.

The Development of Clinical Trials

Historical Controls

Most great advances in therapeutics have been made by contrasting the results of a new regimen with those of previously documented treatment. The enormous benefits of general anesthesia, the reduction of surgical infection rates by asepsis, the cure of many infections by penicillin, and numerous other advances have needed only careful documentation and comparison with previous experience to become accepted.

If a new treatment is immeasurably better than the old, historical controls are not only sufficient, they are the only ones that are ethical. Once it had been shown that penicillin could cure bacterial endocarditis—previously uniformly lethal, not treating all cases with penicillin was unacceptable. Random control trials are justified only if there is a therapeutic dilemma. Ignorance is essential.

The inappropriate use of historical controls can, however, lead to false conclusions. This is particularly true if the results of surgical treatment are compared with previous experience with medical treatment of the same disease. There is a selection bias in such a study; the surgeon operates only on patients who are fit enough to have the operation. The results cannot be compared with those of *all* patients in a previous series treated medically.

An example of this bias was published in the *New England Journal of Medicine* in 1948.[14] Among patients with bleeding esophageal varices caused by cirrhosis of the liver, Linton reported better survival figures for those who were treated by portacaval shunts than for a control group treated medically in previous years. The surgical patients were those who survived long enough to be operated on; those who never became fit for surgery or died before it could be performed were not reported. Linton's conclusions were subsequently repudiated by the Boston Liver Group,[15] who randomized patients fit enough for operation and assigned them to standard medical treatment or to portacaval shunting. The results were not significantly different in the two groups but were vastly-superior to those in a group of patients not fit enough to be recruited into the trial.

Contemporary Nonrandom Controls

Many questions about etiology and epidemiology can be answered only by comparing a group of people subject to certain risks with another group that is not. Sometimes, the evidence from such comparisons is sufficiently compelling to demand acceptance (e.g., the association between cigarette smoking and bronchial carcinoma, or exposure to asbestos dust and mesothelioma). Epidemiological research using case controls can, however, produce more questions than answers; witness the confusion about the connection between diet and atherosclerosis, or between oral contraceptives and breast cancer.

A carefully conducted case-control study showed a significant influence of prolonged use of oral contraceptives on the development of breast cancer in women under the age of 35 years.[16] The authors were careful to minimize biases, but their conclusions are at odds with those of other epidemiological studies and with the absence of a rise in the overall incidence of breast cancer during the years of wide usage of oral contraceptives.

In therapeutics, all contemporary nonrandom comparative studies are suspect because outcomes depend on so many factors. The population sample in the study group may differ from that in the control group with respect to the incidence of risk factors, an uneven distribution of the variables associated with treatment, and variations in the methods of assessment of events. Although the conclusions reached in such studies can be tentative only, they may form the basis for hypotheses to be tested in random control trials.

Normann et al.[17] published an example of such a study. The two surgical departments of Ulleval Hospital in Oslo followed different regimens for the treatment of perforated appendicitis. In one, appendicectomy was completed by inserting a drain into the appendix fossa; in the other, it was followed by two days of peritoneal dialysis. The drainage group recorded 1 death, 6 pelvic abscesses, 1 intraperitoneal abscess, 4 cases of paralytic ileus, 4 repeat laparotomies, and 1 fecal fistula, for a total complication rate of 17 in 77

patients. In the lavage group, the complications comprised 1 death, 3 pelvic abscesses, 1 paralytic ileus, and 1 repeat laparotomy, for a total complication rate of 6 in 78. Firm conclusions about the superiority of peritoneal dialysis are not justified, however, because of the strong likelihood of important undisclosed variables.

Random Control Clinical Trials

Ronald Aylmer Fisher was the first to recognize that many pitfalls in nonrandom trials can be avoided by allocating subjects to each arm of a trial strictly by chance and allowing the investigator no control over the randomization process.[18]

Fisher was a mathematician and biologist who studied physics under James Jeans at Cambridge, but he chose a career in biology. In 1919 he became statistician to Rothamsted Agricultural Experimental Station, where field trials had been carried out since 1843 without ever being subjected to statistical analyses. Fisher undertook the task of analyzing earlier trials and designing new trials free from bias. He wrote widely on the statistical analysis of trials and worked out the exact probability test that bears his name. In 1925 he published *Statistical Methods for Research Workers*,[19] which dealt with the design and analysis of controlled trials. His second book, *The Design of Experiments*,[20] appeared in 1935 when he was Galton Professor at University College, London.

In 1937 Austin Bradford Hill published in the *Lancet* a series of papers that were reprinted in a book entitled *Principles of Medical Statistics*. Its tenth edition is renamed *A Short Textbook of Medical Statistics*.[21] Hill's name has become synonymous with the proper ethical and statistical design of clinical trials. One of his greatest achievements was the organization in 1947 of the Medical Research Council cooperative trial on the treatment of pulmonary tuberculosis by streptomycin.[22] Because the short supply of streptomycin in Britain precluded its being offered to all patients with tuberculosis, a random control trial in which the control group was treated by the best current standard methods was ethically justifiable. Central randomization was used for the first time, and the trial was a brilliant success.

Where Do We Go from Here?

The doctor's duty to each patient must always come first. It is only within the framework of this duty that controlled trials are proper, and numerous measures exist to safeguard the welfare of patients. National and international rules are laid down for the conduct of clinical trials; financial support will not be provided for unethical trials; and lastly, peer review bodies judge and, if necessary, amend protocols of clinical trials to ensure their ethical acceptability.

Ethical principles in surgical research, including the ethical requirements of informed consent for the various forms of clinical trials, are discussed in chapter 60.

Ethical restraints and resistance by patients and surgeons to allowing chance to decide the choice of operation—or the choice of operative versus nonoperative treatment—mean that we will have to rely increasingly on complete, accurate, and honest audit of the outcome of diseases treated in different ways. There must be no exclusions, no excuses, and no concealments.

References

1. Sutherland J, ed. The Oxford Book of Literary Anecdotes. Oxford: Clarendon Press, 1975, p. 253.
2. Ruskin J. The Stones of Venice. Boston: Dana Estes, 1851.
3. Einstein A. Einstein on his theory. The London *Times*, November 28, 1919. (Quoted in The *Times*, November 28, 1985.)
4. Lakatos I. Falsification and the methodology of scientific research programmes. In: Criticism and the Growth of Knowledge, Lakatos I, Musgrave A, eds. Cambridge: Cambridge University, 1970.
5. Popper K. Conjectures and Refutations: The Growth of Scientific Knowledge, 4th edn. London: Routledge & Kegan Paul, 1972, p. 129.
6. McIntyre N, Popper K. The critical attitude in medicine: the need for a new ethics. Br Med J 1983;287:1919–1923.
7. Pearson K. Quoted by Wolpert L.[8]
8. Wolpert L. The social responsibility of scientists: moonshine and morals. Br Med J 1989;289:941–943.
9. Corrigan DJ. Aneurysm of the aorta. Singular pulsation of the arteries—necessity of the employment of the stethoscope. Lancet 1829;i:586–590.
10. Dunea G. Swallowing the golden ball. Br Med J 1983;286:1962–1963.
11. Gaines WJ, Langford HG. Research on the effect of blood-letting in several inflammatory maladies. Arch Intern Med 1960;106:571–579.
12. Murphy TD. Medical knowledge and statistical methods in early nineteenth century France. Med Hist 1981;25:301–309.
13. Westergaard H. Contributions to the History of Statistics. London: PS King & Son, 1932.
14. Linton RR. Porta-caval shunts in the treatment of portal hypertension, with special reference to patients previously operated upon. N Engl J Med 1948;238:723–727.
15. Garceau AJ, Donaldson RM, O'Hara ET, Callow AD, Muench H, Chalmers TC, Boston Inter-Hospital Liver Group. A controlled trial of prophylactic portacaval shunt surgery. N Engl J Med 1964;270:496–500.
16. UK National Case-Control Study Group. Oral contraceptive use and breast cancer risk in young women. Lancet 1989;i:973–982.
17. Normann E, Korvald E, Lotveit T. Perforated appendicitis—lavage or drainage? Ann Chir Gynaecol Fenn 1975;64:195–197.
18. Yates F, Mather K. Ronald Aylmer Fisher, 1890–1962. Biograph Mem Fell R Soc 1963;9:91–129.
19. Fisher RA. Statistical Methods for Research Workers. Edinburgh: Oliver & Boyd, 1925.
20. Fisher RA. The Design of Experiments. Edinburgh: Oliver & Boyd, 1935.
21. Hill AB. A Short Textbook of Medical Statistics. London: Hodder & Stoughton, 1977.
22. Medical Research Council. Streptomycin treatment of pulmonary tuberculosis. Br Med J 1948;2:769–782.

Commentary

Pollock's career-long scholarly interest in surgical history and the conceptual basis for clinical research are reflected in this thoughtful essay, combining philosophy of science with the history of statistics and the evolution of trials. It is reproduced with little change from the second edition.

He speaks from a rich experience in clinical practice. Like many thoughtful surgeons, he has concerns about bias that can creep into clinical trials, even those that are randomized. We will discuss this important issue in a subsequent chapter on clinical trials (chapter 26). Dr. Pollock's highly readable, short book on audit is recommended as a guide to outcomes research (see reference 9 in chapter 56 [Dziuban]).

M.F.M.

SECTION II

Reading and Writing

CHAPTER 7

Appraising New Information

M.T. Schechter, F.E. LeBlanc, and V.A. Lawrence

Every year thousands of articles appear in the surgical literature. While many present the results of careful investigations based on good methodology, many others report studies whose results are either invalid because of defects in their conduct or analysis, or ungeneralizable to other settings because of biases in the way they were executed. This chapter describes a framework within which the validity and generalizability of published research can be appraised and judged. We will examine two frequently published types of research, controlled trials of therapeutic interventions and review articles, according to six easily remembered appraisal criteria:

APPRAISAL CRITERIA

Why?

How?

Who?

What?

How many?

So what?

Controlled Trials

Why? The Study Question

As a critical appraiser, you should always begin by considering the reasons for the study and deter-

mining whether sufficient evidence is presented to justify it. In the absence of clear statements of the purpose of the study and of the study hypothesis at the outset, you may well consider moving on to another article, because such statements are essential for two reasons. First, the design of the study, which includes the population to be studied, the variables to be considered, and the method of analysis to be utilized, depends very heavily on the purpose of the study. Second, you must be able to determine whether the hypothesis was specified in advance (i.e., a priori) or arose out of the data (i.e., a posteriori). The study hypothesis should also indicate whether the study is intended to be hypothesis-generating or hypothesis-testing.

Studies of therapeutic interventions should clearly state whether *efficacy* or *effectiveness* is being considered. Efficacy studies seek to determine whether an intervention results in a specific outcome under ideal circumstances, that is, in properly diagnosed and properly treated patients who are compliant. Effectiveness studies seek to determine whether an intervention does more good than harm in patients under normal clinical circumstances, that is, in patients who are diagnosed and treated, as in the community, and who may or may not comply, as in the community. In general, the outcome measures used in efficacy studies tend to be short-term and specific while those in effectiveness studies are longer term and more global. *Both types of study have their merits. Efficacy studies usually have their place in the early investi-*

gation of new therapies. It is the results of effectiveness studies that indicate whether a given intervention should be adopted. Much of a study's methodology, especially the population to be studied and the outcome to be assessed, will be determined by which approach (i.e., efficacy or effectiveness) is chosen.

Consider a study investigating coronary artery bypass surgery as a treatment for coronary artery disease. To study the *efficacy* of this intervention, one would ideally utilize a treatment group consisting of patients with clearly documented coronary stenoses, all of whom undergo coronary artery bypass surgery. To test efficacy, one would consider short-term outcomes that this intervention is designed to produce, namely increased myocardial blood flow, relief of anginal symptoms, and so forth. In such a study, anyone who was assigned to receive the surgery but did not actually receive it, perhaps because of intervening illnesses, would not be included in the treatment group because any subsequent benefit could not be attributed to the efficacy of the intervention itself.

On the other hand, when one considers *effectiveness*, one is challenging not merely the intervention itself, but the *policy* of using this intervention in the study population. This is sometimes known as the "intent to treat" principle. A study of the effectiveness of coronary artery bypass surgery should consider a wider spectrum of outcomes, including long-term survival, quality of life, and level of function. In such studies, patients who are allocated to receive medical therapy but are given surgery at a later date should be analyzed within the medical group because it is the policies of initial treatment with medical versus surgical therapy that are being compared.

It is important to understand the difference between efficacy and effectiveness studies for two other reasons. Results of analyses from *both* perspectives often are reported and discussed in the same article; they may conflict and lead to different conclusions. Disagreement among colleagues may be due to interpretations from the differing perspectives of efficacy and effectiveness.

How? Study Methodology

You should next endeavor to determine the type of study methodology. The types of study design you are most likely to encounter in relation to therapeutic interventions include (a) *case studies,* which simply report the results of a series of cases treated with a given intervention; (b) *before–after studies,* which compare the patients' condition before and after the intervention, either in entire settings or within individuals; and (c) *controlled trials,* which compare the results in groups treated with experimental and standard therapies. In controlled trials, you should carefully assess how the patients were allocated to the experimental or the control group. Was the allocation truly randomized? If randomization was not employed, could any biases have occurred in the allocation of the patients? Be on the alert for *quasi-random allocation* in which patients are assigned on the basis of some seemingly random process, (birth date, chart number, day of week, etc.). Subtle biases can be introduced in such situations and there is no reason for not using a true randomization.

You should also attempt to determine what type of blindness was employed and carefully assess whether any lack of blindness might have led to an expectation bias that distorted the results. *Single blindness* refers to studies in which only the patient does not know whether the experimental treatment or the "control" therapy was received. When *double blindness* is used, both the patients and the care providers are unaware of the allocation. In *triple-blinded* studies, the patients, the care providers, and those who assess the outcome are all unaware of what treatment was given. In studies of surgical interventions, blinding of the patients and care providers is not always possible, but, at the very least, those who perform the outcome assessment can be blinded to the treatment the patient received.

It is important to determine whether significant prognostic variables were equally allocated to the treatment and control groups. Although most prognostic variables will be equally distributed in large studies employing randomized allocation, maldistribution can occur in small studies. Consequently, it is wise for investigators to use *prognostic stratification,* a method in which patients are first stratified with regard to an important set of prognostic variables, then randomized from each stratum. This method usually guarantees equal distribution of the prognostic variables to the treatment and control groups.

Consider a clinical trial comparing two different treatments for astrocytomas. To make the comparison fair, the groups to which the respective treatments are applied should be comparable with regard to tumor grade, because histological grade is a very important predictor of prognosis in this disease. Since the number of available patients is likely to be small, a maldistribution could occur with simple randomization because an excess of patients with grades III and IV astrocytoma might be allocated, by chance, to one of the treatments. Prognostic stratification would avoid this; that is, patients entering the trial would first be stratified by the grade of their lesion, and then randomized to treatment from within each grade. This would guarantee a more equitable distribution of the grades to the two treatment groups.

Who? The Patient Population

Understanding the type of patient studied is one of the most important aspects of critical appraisal. You must determine whether the type of patient included in an investigation was sufficiently representative to allow the results to be applied to all patients in similar clinical situations or to your patients.

Representativeness can be assessed in a number of ways. Is the source population from which the study sample was drawn clearly described and suitably representative? Are demographic details of the catchment area provided? Was the study sample drawn from a primary, secondary, or tertiary referral center? Did the study sample represent the full spectrum of the disease, or only a small subsample?

Are clear and replicable inclusion and exclusion criteria specified, and do they match the goals of the study? If clear and replicable inclusion and exclusion criteria are not given, you cannot know exactly what type of patient was studied or to which of your patients the results can be applied. The inclusion and exclusion criteria should define a study population that matches the type of patient the investigators intend should benefit from the results. After the exclusion and inclusion criteria have been applied, compare the type of population that remains with the stated goals of the study, to see if they match.

Do the authors account for every patient eligible for the study who did not enter it? This is critically important. Typically, eligible patients (i.e., those meeting the inclusion criteria and not rejected by the exclusion criteria) are approached for informed consent, and some decline. If the proportion of refusals is small (i.e., <10%), it is of limited importance; but *volunteer bias* can occur if a significant proportion of eligible patients do not agree to participate. Participating patients tend to be more motivated, more compliant, and destined for better outcomes than those who decline. Investigators should recruit a minimum of 90% of all eligible patients or provide evidence that those who declined had outcomes similar to those who volunteered; either approach provides some evidence that volunteer bias was not a significant factor.

Finally, determine whether the baseline comparability of the treatment and control groups has been documented. Although randomization of large numbers of patients should produce relatively equal distributions, maldistributions of important prognostic variables can still occur, especially with smaller sample sizes. The investigators should provide an assessment of the baseline comparability of the two groups; if any prognostic variable has been maldistributed, the analysis should take it into account.

What? Intervention and Outcome Measures

This aspect of critical appraisal centers on two questions. What intervention is under study? What outcome measures are being assessed?

Investigators should provide a clear definition of the intervention; without one, you cannot really know what is being assessed. Some measure of *compliance* should also be included, even in trials of surgical interventions if such components of care beyond the surgical procedure as follow-up care, self-care, and adjunct medications require patients' compliance. Examine how noncompliers were analyzed. In effectiveness trials, noncompliers should be analyzed within the treatment arm to which they were randomized; in efficacy studies, it may sometimes be more appropriate to omit noncompliers from the analysis. Investigators should attempt to monitor *contamination* (patients assigned to the control arm who subsequently underwent the experimental intervention), *cointervention* (additional therapies that were made available to patients in either arm of the trial), and all side effects.

All withdrawals (patients removed by the investigators) and dropouts (patients removed on their own volition) should be documented, along with the reasons for departure. *Crossovers* occur when a patient in one arm of the trial receives the intervention assigned to another arm of the trial; for example, in studies of surgical versus medical treatment of coronary artery disease, patients originally assigned to medical therapy may deteriorate and subsequently undergo coronary artery bypass surgery. Determine whether withdrawals, dropouts, crossovers, and poor compliers were analyzed in accordance with the goals of the study. In an effectiveness study of coronary artery bypass surgery, patients initially assigned to medical therapy who cross over and receive the surgical intervention should be analyzed within the medical therapy arm to which they were originally randomized.

To critically appraise the outcome measures aspect of a study, determine whether all clinically relevant outcome measures were used and whether they matched the study's goals. A study comparing two interventions may focus on the subsequent three-week mortality in the treatment and control groups, but an improvement in the three-week mortality with the intervention would not provide any reassurance about the long-term survival of patients. If you are deciding whether to use the intervention, you will want to know if the quality of life is improved for those undergoing the intervention. Was the measurement of the outcomes precise? This may not be an issue if the outcome was length of survival, because the endpoint (death) is clear. But if the outcome measured was severity of pain, quality of life, improvement of clinical signs or symptoms, and so forth, you should determine whether a reliable and valid method was used to gather such information. Those who assess the outcome can usually be blinded to patients' allocations for the purpose of making unbiased assessments. Ascertain whether the process of observation required to assess the outcome could have influenced the outcome.

How Many? Statistical Significance and Sample Size

Determine whether statistical significance was considered, whether the statistical tests used were applied appropriately, and whether the authors considered the methods of analysis and sample size requirements *prior* to initiating the study. The more analyses performed on a data set, the more likely it becomes that a significant result will be obtained by chance. Accordingly, a significant result obtained from a single prespecified analysis is much more meaningful than one derived from a series of analyses suggested by the data. Check for the possibility of the *multiple comparisons problem*, which occurs when investigators consider several different outcome variables and, by so doing, increase the likelihood of a significant result arising by chance. In such instances, the investigators should adjust their alpha level.

Where no statistically significant differences are found between the treatment and control groups, investigators must consider the possibility of a beta (i.e., type II) error and estimate the probability of its occurrence. If a type II error is not considered, you may well ask whether the study was large enough to detect important differences. All too often, investigators conclude that there is no difference between the experimental and control treatments when all they are justified in concluding is that their study failed to detect a difference.

Small sample size frequently leads to trials with weak power to detect important differences in outcome between treatment groups. Freiman and colleagues[1] found that in half the articles reporting no significant differences between the therapies studied, a 50% improvement in performance could easily have been missed. They concluded that type II errors and small sample sizes are ubiquitous in the medical literature. When no statistically significant difference was found, and you know the study was strong enough to have had a good chance of detecting a clinically important difference, you can conclude that the matter is fairly well settled. If the authors do not discuss the power of their trial, you have the right to suspect the study was not large enough to detect important differences.

So What? Clinical Significance

The heading "So what?" reminds you to form some overall conclusion about the importance of the information provided in the article and its relevance to your own clinical practice.

If differences were detected, was their clinical significance discussed? Clinical significance refers to the magnitude of the difference observed between treatment and control groups measured in clinical, rather than statistical, terms. If a statistically significant difference is also clinically significant, it implies that a change in clinical behavior is warranted. For example, a study may observe survival rates of 55% in the treatment group and 50% in the control group. If large numbers of patients are involved, this difference may be statistically significant. If the intervention is exceedingly expensive, however, or entails considerable morbidity, it may be hard to justify using it to obtain such a marginal gain in survival, that is, the difference is not clinically significant.

Assessing clinical significance is a matter of judgment and depends on the severity of the adverse outcome we are seeking to avoid. Consider, for example, an experimental surgical intervention that lowers the mortality in a certain condition from 0.5 under conventional therapy (denoted Pc) to 0.4 under the experimental treatment (denoted Pe). How are we to evaluate the clinical importance of this change?

There are several measures that are of use in assessing the strength of a treatment effect. The first is the *absolute risk reduction*, which measures the difference between the two rates, that is, Pc − Pe. In the example above, one would say that the experimental surgery gives rise to an absolute mortality reduction of 0.10. A second measure, the *relative risk reduction*, measures the absolute reduction as a percentage of the original risk and is given by the following expression: 100% · (Pc − Pe)/Pc. In the example, one would say that the experimental intervention has yielded a relative mortality reduction of 100% · (0.5 − 0.4)/0.5, or 20%. The latter measure is an indicator of the relative impact of new interventions on existing outcomes but can lead to distortions, for example, when rates are low. A 25% relative risk reduction can sound impressive, but less so if it represents only a 0.01 absolute decline in mortality from 0.04

to 0.03. An intuitively appealing alternative to the above treatment measures is the reciprocal of the absolute risk reduction, namely, 1/(Pc − Pe). This has been denoted the *number needed to treat* (NNT),[2] because it represents the number of patients who need to receive the experimental therapy before one additional adverse event is prevented. In the example, the NNT is the reciprocal of 0.1, or 10, indicating that 10 patients would need to receive the experimental surgery in order to avert one additional death (4 deaths expected under experimental surgery versus 5 deaths under conventional therapy).

Were the patients included and analyzed in the study sufficiently representative to allow the results to be generalized to other patients? By considering the source population from which the study sample was obtained, the method by which patients were recruited, the inclusion and exclusion criteria, the possibility of volunteer bias, and the patients actually analyzed, you should be able to decide whether the type of patient studied was sufficiently similar to your patients to make the results applicable to them. A simple rule of thumb is that THE TYPE OF PATIENT INCLUDED AND ANALYZED IN ANY STUDY IS THE ONLY TYPE OF PATIENT TO WHICH ITS RESULTS CAN BE APPLIED.

Was the intervention as performed in the study sufficiently feasible that the results can be generalized to other settings? Is the intervention available in other settings? Were those who performed the intervention highly specialized? If the study involved highly motivated, highly trained, and compliant care providers, questions may arise as to how well the intervention will be performed on a community-wide basis. This is particularly true in studies of surgical interventions performed in specialized settings by highly skilled surgeons who are practiced in the technique under study and supported by highly specialized adjunct care.

Are the outcomes assessed in the study adequate to establish which of the therapies under study does the most good? If six-week mortality was the outcome variable of central interest, you may not consider that the results justify incorporating the intervention into your clinical practice; you may well prefer to await evidence that the benefit is not only a short-term reduction in mortality, but also a long-term improvement in survival, morbidity, quality of life, level of function, and so forth.

In conclusion, the goals and hypotheses (the "why") on which a study is based are inexorably linked to several crucial methodological components of the study design, namely, the source population to be sampled, the inclusion and exclusion criteria, allocation methods, appropriate handling of various events (withdrawals, crossovers, etc.), outcome assessment, methods of data analysis, and interpretation of clinical significance. A clear understanding of study goals and hypotheses is fundamental to good research methodology and astute critical appraisal.

Summary: Controlled Trials

Why? The Study Question

Is sufficient evidence presented to justify the study?
Is the purpose of the study clearly stated?
Is the study hypothesis clearly stated?
Is it clearly outlined whether the study is considering *efficacy* or *effectiveness*?

How? Study Methodology

What exactly is the study design?
If it is a controlled trial, is the allocation truly randomized?
If it is not a controlled trial, are there any biases in the allocation to treatment?
What type of blindness is employed (single, double, triple, etc.)?
Was prognostic stratification used?

Who? The Patient Population

Is the population from which the study sample was drawn clearly described?
Are inclusion and exclusion criteria specified and replicable?
Do the criteria match the goals of the study?
Do the authors account for every eligible patient who did not enter the study?
Is the baseline comparability of the treatment and control groups documented?

What? Intervention and Outcome Measures

What, exactly, was the intervention performed? Is it clearly defined and replicable?
Was compliance with the intervention(s) measured and were noncompliers analyzed appropriately?
Were contamination and cointervention considered?
Were all patients who entered the study accounted for?
Were withdrawals, dropouts, crossovers, and poor compliers analyzed in accordance with the goals of the study?
What outcomes were assessed in the study?
Were all relevant outcomes utilized?
Could the process of observation have influenced the outcome?

How Many? Statistical Significance and Sample Size

Was statistical significance considered in the study?
Were statistical tests applied appropriately?
Did the authors consider the methods of analysis and the sample size requirements prior to the study?
When no statistically significant differences were found, did the authors consider the possibility of a beta (type II) error and estimate its probability?
Was the study large enough to detect important differences?

So What? Clinical Significance

If differences were detected, was their clinical significance discussed? Were the patients entered and analyzed in the study sufficiently representative to allow the results to be generalized to other patients?
Was the intervention, as performed in the study, sufficiently representative to permit generalizing the results to other settings?
Do the outcomes assessed in the study provide an adequate basis for establishing which of the studied therapies does the greatest good?

The framework presented in this chapter for assessing articles about new therapeutic interventions is by no means the only approach that can be taken. The Evidence-Based Medicine Working Group has provided another such framework[3,4] which is summarized in Table 7-1. In this approach, readers ask three fundamental questions: (1) Are the results of the study valid? (2) What were the results of the study? and (3) Will the results help me in caring for my patients? Under the rubric of these three fundamental questions, there are subquestions aimed at elucidating whether basic criteria are met. For example, under the first question regarding validity of study results, there are a number of other questions involving randomization, full accounting of patients and use of the intent-to-treat principle, blindness, baseline comparability, and equivalence of cointerventions. Readers interested in structured critical appraisal are encouraged to utilize any framework with which they feel comfortable.[4]

Review Articles

A review article requires a special type of critical appraisal. Given the volume of medical literature, clinicians and researchers depend on review articles to keep them abreast of medical knowledge across specialty boundaries and within their own areas. The review article is a special type of study or research tool. It should synthesize or carefully evaluate a body of information. Its quality depends on the extent to which evidence is systematically and critically evaluated. You will want to judge the validity and generalizability of review articles carefully, to maximize your knowledge and efficiency in handling the literature. Assess a review article using the appraisal criteria described above[5,6] (see chapter 38).

Why? The Study Question

The purpose or question being addressed by the review article should be clearly stated. You must have a clear statement of the question to give you a frame of reference for choosing types of investigation to review (e.g., using only data from controlled clinical trials for a review of a particular therapy).

How? Review Methodology

For a review, the data are published investigations. You should be given clear information on (1) how published studies were identified (personal knowledge or computerized literature databases such as MEDLINE), (2) inclusion and exclusion criteria used in selecting articles for review, and (3) how methodological validity was assessed. Without this information, you cannot determine how representative the reviewed material is in relation to all the available literature, whether relevant material may have been excluded, or whether selection bias may have been present. In this setting, "selection bias" refers to the degree to which reviewers preferentially choose data that supported

Table 7-1.   Readers' guide to an article about therapy (from the Evidence-Based Medicine Working Group)[3,4]

Are the results of the study valid?

Primary guides

Was the allocation of patients to treatments randomized?

Were all patients who entered the trial properly accounted for and attributed at its conclusion?

Was follow-up complete?

Were patients analyzed in the groups to which they were randomized?

Secondary guides

Were patients, health workers, and study personnel blind to treatment?

Were the groups similar at the start of the trial?

Aside from the experimental intervention, were the groups treated equally?

What were the results?

How large was the treatment effect?

How precise was the estimate of the treatment effect?

Will the results help me in caring for my patients?

Can the results be applied to my patient care?

Were all clinically important outcomes considered?

Are the likely treatment benefits worth the potential harms and costs?

their own opinions. There should be explicit criteria with respect to how published studies, once identified, were included or excluded from review. Articles rejected from consideration should be logged, like patients excluded from a clinical trial. In addition, systematic appraisal of the quality of the studies covered by the review is necessary for accurate conclusions and to determine their generalizability to your own patients. If we are to depend on the reviewers' expertise and ability to read and appraise the literature for us, the review article must describe a systematic process and standardized criteria for judging articles.

Who? The Patient Populations

The review should include information about the types of patient and clinical settings in the published investigations being reviewed. The range of patient characteristics and the spectrum of disease should be described. When such information is lacking, it is difficult to assess the quality of the original data, the reviewer's expertise in collation and integration of data, or the generalizability of the reviewer's conclusions to your clinical setting. If a quantitative assessment is to be carried out by pooling the data, the authors must establish that the populations are sufficiently homogeneous to make such a process valid.

What? Interventions, Outcome Measures, and Synthesis

The interventions and outcome measures used in the individual studies covered by a review article are major factors in the synthesis of data to reach conclusions about a body of evidence. The review should provide adequate information about differences in patient populations among studies, specific interventions, and the limitations and inconsistencies in the data. You must have this information before you can place your confidence in the reviewer's ability to identify good quality data, integrate information from a variety of sources, and explain conflicting results among studies.

If a quantitative assessment is to be carried out by pooling data, the review's author(s) must also establish that the interventions, outcomes measured, and measurement techniques were sufficiently homogeneous to permit such pooling.

How Many? Quantitative Review

Information synthesis may be qualitative (review article) or quantitative (meta-analysis). Critical assessment of both types of review article is similar up to this point. In qualitative reviews, the author(s) should weigh the value of each study according to the appropriateness of the statistical methods it used and its power to detect important differences. Meta-analysis adds an extra quantitative dimension by formally pooling data from several studies. In such analyses, the reviewer should use or derive a common unit of comparison and be able to assess statistical variance in every study used as a source of data for inclusion in the pooling process. The best overall estimate of the treatment effect is not obtained by simply averaging the individual estimates or by combining the number of treatment successes across the trials. Some form of pooling that takes account of individual variances in the estimates is preferable (e.g., the Mantel-Haenszel procedure or other methods of combining contingency tables).

An advantage of meta-analysis is its ability to identify small effects in subgroups that may be statistically undetectable in individual small studies. You should be wary, as usual, of the multiple-comparisons problem, that is, the likelihood of a false-positive result increases with the number of subgroups analyzed.

So What? Clinical Significance

When you read a review article, you should decide whether any summary differences found were clinically significant, whether the combined study patients were sufficiently similar to your own, whether the intervention was feasible and representative in your setting, and whether the outcomes establish which therapy does the greatest good. In a review article, clinical significance rests not only on the validity, magnitude, and generalizability of the conclusions, but also on the identification of unanswered questions. Conclusions are valid only when the review process has been scientific. A good review article directs our attention to a research agenda so that subsequent investigations will maximize methodological quality and will not be redundant or address unresolved issues. The overwhelming breadth of the medical literature compels us to rely on "ghost readers." If review articles are viewed as scientific endeavors in their own right, and their quality withstands critical appraisal, we can be more confident that such ghosts are scientific spirits.

Summary: Review Articles

Why? The Study Question

Is the purpose or question addressed by the review article clearly stated?

How? Review Methodology

Is the method used to select articles clearly described?

Are the inclusion and exclusion criteria for selecting articles clearly stated?

How was the quality of the studies under review evaluated?

Who? The Patient Populations

Are the populations of patients clearly described?

If data have been pooled, did the author(s) establish the homogeneity of the patient populations?

What? Interventions, Outcome Measures, and Synthesis

Is adequate information provided about differences in patient populations among studies, interventions used, and data limitations and inconsistencies?

If data have been pooled, did the author(s) establish the homogeneity of the interventions, outcomes, and methods of outcome assessment?

How Many? Quantitative Review

In qualitative reviews, have the authors appraised the quantitative methods and the power of each study?

In pooled analyses, have the authors combined the results in a way that takes account of individual variances?

In subgroup analyses, have the authors taken account of the multiple comparisons problem?

So What? Clinical Significance

Are any detected overall differences clinically significant?

Were the patients in the combined studies sufficiently representative to permit generalization of the results?

Are the interventions reviewed sufficiently feasible and representative to permit generalization of the results to other settings?

Were the outcomes sufficient to establish which therapy does the greatest good?

Did the authors identify key questions and outline a future research agenda that follows logically from the present state of knowledge?

References

1. Freiman JA, Chalmers TC, Smith H Jr, Keubler RR. The importance of beta, the type II error, and sample size in the design and interpretation of the randomized control trial. Survey of 71 negative trials. N Engl J Med 1978;299:690–694.
2. Laupacis A, Sackett DL, Roberts RS. An assessment of clinically useful measures of the consequences of treatment. N Engl J Med 1988;318:1728–1733.
3. Guyatt GH, Sackett DL, Cook DJ. Users' guides to the medical literature. II. How to use an article about therapy or prevention. A. Are the results of the study valid? JAMA 1993;270:2598–2601.
4. Guyatt GH, Sackett DL, Cook DJ. Users' guides to the medical literature. II. How to use an article about therapy or prevention. B. What were the results and will they help me in caring for my patients? JAMA 1994;271:59–63.
5. Mulrow CD. The medical review article: state of the science. Ann Intern Med 1987;106:485–488.
6. Sacks HS, Berrier J, Reitman D, Ancona-Berk VA, Chalmers TC. Meta-analyses of randomized controlled trials. N Engl J Med 1987;316:450–455.

Additional Reading

Chalmers TC, Celano P, Sacks HS, Smith H Jr. Bias in treatment assignment in controlled clinical trials. N Engl J Med 1983;309:1358–1361.

DerSimonian R, Charette LJ, McPeek B, Mosteller F. Reporting on methods in clinical trials. N Engl J Med 1982;306:1332–1337.

Emerson JD, McPeek B, Mosteller F. Reporting clinical trials in general surgical journals. Surgery 1984;95:572–579.

Fletcher RH, Fletcher SW. Clinical research in medical journals. N Engl J Med 1979;301:1809–1883.

Sackett DL, Tugwell PT. Deciding on the best therapy. In: Sackett DL, Haynes RB, Tugwell PT, eds. Clinical Epidemiology: A Basic Science for Clinicians. Boston/Toronto: Little, Brown, 1985, pp. 171–197.

Sackett DL, Haynes RB, Tugwell PT. How to read a clinical journal. In: Sackett DL, Haynes RB, Tugwell PT, eds. Clinical Epidemiology: A Basic Science for Clinicians, Boston/Toronto: Little Brown, 1985, pp. 285–321.

Commentary

A senior epidemiologist and his team provide us with the methodology they personally use for assessing the many new articles that appear in the surgical literature annually. Their framework can be used to analyze any paper, though it is particularly effective when the subject is a controlled trial. The analysis is based on six easily remembered appraisal criteria. These are demonstrated by example during the course of this chapter.

Over the years, advances in surgery have been made through observation, experimentation, innovation, application, and serendipity. Although the history of surgery is long, the evolution of a scientific approach to surgery spans only 250 years. Understanding the validity and importance of this information requires disciplined and systematic analysis. This insightful chapter presents useful questions and approaches that can sharpen the focus of discussion at a surgical journal club and strengthen critical thinking. John Yancy's "Ten Rules for Reading Clinical Research Reports" (Am J Surg 1990;159:533–539) and his recommended references provide a rich source of complementary material. See also chapter 8 by Rothmund and Stinner, "How I Read and Assess a Scientific Paper."

D.S.M.
M.F.M.

CHAPTER 8

How I Read and Assess a Scientific Paper

M. Rothmund and B. Stinner

This chapter is a focused discussion of how I sort through and evaluate a stack of scientific articles when faced with the need to gain detailed reliable information in a field (for example, when preparing a presentation, making an important decision for my hospital, or writing a scientific paper). It is not about how I browse through and select from the hundreds of articles that cross a surgeon's desk. That task is quite personal. Selecting credible background articles to develop or defend a position on buying equipment or developing a new program is not.

Retrieval systems can help you save time in selecting the appropriate original articles. Review articles provide a more logical, thematic approach than key word searches. Regardless of the search strategy, the result will be a large number of scientific papers claiming solutions for the problem in question. This chapter will focus on the critical assessment of scientific papers assembled in this way, emphasizing the value of their contribution toward solving your problem.

Initial Sorting

Titles

Most authors try to give sufficient information about the content of their article in the title. Some market their work with titles that promise more than is provided by the text. In a review of 45 papers dealing with antibiotic prophylaxis in surgery, 7 titles (15.5%) could be identified as totally misleading.[1] Titles, even those claiming a definite result, should be considered simply as "eye-catchers."

Authors and Institutions

The institution a paper originates from can give weight to credibility. Honorable and well-known institutions usually have some internal reviewing process to guarantee a certain standard of scientific work. The same is true for several principal investigators whose names stand for solid, carefully performed work. The first author may not be the person bearing full responsibility for the quality of the work. The accountable person is sometimes identifiable only by the address given for correspondence. It is a common practice to place the ultimately responsible investigator, often the head of the research unit or department, at the end of the line of contributing authors. Before publishing a paper, highly ranked research journals require a written statement from all coauthors guaranteeing the reliability and authenticity of their work. However, care has to be taken with multiinstitutional publications; all of the material cannot be reviewed and approved by each author, particularly under the pressure of deadlines for preliminary communications or concerning large data sets. Lack of interinstitutional communication and a cumbersome publication process may compound this problem. In general, papers published in highly ranked journals, authored or coauthored by respected experts in the field and generated in known institutions deserve to be taken more seriously, but still need critical evaluation.

Abstract

The abstract of an original article should provide enough information to select a paper for further evaluation. It is not sufficient to use the information presented there when drawing scientific conclusions. Abstracts preceding full papers are more reliable than published meeting abstracts. The latter are written under time constraints, with a primary goal of getting the study accepted for presentation at the meeting. In Evans and Pollock's study, 9 (20%) of the 45 original articles reviewed had abstracts that omitted important information or implied conclusions unjustified by the data presented.[1] Abstracts should be considered as preliminary presentations of the topic; they do not allow a critical examination of the analysis, and they can lead you to the wrong conclusion. The initial sorting process eliminates a substantial number of superficial or unrelated papers. Let's look more closely at the rest.

Close Analysis

General Problems

I use three criteria in assessing a scientific paper for its individual value: correct *methods*, justifiable *conclusions*, and scientific and/or clinical *relevance*. Do not critique the results at this stage; if obtained through proper methods, they reflect the real findings of the authors.

Methodological correctness for laboratory work is usually assured when the presenting authors are experts in their field. Laboratory errors and miscalculation are generally filtered out by the review process. This is much less true for the statistical analyses. In 45 papers submitted to the *British Medical Journal*, only 5 (11%) were considered to have applied acceptable statistical methods at submission, whereas 38 (84%)—but not all—had met good statistical standards at publication.[2] In this review, one major fault was lack of information on the sample size calculation. Trials published in general surgical journals were found to be most frequently deficient in reporting the methods used to generate treatment assignment and the power of the investigation to detect treatment differences.[3] Similar problems have been demonstrated in leading medical journals.[4]

Once the methods are judged to be correct, it has to be decided whether the conclusions drawn are justified. Conclusions are endpoints of mental data processing and may be wrong, even if the raw data and observations are correct. A simple historical example of misinterpretation was the geocentric theory that the sun rotates around the earth (incorrect conclusion based on correct and accurate observations of the daily sunrise and sunset). If you distrust the conclusions, try to draw your own interpretations from the raw data given by the author. If you cannot, do not accept any of the information or interpretations offered in the paper.

If the methods and conclusions are formally correct, a further decision has to be made as to their scientific or clinical relevance. Relevance cannot be inferred from sound methods and conclusions, but is a matter of scientific and clinical judgement. The author can offer an opinion on relevance. Your judgement on this issue may be guided by editorial opinions, but will be the final determinant of the place of the paper in your thinking and practice.

The Magic "P"

Most conclusions given in biomedical papers are strengthened by inferential statistics yielding a p-value. The p-value has a very simple meaning: $p < 0.05$ tells you that there is only a less than 5% chance the null hypothesis being tested is true, for example, that there is no effect, or no benefit for the population from which one has a random sample. This "magic bullet" of biomedical analysis has several important requisites. In addition to the usual requirements of random sampling and random allocation of treatments, there are many methods by which this p-value can be obtained. Some may not be appropriate for the particular data set you are reading about. What appears to be common sense but is generally omitted is the precise definition of the null hypothesis to be accepted or rejected. It is a commonsense rule, too frequently ignored, that precisely defined questions limit the range of possible answers.

The p-values are affected by the magnitude of effects under investigation in the sampled data (this is what they are usually used for), but they are affected much more by the magnitude of the sample, the variability of data, and the particular methodology used to derive them. For adequate assessment of scientific data it is mandatory to see the raw and not the processed data in the article under review. Even with this information, only a crude estimate of the distribution of these data points is possible, and without this information, no conclusions should be drawn. The recommended format for presenting distribution is the estimation of confidence intervals and probable magnitudes of effects[5] (see also chapter 37).

Even if correct, the magnitude of a p-value does not give any indication whether the result reported is clinically relevant. In practice, neither the presence nor the absence of statistical significance has any reliable relationship to the magnitude of a treatment effect or to the extent of clinical importance. If one needs a sample size of 1,000 patients in each group to obtain a treatment difference that is statistically significant, this result may not be relevant in treating the individual patient. Clinical importance is well illustrated by the first controlled clinical trial, conducted by James Lind in 1749. Lind took 12 seamen suffering from scurvy and allocated them to six groups of two persons each. One group was provided oranges and lemons; these two seamen recovered from scurvy—none of the others improved. The clinical importance and relevance of Lind's conclusions are enormous, but if Fisher's exact probability test is applied, it is statistically significant at the 0.05 but not the 0.01 level, which means it is not "highly significant" in the statistical terminology of biomedical research. This conflation of statistical probability with biologic significance is sloppy and confusing language.

Yancey's useful set of recommendations for analyzing clinical research articles deals primarily with statistical pitfalls.[6] These recommendations can be easily applied to the analysis of other areas such as health policy, technology assessment, or laboratory research. Table 8-1 summarizes some of the recommendations for critical analysis from five papers on the subject.

Assessing Completeness and Validity

Peer Review as Insurance

It is reasonable but not completely reliable to infer that a paper published in a well-established journal has passed a sophisticated peer review process, or that the general quality of the journal provides a guarantee of the quality of individual papers. Sixteen percent of the manuscripts published in the *British Medical Journal* between January and June of 1988 were judged to be either inadequately revised or of dubious validity.[2] Surgical journals[3] and medical journals were systematically reviewed using a list of 11 important criteria for design and analysis of therapeutic studies.[4]

In the surgical journals, only 59% of the 11 items were clearly reported, 5% were ambiguously discussed, and 36% were not reported; the results were mirrored in the medical papers (56%, 10%, and 34%, respectively). The reporting was in both cases most deficient in methods used to generate the treatment assignment and in the power of the investigation to detect treatment differences.

Peer review does not eliminate external influences, bias, or error. The personal interests or the interests of a granting institution may influence the amount and composition of published data.[7] The persistent effects or retracted invalid scientific literature may mislead the conclusions of serious authors. A review of 84 retracted articles revealed that, compared to a control group, the subsequent citation of this invalid information was reduced by only 35%, demonstrating an apparent lack of sufficient attention to manuscripts by some authors, reviewers, and editors.[8] This study did not take fraud into account, but it is an important additional source of misinformation for which prevention guidelines are remarkably rare

Table 8-1.   Recommendations for assessing clinical research articles

Reference													
Evans & Pollock (1984)[1]	Title accurate?	Abstract misleading?	Methods reproducible?	Results inaccessible	Discussion reasonable?								
Yancey (1990)[6]	Be skeptical.	Look for the data.	Differentiate between descriptive and inferential statistic.	Question the validity of all descriptive statistics.	Question the validity of all inferential statistics.	Be wary of correlation and regression analysis.	Identify the population sampled.	Identify the type of study.	Look for indices of magnitude-of-treatment effects.	Draw your own conclusions.			
Gardner & Bond (1990)[2]	Objective sufficiently described?	Appropriate study design for objective?	Satisfactory statement of source of subjects?	Prestudy calculation of required sample size?	Satisfactory response rate achieved?	Adequate describing of all statistical procedures?	Appropriateness of statistical analysis?	Presentation of statistical material satisfactory?	Confidence intervals given for the main results?	Conclusions drawn from statistical analysis justified?			
Emerson et al. (1984)[3] DerSimonian et al. (1982)[4]	Eligibility criteria given?	Admission before allocation?	Random allocation?	Method of randomization given?	Patient's blindness to treatment?	Blind assessment of outcome?	Treatment complications?	Loss to follow-up given?	Statistical analyses adequate?	Statistical methods adequate?	Powersize of detectable differences		
Int. Com. Med. J. Edit. (1988)[15]	Rationale for study given?	Selection of observational / experimental subjects given?	Procedures in sufficient details given?	Ethical statement given?	Original data assessable to verify results?	Indicators of measurement error and uncertainty?	Eligibility criteria?	Type of randomization?	Treatment complications?	Type of blinding?	Loss of observation?	Statistical terms exactly defined?	Are new hypotheses clearly labelled?

in academic settings.[9] Even at the highest level of biomedical publication, the peer-reviewed paper in a reputed journal may contain what Evans and Pollock call the "type three error" in which "no data were obtained to support the conclusion expressed."[1]

Rapid Communications and Summary Reports

Some biomedical journals have instituted "rapid communications" to facilitate the publication of very important data in a concise form, usually followed by a more comprehensive report to validate methods and inferences. Substantial numbers of clinical trials continue to be reported only as summaries or abstracts. In these reports, sufficient methodological details to permit informed judgement about the likely validity of the conclusions are generally lacking. Be very cautious about using these presentations to support your own data or conclusions in biomedical work. Half of the studies reported in summary form are never subsequently published in full. Regrettably, study results that have been reported only in summary reports are as likely to be cited as results that are reported in full papers.[10] The only feature that makes a summary report more likely to be followed by a full paper is a large sample size of the population under investigation; this is obviously only loosely associated with valid information.[11]

Publication Bias

A sound conclusion can be drawn only if all actual information available is reported to the scientific community. Underreporting of scientific results has been estimated at a ratio ranging from 1:128 to 1:5, the last appearing slightly optimistic.[12] Selection bias for publication is a multifactoral process involving personal motives of authors, granting agency interests, or simply the fact that a "positive result" appears to be more attractive to reviewers and editors. This subject is discussed further in chapter 9 ("Publications do not always reflect the real world").

Gold Standards

What can we use as a gold standard for validity? Full papers meeting the criteria in Table 8-1 should provide reasonable reliability. Publication bias is lessened when the protocol for a study dealing with a therapeutic approach of major consequence is published before the trial. The published protocol is then open for public discussion and leads to performance of the study and timely publication of results. This sequence has been recommended by the University of Chicago group for innovative therapies such as organ transplantation from living related donors, allowing public review of ethical issues.[13,14] It is occasionally used to initiate large prospective clinical trials.

Conclusion

Reading a scientific paper should be a well-structured, individualized, intellectual process. Neither the stature of the publication nor the character of the "guru" presenting the information guarantees that the scientific claim is true or relevant. *Be positive but skeptical*—these are characteristics of an inquiring but critical reader. *Be economical*—check the title and summary for congruence with your target issue first. *Critically analyze the complete paper*—peer review even in good journals does not guarantee proper methods and adequate conclusions. *Draw your own conclusions* from the raw data given—if this is not possible, don't accept the conclusions of the paper.

References

1. Evans M, Pollock V. Trials on trial. Arch Surg 1984;119:109–113.
2. Gardner MJ, Bond J. An exploratory statistical assessment of papers published in the *British Medical Journal*. JAMA 1990;263:1355–1357.
3. Emerson JD, McPeek B, Mosteller F. Reporting clinical trials in general surgical journals. Surgery 1984;95:572–579.
4. DerSimonian R, Charette LJ, McPeek B, Mosteller F. Reporting on methods in clinical trials. N Engl J Med 1982;306:1332–1337.
5. Gardner MJ, Altman DG. Confidence intervals

rather than *p* values: estimation rather than hypothesis testing. Br Med J 1986;292:746–792.

6. Yancey JM. Ten rules for reading clinical research reports. Am J Surg 1990;159:533–539.

7. Cantekin EI, McGuire TW, Potter RL. Biomedical information, peer review, and conflict of interest as they influence public health. JAMA 1990;263:1427–1430.

8. Pfiefer MP, Snodgrass GL. The continued use of retracted invalid scientific literature. JAMA 1990; 263:1420–1423.

9. Nobel JJ. Comparison of research quality guidelines in academic and nonacademic environments. JAMA 1990;263:1435–1437.

10. Goldman L, Loscalzo A. Fate of cardiology research originally published in abstract form. N Engl J Med 1980;303:255–259.

11. Chalmers I, Adams M, Dickersin K, Hetherington J, Tarnow-Mordi W, Meinert C, Tonascia S, Chalmers TC. A cohort study of summary reports on controlled trials. JAMA 1990;263:1401–1405.

12. Chalmers I. Underreporting research is scientific misconduct. JAMA 1990;263:1405–1408.

13. Singer PA, Siegler M, Whitington PF, Lantos JD, Emond JC, Thistlewaite JR, Broelsch CE. Ethics of liver transplantation with living donors. New Engl J Med 1989;321:620–622.

14. Singer PA, Siegler M, Lantos JD, Emond JC, Whitington PF, Thistlewaite JR, Broelsch CE. The ethical assessment of innovative therapies: liver transplantation with living donors. Theor Med 1990;11:87–94.

15. International Committee of Medical Journal Editors. Uniform requirements for manuscripts submitted to biomedical journals. Ann Int Med 1988;108:258–265.

Commentary

This chapter describes the personal approach of a busy general surgeon and outlines a method that he utilized to read and assess scientific papers in terms of their contribution to important decisions influencing his clinical practice or research. This provides an interesting contrast to the previous chapter written by Schechter, an experienced methodologist. I have concerns related to Dr. Rothmund's technique, as on many occasions I have found that only after I have seen the original data and read some aspects of the discussion will I discard a paper or not review it further. The author emphasizes the unreliability of judging the true contents of the paper based on the title or the abstract. He also underlines many of the statistical inadequacies of papers in the surgical literature. Rothmund highly values peer review, which in my mind may not always be justified. His concluding advice is useful: be positive but skeptical; select papers on the basis of title and abstract, depending on your needs; critically analyze the whole paper, look at the data, and draw your own conclusions. John Yancey's "Ten Rules for Reading Clinical Research Reports" is strongly recommended as a valuable tool for appraising information in the literature.

D.S.M.

CHAPTER 9

Publications Do Not Always Reflect the Real World

M.F. McKneally, S.D. Cassivi, and H. Troidl

The human intellect . . . is more moved and excited by affirmatives than by negatives.
— Francis Bacon, 1621

Introduction

The "literature," a tool used by surgeons and scientists to advance knowledge and to improve practice with a maximum of information and a minimum of error, is not always what it seems. Journal publications rank high in the hierarchy of information sources for decisions regarding health care funding, research endeavors, and, ultimately, improved patient care. Editors and readers of peer-reviewed journals expect authors to maintain objectivity. Authors are required and expected to notify readers, for example, in a footnote on the first page of a report, if they have a financial interest in the company producing an instrument or treatment described, or to identify the company's contribution in subsidizing the research reported.[1] Consumers of the literature expect to be alerted to any potential bias.

There are special venues for biased information or opinion, such as letters to the editor, invited commentary, editorials, or recorded discussion of comments from the audience of a paper presentation. We will develop the argument that bias is subtly present outside these venues as well.

Much of this section discusses the approach to the literature as part of our methodology, including critical assessment and reading and writing techniques. In this chapter we discuss some of the pitfalls and limitations of the literature.

Objectivity of the Literature

From direct personal experience to international conferences to throwaway journals prepared by profit-making publishers and industry, the sources of surgical information are as varied in form as they are in reliability. The peer-reviewed literature, contained largely in journals, is often used as the foundation for the acquisition, maintenance, and dissemination of surgical knowledge.

We use the literature as the basis for teaching students and residents about medicine and surgery, often by unguided forays ("Go look it up in the literature"). These unguided adventures may be illuminating or confusing to the naive reader. To reduce confusion, we may unconsciously introduce bias (as in "Go look up what Wong has written about esophagectomy"). In the way that political convictions guide our selection of newspapers, magazines, or columnists, we tend to select articles, journals, or authors that reinforce our beliefs or our specialty's inclination. Whereas Hans Troidl might direct his students toward articles emphasizing the impoverishment of the quality of life by radical cancer surgery or chemo-therapy, Charles Balch, the director of a cancer center, might select articles emphasizing prolongation of survival by radical surgery. Following this selection, both might use the same critical appraisal criteria in their statistical analyses and inferences, creating an illusion of objectivity and freedom from bias.

Obligation to Publish

One of the fundamental tenets of academia is that acquired knowledge must be disseminated. For some, this is viewed as a moral obligation to publish *all* of our findings in one form or another, thus providing a mechanism for growth of acquired knowledge.[2] In contrast, Claude Organ, the editor of the *Archives of Surgery,* argues that there are too many journals contributing to the proliferation of too much writing about too little information.[3] Indeed, some surgeons publish at a rate that would require them to be writing papers almost continuously. Some who are more skilled in writing than in operating may have more time to publish, based on this imbalance in their capabilities.

The "case report" as a form of publication may be the answer to those who seek a wide dissemination of information. Though often considered low on the hierarchy of evidence-based medicine because of its inherent anecdotal nature, the case report, presented in brief articles or letters to the editor, can have a profound effect on practice, initiate important investigations, or enrich the understanding of disease processes and treatments.[4] Nevertheless, some journals are sufficiently biased against case reports that they maintain a policy of excluding them categorically.

Bias of Omission

The systematic or policy-driven exclusions of some forms of publication such as case reports leads not only to a loss of a certain kind of information but, more importantly, to a systematic bias of omission. The most common form of this bias is the tendency to exclude negative results from the published literature.

Editors and reviewers participate in the development of a filtered view by encouraging the publication of positive results and rejecting negative or suboptimal results. Mahoney[5] conducted an empirical study of the influence of positive results on the opinions of referees. Similar manuscripts were developed and randomly assigned. Some reviewers received only the methods section, while others received a manuscript with the same methods section but results that were either negative, positive, or mixed. It was found that the results section significantly influenced the scores given for methods, data presentation, and publication merit. A simplified summary of Mahoney's findings, adapted from Dickersin's article on publication bias, is presented in Table 9-1. Indirect evidence of bias against the publication of negative results comes from surveys of authors conducting trials in cancer treatment, perinatology, and psychotropic drug therapy.[6,7]

As a corollary, there is an inherent bias toward the publication of small positive trials. This tendency amplifies type I errors of small trials. When the power of a study is small and a *p*-value of 0.05 is accepted as the threshold for statistical significance, 1 of every 20 trials will be a false positive. Over the course of conduct of 1,000 trials, 50 false positive trials might be published. Because of editorial bias toward selecting positive trials, there is less counterbalancing influence toward publication of the 950 negative trials. Thus, the bias toward publication of positive results leads to systematic error. The statistical basis for this effect and the influence of sample size are well described by Mitchell Gail.[8]

An example of this is the small randomized trial of regional postoperative immunostimulation with intrapleural bacillus Calmette-Guerin after resection of lung cancer conducted by one of the authors (MM).[9] The trial indicated a benefit from the innovative treatment. The demonstration that this was a false positive trial required a large multiinstitutional study.[10] The misleading excitement associated with positive results in smaller trials and the cost of the large confirmatory trials underline the need for mechanisms that can accommodate the systematic evaluation of new treatments as an ordinary component of practice. Sir Karl Popper gave us his famous example of the observer who sees four white swans on a lake

Table 9-1. Ratings for the same manuscript in varying presentations

Presentation	No. of reviewers	Mean ratings (0–6, low to high)	
		Methods	Publication merit
Positive results	12	4.2	3.2
Negative results	14	2.4	1.8
Methods only	14	3.4	3.4

Adapted from Dickersin[6] summary of data of Mahoney.[5]

(a small observational study) and then makes the erroneous inference that all swans must therefore be white.

The current enthusiasm for assessment of outcomes among insurers, hospitals, and governments might be used to advantage to develop such a program. An interesting system for large-scale, systematic evaluation without a complex trial structure has been described by Duncan Neuhauser.[11] His proposal is random assignment of patients to sections of the hospital or to health care teams that use different treatment strategies. Subsequent comparisons of outcome are then more credible because of the prior randomization. The natural, inevitable tendency toward publication of positive results in small studies, and negative results in large studies has gradually lead to a cynicism among readers and practitioners that might be countered with a more orderly and general mechanism for treatment evaluation in the practice community.

Also within the category of bias by omission is the tendency of authors to omit publication of mishaps in research or surgical practice. It is a rare experience to read of a clinical error that has been made, though often these "disasters" can be very illuminating.[12] Human nature is such that we would rather suppress our personal foibles than publish them. The potential threat of legal action further reinforces the bias toward publication of good results, and filters out frank disclosure of negative results. It is dangerous to publish a disastrous outcome in an environment that personalizes failure to the surgeon. This has the unfortunate effect of allowing similar mistakes to be repeated unnecessarily. Subsequent meta-analyses will be incomplete and literature reviews will be unbalanced because these negative results or haz-ardous outcomes have been suppressed, leaving their relative weight unknown.

Narrow Pool of Authors

As an example of a surgeon's use of the literature, one might decide to learn laparoscopic appendectomy based on a paper from Germany,[13] or to treat appendicitis nonoperatively, based on a published randomized trial in Finland.[14] The information we give to patients about risk and benefit is often based on the literature, and not necessarily on our own experience, which may not be as quantitatively and critically reviewed as a published series. This particular application emphasizes and, indeed, depends on the importance of unbiased information in the literature. However, as we have explained, the literature seems to be intrinsically biased toward publishing better results than those that are achieved in routine practice.

Surgeons tend to cite the results of experts who publish very large series, such as the experience with esophagectomy of John Wong[15] or the survival results after pulmonary resection of the Lung Cancer Study Group.[16] The implication is that the mortality risk faced by their own particular patient is similar to the low risk faced by the patients in these published series. In contrast, considerably higher mortality rates have been published using Medicare data from nationwide (United States) retrospective studies of lung resection for lung cancer.[17] Institutions performing higher volumes of certain procedures may well be able to achieve better results, as is suggested by Luft et al.,[18] but, nevertheless, this has the effect of skewing the portrayal of reality in the literature. In addition, there is a positive bias toward established views.

Like Pavarotti, who can sing any time and draw a crowd, prominent surgeons are given opportunities to opine in invited commentary, editorials, and observational studies for reasons that might be called "reputation bias."

Academic physicians and surgeons tend to publish far more than their counterparts in community practice because this behavior is reinforced within the social structure of their institutions. Advancement, academic salary, grants, and invitations to appear as a visiting lecturer depend upon publication. Established experts publish the opinions they have expressed in conferences and lectures, emphasizing their own excellent results, at least in part to reinforce their reputation for expertise.

In what could be referred to as a form of commercial bias, it is also in the interest of large centers to publish favorable reports of their experience with various treatments, in order to strengthen their referral network. Emphasis on low mortality, few complications, and a good outcome influence the selection of a topic ("We seem to have unusually good results with this procedure, let's write them up for publication"). The bias toward good results of a given procedure in the literature may be further reinforced by conscious or unconscious exclusion of less successful endeavors.

A far smaller percentage of publications come from community hospitals, although 80% or more of patients are treated there by doctors who do not publish as a part of the pattern of their professional life. Surgeons in a busy practice are not as likely to publish their results because of the lack of incentive in their practice setting (see chapter 3). The literature is impoverished as well as biased by this lack of information from busy clinical surgeons; we feel they should share their experience and thereby strengthen the overall practice of surgery. Data collection for audit and quality assurance provides a mechanism that can facilitate this contribution. Some nonpublishing virtuoso community surgeons, such as Leroy[19] in France, set a very high standard toward which other surgeons could aspire if they were able to share the knowledge and skills of the virtuoso.

The motivation of the author to produce a published document is variable, ranging from altruism to avarice. Some manuscripts are written by authors who wish to become well known, secure an academic position, or accrue patients for their surgical practice. These motives, as discussed above, can lead to a bias toward the compilation and publication of positive results, strengthening the bias in the literature toward results that are better than the real-world experience of the literature's readers.

When surgeons achieve a good result in a "headline-making" area, the tendency toward overemphasis of positive results may be reinforced by reports in the lay press sensationalizing what it perceives as "a good story." Vulnerable members of the public, particularly those with cancer, may be misled to seek imagined cures when small advances are tentatively described in the scientific literature but exaggerated by news reporters. Conflicts of interest may lead surgeons, vulnerable to the lure of self-promotion and notoriety, to be less critical than they should in restraining the press.

Editorial Bias

Through their role as critic and gatekeeper to the literature, editors and reviewers have an immense amount of power and a daunting responsibility. This process of sifting and filtering of submissions is as vulnerable to error as any other step in the course of publication. A memorable example was the elucidation of the Krebs cycle; this work was rejected by a noteworthy journal before it won the Nobel prize after publication in another journal. Important additions to surgical knowledge may be rejected for publication and thus delay their general dissemination. In a similar way, biases against or for a particular author may influence the extent to which published information is accepted.

Editors can also be influenced by current fads and trends. This incursion of subjectivity can be seen when results from private clinics or reviews of nonuniversity practice are for no other reason rated less highly than those from universities. Like the suggestion that the very first patient to undergo a new surgical procedure should be randomized,[20] this reflects a deficiency of familiarity with the real-world context of surgery.

The time to publication has a damaging effect on communication. Some of the best journals take pride in requiring a long time from submission to publication. Semm's paper on the first laparoscopic appendectomy[13] was delayed in publication for one year. It was finally published in *Current Problems in Obstetrics and Gynecology* through the intervention of an American surgeon. A 15-month delay in the review of the landmark studies of breast-conserving surgery by Fisher and his colleagues in the National Surgical Adjuvant Breast Program withheld valuable new information and more appropriate treatment from thousands of patients.[21] Decisions about which journal to submit a manuscript to are too often made on the basis of the known publication delay of one journal over another. This may significantly alter the final audience of the research paper.

Language is also a barrier and leads to ignorance of publications from other countries. The country of origin, or ethnicity of the patient group being studied or of the surgeon presenting the research may provide a source for subliminal or overt societal bias. This particular form of prejudice has been well described by the editor of *Scientific American*, where he demonstrates that a researcher has a much greater likelihood of being published depending on his or her country of origin.[22]

Specialty barriers themselves may prevent recognition of advances. Dissemination of information about changes in the eye of diabetics may not be recognized by endocrinologists or nephrologists who do not read ophthalmology journals.

EDITORIAL BIAS

Editors and reviewers may delay or even suppress publications for unscientific or political reasons:

- Selection of reviewers may influence the editing or even selection of publications.
- Journal policies and journal politics may influence what is published.
- Ultimately, editors or reviewers may simply not have a grasp of the particular novel subject.

Proprietary Bias

Increasingly, proprietary interests have been affecting the content of current publications. The private surgeon in Monaco may not want to publish a "how I do it" article that will give away the basis of an exclusive practice. Similarly, those who have made a substantial investment of money and time developing an instrument of analysis, such as the Apache III program for assessing illness severity, are not inclined to openly publish their findings. In fact, in some jurisdictions, prior publication may preclude the author from obtaining a patent for any components of the research that was published. The tendency toward protection of intellectual property for profit is increasing. This protective bias may be reinforced by contractual imperatives when research is conducted in collaboration with industry. Important findings might be delayed or even suppressed by this collaboration unless contractual safeguards are in place.

This intellectual protectionism seriously undermines not only the timeliness of publications but the very open, free flow of research findings that is so vital to the advancement of surgical knowledge. Given these trends, are we very far from a pay-per-view literature? In contrast, the many authors of this book, who are busy surgeons and experts in their fields, continue to strengthen the professional tradition of altruistic sharing of information.

Reader Bias

Curiously, published work is often ignored. Significant contributions may go unread or may be read but discarded or misunderstood. The inertial force of customary practice, and a free and unfettered approach to the practice of medicine, which distinguishes it as a profession, allows practitioners to say, "Yes, I have seen the evidence but I don't believe it; if this patient were my wife, she would have a radical mastectomy no matter what they say."

In a spirited exhortation on minimizing publication bias, Chalmers[23] identifies this source of bias as sloth. Recommended remedies for sloth, ignorance, greed, hubris, the application of lower standards to practice than to trials, and the bias of reviewers and authors are well presented in his challenging essay.

POTENTIAL BIAS IN THE LITERATURE

- Positive results are favored over negative results.
- Findings, both positive and negative, for different and varied reasons often do not find their way into the literature.
- More than 80% of the surgical workload by "frontline" surgeons is never published.
- Predominance of "experts" over frontline practitioners.
- Clinical disasters are rarely, if ever, published.
- Medico-legal concerns restrict the free flow of information.
- Proprietary interest leads to publication protectionism.
- Outside influences such as professional pressures or personality conflicts can lead to hasty publication either of unknowingly erroneous results or, worse yet, knowingly wrong results.

Solutions

1. We should always be mindful that scientific publications are part of the real world in which bias is a coinhabitant. We as practitioners have to recognize and handle this problem, rather than blindly accepting the literature.
2. Our biases should be identified with our patients, our students, and our readers.
3. Editors should recognize their bias toward the elite. Less highly ranked members of the practice community might be encouraged to publish through policies stated in the journal guidelines. As editors, we are directing our book toward the 80% of surgeons who do not publish, to facilitate the communication of their own experience.
4. Easy access, for example by electronic communication, will facilitate more rapid dissemination of important information and misinformation. Peer-review mechanisms and journal policies will need to be adapted to the age of the Internet.
5. Just as a "white spot" is often reserved on the program of some European meetings to allow unexpected new findings to be featured without displacing other papers, a similar news page of preliminary results might be saved in

our standard medical journals. When an unexpected but dangerous development (such as tumor implants at trochar sites in laparoscopic or thoracoscopic surgery) is discovered, it will then be possible to disseminate the information more widely and more rapidly. An appropriate disclaimer can be offered at the beginning of the news page to emphasize the risks of publishing preliminary or unconfirmed data.

6. There should be a more widespread and accepted policy on retraction and modification as a component of journal publication. Perhaps a page should be available for this purpose, so that the policy seems more welcomed. We have a section for corrections in many journals, but it is usually focused on minor differences in data, misspellings, or misstatements of the titles or addresses of authors. These retraction citations should then be linked to the original article in all electronic and subsequently printed material (e.g., MEDLINE indexes) so that the retraction or correction becomes integrated with the original submission.
7. Financial incentives: When payment for care becomes more directly linked to guidelines and standards of practice, there will be more attention paid to their publication, including timely modifications. This incentive may raise the level of discourse and the extent of participation by practitioners.
8. It is ethically appropriate and useful to society to disclose poor results as well as good results in a nonadversarial setting. Dissemination of information about unsatisfactory outcomes should be protected from malpractice litigation on a contingency fee basis.
9. Negative results should be provided a venue for publication when they are relevant and have sufficient power to support their conclusions.

Conclusion

The scientific literature, when critiqued as a method, has remarkable influence and significant drawbacks. Publications remain an important reservoir of knowledge. We have attempted to give a realistic appraisal of the literature's weaknesses as well as its strengths.

Blind acceptance of the literature can be more misleading than ignorance of it. Understatement in the literature is good science; publication of bad results and discussion of the reason for the results are ethically required, though they may remain legally dangerous. Such publication can prevent future mishaps and should be protected in society.

As consumers and contributors to the literature, we must remain vigilant toward potential bias. Healthy skepticism does not mean cynicism, but our appraisals should be informed and cautious. Just as good surgeons must know their limitations in order to be safe surgeons, readers and contributors must always be cognizant of the literature's inherent limitations in order to make effective and prudent use of it.

References

1. New England Journal of Medicine information for authors. New Engl J Med (printed at the end of every issue of the journal).

2. Small WP, Krause U. An introduction to clinical research. London: Churchill Livingstone, 1972.

3. Organ CH. Personal communication.

4. Guyatt GH, Sackett DL, Sinclair JC, Hayward R, Cook DJ, Cook RJ. Users' guides to the medical literature. IX. A method for grading health care recommendations. JAMA 1995;274(22):1800–1804.

5. Mahoney MJ. Publication prejudices: an experimental study of confirmatory bias in the peer review system. Cog Ther Res 1977;1:161–175.

6. Dickersin K. The existence of publication bias and risk factors for its occurrence. JAMA 1990;263:1385–1389.

7. Troidl H, Bäcker B, Langer B, Winkler-Wilfurth A. Failure analysis—evaluation and prevention of complications; its juridical implications. Langenbecks Arch Chir Suppl (Kongressbericht 1993) 59–72.

8. Piantadosi S, Gail MH. Statistical issues arising in thoracic surgery clinical trials. In: Pearson FG, Deslauriers J, Ginsberg RJ, Hiebert CA, McKneally MF, Urschel HC., eds. Thoracic Surgery. New York: Churchill Livingstone, 1995, pp. 1652–1670.

9. McKneally MF, Maver C, Kausel HW. Regional immunotherapy of lung cancer with intrapleural BCG. Lancet 1976;1:377–379.

10. Mountain CM, Gail MH, and the Lung Cancer Study Group. Surgical adjuvant intrapleural BCG treatment for stage I non–small cell lung cancer. J Thorac Cardiovasc Surg 1981;82:649–657.

11. Neuhauser D. The Metro firm trials and ongoing patient randomization. In: Tanur JM, Mosteller F, Kruskal WH, Lehmann EL, Link RF, Pieters RS, Rising GR, eds. Statistics, a Guide to the Unknown, 3rd edn. Pacific Grove, CA: Wadsworth and Brooks/Cole, 1989.

12. Paul A, Troidl H, Peters S, Stuttman R. Fatal intestinal ischaemia following laparoscopic cholecystectomy. Br J Surg 1994;81:1207–1208.

13. Semm K. Advances in pelviscopic surgery (appendectomy). Curr Probl Obstet Gynecol 1982; 5(10):1–42.

14. Eriksson S, Granström L. Randomized controlled trial of appendicectomy versus antibiotic therapy for acute appendicitis. Br J Surg 1995;82:166–169.

15. Fok M, Wong J. Esophageal cancer: squamous cell carcinoma. In: Pearson FG, Deslauriers J, Ginsberg RJ, Hiebert CA, McKneally MF, Urschel HC, eds. Esophageal Surgery. New York: Churchill Livingstone, 1995, pp. 571–586.

16. Ginsberg RJ, Hill LD, Eagan RT, Thomas P, Mountain CF, Deslauriers J, Fry WA, Butz RO, Goldberg M, Waters PF, Jones DP, Pairolero P, Rubinstein L, Pearson FG. Modern thirty-day operative mortality for surgical resections in lung cancer. J Thorac Cardiovasc Surg 1983;86:654–658.

17. Whittle J, Steinberg EP, Anderson GF, Herbert R. Use of Medicare claims data to evaluate outcomes in elderly patients undergoing lung resection for lung cancer. Chest 1991;100:729–734.

18. Luft HS, Bunker JP, Enthoven AC. Should operations be regionalized? The empirical relation between surgical volume and mortality. New Engl J Med 1979;301:1364–1369.

19. Leroy J. Personal communication.

20. Chalmers TC. Randomization of the first patient. Med Clin North Am 1975;59:1035–1038.

21. Fisher B. Personal communication.

22. Wayt Gibbs W. Mißachtete Forschung der Dritten Welt. Spektrum Wiss 1996;82–90.

23. Chalmers TC, Frank CS, Reitman D. Minimizing the three stages of publication bias. JAMA 1990;263(10):1392–1395.

CHAPTER 10

Computer-Based Literature Searches

P.W.T. Pisters and K.J. Hoffman

The dramatic increase in scientific and medical publications over the past three decades makes it imperative that scientists and clinicians have a focused and defined strategy for searching the scientific and medical literature. The creation of computerized databases has provided increased access to the literature and has facilitated organized approaches to searching the literature. The majority of relatively simple and small searches can be performed directly on-line without the need to leave the office or the home. This is in sharp contrast to the long, tedious hours spent in the library searching *Index Medicus*—a practice quite common less than two decades ago.

This chapter outlines the basic sources of on-line scientific and medical literature and provides generalized guidelines for planning and executing computer-based searches. The appendices (10-1 through 10-6) provide lists of major North American and international providers of on-line scientific data and sites of interest on the World Wide Web.

Sources of Scientific and Medical Literature

The "big four" biomedical databases are MEDLINE, EMBASE, BIOSIS Previews, and SciSearch (see Table 10-1). These databases have different scopes, as described below, and are readily accessible on-line through a variety of search services. DIALOG and Ovid are examples of two such search services that offer access to MEDLINE and other on-line databases (Appendix 10-1).

MEDLINE

MEDLINE is the first database of choice in many health science libraries. It covers about 3,700 international biomedical journals in the fields of medicine, basic sciences, nursing, dentistry, allied health, behavioral and social sciences, and health planning and administration. Journal articles are indexed for MEDLINE, and their citations are searchable using the National Library of Medicine's controlled vocabulary, MeSH (Medical Subject Headings). MEDLINE contains all citations published in *Index Medicus*. Citations include English abstracts when these are published with the articles (approximately 74% of the current file).

In-depth indexing is one of the unique features of MEDLINE. The entire article is indexed, not just the title or the abstract. The MeSH descriptors also include check tags for gender, age groups, human or animal studies, article type, and so forth. In addition to the controlled vocabulary terms, text words or free-text terms may be used

Table 10-1.   Major medical databases.

Database	Years of coverage update frequency	Source documents
BIOSIS Previews	1969–present/biweekly	Sources from over 100 countries; selective indexing of over 8,000 journal titles per year, plus symposia papers and abstracts, reviews, data surveys, notes, bibliographies, keys, monographs, case reports, and letters (when referenced and in a note format).
EMBASE *(Excerpta Medica)*	1974–present/biweekly	Sources from over 110 countries; 4,500 journal titles per year; 3,500 core journals screened cover-to-cover. Books indexed 1975–1980. Reports of drug-related congresses, symposia, and meetings, abstracts, dissertations, and annuals selectively covered. Letters that report original research are indexed.
MEDLINE *(Index Medicus)*	1966–present/weekly (Jan–Oct); monthly (Nov–Dec)	Sources from over 70 countries; 3,700 journal titles per year, approximately 1,700 of which are indexed cover-to-cover. About 31,000 new citations added each month. Some chapters and articles from selected monographs are found in earlier years.
SciSearch *(Science Citation Index)*	1974–present/biweekly	Sources from over 50 countries; virtually cover-to-cover indexing (all significant items) of 4,100 journal titles per year, plus selected multi-authored books, conference proceedings, etc.

for retrieval from the title, abstract, author's address, and other parts of the citation. Exploded tree words, which are the hierarchical arrangement of MeSH, can also be used for retrieval of broad categories of information. Every medical subject heading has at least one corresponding alphanumeric code or tree number that determines its location in the hierarchically arranged *Tree Structures.* In the *Permuted Medical Subject Headings,* each significant word of a MeSH term is isolated, and all of the MeSH terms in which that word exists are listed.

EMBASE

The biomedical database EMBASE is the on-line version of *Excerpta Medica.* EMBASE, a database of international coverage and broad subject scope, offers citations from more than 4,500 journals published in 110 countries. Based in Europe, *Excerpta Medica* covers journals not included in MEDLINE/*Index Medicus.* Citations from all 44

sections of *Excerpta Medica,* the *Drug Literature Index,* and *Adverse Reactions Titles* cover human medicine, basic sciences, pharmaceutical sciences, and drugs. Coverage of the drug and pharmaceutical literature is extensive and comprehensive, with 46% of the citations in this area. Other unique coverage is in the areas of environmental and occupational health and forensic sciences.

EMBASE may be searched by controlled vocabulary, free-text terms, drug trade names, or drug manufacturer names. MALIMET (Master List of Medical Terms) is the controlled vocabulary used to search EMBASE. In addition to MALIMET, broad concepts are indexed with EMCLAS or EMTAGS. EMCLAS is a hierarchical classification scheme of the 46 subject subfiles that make up the sections of the printed *Excerpta Medica.* EMTAGS comprises 220 codes that represent general concepts such as groups, gender, organ systems, experimental animals, and article type. Free-text searching of abstracts, titles, and other elements of the citations is especially valuable because a large number of citations have an abstract.

BIOSIS Previews

BIOSIS Previews, another biomedical database, contains more than 8.3 million citations from the *Biological Abstracts, Biological Abstracts/RRM* (reports, reviews, meetings *[BA/RRM]*), and *BioResearch Index (BioI)*, the major publications of BIOSIS (*BA/RRM* is the successor to *BioI* beginning in 1980). Together, these publications provide comprehensive worldwide coverage of research in the biomedical sciences. *Biological Abstracts* includes approximately 280,000 accounts of original research from 7,600 primary journal and monograph titles. *BA/RRM* includes an additional 260,000 citations per year for meeting abstracts, reviews, books, notes, letters, selected government reports, and other research communications. U.S. patents are also included from 1986 through 1989. Abstracts are available for records from the *Biological Abstracts* portion of the database starting in 1976, and for book synopses in *BA/RRM* starting in 1985. Most *BA/RRM* records do not contain abstracts, and no *BioI* records contain abstracts.

SciSearch

SciSearch is a multidisciplinary database that covers the international literature of science and technology from more than 4,100 journals and approximately 1,400 multi-authored books and conference proceedings. All significant items are indexed, including articles, letters, meeting reports, editorials, and cited references from about 3,300 journals that correspond to the "Source Index" of the *Science Citation Index*. The other 800 journals are from the ISI *Current Contents* publications, including *Current Contents/Clinical Sciences* and *Current Contents/Life Sciences*. Subject access is by natural-language free-text terms from titles of articles in the "Source Index" of the *Science Citation Index*.

SciSearch is distinguished by two important and unique characteristics. First, the indexed journals are carefully selected on the basis of several criteria including citation analysis, resulting in the inclusion of 90% of the world's significant scientific and technical literature. Second, reference citation indexing is provided. This allows retrieval of newly published articles through the subject relationships established by an author's reference to prior articles.

Internet

Although the Internet has evolved in the scientific community over more than 20 years, only recently have resources and on-line databases of interest to large numbers of biomedical researchers become accessible via the Internet. Through tools such as electronic mail (E-mail and listservs), access to remote systems (Telnet), file-transfer protocol (FTP), and menu-driven or hypertext interfaces (such as Gopher and the World Wide Web), the Internet provides new links to colleagues, on-line services, and information.

The traditional on-line services such as a DIALOG, Ovid, and the National Library of Medicine's MEDLARS were among the first resources to become available over the Internet. Although traditional services for searching bibliographic databases are accessible through direct-modem dial or value-added networks (VANs) such as Tynet, Telenet, and Compuserv, a direct connection to the Internet offers advantages such as faster communications, a more reliable connection, and the elimination of a need for a telephone line or modem. Once communications are established through the Internet, using appropriate software, the users interact with the search system just as if the connection was established with a modem.

The World Wide Web is one of the most exciting components of the Internet. The Web was originally developed by and for researchers at CERN, a major scientific research center in Switzerland. It has evolved into a major international network of computers and now offers literally millions of information sites for not only biomedical resources but also general reference, government, business, news, education, entertainment, sports, travel, and weather-related information with an international scope. Navigation of the World Wide Web requires a type of specially designed software known as a web browser that allows mouse and menu-driven browsing of multimedia Web sites. The software also provides interfaces with other Internet services such as E-mail, listservs (mailing lists that send a copy of all messages to each subscriber), and FTPs. Each site on the World Wide Web has a unique address, known as a URL (universal resource locator), that allows anyone with a web browser such as Netscape (Netscape Communications, World Wide Web URL: http://home.netscape.com) to view the contents of the site. Specific mouse-driven pathways at each web site allow viewing and downloading of specific data, image, and even video and audio files.

The National Library of Medicine (NLM) was among the first major biomedical resources to make many of its existing services available over the Internet. The NLM is now using the Internet to offer more than 200 publications free of charge, including fact sheets, biomedical subject bibliographies, AIDS information, systems manuals, and newsletters. Publications may be retrieved in both plain-text format and PostScript format which permits printing of the publication in its original format. In addition, the NLM has made its on-line catalog available over the Internet. The NLM locator (Telnet to locator.nlm.nih.gov) allows menu-driven Internet access to NLMs CATLINE (cataloged records of monographs and serials), AVLINE (audiovisuals), and SERLINE (serials owned by NLM and by member libraries of the National Network of Libraries of Medicine). Together, these databases represent the NLM collection that has been available on-line for many years to MEDLARS users. The NLM has several home pages available on the World Wide Web. In addition to a general information site (http://www.nlm.nih.gov), there is a National Center for Biomedical Information (NCBI) home page (http://www.ncbi.nlm.nih.gov) designed to serve the biotechnology community.

Many hospitals and academic institutions are also establishing World Wide Web sites for dissemination of biomedical information. At this time, there is no formal organization of these Web sites, and thus the user is handicapped in his or her ability to perform a comprehensive subject-specific search on the Internet. The only presently available method to search the World Wide Web requires use of a Web search engine (Appendix 10-6). Although these search engines allow access to 8 billion words found on 16 million Web pages, the capacity to focus the scope of searches using

Boolean operators or other techniques is limited and rather crude (by conventional literature search standards). Appendix 10-5 provides a limited list of relevant World Wide Web sites at the time of this publication. Additional sites are being added literally on a daily basis.

Searching the Biomedical Literature

The basic principles of scientific literature searching are the same, regardless of whether a search is done manually or by computer. The searcher must have a thorough knowledge of what the databases contain, how they are organized, what the access points are, and how to use the vocabularies.

The very nature of a research-level scientific literature search prescribes that it should be as comprehensive as possible. Therefore, a combination of manual and computer-based searching may be desirable. One of the most important advantages of manual over computer-based searching is that manual searching allows inclusion of older materials, whereas on-line databases often cover only relatively recent time periods. However, computer-based searching offers the advantages of speed, currency, more access points, coordinate searching, and access to multiple databases. Since computer-based literature searching is the method most frequently chosen in the health sciences field, this chapter will focus on the principles and techniques of on-line searching.

Who Will Perform the Search?

Computerized literature searching tends to take place in one of three ways: (1) a medical librarian interviews the client and then performs the search alone, (2) the medical librarian and the client work together in planning and running the search, or (3) the client performs the search alone.

Many libraries offer access to on-line databases as well as classes on how to do on-line searching. Novice searchers usually find it beneficial to take one of these classes before embarking on a comprehensive computer-based literature search. Many searchers also enlist the help of a medical librarian or other professional searcher to perform the search for them. Medical librarians have knowledge of the medical literature, and they are also very familiar with on-line searching protocols. An experienced professional can evaluate overall on-line strategy, look for logic errors, pinpoint vocabulary problems, and advise on particularly difficult questions.

Regardless of who performs the search, there are several critical decision points in the search process:

1. Clarifying the information need and search objective
2. Identifying relevant databases
3. Compiling the search terms
4. Formulating basic search logic and planning the search strategy
5. Evaluating the search results

Planning the Search

To clarify the information need and search objective, it is helpful to first write a description or summary of the research topic. The description should be written in the searcher's own words. It is much more efficient to translate something concrete into the vocabulary of the on-line system than to force an unwritten idea into the written language of the system. Next, the summary statement should be divided into separate concepts. And, finally, the searcher should think about what limitations to place on the search. For example, searches can be limited to human or animal studies and by language, sex and age of patients, and publication dates. Examples of known citations that are relevant to the search topic provide an excellent way to help plan the search strategy. By first retrieving known items from the database, the searcher can examine the index terms used and include them in the search strategy (Table 10-2).

Selection of the appropriate database comes into consideration next. There are numerous machine-readable databases, and vendors make frequent updates and enhancements to them to improve search interfaces, coverage, and so forth. Selection of appropriate databases includes several factors: (1) subject scope, (2) publication years of source documents indexed, (3) frequency of file updates and lag time between source publication

Table 10-2.   Steps in planning the search.

1. Write a summary statement describing the topic.
   Example: Articles on the use of doxorubicin in the treatment of breast cancer.
2. Divide the statement into separate concepts.
   Example: Doxorubicin/breast cancer
3. Decide what limitations to place on the search.
   Example: Limit to articles published between 1991 and present; English language only; both human and animal studies.
4. Find relevant citations and examine their index terms.
5. Select an appropriate database. (A different strategy may be needed for each database selected.)
6. Select search terms to describe each concept of the topic.

and on-line access, (4) resources indexed (i.e., types and total number of publications included), (5) geographic origin and language of sources covered, (6) availability of abstracts on-line, and (7) added indexing/access points provided.

Basic Principles of On-line Searching

To perform an effective on-line search, the searcher must understand the key concepts of on-line searching. They include elements such as (1) use of controlled vocabulary, synonyms, free-text, and truncation; (2) exploding MeSH tree categories; (3) use of Boolean connectors; and (4) use of positional connectors.

Database-specific and system-specific requirements will affect the formulation of the search strategy. First, the searcher should determine whether the database uses a controlled vocabulary to index each document. If it does, the thesaurus for that database should be consulted to select the appropriate terms describing the topic. If the database does not use a controlled vocabulary, the searcher will need to make a list of synonyms to describe each concept in the topic. Using more synonyms will usually result in the retrieval of more citations. Also, the thesaurus should be consulted to find out if the database allows searches to be limited by date of publication, sex, age group, animal or human study, or review article. Another technique that the searcher should consider is truncating the search terms selected. Instead of searching several synonyms with the same root, many databases allow searchers to truncate the root in order to retrieve variations of the term. This is a particularly useful technique when searching author names. For example, by entering the name "Silver," followed by the appropriate truncation symbol, a search will retrieve all authors whose names begin with the root "Silver" (e.g., Silverman, Silverstein, Silvers, Silverberg, and so forth).

A primary advantage of on-line searching over manual searching is the system's ability to coordinate any number of different concepts in the same search. Using Boolean logic, search terms can be combined in various relationships. The major Boolean connectors are *AND, OR,* and *NOT* (see Figure 10-1).

AND is used to combine concepts and narrow a search. It will retrieve records containing both terms or sets of terms in a combination. For example, BURNS AND EMERGENCY MEDICAL SERVICES will retrieve articles discussing both "burns" and "emergency medical services."

To broaden a search, the Boolean connector *OR* is used to search for articles containing one or more of the concepts. For example, BURNS OR EMERGENCY MEDICAL SERVICES will retrieve all articles about either "burns" or "emergency medical services."

The Boolean connector *NOT* is used to exclude information. For example, BURNS AND NOT EMERGENCY MEDICAL SERVICES will retrieve all articles on "burns" that are not indexed to "emergency medical services."

Some database services also permit the use of "positional connectors." Positional connectors are special operators used to indicate more precise relationships between certain terms in a reference. They can be used to further limit a search. The positional connector *SAME* is used by some search services to limit terms to the same paragraph, while the positional connector *WITH* is used to limit terms to the same sentence. For example, in the search strategy BURNS SAME EMERGENCY MEDICAL SERVICES, both the word "burns" and the phrase "emergency medical services" must be present within the same paragraph or field; in the search strategy BURNS WITH EMERGENCY MEDICAL SERVICES, both the word "burns" and the phrase "emergency medical services" must be present within the same sentence.

Many databases allow free-text searching. Free-text searching offers several advantages, but it is important to understand the limitations of this search technique. Free-text searching can be most beneficial when an exhaustive search is required on a subject, because free-text searching retrieves all records containing the selected terms even if those terms were not considered sufficiently central to the topic of the record to have been assigned as index terms. Free-text searching is also advantageous when a subject represents a new concept that is not uniquely represented in the controlled vocabulary of the database. Free-text searches can lead to retrieval errors, however, due to unanticipated spelling variations, synonyms, and multiple meanings of words. On-line retrieval studies have shown that computer-based literature searches can be significantly enhanced by selected combinations of indexing terms and free-text words.

There are three main ways to construct a search strategy: (1) the "building block" approach,

Boolean "AND" : Both subjects are present in each article. Use to narrow a search.

INFLUENZA AND COUGH

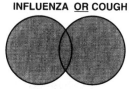

Boolean "OR" : Either subject is represented in each article retrieved. Use to broaden a search.

INFLUENZA OR COUGH

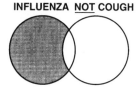

Boolean "NOT" : Retrieves articles on subject "A", not indexed to subject "B". Use to exclude information.

INFLUENZA NOT COUGH

Figure 10-1.   The Boolean operators "and," "or," and "not."

(2) the limiting of a concept through the "successive fractions" approach, and (3) the "citation pearl growing" approach. Searchers will often use a combination of all of these.

In the building block approach, each concept of the search is formulated separately, and the results are combined to reach the final search result. The successive fractions approach is used when the topic covers a broad subject area, but it is necessary to narrow down the subject to make it manageable. A searcher uses the successive fractions approach by running a general search that retrieves a large set of hits and intersecting this set with other concepts until the result is a narrow enough search. And, finally, citation pearl growing is the method used when a searcher begins with a known relevant citation, retrieves it online, and then examines the indexing terms, which can then be plugged back into the search to obtain similar or related citations.

Analysis of Search Results

No matter how carefully planned, most searches require some modification in strategy. It is important to analyze the search results to determine whether the search strategy should be amended. One method frequently used to assess the results of a search is to measure the results in terms of "recall" and "precision." Recall pertains to the ratio between the number of relevant records retrieved by the search compared with the total number of relevant records in the database. Precision pertains to the ratio of relevant records retrieved compared with the total number of records retrieved. When conducting a comprehensive search, high recall is desired, even at the expense of retrieving some irrelevant documents. The search strategy can be modified to achieve a higher recall by (1) using free-text words rather than index terms, (2) including as many synonyms as possible, and (3) reducing as much as possible the number of terms linked by the use of the Boolean operator *AND*. Searches resulting in too many citations can be modified to achieve a higher precision level by (1) using index terms that are at the narrowest level of specificity, (2) using terms that appear in the title field only, or (3) linking as

many terms as possible with the Boolean operator *AND*. Limiting searches by factors such as language, document type, or publication date will not necessarily improve precision, but it will reduce the number of citations retrieved.

Other reasons for poor search results include (1) selection of an inappropriate database for the subject of the search; (2) inappropriate selection of search terms; (3) inadequate attention to synonyms and spelling variations, particularly with free-text searching; and (4) inappropriate use, or lack of use, of Boolean operators and positional connectors.

After the Search: Computerized Reference Management

Once a search is complete and the file has been downloaded, the file can be manipulated in several ways. These include simple viewing or printing of the file with any word-processing or notepad-type software. More important, however, the downloaded file can be imported into reference management software designed to facilitate creation and maintenance of individual reference databases.

Reference management software has become an essential component of any researcher's core software. References of any size can be stored with or without abstracts. The software allows use of a variety of criteria to locate references within the database, including user-defined key words as well as standard criteria such as journal name or author. Reference management programs interact with common word-processing programs to generate automatic bibliographies in predesigned bibliographic formats that fit the specific styles of hundreds of journals. Two popular reference management programs are Reference Manager (Research Information Systems, World Wide Web URL: http://www.risinc.com) and EndNote (Niles and Associates, Inc., World Wide Web URL: http//www.niles.com). Complete and up-to-date information on these programs is available at the Web sites noted above. Figure 10-2 outlines the utility and central role of these software programs in the manipulation of downloaded references.

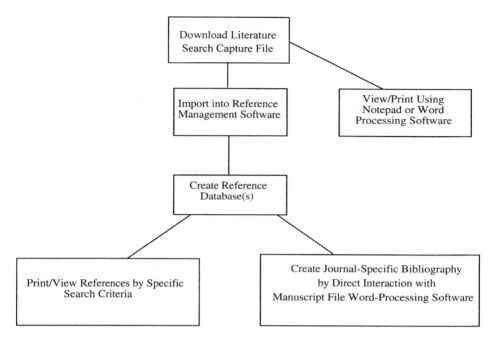

Figure 10-2. The multiple uses of reference management software and central role of this software in reference management.

Conclusion

Computer-based literature searching is a powerful and comprehensive resource. It is important, however, to understand that using this resource may involve trade-offs between efficiency and comprehensiveness. It is strongly recommended that beginning searchers obtain instruction in on-line searching methods or consult a medical librarian. Before starting a search, it is important to learn the fundamentals of Boolean logic and how the use of Boolean connectors will affect the outcome of searches. The searcher should become familiar with the controlled vocabulary of the database that will be searched. Sufficient time should be invested in preparing the search strategy before going on-line: (1) briefly state the search topic in a sentence or two, (2) identify the basic concepts or key words within the topic, (3) list synonyms for each concept, and (4) translate key words into the controlled vocabulary of the database. It is advisable to run the search and then display a few citations to evaluate initial results. If the results are not as expected, the searcher should modify the search strategy and try running the search again. And if, after several attempts, the search results are still unsatisfactory, the searcher may want to seek the aid of a medical librarian.

Additional Reading

Adams CE, Lefebre C, Chambers I. Difficulty with MEDLINE searches for randomised controlled trials. Lancet 1992;340:915–916.

Armstrong CJ, Large JA, eds. Manual of Online Search Strategies. Boston: G. K. Hall, 1988.

Basch R. Secrets of the Super Searchers. Wilton, CT: Eight Bit Books, 1993.

Biarez O, Sarrut B, Doreau CG, Etienne J. Comparison and evaluation of nine bibliographic databases concerning adverse drug reactions. DICP 1991;25: 1062–1065.

Bonham MD, Nelson LL. An evaluation of four end-user systems for searching MEDLINE. Bull Med Libr Assoc 1988;76:22–31.

Chambliss ML. Personal computer access to MED-LINE: an introduction. J Fam Pract 1991;32:414–419.

Curtis KL, Weller AC. Information-seeking behavior: a survey of health sciences faculty use of indexes and databases. Bull Med Libr Assoc 1993;81:383–392.

DeNeef P. The comprehensiveness of computer-assisted searches of the medical literature. J Fam Pract 1988;27:404–408.

Egeland J, Foreman GE. Reference services: searching and search techniques. In: Darling L, ed. Handbook of Medical Library Practice, 4th edn. Chicago: Medical Library Association, 1982.

Farbey R. Searching the literature: be creative with MEDLINE. Br Med J 1993;307:6895.

Feinglos SJ. MEDLINE: A Basic Guide to Searching. Chicago: Medical Library Association, 1985.

Haynes RB, McKibbon KA, Fitzgerald D, Guyatt GH, Walker CJ, Sackett DL. How to keep up with the medical literature. V. Access by personal computer to the medical literature. Ann Intern Med 1986;105:810–824.

Haynes RB, McKibbon KA, Walker CJ, Mousseau J, Baker LM, Fitzgerald D, Guyatt G, Norman ER. Computer searching of the medical literature. Ann Intern Med 1985;103:812–816.

Haynes RB, Walker CJ, McKibon KA, Johnston ME, Willan AR. Performances of 27 MEDLINE systems tested by searches with clinical questions. J Am Med Inf Assoc 1994;1:285–295.

Haynes RB, Wilczynski N, McKibon KA, Walker CJ. Developing optimal search strategies for detecting clinically sound studies in MEDLINE. J Am Med Inf Assoc 1994;1:447–458.

Hersh WR, Hickam DH. A comparison of retrieval effectiveness for three methods of indexing medical literature. Am J Med Sci 1992;303:292–300.

Hewitt P, Chalmers TC. Perusing the literature: methods of accessing MEDLINE and related databases. Control Clin Trials 1985;5:168–177.

Hewitt P, Chalmers TC. Using MEDLINE for perusing the literature: software and search interfaces of interest to the medical professional. Control Clin Trials 1985;6:198–207.

Hewitt P, Chalmers TC. Using MEDLINE to peruse the literature. Control Clin Trials 1985;6:75–83.

Jennings AG. Research or re-search? Why we should read old and foreign literature. Ann R Coll Surg Engl 1994;76:236–237.

Lacroix EM, Backus JEB, Lyon BJ. Service providers and users discover the Internet. Bull Med Libr Assoc 1994;82:412–418.

Largaespada MJ, Pistotti V, Bonati M. How accurate are bibliographic data bases? Lancet 1988;i:538.

Lee JH. Online Searching: The Basics, Settings, and Management, 2nd edn. Englewood, CO: Libraries Unlimited, 1989.

Lowe HJ, Barnett GO. Understanding and using the medical subject headings (MeSH) vocabulary to perform literature searches. JAMA 1994;271:1003–1008.

Marshall JG. Computers: how to choose the online medical database that's right for you. Can Med Assoc J 1986;134:634–640.

McGrath F, Tomaiuolo NG. Practice locally, search globally. Conn Med 1993;57:155–161.

Pinatsis A. Accuracy of bibliographic data bases. Lancet 1988;i:942.

Porter D, Wigton RS, Reidelbach MA, Bleich HL, Slack WV. Self-service computerized bibliographic retrieval: a comparison of Colleague and PaperChase, programs that search the MEDLINE data base. Comput Biomed Res 1988;21:488–501.

Schwartz DG. Techniques for accessing the medical literature. I. Currently available approaches. J Allergy Clin Immunol 1988;82:544–550.

Seago BL. A comparison of MEDLINE CD-ROM and librarian-mediated search service users. Bull Med Libr Assoc 1993;81:63–66.

Searching MEDLINE. Lancet 1988;ii:663–664.

Simon FA. A comparison of two computer programs for searching the medical literature. J Med Educ 1988;63:331–333.

Smith BJ, Darzins PJ, Quinn M, Heller RF. Modern methods of searching the medical literature. Med J Aust 1992;157:603–611.

Wakeford R, Roberts W. Using MEDLINE for comprehensive searches. Br Med J 1993;306:1415.

Walker CJ, McKibbon KA, Haynes RB, Ramsden MF. Problems encountered by clinical end users of MEDLINE and GRATEFUL MED. Bull Med Libr Assoc 1991;79:67–69.

Warling B, Gilman LB. Manual versus MEDLINE searches. Am J Psychiatry 1990;148:686–687.

Wood EH. MEDLINE: the options for health professionals. J Am Med Inf Assoc 199;1:372–380.

Wood MS, Horak EB, Snow B, eds. End User Searching in the Health Sciences. New York: Haworth, 1986.

Wright LC, Sutherland HJ, Jackson JI, Till JE. Comparison of search strategies on CD Plus/MEDLINE. Can Med Assoc J 1991;145:457–464.

Commentary

This chapter was written by a surgical oncologist and the executive director of the research medical library at the University of Texas–M. D. Anderson Cancer Center in Houston. Their practical discussion provides the reader with an excellent description of the current sources of scientific and medical literature available through computer searches, and the authors' evaluation of the four main database sources of scientific and medical literature. The authors emphasize the important role of collaboration with a medical librarian during the earliest phase of the proposed research study. A clear description of the research proposal, and clear identification of key terminology enable the librarian to carry out an effective computer search of the literature.

There are many helpful tips on using the computer for reference management, along with a failure analysis approach. Useful appendices at the conclusion of the chapter allow the reader to obtain practical entry via phone, fax, E-mail, and Internet to the libraries of the world, in addition to providing all of the international MEDLARS centers. I suspect that these appendices will be the most frequently used section of this book.

The references by Hewitt and Chalmers in the bibliography, and Hewitt's chapter in the second edition of *Principles and Practices of Surgical Research* are recommended for further reading.

The authors' brief but clear statement that manual searching gives access to important older material excluded from these databases deserves underlining. Naive researchers sometimes conclude that an observation or idea has never been reported in the literature if it is not available on-line. A pithy and humorous book review by Frank P. Grad, L.L.B., provides a memorable image of this problem:

> Just as the burning of the great library of Alexandria wiped out much earlier knowledge, the creation of computer databases around 1979 or 1980 put earlier materials out of easy reach of researchers. Fortunately, this knowledge is available if [they] leave their computer consoles to browse in the library.[1]

D.S.M.
M.F.M.

1. Grad FG. New Engl J Med 1996;335:140.

Appendix 10-1.   Main Offices of Major Vendors of MEDLINE

Address	Telephone/Fascimile/E-Mail/Web Site
U.S. National Library of Medicine MEDLARS Management Section 8600 Rockville Pike Bethesda, MD 20894	800-638-8480 (toll-free tel) 301-496-0822 (fax) ntsiegal@nlm.nih.gov http://www.nlm.nih.gov
DIALOG Technologies, Inc. Knight-Ridder Information Inc. World Wide Headquarters 3460 Hillview Avenue P.O. Box 10010 Palo Alto, CA 94303-0993	800-3-DIALOG (toll free tel) 415-858-3785 (telephone) 415-858-7069 (fax) Info@www.dialog.com http://www.dialog.com
Ovid Technologies, Inc. 333 Seventh Avenue New York, NY 10001	800-950-2035 (toll free tel) 212-563-3006 (telephone) 212-563-3784 (fax) sales@ovid.com http://www.ovid.com

Appendix 10-2.   International MEDLARS Centers

Country	Telephone	Fax	E-mail
Australia	61-06-273-1180	61-06-273-1180	
Canada	613-993-1604	613-952-7158	cisti.medlars@nrc.ca
China	861-512-8185	861-512-8176	
Egypt	202-355-7253	202-354-7807	
France	33-1-4521-1044	33-1-4658-4057	
Germany	49-221-472-4264	49-221-41-1429	
India	91-11-4362-359	91-11-4362-489	!uunet!nicnet!medlar_!slc
Israel	972-2-758-790	972-2-784-010	
Italy	39-6-4990	39-6-446-9938	
Japan	81-3-3581-6411	81-3-3593-3375	
Korea	82-2-740-8043	82-2-744-0484	cek@sobackhananm.kr
Kuwait	965-533-8610	965-533-8618	
Mexico	525-598-9875	525-598-9959	gladys@redvax1.dgsca.unam.mx
New Zealand	64-4-496-2000	64-4-496-2340	
South Africa	27-021-938-0339	27-021-938-0315	gmilliga@Eagle.mrc.ac.za
Sweden	46-8-728-8000	46-8-330-481	mic%Micforum@mica.ki.se
Switzerland	41-31-301-2572	41-31-301-6556	dokdi@dm.rs.ch
United Kingdom	44-71-323-7074	44-71-323-7018	
Bireme	55-11-549-2611	55-11-571-1919	celia@brm_1.bireme.ansp.br
Pan American Health Org.	202-861-3301	202-223-5971	gamboa@lhc.nlm.nih.gov
Intergovernmental Organization	886-2-737-7690	886-2-737-7664	nsc_51@ + wnmoel_.edv.tw

Appendix 10-3.   International DIALOG Centers

Country	Telephone	Fax	E-mail
Australia	61-2-212-2867	62-2-281-5427	jean_tyan@corp.dialog.com
Bahrain	966-1-477-0477	966-1-476-6337	lisa_parramore@corp.dialog.com
Botswana	27-12-84-3007	27-12-841-3604	michelle_foster@corp.dialog.com
Brazil	55-11-257-2157	55-11-258-6990	claudio_pinto@copr.dialog.com
Brunei	852-868-0877	852-810-5861	wynne_choi@corp.dialog.com
Canada	416-445-6641	416-445-3508	mary_corcoran@corp.dialog.com
Carribbean Countries	52-5-682-2395	52-5-687-7355	claudio_pinto@corp.dialog.com
China	86-21-372-3678	86-21-372-4333	jean_tyan@corp.dialog.com
Colombia	57-1-312-5802	57-1-255-1017	moseresr%dialogvm@mcimail.com
Equador	61-2-212-2867	61-2-281-5427	belinda_benson@corp.dialog.com
Europe	44-71-930-7646	44-71-930-2581	
Hong Kong	852-868-0877	852-810-5861	wynne_choi@corp.dialog.com
India	91-22-218-0831	91-22-218-8175	iipl@soochak.ncst.ernet.in
Indonesia	852-868-0877	862-810-5861	jean_tyan@corp.dialog.com
Israel	972-3-695-0073	972-3-695-6359	claudio_pinto@corp.dialog.com
Japan	813-3439-0123	813-3439-1093	
Kenya	27-12-841-3007	27-12-841-3604	michele_foster@corp.dialog.com
Korea	82-2-220-7272	82-2-796-8811	yamanaka%dialogvm@ciail.com
Kuwait	966-1-477-0477	966-1-476-6337	lisa_parramore@corp.dialog.com
Lesotho	27-12-841-3007	27-12-841-3604	michelle_foster@corp.dialog.com

(continued)

Appendix 10-3.   Continued

Country	Telephone	Fax	E-mail
Malawi	27-12-841-3007	27-12-841-3604	michelle_foster@corp.dialog.com
Malaysia	852-868-0877	852-810-5861	wynne.choi@corp.dialog.com
Mauritius	27-12-841-3007	27-12-841-3604	michelle_foster@corp.dialog.com
Mexico	52-5-682-2395	52-5-687-7355	claudio_pinto@corp.dialog.com
Mozambique	27-12-841-3007	27-12-841-3604	michelle_foster@corp.dialog.com
Namibia	27-12-841-3007	27-12-841-3604	michelle_foster@corp.dialog.com
New Zealand	61-2-212-2867	61-2-281-5427	jean_tyan@corp.dialog.com
Oman	966-1-477-0477	966-1-476-6337	lisa_parramore@corp.dialog.com
Peru	61-2-212-2867	61-2-281-5472	belinda_benson@corp.dialog.com
Qatar	966-1-477-0477	966-1-476-6337	lisa_parramore@corp.dialog.com
Saudi Arabia	966-1-477-0477	966-1-476-6337	lisa_parramore@corp.dialog.com
Singapore	852-868-0877	852-810-5861	wynne_choi@corp.dialog.com
South Africa	27-12-841-3007	27-12-841-3604	michelle_foster@corp.dialog.com
Sri Lanka	91-22-218-0831	91-22-218-8175	lisa_parramore@corp.dialog.com
Swaziland	27-12-841-3007	27-12-841-3604	michelle_foster@corp.dialog.com
Tanzania	27-12-841-3007	27-12-841-3604	michelle_foster@corp.dialog.com
Taiwan	852-868-0877	852-810-5861	wynne_choi@corp.dialog.com
Thailand	852-868-0877	852-810-5861	wynne_choi@corp.dialog.com
Uganda	27-12-841-3007	27-12-841-3604	michelle_foster@corp.dialog.com
United Arab Emirates	966-1-477-0477	966-1-476-6337	lisa_parramore@corp.dialog.com
United States of America	415-254-7000	415-254-7070	
Venezuela	61-2-212-2867	61-2-281-5472	belinda_benson@corp.dialog.com
Zambia	27-12-841-3007	27-12-841-3604	michelle_foster@corp.dialog.com
Zimbabwe	27-12-841-3007	27-12-841-3604	michelle_foster@corp.dialog.com

Appendix 10-4.   International Ovid Offices

Region/Country	Telephone	Fax	E-mail
North Central/So. America	212-563-3006/800-950-2035	212-563-3784	sales@ovid.com
United Kingdom, Ireland Middle East, & Africa	44-(0)-181-748-3777	44-(0)-181-748-2302	info@ovid.co.uk
Continental Europe	31-20-672-0242	31-20-673-8041	info@cdplus.nl
France	33-14-722-4249	33-14-722-4309	nicolasb@ovid.com
Australia, New Zealand, Asia, & Pacific Rim	800-22-6474/800-44-6106 800-44-6106/ +61 (0)-2-231-5086	61-(0)-2-231-5599	aussie@ovid.com

Appendix 10-5.   Representative World Wide Web Sites of Biomedical Interest

Organization	World Wide Web URL
National Library of Medicine (United States)	http://www.nlm.nih.gov
National Cancer Institute (United States)	http://www.nci.nih.gov
University of Pennsylvania Oncolink	http://cancer.med.upenn.edu
Oncolink List of Hospitals and Medical Universities	http://cancer.med.upenn.edu
Nature (the journal)	http://www.nature.com-1
World Health Organization	http://www.who.ch

Appendix 10-6.   World Wide Web Search Engines

Search Engine	World Wide URL
WebWorm	http://www.mcb.cs.colorado.edu/home/mcbryan/www.html
Lycos	http://lycos.cs.cmv
Alta Vista	http://www.altavista.digital.com.edu
Yahoo Search	http://www.yahoo.com/search.html
WebCrawler	http://www.webcrawler.com
InfoSeek	http://www2.infoseek.com
Excite	http://www.excite.com
CU1 W3 Catalog	http://cuiwww.unige.ch/cgi-bin/w3catalog

CHAPTER 11

Facing the Blank Page/Screen

M.F. McKneally and J.A. Bennett

Reading maketh a full man, conference a ready man, and writing an exact man.
— Francis Bacon (1561–1626)

Writer's Block Is a Good Thing

We try to be exact when we write, because writing carries the onus of permanently associating the author with a final product that will be read by an audience of potentially unlimited size and critical powers. This imaginary readership intimidates the writing process in a salutary way, because it reduces the presentation of totally spontaneous, ill-considered rubbish. In this sense, the writer's block that prevents easy generation of the written word is probably beneficial to society. The trait is certainly conserved in the evolution of surgical scholars, as 77% of our authors described blocking symptoms in response to a questionnaire about writing their chapter for the second edition of this book (Figure 11-1).

The contributors who experienced writer's block were all widely published in their fields of concentration. It seems that blocks are the rule rather than the exception, and effective ways have been found to help the writer overcome them. This chapter discusses the problem as experienced by our authors, and provides some suggestions that have been helpful to them and to others who were faced with the task of communicating their ideas in writing. A more extensive discussion of the subject is well presented in the very helpful book entitled *Overcoming Writing Blocks.*[1]

Pathogenesis

The pathogenesis of writer's block has been described as intimidation by the internal critic. Since the skill of writing is developed by trial and error, with a heavy emphasis on correction by the teacher, students of writing develop an internal critic that censors words being selected to express an idea before the words reach the page. This censorship, especially in surgeons, who tend toward perfectionism, can severely restrict the ability to formulate ideas in written words even when the ideas are well developed. The power of the internal critic is actually helpful to the writer if it can be inactivated during the drafting stage and saved for the editing phase.

Getting Started

Starting the flow of words generally requires a considerable amount of preliminary reading and thought, and a locus that separates the writer from interruptions and distractions. The distractions of daily practice and life are extremely tempting be-

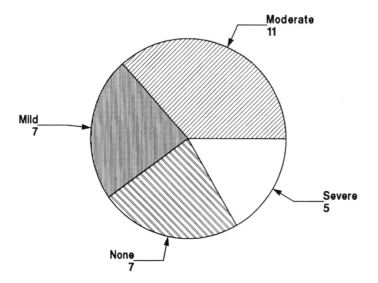

Figure 11-1. Responses of contributors to this book to the question: "Did you have blocking symptoms preparing your chapter?"

cause they are immediate, concrete, circumscribed, and familiar. A ritualized reorganization of the environment seems to be quite helpful and necessary for many writers. Pencil-sharpening, desk-clearing preparations can become significantly elongated into procrastination. Mary

Evans, one of our prolific authors, advises that procrastination indicates inadequate mental preparation for the writing task: she recommends that we not take our blocks too seriously when they occur, but leave the writing task alone for a few more days, reading or thinking about the assign-

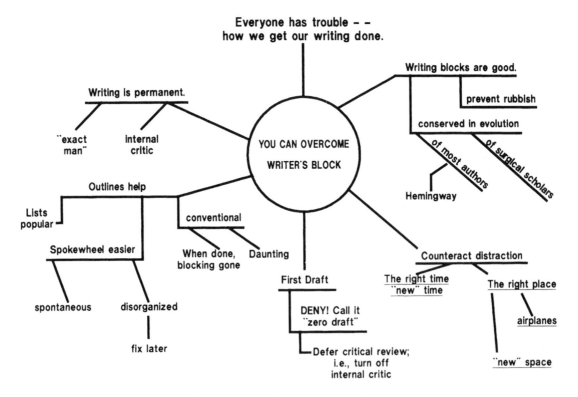

Figure 11-2.   Spoke-wheel outline.

ment more extensively before readdressing the blank page.

The intellectual process of assembling the background information is carried out in many ways by different authors. Popular techniques include keeping a large legal folder or loose-leaf notebook into which are entered references, useful phrases, "single pages with single ideas," any subsequent notes on such ideas, and blackboard brainstorming sessions with coauthors or students; dinner with a friend to discuss the writing project—particularly useful when the friend is a coauthor; or giving a 10-minute lecture to a real or imaginary audience, followed by writing down an outline of the lecture, developed from notes on the blackboard. Presenting the ideas for a paper or chapter to an audience generally unfamiliar with the topic can be helpful for getting started, as well as for clarifying and simplifying the message.

The Outline

Following the prewriting phase, some authors found it most effective to develop an outline, but many of our authors found writing the outline as difficult as writing the first draft. Scattered pages of notes with a separate page for each individual topic can serve as a surrogate or prelude to the outline. This technique has been developed into a popular computer software program (Infoselect; Micro Logic Corp., Hackensack, NJ 07602), that allows the author to summon up notes on various subtopics within the writing assignment by means of a keystroke, and to work on them individually in the way some of us work on randomly scattered pages. A miscellaneous but progressively more structured set of lists replaces the outline for Dr. Mosteller. This chapter was developed using the less intimidating "spokewheel" outline first (Figure 11-2), followed by the more orderly but demanding "conventional" outline (Table 11-1). When the conventional outline is finished, blocking symptoms diminish and writing proceeds more smoothly for many authors. Dr. Neugebauer said, "When my outline is complete, my symptoms disappear and I am happy!" The easier flow of words that comes once the thinking is clarified illustrates Boileau's axiom: Whatever is well con-

Table 11-1.   *Facing the blank page.*

Introduction: Writer's block is a good thing.

    Writing is permanent.
    Audience intimidates.

    Blocking is good.
    Most of us have it.

Pathogenesis? The internal critic.

    Internal critic like our teachers.
    Defer criticism.
    Write a letter, or dictate.

Getting started

    Preliminary reading and thought
    Procrastination and pencil-sharpening

    Collecting information; examples
    Brainstorming

The outline

    Conventional
    Spoke-wheel

    Pages of notes

    Lists

Drafting

    "Zero draft"

    Order
    Key phrases
    Distracting thoughts
    Capturing the right words
    Signposts

Editing

    Reread, rewrite.
    Get critique from others.
    Save "diamond chips."

Environment for writing

    Right time; schedule
    Divide assignment
    Set deadlines
    The right place

How we do it

    David Mulder's list
    Quotes from authors
    End with Francis Moore

ceived is clearly said, and the words to express it flow with ease (*The Art of Poetry*, 1673, canto 1, line 53; Nicolas Boileau-Despréaux, 1636–1711).[2] We are rarely searching for the right word; our search is for the right thought.

Drafting

To get the first draft complete, it is crucial to get the words out past the critic, regardless of how they sound, averting the review or editing process as much as possible. Some writers get started by writing a letter that describes the writing assignment to an imaginary, unconditionally accepting friend. Many speak into a tape recorder, because the critic has far less influence over the spoken word compared to the written word in most people's experience. Our editors prefer to consider the first version the "zero draft," whose principal function is to violate the blank page/screen and provide material for editing and reworking. Since the zero draft is not permanent, you can proceed without interruptions, never seeking the perfect word or spelling or reference until the draft is complete. Some of us put parentheses around incompletely developed thoughts or poorly chosen words, deferring critical review until the whole draft is in hand for editing. Most authors found editing far easier than drafting or outlining. The symptoms of anxiety associated with writer's block seemed to diminish progressively as the manuscript moved from the prewriting phase through first draft, outline, and progressively edited rewrites. (Figure 11-3)

The conventional outline forces an ordered prioritization of ideas, which is very helpful for drafting some writing assignments. The rigid format of an original article on a scientific subject provides a basic outline generic to all such articles. The order in which these main headings are drafted (introduction, methods, results, discussion, abstract) varies with the preference of the author. Many of our authors recommend that, like Alice in Wonderland, we begin at the beginning and continue until the end, then stop! A larger number preferred beginning with some very concrete and simple segment, such as the methods or the tables and figures, which "trick" us into overcoming procrastination. Writing about more exciting and interesting points first energizes the writing process. In this phase, key phrases and words that communicate your ideas effectively should be captured on paper, even in incomplete or awkward sentences if they seem to fit the ideas well, regardless of the flow. As you write, let your thoughts evolve, and accept the fact that the language to communicate the thoughts is also evolving. Remind yourself, "It is not a finished product," and you need not expect the perfect sentence to communicate the drift of your ideas. As you are developing your draft, you will have many thoughts that do not fit the outline or the segment you are working on. It is useful to have a second table or to use an electronic notepad for text memoranda so that well-expressed thoughts can be recorded or reintroduced later. A third tablet or pad of Postit self-sticking removable notes for recording important distractions is useful to keep you from leaving the writing task simply because you remembered another obligation.

Writing assignments travel with us, and the right words or the best fit of ideas often comes at unexpected moments: while driving home, walking the corridors, in the operating room, or sleeping at night. Have a note pad or recorder available to capture these words and thoughts as they appear. Frequent rereading aloud of what you have already written on the topic helps to keep your conscious and subconscious mind focused as you develop the draft. If the process is interrupted, leave signposts in the margin that briefly advertise the upcoming sequence of thoughts. These can be one-word descriptors, short phrases, drawings, or the names of authors of references containing the ideas you wish to discuss. Signposts and reading aloud facilitate reentry into the drafting process at your next sitting.

Editing

In the editing stage, reread the work several times yourself, rewriting where necessary, and then give the draft to others who are experienced in writing. To be sure that you are not misunderstood, you can tell them what you want the written work to communicate and ask if it succeeds. Alternatively,

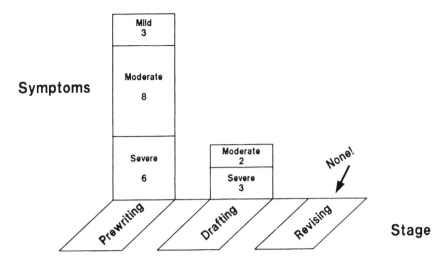

Figure 11-3. When the "zero draft" is done, blocking symptoms disappear.

you can ask them to read it and communicate the main points of the work back to you. At this stage it is important to loosen your ownership over the piece and welcome criticism. Remember that the ultimate objective is to communicate your ideas to the readers. If different words or different arrangements of them accomplish this better than your original attempt, accept the new formulation. It is important that the writing be as reader-friendly as possible. The work is already friendly to you as author, since it is a part of you. The objective input of others is needed to season the work to the tastes of your readership.

Most writers are extremely well informed by the time they overcome their writer's block and move into the editing phase. As you consolidate your material, be sure your familiarity with the subject does not cause you to omit the logical, transitional steps you made in your own thinking. John Bailar advises, "Focus on the message received, not the message sent by the writer. Take pains to be sure that you are not misunderstood." Don't presume that the logic of your readership is the same as your own. You may well have a patterned thought process that is not necessarily communicated in the words you selected to describe your thinking, although it is intuitively obvious to you. Align the readers with your thinking and logic by using connectors such as, "Based on these findings we concluded that . . . ," "It seems reasonable to conclude that . . . ," and "These data support the view . . "; it is easy to be too telegraphic when you are well informed about a subject.

When phrases, sentences, graphs, tables, and ideas dear to your heart are eliminated in the editing process, think of them as diamond chips that can be saved for use in future masterpieces. This will make the editing process easier to handle, and your treasury of unpublished material may provide the impetus or text for further development of your ideas in a subsequent publication.

The Environment for Writing

Most readers of this chapter do not write for a living, and their environment is not ideally suited to the writing process. Making your environment safe for consecutive thinking is a very challenging project. This is particularly true when critically ill surgical patients are part of the environment.

The Right Time

Time has to be created for writing. Ideally, this time should be sufficient to allow you to establish momentum. Writing time should be placed in a fresh, creative phase of your biological cycle. Most of our authors preferred writing early in the morning, but some found it useful to write late at night. "Creating a new time" is very desirable. Ideally, this is done by completing a previous assignment and devoting the newfound time to your next writing assignment. It is important to realize, when you are accepting a large writing assignment, that some other activities in your schedule will have to be eliminated. Without this conscious acceptance and reorganization of time, you will find yourself stealing time to write and resenting the writing assignment. Generally, writing time can be used more efficiently if the assignment is broken down into smaller, more manageable parts. Placement of deadlines for completion of each part helps to sustain motivation, prevent procrastination, verify productivity, and provide a feeling of accomplishment.

The Right Place

The locus for writing is a powerful factor in success. Some authors found that working outdoors or in a new setting, such as a library office or a colleague's conference room, out of the routine venue of daily practice helped to stimulate the writing process and prevent distraction. Airplane trips provide a very satisfactory form of isolated, protected time for writing with minimal interruption.

The ideal writing space should be large enough to allow notes, pads, outlines, and books to be spread out. A dictionary, thesaurus, and appropriate reference books should be within easy arm's reach. Immediate feedback from preliminary drafts keeps the writing process moving. Those who dictate need ready access to transcription, and those who use word processors need immediate printouts, to review their work in progress.

Some writers find it helpful to have inspirational pictures in the environment, such as highly respected and productive mentors, leaders in the specialty, notable writers, thinkers, or family members. It is useful to have space in which to walk, to pace the floor while dictating or thinking about the next iteration of a draft. For many authors, this kind of physical activity is an outlet for the creative tension of writing. Some respondents mentioned the dining room table at home as a practical place for writing. This broad expanse, free of the clutter of the daily routine in the office or laboratory, provides a comfortable and reassuring setting for writing.

Taking control of your writing environment puts confidence and efficiency into the writing process. Periodic changes of position, short walks, and timed small rewards (such as a walk around the block, a cup of coffee, or a 10-minute break to talk to friends or family) will sustain your energy and keep your writing fresh and energized for a longer period of time.

How We Do It

David Mulder's recommendation to surgical residents is as follows:

1. Gather all the reprints about the subject; highlight or underline important points. Choose additional references from the bibliography; read and reread them.
2. List the points you want to make; this will serve as your rough outline.
3. Based on this background and outline, create a long form of the zero draft, triple-spaced. If you dictate, be sure you speak in written language. Mary Evans makes the point that written language is different from spoken language and that "much bad writing comes from a failure to make this distinction!"
4. Revise by cutting, pasting, and deleting from the long zero draft.
5. Stop writing and let the project mature in your subconscious mind for the next several days or weeks, depending on the time pressure.
6. Proceed with the definitive revisions.

Writing in longhand is still popular, particularly for writing the introduction. When the introduction is written and a rough or complete outline is available, many authors prefer to switch to dictation or word processing to accelerate the process. Walter Spitzer says, "Sit down, let it flow, then stand up, pace the floor, and dictate. Consider the first printed draft as zero time. Then go." Ray Chiu advises, "Read extensively. Concentrate on organization and message, and then allow your subconscious to work it over. When you are ready, complete the whole essay rapidly." Mary Evans suggests, "Fill five pages before you stop. . . . Edit five times." In our brainstorming sessions, idea circles on the blackboard or on large, conspicuous pieces of paper seemed to facilitate the creative process.

The computer facilitates outline development for some authors, and a few aggressively expand their outlines into the final text without ever turning to paper. This is the exception. As a general rule, facile word processing alone does not meet all of the needs of our writers. Most need to see the printout and do some manual editing to get "the eagle's view, not the frog's view, of the swamp" (Hans Troidl). The printout shows us where to go on screen for detailed editing. David Fleiszer uses a (paper) pocket notebook for a week while thinking about the assignment, then makes a handwritten outline before he goes on screen. Thereafter he uses a split screen and multiple layers of windows to maintain an overview and to check back on previous material. Some authors find the typing and technical demands of word processing drains the creative energy they need for writing, so they navigate around the computer using more traditional methods. There is a general consensus that technical editing is easier on screen, but conceptual editing for flow of ideas may best be done on paper. David Hackam says the physical sensation of pencil on paper helps him induce the writing process. Once it is started, and the outline is complete, the word processor can sustain the momentum.

Many of our authors identified critical sessions with their mentors who were "liberal with red ink and time" as the most important training for scientific writing. Many felt that their medical school training "militated against good writing" or provided no useful background for writing. Writing essays in undergraduate school or theses in graduate school for Ph.D. degrees was very helpful. Interestingly, some felt that Latin and mathematical training provided pattern recognition and discipline that was very useful in writing. Reading Fowler's *Modern English Usage*[3] and Pope's "Essay on Criticism"[4] were specifically cited as important tools for writers.

Some authors felt that having multiple writing assignments under way simultaneously allowed them to keep the creative process going when progress was slowed on one of the projects. Most authors, however, seemed to feel that juggling more than one writing assignment is detrimental.

Clearly there are many ways to overcome writer's block, and successful authors develop an approach that works most reliably to unlock their creative energies. The inspiration for this chapter was Francis Moore's description of playing the piano wildly to help himself get started writing when he was producing his landmark textbook *The Metabolic Care of the Surgical Patient*.[5] Thirty years later, his response to our questionnaire illustrates the consummate conquest of writer's block, and provides a fitting conclusion for this essay. Dr. Moore writes, "Most of my friends feel that I have written too much in my lifetime, and they would be convulsed with laughter if they thought I were answering a questionnaire on writer's block."

References

1. Mack K, Skjei E. Overcoming Writing Blocks. Los Angeles: Tarcher, 1979.
2. Bartlett J (Kaplan J, ed) Familiar quotations, 16th edn. Boston: Little Brown, 1992, p. 280.
3. Fowler HW. A Dictionary of Modern English Usage, 2nd edn. Gowers E, rev. New York: Oxford University, 1983 (paperback with corrections).
4. Pope A. An essay on criticism. In: Pope: Poems and Prose. Grant D, ed. New York: Penguin USA, 1985, pp. 14–35.
5. Moore FD. Metabolic Care of the Surgical Patient. Philadelphia: Saunders, 1959.

Commentary

This is a practical chapter produced by two senior surgical scientists, based on their own experience and a survey of some of the authors of the second edition of this book. We all face an enormous hurdle when attempting to clearly express our thoughts in a written form. One of our senior authors had difficulty meeting the deadline for this textbook because he wanted his chapter to be the "Mona Lisa" in his particular area of research, a definitive and memorable contribution. Meeting with a surgical colleague focused his attention on critical aspects of what was required. They created an outline that was simple but not superficial. Like a well-drawn sketch, the outline led to a completed work in a reasonably short time. This emphasizes the important role of the outline in overcoming writer's block. Several leading medical writers share valuable tricks they use to overcome writer's block. The authors favor the spoke-wheel outline which is illustrated in the chapter.

The importance of creating the environment for writing was driven home for us when the editors worked together away from the pressures of administrative or surgical tasks; productivity increased dramatically. Similarly, when working with a colleague to develop a paper or an idea, the results are often synergistic and usually considerably more satisfying. Read this chapter to warm up your writing arm the next time you are trying to communicate the results of your research.

D.S.M.

CHAPTER 12

Getting Your Abstract on the Program

B.A. Pruitt Jr. and A.D. Mason Jr.

An abstract should be a concise distillate or synopsis of the work being reported and must emphasize what was done, how it was done, the results obtained, and how the author interprets them. In most instances, the organization or publication to which the abstract is submitted defines its length (usually one standard-size, double-spaced typewritten page, i.e., approximately 200 to 250 words), and that limit is inviolable. This required brevity precludes all extraneous material.

Recently, what are called structured abstracts have been increasingly used for papers to be presented at professional meetings, and particularly for publications reporting the results of clinical research.[1] Such abstracts typically include specific, concise statements about the objective of the study, the experimental design and setting, the demographic characteristics of the study subjects, and the intervention or interventions made. Outcome measures, results, and conclusions are also succinctly presented.[2] In the name of simplification the *New England Journal of Medicine* reduced the required sections to background, methods, results, and conclusion, and permits the methods and results to be combined.[3]

Mechanical and technical factors, as well as presentation and content, determine the strength and attractiveness of an abstract. If the source of the abstract is to be "blinded" to the reviewer, the originating institution should not be surreptitiously identified in the body of the abstract. A dot matrix printer should not be used to prepare an abstract since most reviewers find a typed abstract easier to read. A grammatically correct abstract, free of typographic errors, jargon, and colloquialisms, will be viewed with favor but requires meticulous proofreading of each successive draft—capricious word processors have been known to drop out words, phrases, and even entire sentences. Acronyms should be used sparingly (never in the title) and only if widely accepted. Each acronym must be presented in parentheses after its first citation in the abstract. Data tables should be easily read, with entries kept to the essential minimum, units of measurement defined, the number of entries or observations stated, and levels of statistical significance defined and indicated by conventional symbols.

Format

The format of an abstract is usually that of a scientific report or presentation: title, introduction, materials and methods, results, discussion, and conclusions. An interesting or even clever title can enhance attractiveness, but cuteness is to be avoided at all costs. It is sometimes appropriate for the title to be presented as the question addressed by the reported research, thus reducing or even eliminating the need for an introduction. In general, the introduction should be limited to a sentence or, at the most, two sentences that establish the importance of the problem addressed and the rationale for the study.

The abstract should emphasize results and materials and methods, in that order of importance. Materials and methods should be described in generic or categorical terms, with specific details of data processing, experimental procedure, and fine points of technology or technique left for the presentation or publication. Control or comparison groups or proposed models should also be described in general terms, but with sufficient detail to verify relevance and appropriateness. All the information contained in these two sections must be covered in the presentation and the final publication. The abstract itself must focus on the results of greatest importance and widest applicability and provide the basis for any conclusions drawn. The materials and methods and results sections of an abstract are customarily written in the past tense, but in the other sections the present tense can be used, as appropriate.[4]

The discussion should focus on the present study and explain in concise fashion the applicability of the results to the problem addressed, omitting needless reference to the work of others or even the author's previous work in that field. The word *significant* should be applied only when a difference has been statistically verified.

The conclusions section should consist of one or, at the most, two sentences and should be confined to the work being reported. In the conclusions section, hypotheses should be clearly separated from facts,[5] and one should not make unwarranted extrapolations of the findings beyond the point supported by the data presented. In the case of a clinical study, the conclusions should make clear how the results influence patient management or outcome. In the case of a laboratory study, the conclusions should explain the importance of the findings to understanding of biologic processes and disease mechanisms or, if relevant, clinical application.

Study Design

It is obvious that the potential quality of an abstract is directly related to the quality of the study being reported. Any clinical or laboratory study should be conducted according to an experimental design that will permit appropriate statistical assay and answer the question being asked. A priori statistical comparisons reported in the abstract must be comparisons that were planned before the study began: a posteriori comparisons should be clearly identified. Serial comparison of multiple nonindependent test groups by means of t-tests without appropriate adjustment is considered to be a fatal flaw by many reviewers. The attribution of a trend to data that approach but do not reach a level of statistical significance is apt to be regarded by reviewers as wading by the "no swimming" sign. In the preparation of an abstract reporting a chronologically lengthy series of cases, one should keep in mind improvements in general care and changes in treatment modalities that have occurred across time and then stratify patients within appropriate time segments.

Topic Relevance

The acceptability of an abstract will be enhanced if the abstract topic is related to the subject of the meeting, conforms to the interests of the membership of the sponsoring organization, and deals with a subject that has not been featured at recent meetings of the organization to which it is being submitted. Topics of clinical relevance and significance will be most favorably considered for programs in which clinical medicine is emphasized. Similarly, laboratory studies will be most favorably reviewed for programs in which research and the understanding of disease processes are emphasized. An abstract addressing a nonexistent, archaic, or even a recently well-covered problem or one that could be perceived as a reinvention of the wheel will elicit little enthusiasm on the part of reviewers. Single case reports are similarly lightly regarded unless the information presented illustrates a general principle or reports a spectacular result of importance to an entire class of patients. Negative studies will, in general, receive little consideration unless they refute established dogma, break icons, gore oxen, or dispel myths.

Things to Avoid

There are certain features of an abstract that are likely to dampen the enthusiasm of all but the most inexperienced reviewers.[6] Although brevity is essential, an abstract should not read like a telegram. The abstract should not represent merely a review of the work of others or address a self-created straw man. In the introduction, one should avoid sentences that begin "The following experiment was performed to . . . ," since it should be obvious from the introduction and body of the abstract why the experiment was performed. In the discussion section, space should not be devoted to things "not done" or "not found," and one should consider only the data that were generated in the study being reported. There should be no surprise endings with conclusions unrelated to the information provided in the abstract or not supported by the data presented. The conclusions can usually be stated without a preamble such as "The results of this study showed. . . ."

The abstract should not intermix materials and methods with results or conclusions; the integrity of each section should be maintained. The abstract should not promise any answer that is not provided, and the authors should not request carte blanche for "work in progress" or "to be done." Vague generalizations regarding data to be presented, results to be discussed, experience to be reviewed, or techniques to be described should be avoided. References to a nondescript "extensive experience" or self-denigrating comments regarding a "limited" or "modest" experience will not excite the enthusiasm of reviewers. It goes without saying that the abstract should contain only information at hand, since subsequently generated data may significantly alter the results and interpretation of the research and necessitate an embarrassing withdrawal of an accepted paper. Important research results are not so perishable that one cannot delay submission until the research is completed.

Reviewing and Editing

In an abstract, it is much more difficult to describe the key aspects of a study than to write the paper for publication. A first draft is never submittable, and even the final draft should be reviewed by each coauthor as well as selected peers. Even in these antipaternalistic times, it is a courtesy to offer the department chairman the opportunity to review the abstract, particularly if he or she will have to answer to colleagues for the results and conclusions. Good abstracts are made better by rewriting, and the need for this "aging" process speaks against writing the abstract the night before the submission deadline. Though robust results often speak for themselves, even the best are enhanced by an outstanding presentation; the fate of a report of more fragile results frequently hinges on the quality of the abstract.

The Rejected Abstract

Because more abstracts are submitted to program committees than can be accepted for presentation at professional meetings, almost every author will receive a rejection notice sooner or later. When you have recovered from the emotional impact of being rejected, you must decide whether to attempt resuscitation of the failed abstract.

An understanding of the sorting and selection process followed by a program committee is helpful when you are performing such a triage. The committee will unanimously approve 10–15% of every batch of abstracts and reject 20% or so, with equal enthusiasm. Abstracts prepared hurriedly at the last minute, and those reporting marginal modifications of previously published material usually fall into this ill-fated 20% and are best left to die unmourned. The reasons for the rejection of the remaining 65–70% vary, and some of this material will deserve rescue.

Postpone revision of your potentially viable abstract for a few weeks; you may be asked to serve as an invited discussant of similar papers accepted for presentation. By the time of the meeting, if your series is larger than the one to be reported in an accepted paper, or if you can present a different and well-supported conclusion, you may be able to savor the pleasure of being one up.

Diagnosing and Correcting the Problem

Rejection may reflect a surfeit of recent papers on your topic at meetings of the society you chose or in the literature. As an author, you will usually be aware of such focused increases in publication density; but if you are in doubt, a search of the literature, by title, over the past five years, will

Table 12-1. Abstract "detractors."

1. Typographic, grammatic, and spelling errors
2. Use of jargon and colloquialisms
3. Failure to define acronyms
4. Failure to define units of measurement or identify numbers of cases, experimental subjects, or observations
5. Extensive review of the work of others
6. Excessive experimental detail
7. Needless reference to earlier work of author or other investigators
8. Inclusion of what was "not done" or "not found" in the discussion
9. Intermingling of hypothesis and facts
10. Unwarranted extrapolation of findings
11. A surprise ending
12. Promises of work "to be done"

usually clarify the situation. If your subject is faddish or a commonly encountered surgical problem, undertake a revision of your abstract only if your results illuminate significant pathogenetic factors, validate a new treatment, or significantly enhance understanding of the area you have studied. Even if you think that your abstract does fit into one or more of these categories, you should honestly try to identify why these sterling qualities were not perceived by the program committee.

Some abstracts fail because they are messy. Organization, neatness, grammar, and spelling really do count; careful revision and reorganization will sometimes reveal the prince within the toad. Every sentence should be reviewed for clarity and economy of wording.[7] Invite uninvolved col-

Table 12-2. Abstract "enhancers."

1. A clever, specific, and concise title
2. Conformity to interests of program committee and sponsoring organization
3. Emphasis on new or unique findings and observations
4. Grammatically correct, error free typescript
5. Easily read, minimal entry data tables
6. Properly defined and appropriately applied statistical assessment
7. Definition of all measurement units
8. Identification of number of cases, experimental subjects, and observations
9. Use of graphic display to emphasize important relationships
10. Use of "typeset" format

leagues to review your abstract and correct any deficiencies they find. Shear away the "detractors" listed in Table 12-1 and incorporate as many of the "enhancers" in Table 12-2 as possible.[8] In addition to the listed abstract "detractors," common reasons for the rejection of abstracts of papers being considered for presentation at professional meetings include prior presentation or publication of the paper, too little data, inadequate controls, insignificance of the research question, and lack of conformity with abstract requirements. Presenting your data in a table will often rid your abstract of a jumble of abbreviations and wordy descriptions. A graphic display, easily produced by desktop publishing and computer enhancement techniques, is even better; a picture worth a thousand words can be put in the space required for sixty. The same techniques allow you to employ stylish arrangement, font selection, and laser printing to enhance the appearance of your abstract. Significantly higher acceptance rates are reported for such "typeset" abstracts.[9] While the necessity for such embellishments may be inversely related to the importance of the content of your first submission, the extra effort is almost certainly desirable for your revised abstract.

If there were few observations in your original abstract, make every effort to buttress your new one with more data, even if gathering them entails some delay. The new material should include supplemental observations that confirm an initially tenuous hypothesis or logically extend your original data. Next, review your conclusions to ensure that they are appropriately supported by the data you have presented and that they relate your results to a topic that interests the organization to which you are submitting your abstract.

Accepting a Second Rejection

If your diagnosis of the cause of your abstract's rejection is correct, these prescriptions may save it. If, however, a second rejection ensues, consider your abstract moribund and move on to more fruitful endeavors. At such a time, you may find it comforting to remember that almost every successful scientist has, tucked away somewhere, a copy of an abstract that only he or she still cherishes and believes to be important.

References

1. Schwartz RJ, Jacobs LM, Gabrum SG, Bennett-Jacobs B. Continuous quality improvement applied to a scientific assembly; the history of the Eastern Association for the Surgery of Trauma. J Trauma 1993;35:544–549.
2. Rennie D and Glass RM. Structuring abstracts to make them more informative. JAMA 1991; 266: 116–117. Editorial.
3. Relman AS. New information for authors—and readers. N Engl J Med 1990;56:323.
4. Warren R. The abstract. Arch Surg 1976;111:635–636.
5. Baue AE. Writing a good abstract is not abstract writing. Arch Surg 1979;114:11–12.
6. Pruitt BA Jr. Improve your next abstract. Presented at the Seventh Annual Meeting of the American Burn Association, Denver, March 20–22, 1975.
7. American Association for Laboratory Animal Science. How to Prepare an Abstract. Cordova, TN:AALAS, January 1990.
8. Pruitt BA Jr. Tips on how to write abstracts, for newer members of the American Burn Association. Presented at the 21st Annual Meeting of the American Burn Association, New Orleans, March 30, 1989.
9. Koren G. A simple way to improve the chances for acceptance of your scientific paper. N Engl J Med 1986;315:1298. Letter.

Commentary

Reviewers judged this to be one of the most effective chapters in previous editions of this textbook. It provides practical information and advice that will advance you toward your goal of getting on the presentation program. The list of abstract detractors and abstract enhancers is invaluable for authors whether they are preparing their first abstract or are seasoned investigators like Drs. Pruitt and Mason. This concise essay should be required reading for residents before they bring their abstract to senior colleagues for review.

D.S.M.

CHAPTER 13

Writing a Scientific Paper

A.V. Pollock and M. Evans

Anybody who suggests that writing a scientific paper is easy has never written one. Even more bizarre is the belief that the gift of writing is given to some people and not to others, so if you don't have the gift there is no point in trying hard. Both these statements are false. Be assured that to produce good scientific writing is always difficult. It always takes a long time, and it always needs revision after revision after revision. But you have done a nice bit of research, and you did not find that particularly easy or quick. No, you were meticulous in drawing up your protocol, following it, and analyzing your results. You must not be surprised that the writing up of those results is no easier than the research itself.

General Aims

What are you aiming at? Well, above all you aim to tell the truth as you found it (and a pox on modern-day philosophers who proclaim that there is no such thing as truth). You try to be as accurate as possible—you do not conceal data that are out of line, and you disclose any faults and errors in the performance of your research. For instance, it is far better to write that you dropped and broke the flask on your way to the bench than merely to write that that result was not available.

You will find that a lot of teachers ask you to write well enough to be understood. We think that it is much more important to write in such a way that it is impossible for your words to be misunderstood. And, finally, you will aim at an elegant presentation. It should not need saying that every bit of the manuscript (including tables and references) must be double-spaced. Some computers default to 1.5 line spacing; this makes the job of the copy editor much more difficult.

Above all you must read the "instructions to authors" of the journal to which you intend sending the manuscript, and you must consult a recent issue of that journal. Editors have better things to do than put contributions into house style.

You must obey the rules of composition at all times, but try to impart personality into the discussion. This is when you can display some elegance. Avoid hedging and too much use of "may" and "might." On the other hand, do not be over-presumptuous. Modest conclusions may be more effective than bold claims that the research that you are reporting will transform the diagnosis or treatment of some disease. Take a hint from writers such as Alexander Fleming who concluded that "Penicillin, in regard to infections with sensitive microbes, appears to have some advantages over the well-known chemical antiseptics"[1]; or Watson and Crick: "It has not escaped our notice that the specific pairing we have postulated immediately suggests a possible copying mechanism for the genetic material."[2]

You must, when you report your research, use the IMRAD formula: introduction, methods, results, and discussion. When you have finished you must write an abstract and give the paper a title. Because the abstract always comes before the introduction in a scientific paper, we are going to consider it first, but you will write it only when you have finished writing and editing the text.

Abstract

More and more journals are adopting the structured abstract, but whether the journal that you are going to send your paper to uses the structured form or not you must be absolutely sure that *the whole message of your work comes across in the abstract*. It is sad but incontrovertible that the part of a research paper that is most likely to be read is the abstract.[3] No editor of a medical journal is naive enough to believe that all his readers will go through each issue, article by article, and word by word. It is probable that they will scan the list of contents for subjects that interest them, then look at the abstract to see if the paper has the potential to add to their knowledge. If the abstract lacks vital information, their interest will wane and they will go and browse elsewhere.

Probably the most popular places for browsing are the computer databases such as MEDLINE, which publish only abstracts. When one is seeking information, these are the places to start, and vague or incomplete abstracts will merely be overlooked. This could be one explanation for the fact that only about half of all published papers are ever cited.[4]

From ignorance rather than design, those who practice medicine in the developed world may not consider fully the needs of colleagues in the Third World. There are many centers in which the only journals that are available are abstracting journals. Indeed it has been said that there have been occasions when patients were treated solely on the basis of information given in abstracts.

All the more reason, then, for abstracts to be clear and succinct, and answer all of Bradford Hill's questions:

1. Why did you start? (Introduction).
2. What did you do? (Methods).
3. What answer did you get? (Results)
4. What does it mean? (Discussion).[5]

Prompted by the ever-increasing number of papers published each year (over two million in about 20,000 journals), a working group was set up at McMaster University in Canada to improve the quality of information in abstracts.[6] This group was greatly helped by Edward J. Huth, then editor of *Annals of Internal Medicine,* who became the first editor to introduce the "structured abstract".[7] Within the next couple of years other journals adopted the general format, though not necessarily with the same headings.[8]

Structured abstracts help not only the readers but also the authors, because they remind them what the essential data are and in which order they should be put. The following are the headings and required content of a structured abstract. Each heading should start a new paragraph, and all except the last two may be written in note form. All numbers should be written as numerals, even if they are less than ten, and abbreviations may be used if they are spelled out first. References should not be given.

Objective. This should give, usually in one sentence, a precise statement of why the study was done. It should be possible to make a connection between the conclusion and the objective.

Design. This should provide a few words describing the type of study (for example, "double blind trial," "prospective randomized controlled trial," "retrospective analysis," "open study") and whether the study was from a single center or was multicentric.

Setting. So that readers can assess the applicability of the study to their own circumstances, this paragraph should state whether the setting was the community, a university department, a district hospital, a regional or tertiary referral center, or private practice.

Subjects or material. The total number of patients, subjects, or animals should be given, together with a note of whether they were selected (and if so, how) or consecutive. This will give the reader an idea of the generalizability of the results.

Interventions. This should include a description of any intervention including, for example, the

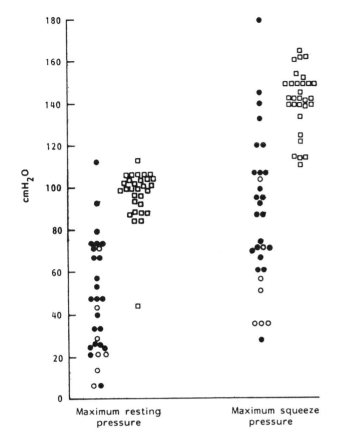

Figure 13-1. Maximum resting ($p < 0.005$) and maximum squeeze ($p < 0.01$) anal pressure (cm H_2O) after restorative proctocolectomy compared with controls. ●, Patients with good function; ○, patients with poor function; □, controls. Reprinted with permission of Butterworth & Co., publisher, from Keighley MRB, Yoshioka K, Kmiot W, Heyen F. Br J Surg 1988;75:997–1002.

technique of an operation or the duration and dosage of a drug regimen. Generic names are preferred, but trade names may be given as well in case there is some difference in the formulation from country to country.

Main outcome measures. Methods by which patients were assessed or the success of experiments judged should be mentioned.

Results. The main results should be given, together with a note of the fate of exclusions and withdrawals. Numerical results should be stated as "mean (SD)" or "mean (SEM)" in the case of normally distributed data, and median (range or interquartile) if the data are skewed; 95% confidence intervals (CI) and the level of significance should be indicated. If the differences in the main outcome measures between two (or more) groups are not significant, the 95% CI for the difference should be given and any clinical inference stated.

Conclusion(s). Only those conclusions supported by the data that are presented should be given, followed by a short statement on the possible clinical applications of the work, bearing in mind the limitations of the study (for example, size of sample, number of withdrawals, or length of follow up).

It should be possible to put the whole abstract on one double-spaced sheet of A4 or quarto paper, and no abstract should contain more than 400 words, because that is the limit set by MEDLINE.

Quite apart from being of immense help to readers and speeding up the refereeing process (thereby shortening the time from submission to publication), structured abstracts help authors to know what is expected of the design, conduct, and analysis of a research project.

Title

The generation of a good title is important. It must above all allow people who merely glance at the contents of a journal or the screen of a

Table 13-1. Percent graft survival after first cadaveric renal transplantation.

Months postoperatively	Age	
	<55 years ($n = 444$)	>55 years ($n = 63$)
1	90	90
3	77	80
6	70	77
18	65	70
24	65	65
36	60	65
55	55	60

MEDLINE search to know what your paper is about. It is only when you are senior enough to be asked to write review articles that you can afford to put in coy titles. There is no place in the title of a research paper for wit or double entendre.

Introduction

It is only when you are writing a thesis for a higher degree that you are allowed to put in more than a few sentences in this section. In a research paper the introduction must set out what you aimed to achieve, and why you pursued the goal in that particular way. It is not a review of "the literature." It is usually an only slightly protracted version of the opening sentences of your experimental protocol.

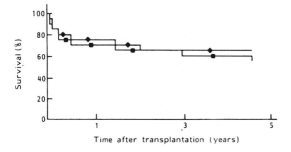

Figure 13-2. Actuarial graft survival for 5 years in 444 under-55-year-old (■) and 63 over-55-year-old (◆) first cadaver renal transplant recipients. Reprinted with permission of Butterworth & Co., publisher, from Lauffer G, Murie JA, Gray D, Ting A, Morris PJ. Br J Surg 1988;75:984–987.

Methods

The methods section can be a slightly edited version of your protocol. Unless you have been using an esoteric test or intervention, it can usually be condensed into a few sentences and referenced. Make sure that the description of the methods that you used (including the statistical tests) is clear enough to ensure that the work can be replicated.*

Results

The results section is, of course, the most important part of the paper. You have tabulated your data, but these tables obviously must be simplified for publication. You must decide whether the simplification is best done as tables or as graphs. On the whole there are only two absolute indications for a graph rather than a table: when you want to present a scattergram (see Figure 13-1), and when you want to present a complicated life table. A life table that is simple and has few measurements is probably better given in tabular rather than graphic form (compare Table 13-1 with Figure 13-2).

When you are preparing the artwork for a graph (for which there are many computer programs), do observe the fundamental rules enunciated by Tufte[9]: above all else, show the data; maximize the data-to-ink ratio; erase non-data ink; erase redundant data ink; revise and edit. Good graphs use as little ink as possible, consistent with getting their message across. Tufte used the concept of "data ink" to describe ink on a graph that cannot be erased without losing the meaning of the graph. Non-data ink can be erased without loss of information. Compare Figure 13-3 with Figure 13-4. The former is eminently suitable for the annual report of a business, but by

---

*When laboratory experiments require novel or complex methods, they should be clearly presented in this section. For sequential investigations it is useful and economical to publish a clear account of your methods separately and cite the publication. Rarely, a methods paper may be prepared and made available on request. It is misleading to other investigators if the description is oversimplified to meet publication requirements. M.F.M.

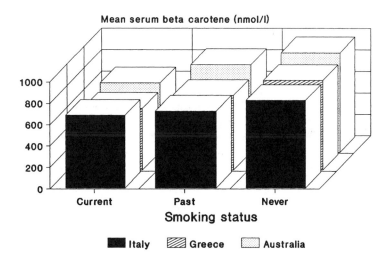

Figure 13-3. There is too much non-data ink.

erasing all the non-data ink (Figure 13-4), the concentrations of beta carotene in the various countries in smokers and nonsmokers are much more easily found. The three-dimensional layout in Figure 13-3 is acceptable for a slide for verbal presentation, but not for a figure for publication.

A figure that shows means and standard deviations (or standard errors) of a variable over a period of time is not as accurate as a table that gives the actual figures. Compare Figure 13-5 with Table 13-2; the figure shows immediately that there is a difference, but the size and significance of that difference is better appreciated in the table. On the other hand, when the size of the difference is unimportant, a graph such as that shown in Figure 13-6 is excellent and easily allows the reader to speculate on the reason why some measurements went down after a meal and others went up.

There are four absolute rules about tables:

1. Tables must not repeat results that you have already detailed in the text.
2. Each table must stand on its own and not require reference to the text to explain it—it must have a title and it must not have abbreviations. The numbers must add up.
3. Each table must disclose whole numbers, with or without percentages; percentages alone are not acceptable.
4. Tables, like everything else in the manuscript, must be typed double-spaced; you must not rule vertical lines, since they would only have to be removed by the editor.

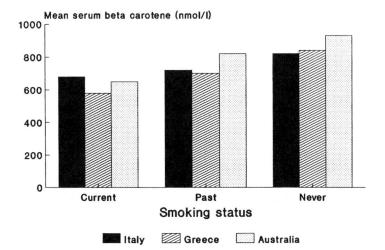

Figure 13-4. All non-data ink has been erased.

Table 13-2. Natural killer cell activity against K562 before and after operation; values are expressed as mean (SEM).

	Activity			
	Control group (n = 15)	Interferon α group (n = 15)	t value	p value
Before operation	38 (6)	41 (6)	.35	>.50
Postoperative				
day 1	15 (4)	33 (5)	2.81	>.01
day 3	16 (5)	36 (5)	2.83	>.01
day 5	16 (5)	30 (5)	1.98	>.05
day 10	22 (4)	22 (5)	0	1.0

Discussion

It is the discussion section in which it is so tempting to let yourself go and show what a tremendous amount of reading you have done. A new syndrome—the MEDLINE syndrome—has become recognized in recent years. It is not necessary to mention every paper that your search has

identified. Be selective (and that does not mean biased) and on no account quote a paper that you have not read in the original.

Try to contain your enthusiasm. Editors like concise contributions and will give you no credit for a discussion that is twice as long as the rest of the paper put together. Don't repeat your results, but comment on them in the light of substantial contributions from other workers. And, finally, conclude circumspectly, but make sure that you do not commit a type III error[10]: "The conclusions drawn are not supported by the data presented."

References

1. Fleming A. On the antibacterial action of cultures of a penicillium, with special reference to their use in the isolation of *B. influenzae*. Br J Exper Pathol 1929;10:226–236.
2. Watson JD, Crick FHC. Molecular structure of nucleic acids. A structure for deoxyribose nucleic acid. Nature 1953;4356:737–738.
3. Lock SP. Structured abstracts. Br Med J 1988; 297:156.

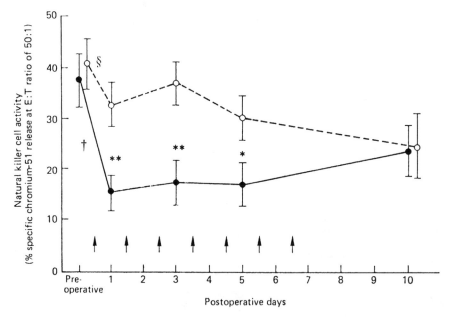

Figure 13-5. Natural killer cell activity against K562 levels before and after surgery. ●———● control group; ○———○ r-HuIFNα (2 megaunits/day) (n = 15 for both groups). r-HuIFNχ versus controls, *P < 0.05, **P < 0.01, § Preoperative versus postoperative: ●, P < 0.01; ○, n.s. E:T, effector:target ratio. Reprinted with permission of Butterworth & Co., publishers, from Sedman PC, Ramsden CW, Brennan TG, Giles GR, Guillou PJ. Br J Surg 1988;75:976–981.

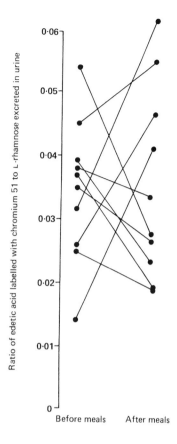

Figure 13-6. Ratio of edetic acid labeled with chromium-51 to L-rhamnose excreted in urine. Reprinted with permission from Bjarnson I, Levi S, Smethurst P, Menzies IS, Levi AJ. Br Med J 1988; 297:1629–1631.

4. Lock SP. How editors survive. Br Med J 1976; 3:1118–1119.
5. Hill AB. The reasons for writing. Br Med J 1965; 2:626–627.
6. Ad Hoc Working Group for Clinical Appraisal of the Medical Literature. A proposal for more informative abstracts of clinical articles. Ann Intern Med 1987;106:598–604.
7. Huth EJ. Structured abstracts for papers reporting clinical trials. Ann Intern Med 1987;106:626–627.
8. Haynes RB, Mulrow CD, Huth EJ, Altman DG, Gardner MJ. More informative abstracts revisited. Ann Intern Med 1990;113:69–76.
9. Tufte ER. The Visual Display of Quantitative Information. Cheshire, CT: Graphics, 1983.
10. Condon RE. Type III error. Arch Surg 1986;121: 877–878.

Commentary

This chapter contains the advice of two authors whose wealth of experience is immediately evident in the content of the chapter. They properly emphasize the importance of your abstract, which is too frequently the only component of the work that is read and cited. They clarify the distinction between an abstract of your scientific paper and the abstract sent to entice a program committee to accept your work for presentation at a meeting. The value of a structured abstract is emphasized. Regardless of the format, it is essential that the entire message of your scientific work be presented clearly in your abstract.

Important information is provided about artwork for graphs; the reader should also be aware of the chapter by McGovern et al. (chapter 21), in which more details about the preparation of slides and other visual materials are presented. I personally like the advice quoted from Tufte, and the concept of "data ink" presented in his classic book *The Visual Display of Quantitative Information.* This is a text that I go back to time and time again when looking for new methods to present clinical or research data.

The discussion section of a scientific paper is the place for the research work to answer the Bradford Hill question "What does it mean?"; or as my former chief Professor Frazer Gurd put it bluntly as I emerged triumphantly from the lab, "So what?" Combining this paper with "Facing the Blank Page/Screen" (chapter 11) should provide constructive help for preparing a scientific paper.

The International Committee of Medical Journal Editors has recently reissued its *Uniform Requirements for Manuscripts Submitted to Biomedical Journals,*[1] summarizing the criteria of over 500 journals. This source document simplifies manuscript preparation for most major journals.

D.S.M.

1. International Committee of Medical Journal Editors. Uniform requirements for manuscripts submitted to biomedical journals. New Engl J Med 1997;336:309–315.

CHAPTER 14

Where Should You Publish Your Paper?

M. Rothmund, D. Bartsch, and W. Lorenz

Introduction

In contrast to a recent cartoon from *The New Yorker* (Figure 14-1), when most surgeons see a patient and make a diagnosis, they do not think about a journal in which a manuscript may be published or even about preparing the manuscript itself. However, the clinical challenge of a particular patient often inspires related research at the laboratory bench or by the design of clinical trials.

Authors often think about where clinical or experimental material should be published only after they have reviewed their raw data and have interpreted the results. Writing the first draft of the manuscript probably begins after the first author has discussed the selection of an appropriate journal with fellow authors and especially with the senior investigator. Scanning the *Current Contents Journal Citation Reports* may assist in deciding upon a journal. Every journal has specific "instructions for authors" concerning text and bibliography, which will be essential in preparing the final draft. The journal should have been selected on the basis of features such as scope, specialty, reputation, and impact factor, but also on the characteristics of the manuscript, for example, quality, content, or format. The following chapter will cover all of these considerations and will also discuss the special concerns of non-English-speaking authors, as well as the issue of electronic publishing.

What Is Your Manuscript Like?

When you are selecting a journal, you should know quite precisely the features of your manuscript; this is easy as far as content and format are concerned. Usually you first identify a journal related to the topic and specialty of medicine you are addressing. Then you might consider whether your work is clinical, a clinical trial, experimental data, or a report on a new surgical technique, and whether it is patient related or basic science. This is important because some journals publish exclusively or mainly clinical work, whereas others are more devoted to publication of experimental data. Only a few are willing to publish manuscripts from both fields. The journal should also be chosen to suit the format of your manuscript. Is it a collective review, a case report, or an original paper, for example, a manuscript following IMRAD organization (introduction, materials and methods, results, and discussion)? Almost all journals prefer original papers because these have a strong influence on the journal's reputation and impact factor. The majority of reviews are published by request only, and few journals will publish reviews that have not been solicited by them. Unfortunately, most journals have limited space and they therefore avoid case reports, which are considered to be of minor scientific value. Hence, you should determine whether the journals in your field con-

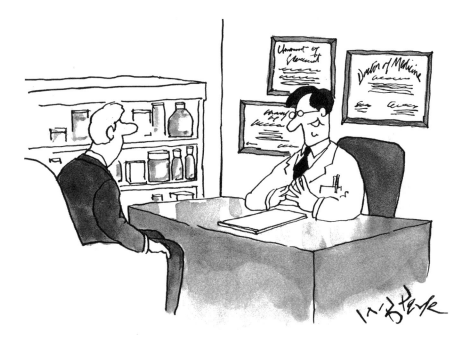

*"Mr. Wilkins, I believe that your condition is going to get us both
into the 'Journal of the American Medical Association.' "*

Figure 14-1.

tain case reports (often indicated in the "information to authors" section of the journal).

The most important aspect of your manuscript is its quality. In order to avoid being biased toward your own work, let others such as senior investigators or friends working in the same field take a look at your manuscript. They should put it in one of the quality categories indicated in Table 14-1.[1]

If the manuscript meets the criteria of category 1 you should hasten to send it to the best journal in your field. This journal should also be able to publish your material within a short period of time. In this case it would also be wise to let the editor know in your covering letter about the impact the information in your article may have on your specialty. For general clinical research, the appropriate journal would certainly be either number 1 or 2, as indicated in Table 14-2, that is, the *New England Journal of Medicine* or *Lancet*.

Most of us will never produce and publish such a paper. If we are bright, keen, hardworking, and

lucky we might be able to write a manuscript that qualifies for category 2. Most papers are suited to the other categories. The plethora of medical journals suggests that it should be possible to get your manuscript published unless it is entirely inadequate. Some authors resubmit a rejected manuscript over and over, from one journal to another, until the article is finally accepted. In a publication from the field of dermatology addressing this issue of resubmission, the authors wrote, "There are 32 dermatologic journals indexed in the *Index Medicus*. We feel that a paper is not really rejected until you have a letter from at least 32 editors."[2]

There is a better way to deal with the rejection of your manuscript. You should use the review, which is usually competent, accompanying the rejected manuscript to improve your work so that it may be accepted by another journal of similar quality.

Journals tend to shun papers that contain negative results (for example, a manuscript that reports

Table 14-1.   Categories of surgical publications.

1. Original and exciting discovery that may have a profound effect on the practice of surgery
2. Clinical trial or experiment whose results will change, though perhaps not revolutionize the practice of surgery
3. Carefully compiled observation suggesting that current surgical practice should be revised
4. Describes modification of diagnostic or therapeutic approach, having assembled a small collection of unusual cases or having reviewed your own experience
5. Superficial review of your institution's experience of a common surgical condition

Ludbrook J, Aust N Z J Surg (1991).[1]

Table 14-2.   Internal medicine journals ranked by impact factor.

		IF[a]	CH[a]
1	New Engl J Med	22.673	6.2
2	Lancet	17.332	6.3
3	Ann Intern Med	9.887	7.0
4	JAMA-J Am Med Assoc	6.863	6.3
5	Diabetes	6.260	6.1
6	Diabetologia	4.988	5.8
7	Brit Med J	4.411	7.2
8	Arch Intern Med	4.137	6.9
9	Medicine	3.900	>10.0
10	Annu Rev Med	2.829	7.2
11	J Vasc Res	2.768	2.2
12	Diabetes Care	2.755	4.4
13	Am J Med	2.703	8.7
14	J Lab Clin Med	2.244	>10.0
15	Eur J Clin Invest	2.224	6.2
16	Who Tech Rep Ser	2.179	9.7
17	Q J Med	2.069	8.7
18	Maturitas	1.975	5.8
19	Mayo Clin Proc	1.814	7.8
20	J Clin Epidemiol	1.641	4.2
21	J Intern Med	1.622	3.6
22	Brit Med Bull	1.577	9.2
23	Adv Internal Med	1.475	6.5
24	Brit J Gen Pract	1.402	2.8
25	Lupus	1.293	2.2
26	Prev Med	1.288	7.0
27	Diabetic Med	1.277	4.1
28	Can Med Assoc J	1.243	9.1
29	Med J Aust	1.174	6.4
30	Ciba F Symp	1.145	7.2
31	Ann Med	1.129	3.4
32	Med Clin N Am	1.083	8.4
33	Aust N Z J Med	1.000	6.1
34	Clin Investigator	0.963	2.2
35	J Roy Coll Phys Lond	0.932	4.8
36	DM-Dis Mon	0.917	5.6
37	J Fam Practice	0.904	6.2
38	Am J Med Sci	0.897	>10.0
39	Klin Wochenschr	0.889	8.3
40	J Gen Intern Med	0.862	4.4
41	Med Clin-Barcelona	0.801	4.1
42	J Pain Symptom Manag	0.773	3.7
43	Harvey Lect	0.750	>10.0
44	S Afr Med J	0.742	8.4
45	J R Soc Med	0.697	5.7
46	Am J Prev Med	0.617	4.9
47	Deut Med Wochenschr	0.605	7.0
48	New Zeal Med J	0.545	6.2
49	Support Care Cancer	0.519	
50	Presse Med	0.503	6.7

[a]IF, impact factor, CH, cited half-life.

that the effect of substance X on serum levels of Y could not be demonstrated, as you or others might have predicted), even though negative results are sometimes as important as expected ones. Even if the study was well designed and carried out, and the manuscript is well written, it will probably end up in a journal category several ranks below the one you expected simply because the positive effect could not be observed. In the future, the limitless capacity of the Internet might allow electronic publication of negative results.

What Is the Purpose of Your Publication?

The publication of your manuscript will probably have more purpose than the purist's goal of informing the scientific community about your data. You may want to demonstrate to the community that you are a great scientist in order to increase the chance for renewal of your grant or to promote your academic career (a clinical trial that makes the principal investigator famous is a "good trial"), or you might just want to advertise for referrals.

If your goal is only to inform, you can take your time with the manuscript. You should not worry about which journal in which to publish, as long as it is listed in one of the literature retrieval systems such as *Current Contents* (*Current Contents/Life Sciences* or *Current Contents/Clinical Medicine*), or *Index Medicus* (available with MEDLARS or MEDLINE). It would be beneficial to choose the journal that might best address your target group. If you want to let your surgical colleagues know that your scalpel prowess surpasses that of most others, or that you have found and tested a new surgical method, then you should think of a surgical journal of the respective specialty. Recently, the endocrine surgeons of the Mayo Clinic reviewed their data on surgical treatment of Graves's disease in children and observed excellent results that questioned the priority of conservative treatment preferred by pediatricians. When asked why they published their results in a surgical journal for a supportive audience instead of in, for example, *Pediatrics,* they argued that the manuscript would likely have been rejected by the reviewers of this journal.

If your work describes a diagnostic method or deals with the pathophysiology or overall treatment of a certain disease (surgical and nonsurgical), a general medical journal should be favored. If the subject of your article is a highly specialized aspect of surgery, a select journal sponsored by one of the large specialty associations or societies should be chosen, for example, *Surgical Endoscopy* for laparoscopic techniques. These society-sponsored journals usually have a high circulation rate.

The selection of the appropriate journal for your article might also depend on the time between submission and publication. Journals tend not to divulge the length of time they require for editorial review and printing. However, a rough idea may be derived from the frequency of the journal. The publication lag of a monthly journal is usually shorter (6 to 8 months) than that of a quarterly journal (9 to 12 months). Colleagues experienced with the particular journal you are considering may be helpful. Some journals publish the manuscript receipt date or even the date of acceptance after revision.

An important purpose in publishing an article might be medical "advertisement." If you have developed a new operation, have modified the surgical approach to a disease, or you have achieved excellent results performing a demanding procedure (for example, 100 consecutive Whipple operations without mortality), and you want to inform internists about your results to increase your referrals, then you should publish the manuscript in a general or internal medicine journal.

Alternatively, publishing in a surgical journal will not increase your caseload but might foster respect among your colleagues—or cause possibly negative reactions such as professional jealousy. Publishing in a surgical journal may also serve to educate, provided the manuscript is well written, honest, and detailed, and the author is courageous enough to report not only his or her brilliant results but also the problems, pitfalls, and complications that were encountered and how they were resolved.

The Prestige Factor

Assuming that your manuscript is considered to be at least interesting by your peers or the senior investigator, you would of course want to publish in the best journal possible. The "best" journal may have many different features that make it a fine publication, but the most important criterion for journal quality in the medical community is the "impact factor" (IF). Published by the Institute for Scientific Information (ISI) in Philadelphia, the IF is a number calculated from the number of citations from a particular journal that appear in biomedical journals each year. Mathematically, it is defined as the mean number of citations from a specific journal divided by the number of articles published by the journal. In other words, the IF approximates the number of times an article published in a particular journal will be cited, on average, in the 2 years following the publication of this article. "Citation half-life" indicates the time lag between the publication of articles in a specific journal and their citation in other articles.

Politicians use the IF to evaluate medical and other faculties, while grant-providing organizations use it to assess the scientific performance of a department, a group of investigators, or a single scientist, even though the IF is related to only a single journal. For the assessment of a particular person, the *Science Citation Index* is probably much more appropriate because it tells how often the articles published by a certain author are quoted by others. Rating a person by the IF is only an approximate, less-encompassing evaluation based on the sum of the IFs of the journals where he or she published articles during a certain time period.

There are several factors that affect the IF of journals, as follows:

1. The IF is influenced by the specialty the journal covers. In the fields of biochemistry and molecular biology, there were 62 journals with an IF of more than 2 in 1992. Only 8 in the field of surgery fulfilled this criterion, and none in orthopaedics, otolaryngology, traumatology, geriatrics, or rehabilitation medicine. Since only articles that are cited within 2 years after publication contribute to the IF, journals publishing short-term studies are favored, and clinical journals are considered less valuable.[3] The best clinical journal in surgery, *Annals of Surgery* (IF for 1994: 4.166) will never be able to compete with the *New England Journal of Medicine*, which ranked number 1 in general and internal medicine (IF for 1994: 22.673), or with basic science journals such as *Clinical Research* (IF for 1994: 57.778) or *Cell* (IF for 1994: 39.191). Therefore, determining the "importance" of journals by using the IF can be accomplished only within a given specialty.
2. Since the IF is calculated by dividing the mean number of citations by the total number of articles published in a particular journal, it follows that a journal containing few articles (source items) would have a higher IF than a journal containing many articles, if both journals had the same number of citations. It was recently shown that the internal ranking of biomedical research journals (basic science and clinical), performed by 50 NIH scientists, differed enormously from the IF ranking, mostly because the scientists did not refer to the average number of source items appearing in the particular journal.[4]
3. The IF certainly favors English-language journals. The first non-English surgical journal and the first non-English general and internal medicine journal to appear in the ISI ranking both were listed at number 39 in 1994 (Tables 14-2 and 14-3). It is probable that they would have ranked somewhat higher if they were English-language publications.

As long as these points are kept in mind, the IF is a very useful method to assist in choosing a journal for publication.

Table 14-3.   Surgical journals ranked by impact factor.

		IF[a]	CH[a]
1	Ann Surg	4.166	9.8
2	Am J Surg Pathol	3.775	5.7
3	J Neurosurg	3.296	9.2
4	Transplantation	2.929	4.8
5	Arch Surg-Chicago	2.402	8.9
6	J Thorac Cardiov Surg	2.389	8.2
7	Endoscopy	2.096	4.9
8	Surgery	2.038	9.2
9	J Vasc Surg	1.972	5.3
10	Am J Surg	1.927	9.5
11	Surg Endosc-Ultras	1.854	2.9
12	Brit J Surg	1.778	7.4
13	Neurosurgery	1.670	6.7
14	Ann Thorac Surg	1.651	5.1
15	World J Surg	1.507	6.4
16	J Bone Joint Surg Am	1.462	>10.0
17	Laser Surg Med	1.429	5.0
18	Surg Clin N Am	1.428	8.9
19	Surg Gynecol Obstet	1.302	>10.0
20	J Bone Joint Surg Br	1.264	>10.0
21	J Surg Res	1.205	6.2
22	Plast Reconstr Surg	1.174	9.6
23	Curr Prob Surg	1.040	6.9
24	Clin Transplant	0.891	4.4
25	Transplant P	0.885	4.6
26	Head Neck J Sci Spec	0.855	6.7
27	J Pediatr Surg	0.846	6.4
28	Clin Orthop Relat R	0.844	8.8
29	Arch Otolaryngol	0.836	>10.0
30	Eur Surg Res	0.795	7.5
31	Cleft Palate-Cran J	0.785	7.8
32	Acta Neurochir	0.748	6.5
33	Ann R Coll Surg	0.740	7.5
34	Eur J Vascular Surg	0.721	3.6
35	J Dermatol Surg Onc	0.718	6.6
36	Otolaryng Head Neck	0.714	5.9
37	Oral Surg Oral Med O	0.703	9.8
38	Can J Surg	0.658	8.5
39	Chirurg	0.657	4.1
40	Surg Neurol	0.625	9.7
41	Semin Surg Oncol	0.618	4.7
42	Theor Surg	0.606	3.8
43	Am Surgeon	0.581	7.5
44	Hepato-Gastroenterol	0.577	4.8
45	Brit J Plast Surg	0.558	9.8
46	Langenbeck Arch Chir	0.556	6.2
47	Skull Base Surg	0.552	
48	Brit J Neurosurg	0.534	4.4
49	Eur J Surg	0.534	2.3
50	Pediatr Neurosurg	0.532	4.9

[a]IF, impact factor, CH, cited half-life.

To send a manuscript to a certain journal because you know a member of the editorial board personally is not a good idea. Almost all journals have adopted the peer review system, most in a blinded manner (the reviewers know about the authors, but the authors do not know the reviewers), a few in a double-blinded manner (the reviewers are also not aware of the authors). Even if he or she so desires, this system does not allow a member of an editorial board to force the publication of an article that is not recommended for acceptance by the reviewers (which are usually two or three in number). Reviewers rarely disagree in their judgement of an article. In these rare cases the editor will often ask another person to review, and if this does not lead to a decision, most editorial boards will hold a deciding conference known at the *British Medical Journal* as the "hanging committee."[5]

Submitting Your Manuscript to the Wrong Journal

If one does not follow the above recommendations, and the manuscript is unwittingly submitted to the wrong journal, there are several possible outcomes. The first is the least troublesome: the editor realizes the mistake and returns the manuscript immediately to you with the comment that your manuscript is outside the scope of the journal. The situation is worse if the manuscript is rejected after several months of reviewing, and is even worse if you receive an incompetent or unfair review because the editorial board of the journal is not familiar with the work. This may lead to an unjustified rejection or to a comment that does not provide appropriate suggestions for improving your article. Alternatively, your paper may be accepted despite the fact that it needs improvement, as determined by competent review. The worst situation occurs if your paper is accepted by an entirely inappropriate journal, and you soon discover that it has been printed in a publication that your peers do not read.[6]

Special Concerns of the Non-English-Speaking Author

Few would argue with the fact that English is the current lingua franca of international science. Studies by the ISI have shown that the majority of all scientific literature is written and published in English and that English-language literature is by far the most cited. According to the IF, an English-written publication will be cited, on average, 3.7 times, whereas German, French, and Japanese publications will be cited, on average, only 0.6, 0.5, and 0.5 times, respectively. Thus, an English-written article meets with a more than six times higher response than, for example, a German-written article.[7] This language barrier in medical research has three important consequences. First, authors not reading and writing English risk being simultaneously unaware of and overlooked by mainstream international research. Second, English-speaking authors risk being ignorant of significant findings reported in foreign languages. Third, it is still a fact that in some countries, for example, Russia, Germany, and France, most physicians read journals written in their native language almost exclusively. Therefore, the most important step for the non-English-speaking author or the author who does not speak English as a first language is to decide the purpose of his or her manuscript. Is the goal to promote one's academic career by contributing to international medical science, or is it to achieve national reputation? The only way to get around this problem is probably "double" publication, that is, domestic and international. However, this could be construed as ethically dubious and might cause the rejection of a manuscript. If the paper is published in one language and is subsequently submitted in another language to another journal, this journal must be notified that the study was previously published in a different language.

Another significant problem for some non-English-speaking authors is their inadequate knowledge of the English language. If you want to address an English-language journal you must be able to read and write medical English. It is not feasible to write the manuscript in your native language and then have it translated into English by a commercial translator. This is expensive and involves a significant danger in that the meaning and message of your manuscript may be altered or lost in the translation, simply because most translators lack comprehension of your medical specialty. If you are not very familiar with the English language you should choose an English-language journal that provides editorial assistance in optimizing your English style, for example the *World Journal of Surgery*. It is obviously very important to prepare your manuscript in the best English style possible.

Researchers are under great pressure to publish their work. More than ever before, careers and funding depend on publications ("publish or perish!"). Journal offices receive mountains of manuscripts. A few are of great scientific value, some are poor in quality, and most are average. Manuscripts in the first two categories are generally easy to spot, but editors spend a great deal of time deciding which of the average manuscripts merit publication. Undoubtedly, good writing style and attention to detail can improve the chances of an average manuscript being selected for publication. The author for whom English is not a first language must be especially careful to write a concise, clear, and easy to read paper. Editors do not enjoy rewriting manuscripts because of poor English, nor do they have the time. Therefore you should ask one or more colleagues who are familiar with the English language to review the manuscript and to point out areas that require clarification. Any ambiguities can then be eliminated before the paper is submitted.

In 1994, one-third of the articles published in the *New England Journal of Medicine* originated from non-English-speaking Europe.[8] This fact might be an incentive for non-English-speaking authors to choose the more laborious route of publication—in English-language literature.

Electronic Publishing

In the early 1970s, it was predicted that by the end of the century the traditional paper journal would have been replaced by the electronic journal. Of course, this prophecy has not yet been fully realized, but many physicians now use E-mail as well as the Internet, and it is likely that electronic publishing will become critically important in medicine.

What will be the advantages of electronic publishing via the Internet? First, the volume of information that can be published becomes essentially infinite. The number and length of articles is of little concern on the Internet. Reams of raw data from experiments can be added to papers, and perhaps case reports and negative findings will be much more acceptable for publication. Second, the speed of information exchange will continue to accelerate incredibly; in theory, articles could be delivered to the journal, edited, refereed over the Internet, and published in a single day. Third, targeted access will allow the reader to preselect topics on a need-to-know basis. Fourth, interactivity between the electronic journal and the reader will allow instant comment by the latter on the published material for the benefit of both editor and reader. Fifth, the availability and circulation of the journal will be enhanced. Readers and libraries, currently submerged by costs and the sheer weight of published material, may welcome the potential that easy access to information without the need for physical storage implies. Sixth, an electronic journal distributed via the Internet would be much less expensive than the classical paper journal.[9]

For about 15 years, physicists have been communicating preliminary results ("preprints") via the Internet. The Los Alamos National Laboratory computer has become a vast repository for physics manuscripts. The physicists submit and replace their preprints and make changes whenever they want. This system functions like an electronic journal which allows individual communications to be consistently revised by the investigators. Such a publication system is probably not desirable for medical publishing. Electronic publishing of medical preprints bypasses peer review and increases the risk that the data or interpretations of a study will be biased or even wrong. Such a system could also invite manipulation or possibly fraud. The comments of multiple, anonymous users of the Internet is no replacement for peer review. The wide distribution of unedited medical preprints could have an immediate and disastrous effect on the public health.[10,11]

To date, however, most physicians haven't even dipped their toes into the world of electronic communication. In the future, when the Internet is widely used by physicians, new medical information will most likely be best transmitted through this medium. A fertile marriage between the traditional paper journal and its electronic counterpart could result in a system that involves the publication of abstracts in a paper journal that describes the full article that appears simultaneously on the Internet, with both forms of the article having received an appropriate peer review. Such a system would provide easy and precise access to evaluated research results for all interested readers. The availability of information has been and always should be the primary purpose of medical publishing.

References

1. Ludbrook J. Where should I submit my surgical manuscript? Aust N Z J Surg 1991;61:329–331.
2. Arndt KA. Information excess in medicine. Arch Dermatol 1992;128:1249–1256.
3. Hanson S. Impact factor as a misleading tree in evaluation of medical journals. Lancet 1995; 346:906.
4. Foster WR. Impact factor as the best operational measure of medical journals. Lancet 1995;346: 1301.
5. Lock S. A Difficult Balance. Editorial Peer Reviews in Medicine, 3rd edn. London: British Medical Journal, 1991.
6. Day RA. How to write and publish a scientific paper. Philadelphia: ISI, 1975.
7. Garfield E, Welljams-Dorof A. Language use in international research: a citation analysis. Curr Contents 1990;33:5–17.
8. Kassirer JP. My years at the journal—so far. New Engl J Med 1995;333:654–655.
9. Young AE. The future of surgical journals in the electronic publishing era. Br J Surg 1996;83:289–290.
10. Kassirer JP, Angell M. The internet and the journal. New Engl J Med 1995;332:1709–1710.
11. Long M. The future—electronic publishing. In: Hall GM, ed. How to Write a Paper. London: MJ Publishing Group, 1994, pp. 107–112.

Commentary

The authors present a practical approach to the process of selecting a journal for your manuscript as a series of questions: What is the quality? What is the purpose of your publication? Where will it best serve your particular intents? Which journals are most prestigious, or have the greatest impact factor?

The section on the special concerns of the non-English-speaking author outlines three important consequences of publishing in a language other than English. Perhaps the most important is the observation that North American authors are frequently ignorant of significant findings reported in foreign-language journals. The authors make valuable suggestions about this problem and also raise the issue of the ethics of double publication (when the same article is published in two different languages, for domestic and international consumption). We favor the view that this form of double publication is a solution, not a problem.

The authors take us into the future of electronic publishing. This section combined with the chapter by Pisters (chapter 10) on computer-based literature searches will challenge surgical investigators to accelerate their entry into the world of electronic communication.

D.S.M.
M.F.M.

CHAPTER 15

What to Do When You Are Asked to Write a Chapter

B. Lewerich and D. Götze

When you receive an invitation to contribute a chapter or section of a book, allow yourself 10 minutes to feel flattered. Then, read the letter again and try to figure out exactly what the editor or senior author wants you to do. Most invitation letters are rather vague because, for understandable reasons, the inviting editor does not want to give away too much information about the project before gaining a prospective author's agreement to participate. Before you answer the invitation, ask yourself a few specific questions and try to answer them honestly.

Do I really have the time to take on another obligation?

Is it likely that I will be able to complete the required work by the stipulated deadline?

Do I want to write about the topic suggested, or will the editor permit me to alter it in some satisfactory way?

Accept the invitation only if you are able to answer "Yes" to all these questions. A good friend may feel offended if you reject such a request, but your friendship will suffer much more if you have to ask for repeated extensions beyond the deadline. Be aware that experts in delaying contributions soon earn a "special" reputation among editors and publishers.

Before you agree to write a chapter for a book, make sure you ask the inviting editor at least the following questions:

What kind of readership do you want to reach?

What is the complete outline of the book like? (Ask for as much detailed information as is available.)

How many pages will the publisher allow for my chapter?

How many figures and how many tables am I allowed to use?

How many references are allowed?

Must I prepare camera-ready figures?

Is the use of color figures permitted?

Has a sample chapter been prepared, which would help to clarify any further questions?

Since some editors feel that their job is finished when the outline of the book has been drawn up and the authors have been invited, ask your editor for a detailed explanation of how your chapter should be structured.

The more detailed the editor's advance instructions are regarding your chapter, the less difficulty there will be in incorporating your contribution into the book, and the fewer revisions you will have to make. As indicated above, an editor is well advised to send participating authors a sample chapter at the beginning to give them some idea of what their work should look like. It can be taken as a general rule that the less specific and the less strict a book editor is in approaching authors, the less acceptable the book will be.

When you have received answers to all the foregoing questions, start work as soon as possible. Good authors have many demands on their time and energy. Do not postpone writing the article until two days after the deadline. The excuse that you can work only under pressure is a very bad one. Grapes and cheese produce excellent results when put under pressure, but brains behave differently.

There are several things you can easily do as soon as you agree to prepare a contribution:

Develop your own manuscript outline and check it with the editor(s) to make sure you really understand your assignment.

Start a bibliographic search and collect relevant reprints. Speak with other experts for fresh ideas or to learn about recent work you are not aware of.

Look into other books on the subject to see whether a similar contribution has been published before.

Think about how your contribution could be better.

At an early stage, start developing sketches of the figures you are going to use.

If you want to use figures that have already been published, seek permission for their reproduction from the author or publisher, now.

Obtain author's instructions for the preparation of manuscripts from the editor or publisher to avoid inconsistencies of format within the book as a whole.

Technical Considerations

Type the text of your contribution double-spaced with broad margins on both sides to allow space for the editor's and the copy editor's corrections. The compositor will have fewer difficulties when your text is not crammed together too closely.

Most authors use word processors to produce their papers, and some books are produced by turning authors' diskettes over to a conversion company, which uses computers to print the material, rather than the labor of compositors. If the publisher has not already sent you infor-

mation as to whether diskettes are to be used for typesetting the book, you should ask which programs are preferred. Some publishers have designed special software to make your secretary's work easier.

Attach figures, diagrams, and tables on separate sheets. These parts of the book are handled separately in the production process, and providing separate sheets will make things easier for the compositor or printer.

Make sure that each page and each figure carries your name. It may happen that some figures will get mixed up, but yours never will.

See that all your figures and tables are cited in your text by number. The book editor may change the numbering, if necessary, but your material and its sequence can always be identified.

Be sure that the way you cite references complies with the instructions given by the publisher. Be even more careful about giving correct page numbers, volume numbers, and publication years.

See that all the references listed at the end of your chapter are mentioned in the text, and vice versa. Make sure that all references are complete, with names of all authors, title, publication date, volume, and pages. If books are quoted, supply authors' names, editors' names where appropriate, book title, pages referred to, publication date, and publisher's name and location. Ask your editor or publisher which citation system you should use (e.g., Vancouver or Harvard guideline for the preparation of manuscripts). Regardless of how the references will appear in the printed book, in your manuscript they must be double-spaced, like the rest of the text.

No one else can verify the sources you have used as well as you can. Readers who order a reprint of a paper you have referred to will be anything but pleased when they receive a photocopy of an article on water pollution, when your article was about surgery of the pancreas.

A final important rule to be heeded when you are involved in the writing of a book is this. *Do not tell the readers what you know about the subject; tell them what they should know about it.*

When you have delivered the complete manuscript to the editor or publisher, you are not quite clear of your commitment, yet. Your manuscript will be checked by the editor and publisher for its content, consistency, completeness, and clarity. You may get your manuscript back, marked with queries and flags. Even if you consider the queries inappropriate, try to answer them as clearly and positively as possible. If someone has misunderstood a point, do not attack the messenger; accept the opportunity to explain the point more lucidly. In most instances, this will improve the book's readability, promote readers' understanding, and facilitate production. Make sure to adhere to the deadline set for the return of the revised manuscript. The manuscript that comes in last sets the pace for the whole publication.

When the final copyedited manuscripts of all contributors are in the hands of the publisher and everything is ready for composition, the publisher will notify you of the date on which you can expect to receive galley and/or page proofs so that you can plan time for proofreading. If you will be unable to do the proofreading at the indicated time (you may be on holiday, at a congress, etc.), let the publisher and editor know immediately so that an alternate date can be arranged.

When you receive the proofs, do the following:

Check them carefully for correct spelling, completeness, correct structuring (headings, sections, paragraphs), and optimal arrangement of text, figures, and tables.

Respond to *all* queries even if you think some of them require no comment.

Do not add new material (text, figures, or tables), because this may necessitate a complete new "paste-up" of the whole book. This will not only delay publication but probably will cause you to be billed for the extra costs so incurred.

Return proofs by the requested time (usually 48 hours after you received them). Publishing a book is a team effort that involves not only the author(s), editor(s), and publisher, but also the less visible and equally important compositors, printers, and binders. If anyone's work is not delivered on time, the schedule of everyone else is disrupted, progress comes to a halt, publication is delayed, and costs soar, sometimes astronomically.

Conclusion

Do not agree to contribute to a book unless you honestly believe you will be able to complete the task by the stipulated deadline. Moreover, do not agree until you have received, from the editor, a detailed outline of the planned book, as well as sufficient information about the intended readership and the type of material desired. Write exactly what you have been asked to write. Show understanding toward your readers and mercy toward your coworkers in the production of the book.

Commentary

I advise young surgeons against writing book chapters until they become quite senior and experienced. They can make a much better investment of their energy and thinking skills by writing peer-reviewed articles and grant applications. Academic departments and societies give far less credit for book chapters than for original articles because chapters are not peer reviewed at the same level.

Senior academicians should write chapters preferably with younger members who can benefit from their tutelage and mentorship, which provide the balance, judgment, and wisdom lacking at the early stage of a career. They can avoid pontification, hazy recollection, and bias by critically reviewing the material with their younger coauthor. This two-way street becomes a productive experience for all concerned, including the readers of the chapter.

Never write a chapter out of a sense of obligation to help a colleague fill a gap in his or her book, and never promise a chapter you can't deliver.

Be careful not to invest your energy in a book that will not come to publication. Publishers like to look for trendy topics and invite rising stars who have written important papers within these domains to organize a book. This entrepreneurial approach provides an opportunity for you to waste your time and energy writing a chapter that never reaches publication.

M.F.M.

CHAPTER 16

Organizing Your Reference Material

R. Lefering and E.A.M. Neugebauer

As both a scientist and a physician, you have to deal with a seemingly endless stack of new papers, articles, and other important literature from journals, the library, your department or clinic, from companies or colleagues aware of your field of interest, and from computer searches. In order to get efficient use of and maximum benefit from this information, you need to organize your reference material.

The availability of information has two complementary aspects: storage and retrieval. The only reason for storing material is to have the ability to retrieve it later, and the amount of effort invested in proper storage determines the ease of retrieval. Conversely, retrieval needs should determine the type of storage used. Both of these aspects will be discussed here, from the viewpoint of an individual user as well as from the departmental perspective. At the end of this chapter, you will find criteria that may be helpful in selecting the appropriate software for literature organization.

Individual Literature Organization

After having examined an article carefully, consider whether this article is worth storing, or is ready for the trash can. Articles you have decided to read will usually contain some useful remarks or comments and should be stored. For articles of minor importance, if the original can be easily reaccessed (for example, if the journal is in your library), it may be more efficient not to store these papers but to copy them when needed.

The amount of effort devoted to storing papers you have amassed is related to the frequency and type of retrieval requests you make, and to the average amount of time needed to make a successful retrieval from your collection. If you decide to use one of the systems described below, weigh the number of your real requests (not the possible ones) made using such a system against the time and effort needed to input information and update your system.

Literature Storing and Retrieval Systems

A Single Stack of Paper

This system is included only to familiarize you with cost-benefit analysis for measuring the usefulness of a storing and retrieval system. The "cost" is the effort involved in adding each new paper to your collection. In this example, the cost is nearly zero because putting a paper on top of a stack requires no work. The benefit can be measured by the system's ability to meet different types of requests, as listed in Table 16-1. Retrieval operations could be divided into two main areas: (1) looking for a certain paper, probably with incomplete knowledge of the specific reference; and (2) getting an overview of a certain scope. The ability to execute these operations and the time required to do so determine the benefit of a literature storage and retrieval system. A simple stack responds very poorly to any type of request. But as long as your collection is small, this type of storage may be the most effective one.

Paper-Based Systems

The usual way to organize literature involves paper-based systems. Typically, you identify the different fields or topics that cover your domain of interest. If the number of articles in a certain field is small enough, you can organize them as a stack; when the number is large, alphabetic storage by the author's name is more appropriate.

There is no generally accepted rule for choosing an optimal classification system for medical literature. Some people like to organize their literature by organ systems or diseases, but other categories, for example, animal studies, surgical techniques, X ray, statistical methods, and so forth, may be more suitable. Others prefer to store all material for a specific paper or lecture—figures, slides, and bibliography—under its own category.

Problems arise when papers could be filed under several headings. A paper describing the diagnostic value of ultrasound for detecting stones in the common bile duct could be stored under "ultrasound," "diagnostic tests," or "gallbladder diseases." You could file a copy under each heading (which requires additional effort in storing) or choose the most relevant heading and face additional effort when the time comes to retrieve the article.

There are two guidelines for the selection of your individual system of headings. First, choose headings with as few overlaps as possible. This will minimize the problem of double storing described above and enhance the effectiveness of retrieval. Second, be sufficiently specific but avoid excessively narrow categories. Restrict the number of headings as much as possible.

Paper-based systems have very clear advantages

Table 16-1. Differences of literature organizing systems to meet certain retrieval requests.

Task	Stack	Paper-based	Card-index	Computer-assisted	Computer-assisted with keywords
Retrieve a *certain* paper					
with complete citation	$-^a$	$+^b$	$++^c$	$+++^d$	$+++$
with author known	$-$	$+$	$++$	$+++$	$+++$
with coauthor known	$-$	$-$	$-$	$+++$	$+++$
with title (word) known	$-$	$-$	$+$	$+++$	$+++$
about a certain topic	$+$	$++$	$++$	$++$	$+++$
other (year, journal, etc.)	$-$	$-$	$-$	$+++$	$+++$
Retrieve *all* papers					
of a certain author	$-$	$+$	$++$	$+++$	$+++$
with a certain title-word	$-$	$-$	$+$	$+++$	$+++$
about a certain topic	$-$	$++$	$++$	$++$	$+++$
other (year, journal, etc.)	$-$	$-$	$-$	$+++$	$+++$

[a] $-$, Impossible or very time-consuming.

[b] $+$, Possible but with restrictions.

[c] $++$, Performable within reasonable time.

[d] $+++$, Very quick and easy.

for those who are uncomfortable with computers, especially if no research support staff is available. They offer a cost-effective solution with little time needed for storage and adequate retrieval results.

Card-Index Systems

Since working with condensed and relevant information is much more comfortable than handling a stack of original papers, people often use cards containing the particulars of an article as well as individual remarks and comments. This approach requires considerably more effort than a simple filing system, and the improvement in retrievability is small (see Table 16-1). In addition, you will have to establish a procedure to find the original article. One commonly used procedure is to number every paper and store the originals in sequence. This allows the quickest retrieval. Another procedure is a "signature" system with predefined headings as described in paper-based systems.

Computer-Assisted System

Many boring tasks are now assigned to computers, including time-consuming searches of specific topics (see chapter 10). Computers are also used to manage personal literature collections, replacing card-index systems. The act of storing an article is comparable to filling out a filing card, but retrieval of information is remarkably easier, even if you store only the citation without keywords or comments (see Table 16-1). All stored items, or any combination thereof, can be used as search criteria.

As described for card-index systems, you will have to establish a procedure to identify the original paper in your files from the information stored in the computer. This requires maintaining two systems: the references in the computer and the originals. Changes in one of them require the same changes in the other, or retrieval operations will not be successful.

The time needed for storing articles in your personal database should not be underestimated. The widespread use and accessibility of large medical databases such as MEDLINE, EMBASE, or Current Contents on Diskette offer the possibility of reducing this time because many programs can read the specific formats and import selected references (see the criteria for selecting the appropriate software at the end of this chapter). If research staff is available, the storage of selected articles can be delegated as a routine task.

Computer-Assisted System Using Keywords

The computer-assisted system can be used without knowing anything about a paper beyond its author(s) and title. This may be an advantage if you are short on time, but the retrieval options are limited. Your list of papers dealing with a specific subject, such as "meta-analysis," will be incomplete because many relevant articles will not contain your search word in their titles (for example, Peto's paper entitled "Why do we need systematic overviews of randomized trials?"[1]). Methodology is rarely mentioned in a title; if you are looking for an example of the application of discriminant analysis, searching title words will not be very fruitful. A successful search for special topics requires a short examination of each paper to enable you to attach a few keywords covering the main issue(s). These keywords and a certain amount of discipline in choosing them will result in an effective retrieval. Some computer programs allow keywords to be arranged hierarchically; for example, a search for papers dealing with "bacteria" will also yield all entries with the keywords "*E. coli*," "*Streptococcus*," and so forth.

The task of providing a broad overview about a certain topic may be more efficiently served by the big commercial medical databases (MEDLINE, etc.) which have, in addition, the advantage of containing the most recent publications. The combination of a MEDLINE search together with quick subsequent identification of those articles contained in one's personal file is the most efficient strategy.

Consider Dr. Readsalot who has collected his literature in files divided into many small fields. He chose this method because he didn't want to have to look through a large file if he needed a certain piece of information. Many of his papers could be classified under several headings, and he always chose one field as the main topic. Gradually, he came to realize that his files on a specific topic did not include all the relevant literature he had stored, so he decided to switch to a computer-assisted system. To start, he prepared a checklist of his requirements and visited some of his colleagues who used computers to organize their literature. When he had chosen an appropriate system, his next decision was whether to use keywords. He soon realized that attaching keywords retrospectively to all his old papers would consume an enormous amount of his time, even if the input of basic reference data could be done by someone else. Consequently, he decided not to use keywords.

The typical procedure Dr. Readsalot follows when adding papers to his system is the following:

1. Scan the article and assign it to a field of interest.
2. Mark this field as a label on the paper itself.
3. Add the paper to the stack of other papers awaiting registration.
4. After the information has been stored in the computer, the paper is immediately filed in the place indicated by the signature.

When papers registered in the computer are filed together with papers that are not, marking the articles available in the computer is useful. Note that, to Dr. Readsalot's advantage, the old filing structure did not have to be reorganized. Dr. Readsalot learned the search operations of his software without much difficulty. He can now use his more effective system and feels pleased at the growing power of his database.

How to Develop a Literature Storage System

The following list summarizes the basic approach to developing a practical literature storage and retrieval system.

- Keep only those papers you probably will use; throw away the rest.
- Organize the remaining literature by different topics or headings.
- When the time required for searching or the number of unsuccessful searches becomes intolerable, change to a computer-assisted system. Card-index systems produce poor results compared with computers.

- Compare the expense (time) required to summarize the content of a paper and assign some keywords, with the benefit to be derived when you need a high-quality search on specific topics.

Note that the increasingly common ability to find a paper via computer searches will lower the importance of individual literature collections.

Departmental Literature Organization

A joint system for the common use of all collaborators in a department or unit will never have all the advantages of an individual collection but may offer several additional advantages in some cases. A collaborative system has limited justification if there are only two or three colleagues; individual literature systems and personal communication will yield better and more immediately relevant answers, helpful remarks, and advice. If the areas of interest of the group have little overlap, a joint literature administration will likely yield no benefit. If the unit is large, an enormous effort is required to keep a joint system up-to-date. Shared systems are generally more vulnerable to piracy and incompleteness than private systems, especially if access is not limited. Each member of the unit will understandably give priority to keeping his or her own system current.

What are the benefits of a joint system, if it won't replace individual ones? First, it will provide complete documentation of the literature available within your department, save some trips to the university library, and speed up your work. Second, those colleagues who do not store their references on a computer will gain the advantages of electronic searching if the central database is computerized. Third, a central system will relieve everyone from holding a large number of papers classified somewhere between "important" and "of no interest." Knowing that these kinds of "perhaps" papers are still retrievable if you need them can help you to concentrate on more important things. Finally, should one of your colleagues leave, his or her references will not be lost to the department.

You should have no illusions about the time and

cost of maintaining such a system. Keeping it current requires several hours per week; this is preferably the responsibility of a special librarian or research secretary who facilitates access to the literature.

The system installed in our research department, comprising five collaborators working in related fields, will serve as an example. We have introduced a paper-based joint filing system that is independent of each member's personal literature files. We have agreed on 11 different headings such as "pain," "quality of life," "meta-analysis," and so on. Each team member scans new articles as they arrive. If a paper is worth storing, it is assigned to one or more of the predefined headings. We make a separate copy for our own files if it is a very important paper. If there is any doubt about storing an article and we believe a colleague might make a different decision, we send it to the colleague for review. At our library the papers are copied and filed according to their assigned heading(s). This procedure helps to keep one's personal literature files lean and offers the possibility of finding additional important articles by scanning through our joint literature files. It is also an effective tool for students or clinical colleagues who seek a basic set of important papers about a certain topic.

Criteria for Choosing Literature-Organizing Software

Many programs are available, ranging from low-cost public domain software to systems for huge libraries, and are continuously changing and improving. We cannot provide a complete list of current programs and do not wish to favor particular products, but we can present some options to consider when you are making choices.

Fields

The different components of a reference will be stored in "fields"—one field for the title, one for the author(s), and so on. Write down the complete reference when you want to store it. Does the program you are considering provide fields that are adequate for your needs? The fields in some programs are fixed, that is, their names and lengths cannot be changed; other programs allow adaptations to be made by the user.

Search

Before you test a program, define some typical patterns of searching you will want to use on your database. Don't forget to ask about the program's ability to find a certain word within different fields and to incorporate previous search results.

Duplicates

The capability to identify duplicates is a very helpful tool for assisting data input, but if the program recognizes only completely identical entries, it is worthless. Identification of duplicates using only year, journal, and pages is a very useful tool.

Keywords

Storage of some keywords is offered by nearly every program, but if you really want to work with keywords, look for the capacity to define a catalog of keywords or to structure them hierarchically.

Output

Several output formats should be available for different purposes, and it is advantageous to have them adjustable to meet your requirements. Some programs have the feature of being able to create a reference list from the database, which is very helpful when you are writing a paper. This list can be produced in the format required by the journal you have selected, or stored in a file that can be transferred to your word-processing system.

User Friendliness

It is a big advantage, especially for those who do not work with the software every day, when the information presented on the screen is largely self-explanatory. It should be easy to perform standard operations such as search procedures without having to study big handbooks. A context-sensitive help function should be available also.

Protection

If you have reason to fear abuse of your literature data bank, or if you want to restrict the use or manipulation of your data, choose a program with protection mechanisms such as passwords.

Volume

Try to estimate how much data your system will have to handle. Will the performance of the system still be satisfactory a few years from now? How long does it take the program to perform an operation such as performing a special search within a large database?

Import of data

If you want to take over an existing database or insert data from other databases (e.g., MEDLINE), look for a program with this capability. An additional module is often available.

Tasks

In addition to administration of literature, some programs can be modified to execute other tasks, such as organizing your books, slides, or lectures.

It is a distinct advantage if the system that is familiar to you is usable for other purposes.

Testing

The manufacturers of large software programs often distribute a low-cost test or demo version that may help you to decide how practical or valuable it would be in meeting your requirements. It is much better if you have the opportunity to watch colleagues work with the system and ask them for their evaluation of it.

References

1. Peto R. Why do we need systematic overviews of randomized trials? Stat Med 1987;6:233–240.

Commentary

The biomedical literature increases each year, and the availability of copying machines and computer-assisted literature searches seems only to add to a continuously increasing flow of papers across your desk. Even if you are quite selective about what you retain, let alone what you read, large piles of paper accumulate around you; someday you will want to return to it. Dr. Lefering and Prof. Neugebauer offer some helpful ideas about the management of material for future reference. We can profitably review our own reference storage and retrieval capacities and benefit from their suggestions.

B.M.

CHAPTER 17

Reviewing Books and Refereeing Scientific Papers

J.R. Farndon

Experience is fallacious and judgement difficult.
—Hippocrates: Aphorisms, I

In reviewing articles or books, influential judgments are made about the scientific worth and value of colleagues' written work. This should be done with a more than adequate background knowledge and a desire to be fair and just. Hippocrates correctly tells us that experience alone is fallacious and any reviewer must also agree that "judgement is difficult." From the perspective of the journal using referee comments to decide upon the fate of a paper or deciding whether to publish a book review, other criteria must obtain. One hundred years ago the editorial columns of the *New York Medical Journal* were "controlled by the desire to promote the welfare, honour and advancement of the science of medicine, as viewed from a standpoint looking to the best interests of the profession. Nothing is admitted to its columns that has not some bearing on medicine, or is not possessed of some practical value." These parameters have probably changed little since 1892 and apply equally to specific surgical disciplines.

The review process is dynamic and varies in certain details when applied to journal articles or books. It is dependent upon reviewer characteristics, the work being reviewed, and the ethos and criteria stipulated by the journal.

Book Reviews

Most surgical journals receive copies of newly published books each month with an invitation to review them. The unwritten and unspoken desire is that a favorable review will be published and read by all subscribers to the journal who will flock in their thousands to buy a copy of the tenth edition of *Buggins' Laparoscopic Surgery of the Left Kidney*. This is not quite how things happen.

First, the journal will be selective in which books it sends out for review. Publishers appear to use a scatter bomb technique and send all newly published surgical textbooks to all surgical journals. Each journal is likely to have a review editor who will decide whether the book should be reviewed. *Laparoscopic Surgery of the Left Kidney* is unlikely to be reviewed in a plastic surgery journal, for example, but would probably be reviewed by the *Euroland Journal of Urology*.

Second, the journal will have instructions to book reviewers that will stipulate requirements of the review and the format of submission. There is usually a word limit that must be followed. It is advisable for potential reviewers to be aware of the style of book reviews. Some journals will have a cold clinical approach and will not allow a light-hearted or jocular approach. This detail may not be stated in instructions but is clear on reading copies of previous journal issues. Be sure to do so and avoid wasting your time writing an inappropriately styled review.

Third, most journals designate two to four pages toward the end of each issue for book reviews. These pages tend to be lighter reading (along with correspondence columns) after the more strenuous pages of scientific articles, but one should not assume this as fact.

How to Begin

When you receive the book and the review instructions, examine both carefully. Decide whether the book needs to be read. It will be easy to read a 100-page text on undergraduate surgery; it would be impossible for most to *read* 2,700 pages of postgraduate text. A strategy must be adopted that will allow the foundation of an opinion. In a larger work, especially if it is multi-authored, care must be taken that the whole work is sampled such that strengths and weaknesses can be identified.

The heading or title of the review may be given by the journal and, in any event, should include the title of the book, the author(s), the publisher, the number of pages, whether it is illustrated or not (color or black and white), and the cost. The ISBN is sometimes given; it is a useful component of the heading. The journal may allow a superscript eye-catching headline title such as "indispensable for surgeons." The review editor will decide or advise on this last point.

Before embarking on the task, read the preface of the book carefully and in full. Note whether this is a new book or a subsequent edition. If dealing with the fifth edition try to obtain the first and fourth for comparison. In the preface, read about the target readership, (e.g., surgeons interested in the left kidney) and whether readers are expected to be at undergraduate or postgraduate level. Be sure to see if the aims and objectives of the book are set out clearly. See if the authors state how the fifth edition is better than the fourth and, hopefully, the first. Is the book to be national or international? These points are essential parameters on which to base the review. If they are not determined, it may not be worth going on to the next page.

What Next?

Try to find time away from distractions to study the book in as much detail as you can. As the reviewer you must then construct a short descriptive article covering the main points of the book (Table 17-1). This information may influence a reader of the review to buy or consult the book, or acquire it for a department library.

It is easy to praise outstanding works but "judgement is difficult," especially when dealing with mediocrity. Let it be hoped that reviewers never have to deal with a poor product. Publisher astuteness and shrewdness should prevent poor books being produced.

If defects are found then these should be described. If major deficiencies are present these should be checked by a colleague to be certain that they are appropriately and correctly identified. Remember that the production of a book will have taken much hard work; level your criticisms with diplomacy and humanity. Remember that authors are often reviewers. Do unto others as you would have done unto you!

Table 17-1.   Some helpful questions for book reviewers.

Is the book pitched at the appropriate level?

Is the content national or international? (i.e., applicable to the specified audience)

Is the text clear and well written?

If a multi-authored book, is the editorial direction sufficient to unify style, content, and illustrations?

What is the quality of the illustrations?

Is the book worth the price?

If a new book, does it fill a market niche or requirement?

If a subsequent edition: has it aged?
is it still appropriate?
has it been brought up to date?

What about the fabric of the book and the quality of paper and covers?

How does the book compare with its nearest competitors?

Is It Worth It?

There is usually little inducement for undertaking a review. A few journals pay a nominal sum, averaging about $1.23 for each hour spent on the task. Most journals make a donation of the book to the reviewer or the department library. As the reviewers for the *New York Medical Journal* did 100 years ago, your work is done "to promote the welfare, honour and advancement of the science" of surgery.

A Unique Solution

Instead of writing just a preface to their book *The Parathyroid Glands and Metabolic Bone Disease*, Albright and Reifenstein wrote a "Preface and Critical Review Combined":

> On starting to write the preface, it occurred to the authors that it might be well to incorporate their own critical review. The thought existed, it must be admitted, that, by pointing out the shortcomings in particular, the wind might be taken out of the sails of those of the reviewers who will be impressed largely by the faults of this work. In other words, we are incorporating a little prophylactic criticism.[1]

Refereeing Scientific Papers for a Journal

Most will remember the thrill and pride of receiving the first letter of acceptance of their first surgical article. This meant that the editors of the journal and a process of peer review accepted the work as worthy of publication and dissemination in the world literature. For a few, one or more of those papers would be the initiation of nominal immortality (e.g., Zollinger-Ellison syndrome, Blalock procedure, etc.). For most it would be a pleasure that the work had been "admitted to its columns" and judged to have "some bearing on medicine or is possessed of some practical value."

The number of journals available to receive articles increases week by week. In addition to those that appear in line with new technology, others arrive with new organ-specific titles that mirror growing specialization. Most surgical journals, however, will employ similar peer review processes. Journals may have rejection rates as high as 70%. How are papers rejected and, more importantly, what criteria are used to identify "successful" papers?

The editors in charge of running a journal are likely to be surgeons in day-to-day practice, with a special interest in publication. They will be supported and guided by an editorial board that defines the scope of the journal and guides publishing strategy. These should be described in some preface piece in each issue of the journal. The stated strategy might allow editors some preliminary control over whether to reject or accept papers, for example, it may be policy not to carry case reports or review articles.

Working behind this editorial team will be a panel of referees that should be compatible with the circulation and strategic aims of the journal. For example, a journal that says it is "European" should have appropriate editorial and referee membership; an international journal should have global representation. This is not always readily achieved. The panel of referees is charged with the peer review process.

The Current Climate of Publication of Surgical Research

In an editorial in April 1996 Richard Horton described a study he had undertaken examining the work published in one issue of nine surgical journals. Excluding letters and book reviews, there were 215 articles of which 175 contained original research. Only 12 papers (7%) reported results of a randomized trial, case series comprised 80 papers (46%), and experimental work 31 papers (18%). Horton asked "Does surgical research have a future?" and stated "Only when the quality of publications in the surgical literature has improved will surgeons reasonably be able to rebut the charge that as much as half the research they undertake is misconceived."[2]

There are acknowledged difficulties in evaluating new surgical procedures,[3] but understanding the principles of observational epidemiology not only helps critical appraisal of research reports but guides design and execution of studies that will be scrutinized by our peers.[4]

The Unbiased Referee

In acting as a referee, remember that surgeons contribute low proportions of articles describing randomized controlled trials. This may reflect a lack of expertise by surgeons in clinical trials, lack of funds for surgical trials, methodological problems peculiar to surgical trials, or a need for adoption of other research designs to assess surgical therapies.[5] Bias must not be introduced during review because a study does not conform to the format of a prospective, double-blind, randomized trial. Inevitably, flaws will be detected and should be reported fairly. Between 1988 and 1994, 364 surgical trials were reviewed, and less than 50% made comment about an unbiased assessment of outcome, gave an adequate description of the randomization technique, or provided a prospective estimate of the sample size. Economic factors were described in only 6.5% of the trials, and only 2% attempted some measure of the effect of the intervention on the quality of life of patients.[6] Against this background a referee should weigh and report the strengths and weaknesses of a study in context, remembering that "experience is fallacious and judgement difficult"!

The Referee Process

If asked to be a referee, it is likely that you are nationally or internationally recognized as an expert in a particular field, and you have been "noticed" by an editorial board. After you have allowed your chest to deflate from pride remember that an expert is someone who knows everything about very little. Be pleased, but keep a sense of perspective.

You are likely to be one of a pair or triplet of referees, so you are not alone. A good journal will cross-circulate referees' comments with the resulting decision on publication. Differences of opinion occur (Table 17-2).

Note the skewed distribution toward rejection, as well as the discord. Learn from this process. Go back to your own comments, balance and

Table 17-2. Referee concordance for pairs of referees for a sample of 200 papers (80 accepted) submitted to the *British Journal of Surgery*.

Referee 2	Referee 1			
	Accept	Minor faults	Major faults	Reject
Accept	1	3	4	5
Minor faults	–	5	20	13
Major faults	–	–	19	19
Reject	–	–	–	22

measure them against those of your coreferee with respect to agreement or discord. Discord is resolved by third or fourth referees and the advised judgment of the editors. Measure your own accuracy by the editors' final decision. Remember that rejection rates vary from journal to journal, and standards of quality of publication vary. This variation in "quality" is measured to some extent in performance figures such as "impact factor" and "citation index." These indices are important to editors and publishers; referees indirectly affect these by their integrity, incisiveness, and critical powers.

What to Do Next?

Take the duty seriously, set time aside to carry out the work and return the paper with your comments as soon as you can. Editors will often advise on the time frame; stay within it. If it were your paper you would like it in print next month!

Read the referee instructions *carefully* and follow them *exactly*. Most journals will guide you on the parameters to be assessed. Table 17-3 provides an example from *Surgical Endoscopy*, published by Springer-International.

Novelty

Most journals do not want to publish material that is not new or innovative (Table 17-3, question 1). As an expert you will be expected to be *au fait* with current bibliography (Table 17-3, question 4) and thereby able to assess the novelty factor. You must advise editors if you suspect dual publication.

Table 17-3. Example of referee guide to assessment of a paper.

	yes	no	n/a		yes	no	n/a
General				**Results**			
1) Does the paper contain new findings or ideas?	—	—	—	8) Is the opinion of a statistical consultant needed?	—	—	—
If no, does it present old material better?	—	—	—	9) Are the results clearly presented (e.g., are the important results highlighted)?	—	—	—
2) Are the findings or ideas important to the academic medicine community?	—	—	—	10) Are the tables and/or figures useful?	—	—	—
3) Is the material clearly presented, without excessive jargon?	—	—	—	Which, if any, could be deleted?			
4) Are the major relevant recent references included? Please specify omissions	—	—	—	_____			
				_____			
Introduction				11) Would the figures reproduce well?	—	—	—
5) Is the objective of the paper, or the purpose or hypothesis of the study, clearly stated?	—	—	—	12) Is color necessary?	—	—	—
				13) Do the tables and/or figures agree with the text (in general and specifically)?	—	—	—
Methods				**Discussion and Conclusions**			
6) Are the sample and sampling method adequately described?	—	—	—	14) Are the conclusions or generalisations adequately supported by the paper's findings or arguments (e.g., does the author exaggerate their importance)?	—	—	—
7) Is the research design adequate to achieve the objective of the study? (Consider, for example, definition of variables, sample selection, sample size, data-collection instruments, length of study.)	—	—	—				

Style

The clarity of the written style is important (Table 17-3, question 3), and editors appreciate advice on appropriateness of tables and illustrations (Table 17-3, questions 9–13). Note whether any duplications occur. For example, it is unnecessary to present the same data in text, table, and graph. Is the text clear and is the English of good quality?

Scientific Validity

This is the most important area (Table 17-3, questions 5–8, 14), and your criticisms here need to be sure and justified. If you are not sufficiently adept at statistical methodology but "sniff a rat," advise the editor to obtain a statistical opinion. Most surgical journals have a statistical adviser. Remember that statistical methods applied to

some retrospective or observational studies are not appropriate.

You must be sure that any conclusions are justified. The escape into print of inappropriate or unjustified conclusions has allowed authors to "get away with it" despite subsequent letters invalidating the conclusions and berating the incompetence of the editors for not spotting biases and flaws in the work. Few researchers find and quote correspondence. As a referee you are an important guard of the integrity of surgical science—keep your visor down and your sword at the ready.

Other Issues

Examine the title and give advice on revision if necessary. Questions as titles and "snappy" titles should be avoided. Compare, for example, "Should cholecystectomy be carried out through a mini-open incision or by laparoscopy?" or "Laparoscopic cholecystectomy is the business," with "A prospective randomized trial comparing mini-open with laparoscopic cholecystectomy."

How many authors are there? There is a trend toward increasing the number of authors for an article, and this does not appear to be due to an increase in the complexity of work that needs wider collaboration. It is reasonable for a referee to question the contribution of authors, with respect to either the work or the writing tasks.[7]

Examine and comment on ethical issues. Should an ethics committee have been approached to agree to the study? If animals were involved did their handling and management, and the experimental procedures performed follow national guidelines as well as the regulations of the hospital, institute, or university?

Relatively new issues covered in surgical publications include health care policy, quality of life issues, and economics. Relevant specialty guidelines need to be understood and cited by authors and peer reviewers.[8]

Editors will expect a final decision concerning the reviewed paper. This is usually noted by the reviewer in a section "not for transmission to authors," as follows:

Accept as is. Outstanding.
Accept with minor modifications.
Accept with major modifications.
There are major deficiencies. Probably reject.
Beyond redemption. Reject.

Reviewers must summarize their feelings about a paper by choosing one of these categories. Very few articles will qualify for "accept as is"; overall rejection rates for popular journals can be as high as 60–70%. There is often a space on a review form that will allow transmission of confidential comments to the editor. In this section, criticisms can be free flowing. Conversely, remember that in "comments to authors" you should not state anything regarding the quality of the article or whether you think the article is worth publishing. Remember that your comments should help authors reconstruct a better article. Make suggestions in an objective, caring way. "Do unto others as you would have done unto yourself!"

Conclusion

A reviewer is an indispensable aid to an editor, and all good reviewers should aspire to becoming an editor. "Editing is Fun" according to Richard C. Bennett, Editor Emeritus, *Australian and New Zealand Journal of Surgery*.[9]

To make the life of reviewers and editors easy, refer authors to other chapters of this book for guidance in methodology and reporting. Submissions might become so exemplary that reviewers and editors would become defunct!

References

1. Albright F, Reifenstein EC. The Parathyroid Glands and Metabolic Bone Disease. Baltimore: Williams and Wilkins, 1948, p. 1.
2. Horton R. Surgical research or comic opera: questions, but few answers. Lancet 1996;347:984–985.
3. Stirrat GM, Farrow SC, Farndon JR, Dwyer N. The challenge of evaluating surgical procedures. Ann R Coll Surg Engl 1992;74:80–84.
4. Hu X, Wright JG, McLeod RS, Lossing A, Walters BC. Observational studies as alternatives to randomized clinical trials in surgical clinical research. Surgery 1996;119:473–475
5. Solomon MJ, Laxamana A, Devore L, McLeod RS. Randomized controlled trials in surgery. Surgery 1994;115:707–712.
6. Hall JC, Mills B, Nguyen H, Hall JL. Methodologic standards in surgical trials. Surgery 1996;119:466–472.
7. Epstein RJ. Six authors in search of a citation: villains or victims of the Vancouver convention? Br Med J 1993;306:765–767.
8. Drummond MF, Jefferson TO. Guidelines for authors and peer reviewers of economic submissions to the BMJ. Br Med J 1996;313:275–283.
9. Bennett RC. Editing is fun. Aust N Z J Surg 1990;60:931–933.

Commentary

Farndon emphasizes that reviewing a book and refereeing a scientific paper are two distinctly different tasks. A book review asks the reviewer to examine a completed work. It is hoped that the contributors, editors, and publishers have guaranteed a high level of quality. The reviewer's task then is to determine the book's target audience, its strengths and weaknesses, and whether it would be a useful addition to your own library. It is helpful to compare the text to others in its field, to provide the reader with an assessment of this new text.

Refereeing a scientific work is a very responsible undertaking. I agree completely with the aphorism with which Farndon begins the chapter, that experience is fallacious and judgment difficult. The primary prerequisite of a reviewer is to be fair and just. It is proper to criticize the work on a scientific basis, but always with a constructive purpose in mind and a high degree of intellectual humility. Remember that the non-English-speaking author may have presented an extremely good idea that may be misunderstood because of a language barrier. When a paper is poorly written according to the reviewer's standards but contains valuable ideas or information, the reviewer should provide helpful advice to the author for revision. This is particularly important for authors from other countries or cultures. Be sure to word your remarks so they will stand up to public scrutiny. It is easy to be hypercritical, and you should perhaps think that your commentary may be published and subject to the critique of other readers.

Farndon's vast experience as editor of the *British Journal of Surgery* and consultant for the *World Journal of Surgery* makes this chapter an especially useful contribution to this edition of the text.

H.T.

Speaking and Listening

CHAPTER 18

The 10-Minute Presentation

A.V. Pollock and M.E. Evans

You have finished your research project. Now you want to tell people about it. There is no better way than to present your work at a scientific meeting, after which you can think about writing it up for publication. Most scientific societies aim to present four papers an hour, so the presenter has 10 minutes, and each paper is followed by 5 minutes of discussion.

PREPARING A 10-MINUTE PRESENTATION

1. Writing the abstract
2. Preparing the talk: IMRAD
   —Introduction
   —Methods
   —Results
   —Discussion and conclusion
3. Visual aids support and speed your message
   —Overhead projection
   —Slides: appropriate, accurate, legible, comprehensible, well executed
4. Techniques of presentation, appearance, and manners

The first thing you must do is write an abstract (see chapter 12). The society that you have chosen probably has its own rules about the structure of abstracts, and you must abide strictly by those rules. The universal rule remains that the abstract must be a complete abbreviated statement of the aim, methods, results, discussion, and conclusion of your work. You must take as much care in the preparation of the abstract as you did in carrying out your research. You should edit it several times and show it to a friend or two. Make sure that what you have written can not only be understood, but also cannot be misunderstood.

When the letter of acceptance of your paper arrives, waste no time. Start to prepare your talk. Obviously the prime consideration must be scientific reliability, but it is wise to remember that there are differences between the spoken and the written word. Both must, of course, be intelligible. Both must be honest and accurate. But whereas a reader can select and concentrate on parts of a paper, you have got to hold an audience's attention for the whole of your presentation. It is not a bad rule to say what you are going to say, say it, and then say what it is that you have said.

The presentation must to a greater or lesser extent follow the IMRAD pattern (introduction, methods, results, and discussion and conclusion). Sometimes you must spend more time on one of these aspects, for example, if you are describing a new method or if your results point to a new interpretation of phenomena. You will, however, always be guided by the need to never be obscure, never be boring, and never come to conclusions that are not justified by your work. Don't hedge. If your results suggest a certain conclusion, it is better to come straight out and say, "In our opinion these data support the hypothesis that. . . ." This is always more acceptable than to reach such a woolly conclusion that nobody can contradict you.

If you are going to get your message over in 10 minutes you have got to take a few short cuts. One of these is to use overhead transparencies (acetates) and slides intelligently and not to show them merely to remind you of what you want to say.

Overhead Projection

There are few indications for the use of overhead transparencies in preference to slides, and none at all when you are giving a 10-minute presentation. Overheads can sometimes be used to good effect if you are giving a review lecture. Their merit is that you can use overlays and you can reveal information as you discuss it. They should be printed on acetate in Helvetica 18 point, using no more than 12 lines and no more than seven words in each line. See also chapter 21.

Slides

The quality level of slides at surgical meetings has improved enormously in the past 20 years, but you still find people who put up a slide that resembles a railway timetable. They generally say, rather demurely, "This slide may look a bit complicated," when they ought to say, "I should never have made this slide."

Slides provide background, evidence, and illustration.[1] They must be appropriate, accurate, legible, comprehensible, and well executed. Occasionally one sees a slide that is also interesting and memorable, but that is rare. Most slides should be in "landscape" format (wider than they are high), and the proportion of width to depth is always 1.59:1 (35:22). This proportion is close to the "golden rectangle" of aesthetics, which has a proportion of 1.62:1.

What is the place of dual projection? It is certainly not to allow you to present twice as many slides in your 10 minutes (don't forget that it takes 5 seconds to read even a well-designed slide). It is an obvious courtesy to an audience whose first language is not English to present at least the most important slides in the language of the country you are in, and occasionally it may be acceptable to have one screen showing a photograph or line drawing while the other shows data in tables or graphs. If you do have dual projection, make sure that both projectors can be advanced simultaneously. That generally means that you will have to have some blank or duplicate slides.

There are four kinds of slide that you may need in a 10-minute presentation:

- Photographs (particularly portraits and photomicrographs)
- Line drawings (particularly to show details of an operation or an experimental method)
- Graphs
- Slides with nothing but words on them

The first two of these do not depend on computers or word processors, but they do require a good camera and a good artist. Slides that are made by photographing electrocardiographs and charts such as temperature charts always show too many irrelevant lines. They should be redrawn to eliminate the unnecessary lines. Radiographs should be of good quality, and it is sometimes necessary to point out lesions by using arrows. Ultrasound images should always be accompanied by line drawings.

There are many computer programs that will make graphs and word slides, including Powerpoint and Presentation Express. With these programs, however, we find that it is easy to produce slides that have too many colors and too jazzy a background. The most attractive word slides are made by using a word processing program in a computer. The font should be 24 point and sans serif (Helvetica is suitable), and printed by a laser or ink jet printer in bold italic in landscape format on standard size white paper.

The resulting art work is then photographed using Kodalith film to produce negative transparencies. These are mounted and projected as white letters on a black background, or they can be judiciously colored with a felt-tipped pen. It is most important not to overdo the color. We find that light blue, yellow, and orange are good colors. Red and green do not project well. Above all, however, remember that you are aiming at legibility above all, and a lot of color and a fancy background both detract from legibility and distract the audience from the information on the slide.

Graphs

Tufte wrote the definitive work on the visual display of data.[2] He demanded the following:

- Graphs must not lie.
- The data must be shown.
- The data-to-ink ratio must be maximized.
- All non-data ink must be erased.
- Redundant data ink must be erased.
- Lettering must be horizontal, not vertical.

The data-to-ink ratio is the ratio of the parts of the graph that disclose the data to the total amount of ink used to make the graph. For example, you should never make a slide from a graph drawn on graph paper, because the squares of the graph paper do not help in understanding the data, they merely overcrowd the slide. A large amount of data can be shown most effectively by a scattergram, which should include a mean and standard deviation if the data are normally distributed, a median and interquartiles if they are not, or a correlation line when that is appropriate. For the graphic display of proportions, bar diagrams and pie charts are suitable, but life tables should always be drawn in steps. In graphs for a 10-minute presentation it is allowable to use percentages without whole numbers, but there should be some measure of the confidence that the data can command, such as 95% confidence intervals. There should always be a denominator.

It is inevitable that you will use a computer to make your graphs. There are several programs to choose from, two of the common ones being Harvard Graphics (Software Publishing Corporation, Santa Clara, Calif.), and GraphPad (GraphPad Software, San Diego, Calif.). Whatever you do, make sure that you follow Tufte's rules.

Technique of Presentation

Should you read from a manuscript, or should you take to the lectern only a few jottings to remind you? This is controversial. On the one hand, proponents of reading from a manuscript claim that it eliminates inaccuracy and allows accurate timing. On the other hand, there are those who find that a presentation that is spoken is more likely to be lively and interesting. The rule must be to follow the custom of the society to which you are making your presentation. Whichever method you use, you should know enough about your subject to not need a manuscript. If it falls on the floor you should not have to tolerate the embarrassment of trying to retrieve it.

Personal Appearance and Manners

Burkhart wrote the following description of an inept lecturer: "Verbosity overtakes conciseness; disorganised presentation overtakes clear thinking and careful preparation; mumbles overtake articulateness; and, worst of all, you can't read the slides beyond the third row."[3] You should make sure that the audience is concentrating on your presentation, not your appearance. You should therefore dress conventionally. You should keep still so that nothing distracts attention from your words and your slides. It is a good idea to ask a friend to video record you during a rehearsal of your presentation. This will alert you to little irritating mannerisms that you must correct. When you watch an experienced television presenter interviewing somebody who has never been televised before, you cannot fail to notice that the interviewer keeps still whereas the tyro waves his or her arms about. You can make a good presentation and avoid being boring by modulating your voice. You do not need gestures.

There is no place for jokes in a 10-minute presentation, nor is it your place to be rude about a previous speaker or anybody else. During question time it is not unusual for somebody in the audience to make disparaging remarks about your work. However vexed you feel and however unjustified the criticism, you will gain a lot more sympathy from the rest of the audience by thanking the questioner for his or her observations.

The ideal speaker does not wander about the platform as if searching for a way out and does not wave the arms (or the pointer) about for emphasis. What a good speaker does is to establish rapport with the audience by being enthusiastic about the subject and, if necessary, by referring to a previous speaker's talk. The presentation will have a beginning, a middle, and an end.

Although speakers who follow all these rules make it look easy, you can be sure that they have taken a lot of trouble to make their manuscripts and slides accurate; they have rehearsed with their slides in front of a critical audience of colleagues; they have changed the order of their slides several times; they have not memorized their speech like an actor, but will always have room for a spontaneous remark.

It is just as important to present your work in a polished form as it is to conduct your research carefully. Making a presentation is an integral part of any research project, and it can be a stimulating exercise.

References

1. Evans M. Use slides. In: How to Do It, vol. 2, 3rd edn. London: British Medical Journal, 1995, pp. 117–127.
2. Tufte ER. The Visual Display of Quantitative Information. Cheshire, CT: Graphics, 1983.
3. Burkhart S. Do as I say, not as I do? Br Med J 1983;287:893.

Commentary

Few writers and speakers of the English language have done more to improve the quality of presentation of scientific data at surgical meetings than the scholarly surgeon Alan Pollock and the medical editor Mary Evans. Their appearance on a list of speakers or writers promises clear, lively, and pleasant communication—a real treat.

Reference 2 in this chapter, Edward R. Tufte's book *The Visual Display of Quantitative Information* is a beautiful work; every scientist should own a copy of this masterpiece.

B.M.

CHAPTER 19

Asking and Responding to Questions

A.S. Wechsler

Scientific societies usually afford authors the opportunity to present their work in the format of a 10-minute talk. A program committee has invariably reviewed the work on the basis of submitted abstracts and has chosen it because it will inform the audience or provoke discussion. Members of the audience are encouraged to ask the speaker questions at the conclusion of the talk, and those who are knowledgeable about the work or the field have an obligation to make constructive comments and pose appropriate questions.

Asking Questions

Critical discussion is a source of important new knowledge. The program director frequently encourages younger members of the audience to comment on work that touches on their own investigations. Commenting in this context increases the knowledge of other members of the audience and directs attention to the speaker. Depending on how a comment is made, it may be favorable, constructive, or detrimental. We offer some fundamental philosophy, in the form of the following list of "dos and don'ts":

Do

1. Do be sure you understand the data before you comment.

2. Do formulate a question that clarifies or contrasts the data, or puts the data into perspective.
3. Do write your question out in advance.
4. Do initiate discussion that is likely to be of general interest.
5. Do feel a responsibility to participate if the field is within your area of expertise or close to your own work.
6. Do remember that criticism can be politely raised in the form of a question.
7. Do put yourself in the speaker's position.
8. Do, if you wish, bring a simple, highly pertinent slide, but prearrange for its projection to avoid creating a delay in the flow of the program.
9. Do know and follow the rules of the meeting.
10. Do let the chair know, in advance whenever possible, that you wish to discuss the paper.
11. Do feel comfortable about referring to a specific slide used by the speaker.
12. Do realize the importance of the discussion to the science, the speaker, and yourself.
13. Do prepare yourself in advance by carefully reviewing the abstract(s) prior to the meeting.

Don't

1. Do not take more than your fair share of the session time.

2. Do not personalize your comments; deal with the scientific data only.
3. Do not use your comments for self-glorification.
4. Do not waste time with excessive compliments.
5. Do not ask incriminating questions.
6. Do not set up a series of questions to make your point.
7. Do not bring a handful of slides.
8. Do not give another paper.
9. *Do not even consider using a public forum to vent personal animosity or attempt to embarrass another scientist.*
10. Do not entertain your colleagues with tutorial comments as an alternative to standing and contributing to the quality of the session.

Responding to Questions

The program moderator will usually organize this facet of a presentation and should protect speakers from excessively long, abusive, or inappropriate forms of commentary. You, as a speaker, will have to do some thinking on your feet, but thoughtful preparation will pay off. We offer some helpful advice:

Do

1. Do jot down critical aspects of questions, as they are asked.
2. Do try to anticipate questions by talking with your peers and others prior to the meeting.
3. Do remember that the knowledge gradient is in your favor for your focus paper and do not

be disconcerted by the sudden appearance of an "expert" in the audience.
4. Do recognize each questioner visually, or by name.
5. Do give the shortest answer possible.
6. Do answer the question specifically, and do not use it as an opportunity to speak about marginally related topics.
7. Do prepare a couple of slides you think you may need, but keep them simple.

Don't

1. Do not waste time thanking questioners excessively.
2. Do not belittle the question or the questioner, no matter how off-the-mark the question may be.
3. Do not be afraid to admit a lack of knowledge or data.
4. Do not promise to do the suggested experiment next year.
5. Do not be afraid to ask for clarification of a confusing question.
6. Do not use the question period as an opportunity to show how much you know.

Commentary

Often the most helpful part of a scientific meeting is not the presentation, but the discussion that a speaker's data and the message provoked. This is especially true when new or controversial information is discussed. Professor Wechsler's clear dos and don'ts should set the standard for discourse at

CHAPTER 20

The Longer Talk

J. Alexander-Williams

The conventional maximum time for oral presentation of a scientific paper is 8 to 10 minutes. Anything longer than that can be defined as "a longer talk." A longer talk is usually by invitation and is a review. It may be an eponymous lecture or designated by such terms as *state of the art* or *quadrennial review*.

You are usually asked to deliver a longer talk because you are considered to have a balanced view on the subject or have made an important personal contribution. However, sometimes you are asked at the last minute because the first or even second-choice speaker has withdrawn. Generally, but not always, it is an honor to be invited, and usually you have your expenses paid for travel, registration, and accommodation. If you are the star attraction of the meeting or are sponsored by a member of the biomedical industries, you may also receive an honorarium.

Shall I Accept?

The first reaction to the receipt of an invitation to give a longer talk is one of honor to be so selected. Your feelings may soon be tinged by the pervasive doubt as to whether you have the qualifications or the time to do justice to the invitation.

The decision to accept or reject such an invitation warrants careful consideration. First, answer the following three questions:

DECIDING TO ACCEPT AN INVITATION TO SPEAK

1. Can I make a success of it?
2. Have I time to prepare adequately?
3. What's in it for me?

If you grade your answer to each of those three questions on a 1–3 scale, you need to have a total of more than 5 points and preferably more than 7 points before accepting. Before answering the second question remember that those in our profession who are invited to give longer talks almost invariably do not have sufficient time to prepare them adequately. Those of you who have scored 4 or fewer points on my scale should decline and read no further.

It is advisable first to give a tentative reply and ask for further details. Find out all the details of the meeting at which you will be speaking; find out who else will be giving papers and on what subjects and find out how your contribution fits into the overall pattern of the occasion. Make sure that the material that you have to offer will be able to excel in the context of the meeting and of the other speakers. If it won't, then draft a definitive, polite letter of declination. Do not miss the opportunity of suggesting an alternative talk on a vaguely related subject in which you know that you can excel.

Before you make a definite answer to the question "Do I have time?" consider whether the talk is a repeat of one that you have already given, a reconstruction of a number of subjects on which you have already lectured, or a totally new lecture that you have never given before. Repeating a lecture you have already given will involve a little time spent in revision of not only the text but also the illustrations. A reconstruction of previous related talks will take longer and involve a fundamental rearrangement of the arguments. A totally new subject will require a lot of time spent on the literature, research, writing, and revision. Always remember all the other things that you have planned and want to do, realizing some of them will have to be sacrificed if you are to accept the invitation to give a longer talk. Some of you will wonder why anyone ever agrees to give a longer talk; you are right to wonder.

Planning

Once you have accepted—and most of us are sufficiently egotistical to do so—you have to go through the three phases of planning: the text, the illustrations, and practicing the delivery. The key points of planning are (1) know the audience, (2) know your message, and (3) structure the talk.

Then it is a good idea to divide the talk into three parts: (1) introduction, (2) evidence, and (3) con-clusions. You should plan to spend about one-third of the talk on each. Start by planning a talk for much less time than you have been allocated. Aim at 20 minutes when you have a half-hour slot in the program, and 45 minutes if your allotment is 1 hour. Your hosts will love someone who finishes short of the allotted time (Figure 20-1).

For tyros who are concerned about keeping within the time limits, I suggest using three pale primary colors as a background for the illustrations of the three parts of the talk. The color changes are a help in accurate timekeeping.

When structuring your talk, it is essential that you define a number of stepping stones in the argument you are putting forward. Too many stepping stones can be disruptive to the argument, but, as long as the steps are logically progressive and do not deviate from the main theme, they should form the basis of the structure. An example is cited in Figure 20-2.

Once the steps of the argument have been developed, make copious notes. You can do this by having a small notebook and a pencil ever with you. I find it better to keep my notes on small cards with a hole punched in one corner and secured by a string and tabs. This means that I am able to rearrange the order of the arguments.

Always keep these note cards or pad with you. Jot down ideas whenever they occur. Have the cards or pad beside your bed at night in case you

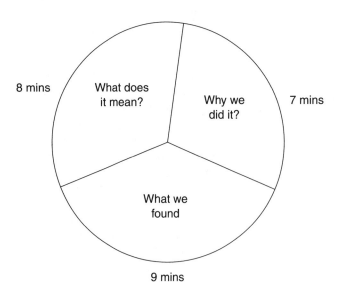

Figure 20-1. Plan for a 30-minute invited lecture.

Some surgeons report better survival results for large bowel cancer than do others.

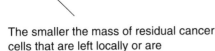

The smaller the mass of residual cancer cells that are left locally or are disseminated, the better the prognosis.

There are likely to be smaller masses of residual cells if the tumour is handled gently; the veins are tied first and all potential tumour bearing nodes are removed.

The scientific evidence will be reviewed to support or refute: no-touch isolation technique, high I.M.A. ligation, mesorectal excision and laparoscopically assisted resection.

Figure 20-2. Logical steps in the argument.

wake up with a good idea. When necessary plan one or more computer literature searches to support or illustrate your arguments.

Illustrations

Remember that "A good picture is worth a thousand words" and "Many a good story is ruined by bad slides."

The Essence of Good Illustration Is Simplicity

It is only the complete professional who can successfully mix media in a presentation. I have observed some—even experts—who have had things go disastrously wrong. Choose one medium of illustration. For a small audience, a blackboard, white board, or flip chart may be appropriate. For an audience of up to 50, overhead transparency projection is cheap and cheerful. For larger audiences there is at present no reasonable substitute for slide projection.

Disasters can occur even if you use one simple medium. My advice is not to try to mix clips of video projections into lectures, but, rather, illustrate with slides.

Keep It Light

It is also unwise to have dark and light periods in a talk, as happens when slides are switched off for a while and the house lights come on. It is better to keep a constant level of light and to keep it as brightly illuminated as possible, compatible with good visibility of your slides. Your slides must be so clear that they are easy to read in the half-light. Never have less than half-light because it promotes audience somnolence.

Avoid Disasters

I have ten commandments to ensure that you avoid the common disasters.

1. Avoid double projection, it causes four times as many problems as single projection. Dou-

ble projection is rarely or never necessary. If you wish to show two slides side by side have them remade into one slide with one image on each half.

2. Use no more than three colors. Multicolored slides decrease legibility. One dark tone on another projects badly.

3. Use no more than 32 words on a slide; under exceptional circumstances you may use up to 40. If, when you hold the slide up to the light, you cannot read it with the naked eye, there are too many words on the slide.

4. Do not print in capital letters only. Upper and lower case letters are easier to read.

5. Never make slides by photographing illustrations from textbooks or papers. When drawings are needed for illustration, use simple line drawings not halftone drawings.

6. Always project slides in the horizontal, or landscape, format. If you use vertical, or portrait, format, the punch line or caption of your slide may not be included on the screen.

7. When traveling far or by air avoid glass-mounted slides. Not only are they heavy, but however carefully you look after them, the glass may crack or shatter.

8. Do not number your slides. You may well want to alter the order of the presentation of your argument, or you may decide to delete a step in the argument; numbered slides may confuse your audience.

9. Do not date your slides unless you can cheaply make new slides for every talk. It is amazing how quickly dated slides appear to become out of date. Even a discreet institutional logo in one corner of the slide with the date written small could well alert a hawk-eyed audience to the fact that you are presenting old data.

10. Date and number the slide mount. It is particularly useful to have a label or part of the mount surface on which you can write the slide number in pencil. When you have completed the final rehearsal of your talk, then, and only then, should you number them. This may avert the disaster of the projectionist inadvertently inverting an uncovered carousel, tipping out your slides, and reducing them to random order.

RULES FOR ILLUSTRATIONS

- The essence of good illustration is simplicity.
- Keep the room light, compatible with good visibility of your slides. (Darkness promotes audience somnolence.)
- Avoid double projection.
- Use no more than three colors.
- Put no more than 32 words on a slide.
- A mixture of upper and lower case letters is easier to read.
- Never make slides by photographing illustrations from textbooks or papers.
- Always project slides in the horizontal, or landscape, format.
- When traveling far or by air avoid glass-mounted slides.
- Do not number your slides.
- Do not date your slides.
- Date and number only the slide mount.

Rehearse On-Site

To rehearse on-site, it is often necessary to arrive well before your scheduled talk begins so that you can rehearse during a break in the program. If at all possible have the rehearsal in the hall where you will be giving the lecture. This will allow you to make sure that the slide format fits the screen and that the illumination can be set sufficiently high to help the audience avoid sleep, and sufficiently low for all your slides to be readable.

Always test the microphone. If you are provided with a neck or lapel microphone you will be able to move away from the podium should you wish. However, if there is a fixed microphone on the lectern, speak to it in a normal tone of voice and have someone tell you how far away you should be from the microphone to give perfect audibility. The only thing that is worse than a lecturer too far away from the microphone is one who struts about, causing the sound to vary from deafening to inaudible. Perhaps worse still is someone who has his or her mouth so close to the microphone that the consonants and sibilants crackle and splutter. A few seconds of rehearsal can save a lot of embarrassment.

You can probably guess from my list of disasters that all of these have befallen me in the last 30 years "on the circuit."

Delivery

Dress appropriately. Even if the meeting is in the tropics, you can be reasonably sure that the lecture hall will be air-conditioned. Whatever you may wear around the pool, a Hawaiian shirt and Bermuda shorts are not appropriate for the lecture. I think that long sleeves, long trousers, and a tie are the minimum requirements, even in the tropics. In most circumstances a suit should be worn. It is amazing how some hosts are upset or even insulted by a shabbily turned out lecturer. Other points of delivery style that I think are obligatory include standing still, whether you are in front of a lectern or standing free on a stage, and the avoidance of fidgeting with the hands or shuffling the feet. A few gestures, however, may help with emphasis.

The Start

Start slowly and gently. Try to appear at ease and humble, even if you are neither of these. With your first experiences of the longer talk, you are certain to feel nervous and often in awe of your audience. In the first edition of this book, a famous American surgeon, Edward D. Churchill, was quoted as giving his antidote to stage fright. He taught himself to stand silently for a few seconds in front of the podium, during which time he did two things. First, he reminded himself that, as the speaker, he was in charge of the occasion. Second, he looked out over the assembly and, in his mind's eye, tried to visualize the members of the audience dressed only in their underwear. I have never tried this second piece of advice because I think it might make me giggle, which is never a good way to start. However, I strongly advise 2 or 3 seconds spent silently regarding the audience, followed by a simple and humble greeting of "Good-morning" or "Good-afternoon," or whatever is appropriate. Many people start the longer talk with an effusive thanks to their hosts for the invitation. I think that this can be over done. An obsequious expression of thanks often sounds to me as if the speaker is congratulating his or her hosts on their wisdom and perspicacity in inviting someone so worthy. Also, if you are over effusive you could well embarrass a sensitive host.

The Opening Slide

An eponymous lecture often begins with a picture of the "name." This often works well and is sometimes obligatory. I do not like lectures that begin with a slide of the beautiful or luxurious place in which you work. I have a rule that says "Never show a picture of a prestigious hospital from the air—it may aid terrorist bombers!" Because I had the privilege to work in a very old and, in some eyes, decrepit hospital, I would sometimes start with what I described as a "sympathy slide."

A Text

I think it best to begin with a text, as in a sermon. To find a suitable text requires thought and a little imagination. It is helpful to have available a book of quotations. An example that I have used in a longer talk that considered the advantages and disadvantages of intraperitoneal drainage following biliary or colonic surgery is a paraphrase of Hamlet's soliloquy: "To drain or not to drain, that is the question." A good text is one that summarizes in a phrase the main message of the talk. In the days or weeks before your lecture, consider many suitable texts and write them down on your cards or pad.

Practice Helps to Perfect

Peer criticism of your delivery by an informed, sensitive colleague is a boon. Performing in front of a video camera followed by self-criticism of the replayed tape is valuable and increasingly available.

Fallback Strategies

At some time in your lecturing career you will certainly have something go wrong with your organization or the facilities. The wise lecturer anticipates these catastrophes and is ready with an alternative for most eventualities. Can you give your talk without any visual aids? Think how you would manage with only a blackboard or flip chart if there is a power failure or the only projector bulb fails. Think how you would manage if discipline is so bad that the previous speakers have left you with only 10 minutes to give your 40-minute talk. It does happen, it has happened to me! Reduce your message to the absolute essentials in a form that you can convey in the minimal time, with minimal data and no visual aids. Such an exercise is good discipline and helps you to focus your message. It may turn a catastrophe into a triumph.

End Well

Study the great musical composers and the great orators. A longer talk should end with a clear message and a resounding climax. Deserve your applause by making the climax demand it. You may not achieve a standing ovation or cries of "Encore," but you should plan the end as if you expect no less. The end should be planned and practiced at an early stage in your preparation. It is unwise to leave it until the last minute, yet many lecturers do. You have probably heard a longer talk in which the lecturer had to skip rapidly through or omit the last few slides because of poor time-keeping and then finished with a deflatory, "Well, I think that is all I have time for." Such an end deserves no applause. Also avoid statements such as "time does not permit. . ." or "Chairman, may I have just a few more minutes." If your planning and timekeeping have been done well you should have plenty of time to vary the pace of the main body of your talk with quieter passages. The slower passages lead to a final crescendo at a time when the audience wishes that you would continue. Study the great composers, study the great communicators. Wonder how they do it. Analyze their techniques and copy them. You will be a great success and will have earned the applause and also the approbation.

Commentary

I use invited lectures as a curriculum for my continuing medical education by choosing topics or aspects I want to read or learn more about. This makes the preparation and the lecture more fun for me and, I believe, more fun for the audience. It is particularly effective to tell about calling or visiting someone whose work you are citing, and to introduce the human aspects of the authority to enliven the citation. For example, before giving an invited lecture titled "Immunotherapy of Cancer" to the Western Thoracic Society Association, I visited Steve Rosenberg at the National Cancer Institute in Bethesda. I talked to him, his residents, his lab people, and his patients. I took some photographs for supplementary slides. I learned and the audience learned through me about the current status of the field.

When you make up your slides don't forget that 11% of the population is red-green colorblind. See chapter 21 by Kevin and Leo McGovern on "Slides, Transparencies, and Videos."

M.F.M.

Commentary

I feel that a longer talk should always include new information combined with entertainment and humor. The beginning and the end are especially important; I prefer to use pictures or scenes that suggest a view of the future, or the larger framework around the topic. Finally, don't embarrass yourself or your host by giving a boring talk or making the host or the audience the target of your humor.

H.T.

CHAPTER 21

Slides, Transparencies, and Videos

K. McGovern and L. McGovern

Introduction

In recent years, the technology for processing and displaying information has progressed so dramatically that there seem to be no boundaries on the preparation and presentation of information. These technologies can magnify confusion, and have their own pitfalls. Good, basic techniques in preparing visual materials, and a reasonable understanding of the technology are even more essential to clear and effective communication.

This chapter is designed to be a practical "how to" guide on preparing effective slides, overhead transparencies, multimedia interactive computer-based media, and videos.

An important first step is to select a deliverable medium that portrays your topic most effectively. Video is well suited for showing a surgical technique, but not for describing statistical analysis. The size of your audience will help you determine what medium to select; a presentation using transparencies or a computer-based interactive program is applicable for an audience of 25 people, and a slide presentation is effective for an audience of 100 to 200.

Slides and Overhead Transparencies

The rule of thumb for designing slides and overheads is "6 by 6 by 6." No more than *six lines per slide*, no more than *six words per line*, and the hardcopy slide has to be *readable from six feet away* (at a size of 8.5″ × 11″).

The style of your slide will vary depending on your personal taste, but it is important that it be readable and pleasing to the eye. The color blue is typically considered to be conservative; bright colors such as bright green, orange, and pink are not recommended. Black and white are good colors for text with a consistent font style that is easily read, such as Times Roman or sans serif fonts.

Slide and Overhead Preparation Rule of Thumb

Use the following recommendations as your guide:

- 6 × 6 × 6
  No more than 6 lines per slide
  No more than 6 words per line
  Readable from 6 feet away
  (projected at 8.5″ × 11″)
- Colors
  Blue (conservative), deep green, purple, white, and black
- Font
  Readable and clean, i.e., Times Roman or sans serif at 16 to 36 point size.
- Illustrations and Photographs
  Enhance the efficiency in facilitating learning

Using Color Photos and Illustrations to Enhance Your Presentation

Color photographs and illustrations are highly recommended because they enhance instructional presentations. They have the following advantages:

- Facilitate the accuracy and standardization of the message being communicated
- Illustrate, clarify, and reinforce oral and printed communication, quantitative relationships, specific details, abstract concepts, and spatial relationships
- Provide concreteness (realistic detail) in the learning situation
- Present the learner with the opportunity to process the information (accept, reject, query)

Traditional 35-mm slides and overhead transparencies are relatively simple to create, readily available, and, in most cases, inexpensive.

Multimedia Presentation

While an effective presentation can be made with simple charts, static illustrations, and photographs, a dazzling presentation can be made with readily available software (Table 21-1) that will run on your PC or Mac. This type of software is relatively easy to use and offers a number of visual effects that will intensify your presentation, including animation, video clips, and audio. Many products come with ready-made templates for slide presentations, making it easier to create a professional graphic presentation. The presentation can be displayed through a standard television or a video projector with an additional piece of hardware called a VGA-to-TV converter. It can also be displayed through an overhead projector with the use of an LCD projection panel.

When selecting a presentation software product, important features that you will want to consider include the following:

Usability. The learning curve is important because presentation software can be complex, and you will use it only sporadically. Are the commands easy to find and easy to understand? Is a demonstration of the tutorial available and is it explanatory? Are there customization tools? Look for a generous selection of ready-made templates. As you get more adept with the software, you will become more creative with it.

Outlining and Charting. An outliner should be directly linked to the slide viewer. You will want to format and edit the graphics of your slides in this mode so you can make global changes in your presentation without changing each slide. The outlining mode allows you to bring in text from many word processor programs which are typically easier to use for editing text. You will want a decent selection of the most useful chart types.

Table 21-1. Comparison of presentation software.[a]

	Transitions and animations	Interactivity	Media synchro & editing	Graphics	User interface	Overall value
Harvard Graphics	4	5	3	4	5	4
Freelance Graphics	4	5	3	3	4	4
Charisma	3	5	3	5	3	3
Persuasion	3	5	3	4	2	3
PowerPoint	3	5	3	4	5	4
WordPerfect Presentation	2	5	3	4	4	3

[a]Ratings key: 5, excellent; 4, very good; 3, good; 2, fair; 1, poor.
New Media News (Boston Computer Society, May 1995, p. 66).

Look for the latest in multimedia chart technology such as animated chart builds and three-dimensional charts.

Synchronizing Events. For a multimedia presentation, perhaps the most fundamental aspect of the presentation is how precisely and easily you can control the events in each slide. Typically, the software gives you a Gant-style timeline to give you an overview of the presentation and the order in which the components in your slides will change (e.g., revealing text or animating a bar graph).

Important Features to Look for in Presentation Software

The following features are essential for good presentation software:

- Usability
- Outlining and charting abilities
- Synchronizing capabilities

There is a wide selection of presentation software available on both Windows and Mac platforms. For Windows you will find Harvard Graphics, Freelance Graphics, Charisma, Persuasion, PowerPoint, and WordPerfect Presentation; for the MacIntosh, Persuasion and PowerPoint are good traditional presenters that will fill the needs of most presentations. These all have good outliners, charting, templates, and help features. According to a recent comparison of available presentation software by *New Media* magazine, PowerPoint for Windows and the Mac appears to be the best overall presentation software product at the moment.

Video

The most important step in preparing for a video program is establishing clear objectives and a well-organized outline. Once the exact concept is decided, support materials can be identified and sought out.

When beginning a concept outline, you should consider three main teaching points to form the program. These main teaching points will make up the framework of the program and be the basis

of the information that is contained within the video. Most video presentations should be shorter than 15 minutes in length, so it is important that the objectives are clear and concise.

Surgical Video

A surgical video ideally consists of three sections (Table 21-2). The first part should include *appropriate background materials* such as etiology, prevalence, historical features, pathology, symptoms, medical management, surgical variations, and so forth. You can visualize these scenes with video graphics, on-camera presentations, clinical slides, and relevant surgical scenes. The second part should consist of *clinical problems and solutions.* The clinical material may include case histories, X rays, or laboratory studies of the cases you are presenting. Key operative techniques may be enhanced with medical illustrations. This section is the main part of the video and will consist primarily of operative scenes. The final part is the *conclusion.* The major points covered in the program, important objectives achieved through the program, and observations concerning future developments should be summarized here. Video graphics, on-camera presentation, or clinical slides and video clips can be used as visual references.

Once the objectives and outline have been spelled out, a production schedule should be made. Allow at least 1 month for taping, editing, revisions, and narration. This will ensure that the program is at its best before it is presented. Taping the surgery requires some preparation in order for the day of the shoot to proceed smoothly.

Once a suitable patient and day are identified, schedule the production company and notify appropriate hospital personnel, including security, public relations, and the appropriate operating room staff, that a professional video team will be in the hospital. This is best done by a short memo as well as verbally.

Brief the production staff to avoid unnecessary camera movements and lost shots of important techniques. The briefing should include the specifics of the technique to be demonstrated, the possibilities of variations that could be encountered, and the pertinent teaching points to be demonstrated. Since close communication and

Introduction	Clinical problems and solutions	Conclusion
Etiology and prevalence	Case history	Major points
Historical features	X rays	Important objectives
Variations of pathology	Laboratory studies	Observations concerning
Symptoms	Anatomical illustrations	future
Medical management and/or surgical variance		

Table 21-3. Example of revision form.

cooperation between the cameraperson and the physician is necessary to ensure a good product, a strategy should be discussed as to how to achieve these goals. The cameraperson needs to bear in mind that the physician is the best judge of what is important in the procedure, and should be ready for direction concerning where and when to shoot. Advance warning will ensure that the camera is in position and rolling at the times important techniques are demonstrated. The cameraperson will exercise his or her own judgment in filming routine techniques such as incisions, dissections, suturing, and lengthy closures to reduce editing.

Following are some recommendations that have helped us to enhance and compliment the quality of the video: (1) Avoid obese patients to allow for good exposure and to secure an unobstructed view of anatomical details. (2) When possible, multiple cases should be scheduled on the day of taping so that as much documentation as possible can be obtained in a single trip. (3) Keep in mind that taping an operative procedure can add as much as 1 hour to the case. If everyone in the operating room is aware of this, there will be less rushing toward the end of the procedure, and important details can be recorded appropriately. (4) The surgeons should avoid, as much as possible, blocking light on the operating field, and should try to keep hands, shoulders, and heads from blocking the view of the operating field. Longer instruments can help to keep the view clear for the camera. (5) It is essential that gloves, towels, and so forth be kept as free from blood as possible. (6) Colored linen, gowns, and hats should be uniform to minimize light reflections and give a more pleasing photographic result. (7) Large instruments such as retractors should be covered or satin finished to avoid glare; fine-tipped suckers will minimize visual blockage.

Endoscopic Surgery Videos

For endoscopic videos, you will not require the expertise of a professional video crew. However, it is important that you begin the project with the highest quality video format available to you. There are a number of standard video formats available, but only a few will maintain the utmost quality that is demanded by today's savvy audiences. VHS (vertical helical scan) is the most common video standard available, and it plays on most household VCRs (video cassette recorders). This is probably the format in which your tape will be distributed or projected, but it is not advisable to begin your video on this format. Videotape tends to lose quality as it progresses from generation to generation. Super VHS is a higher quality version of standard VHS and is widely available with most endoscopic equipment. Super VHS is an adequate format to maintain quality through the editing process, especially if it is edited to a higher quality format. The 3/4″ Umatic format is a higher quality format than VHS but is becoming obsolete as video technology pushes toward smaller formats. Umatic also comes in a higher quality Super Umatic format as well. Professional formats such as Beta Cam, Beta SP, and MII will insure the highest resolution in the final product.

Editing and Narrating

Once the procedure is shot, there are typically three editing stages that the tape will undergo.

The first is called the rough cut. In this stage the editor will cut out all redundancies, missed or blocked shots, and unnecessary camera movements. The tape is typically cut down to 30 minutes at the rough cut stage and sent back to the surgeon for review with a time-code window.

The second stage may comprise a number of revisions as fine tuning adjustments are made. The use of time coding will enable an organized approach to the revision process. The time code consists of the numerical definition of the frames that were recorded on the tape during the shoot. There are 30 frames per second of video, and the time code is displayed as frames, seconds, minutes, and hours. The frame numbers will not change as the tape is edited, so do not be alarmed when the revised time code does not flow in numerical progression. The surgeon can easily identify sections to be deleted or moved by the numbers displayed on the screen. The production staff should provide a form for the physician to utilize when selecting scenes to be revised (Table 21-3).

During this editing phase, the surgeon should identify the collateral visuals that will be included in the tape, such as medical illustrations, X rays, CAT scans, and video graphics. Medical illustrations require additional time to create, so plan to have them produced well in advance. It is helpful to give the medical illustrator an example of the illustration you have in mind, using scenes from the video or from the literature.

If you plan to do an on-camera introduction or conclusion, you can avoid losing the attention of the audience by limiting your talk to no more than 2 minutes. The rule of thumb is approximately 2 minutes per double-spaced page of script. The on-camera presentation should be memorized even if a TelePrompTer is available, so that it will be familiar and delivered smoothly. Always look directly at the camera as if you were speaking to an actual person. Avoid wearing patterns, stripes, or bright colors such as red or white. Try to make the last few words of your introduction lead into the section that follows it. Try to be relaxed and natural. Use a conversational or informal tone and manner, as if you were telling a visiting friend about the procedure. While all of these suggestions will keep your audience attentive and interested, acting naturally will also keep the focus off of you and on your subject.

The third stage is the narration and final edit. This can begin once the final revisions have been made to the video. By this time, you should be very familiar with the content of the video, and the narration should go smoothly. You will want to schedule at least 1 hour with the audio visual department or production company for completion of the narration. This will allow you to review the tape prior to the narration and to finalize your thoughts. The production staff will outfit you with a lavaliere microphone and a video monitor. During the actual narration, you will view the latest revision of the program on a monitor and comment while the tape is running. If you stumble or get ahead or behind yourself, ask the video technician to stop and back up to a convenient spot, such as a change of scene, and begin again. When the narration is finalized, the production company

Revision Form

Edit number from	To	Comments
Example: 1:00:05:12	1:00:14:06	Delete clamping vessel

will begin the final editing process. Once the final editing is complete, you will receive a review copy to verify that the program has been edited correctly.

Video Presentations of Nonoperative Aspects of Surgery

As computer animation becomes more capable of accurately showing things such as disease processes and drug interactions that cannot be seen with the human eye, video is becoming an ideal way to present information about the basic science background, critical care, infectious complications, and other nonoperative aspects of a surgical subject.

These types of presentations require a more traditional filmmaking technique. But as with all educational presentations, the first step is still defining clear teaching objectives. When you have decided on the topic and your objectives, develop the video script. Start with an outline and weigh the topics to be covered against the amount of time you think it will take to present them in the final product. You may want to solicit the help of a medical writer who has experience in writing video scripts. The scriptwriter will follow your direction on the information to be included, while balancing the time each subtopic receives and matching each statement with a visual concept.

The final video may consist of clinical scenes in the operating room, the ICU, trauma rooms, or on the patient floor. Typically, video graphics and, in some cases, computer animation will be included. It is important that you notify the appropriate hospital personnel of your filming schedule so that they will be prepared on the day(s) of the shooting. You may also need to ask some of the staff to be a part of the video. It is important that you gain the proper releases from all who appear in the tape (Table 21-4).

When the filming is complete, the production company will begin the editing process. Unlike the surgical video, these programs typically only go through one or two edits. The first edit you will see should be in its near-complete form. Review it for accuracy and make comments, using the time code. The next edit will complete the program.

Table 21-4.   Example of release form.

Release Form

I, _____ , hereby authorize **COMPANY** of **CITY/STATE,** to record my voice and picture for an educational videotape entitled:

_____

I acknowledge that **COMPANY** owns all rights to the aforementioned work and may licence another company to distribute it

Signature: _____

Date: _____

Parent or Guardian signature required if under 18 years old

Please type or print

Social Security Number: _____

Address: _____

Phone: _____

A clear definition of objectives, close cooperation and communication throughout the creation of the presentation, attention to detail, and presentation of the material in a well-organized manner will enable you to develop a presentation that will be memorable and educational for your audience and satisfying to you.

Commentary

With the increasing capacity of laptops and the increasing user-friendliness of presentation software, computer-based presentations should become the medium of choice for most speakers. The ability to edit, add new material, rearrange material, and, especially, to include video, animations, and sound make this medium superior to slides and overheads for most presentations. I have found computer-based (interactive) presentations very suitable for large audiences (more than 200).

A Viewpoint on Informatics in the Next 5 Years. The broad areas in which we will see major changes over the next 5 years include the use of telecommunications in clinical medicine, the use of computers in teaching and training (including virtual experience), and the establishment of peer-reviewed electronic journals that can be accessed via the Internet.

1. Telecommunication technology has advanced to the point where telemedicine is feasible and probably cost effective. Domains such as radiology and pathology lend themselves particularly well to remote diagnosis. Increasingly, the use of remote expert consultation for clinical conditions will become commonplace. This will be facilitated by the live transmission of breath sounds, heart sounds, overall images of the patient, skin rashes, and endoscopic procedures (including otoscopy and fundoscopy), along with the opportunity for local physicians to discuss the case with a remote expert while the patient is immediately available. Telemedicine will be a boon to the health care of individuals in remote areas and in developing countries, where expert advice may be difficult to obtain. Beyond this, one can envision a day when patients will be able to obtain expert advice directly from their homes via interactive TV. As this kind of data becomes digitized, it will form large banks of clinical information available for clinical research. Evidence for "evidence-based medicine" will take on an entirely new dimension.

2. Teaching and training will change dramatically over the next 5–10 years. Highly interactive teaching programs will incorporate text, narratives, animation, audio, video, and other modalities. These programs will support both the presentation of teaching materials and the assessment of the learner. They will be applicable to undergraduate and resident teaching as well as continuing medical education. Even with current technology, it is quite feasible to have a physician take a refresher course based on interactive multimedia at a university center many miles away without the physician ever leaving home. A computer, telephone line, and Internet connection are all that are needed. In the near future, direct satellite links will make these connections simpler, much faster, and quite affordable.

Virtual reality is soon to become a major force in the domain of training. Virtual clinical encounters with patients will allow students to develop interviewing skill as well as diagnostic and therapeutic skills never before attainable. These virtual patients (with a curriculum of problems) will allow the student unlimited practice rather than the restrictions of being subject to chance availability of patients with a random set of problems. The student will be able to "back up" and try different approaches with the same virtual patient in an effort to achieve excellence in interviewing. Students will also have "expert" assessment of their performance and built-in "coaching." Diagnostic and therapeutic skills can be honed in comparison to the experts in the nonthreatening environment of virtual reality. Further, the development of excellence in procedural skills, (e.g., endoscopy and surgery) will no longer depend on the availability of "willing" patients but will be brought to a relatively high level before real patients are approached. Unusual or rare situations can be encountered by the "average" physician in a virtual encounter to improve patient care and avoid complications. This broad area will be subject to a great deal of pedagogical research to determine the best new ways of teaching and learning.

3. The third area in which major changes will be seen is journal publication. The Internet has developed to the point where peer-reviewed web sites are now beginning to appear. This mode of disseminating information facilitates wide distribution of information in a timely manner. Not only will journals continue to change in this way, but expensive textbooks, generally accepted to be largely out-of-date by publication time, may become obsolete. Electronic journals and textbooks will begin to blend with teaching and training programs as each begins to incorporate multimedia in an interactive fashion.

D. Fleiszer

Commentary

Surgical meetings and most other scientific conferences tend to be dominated by visual presentation of information. Illustrating the ideas you wish to communicate with well-chosen spoken words as the only medium can be as powerful today as it was in the centuries that preceded the current era of technological sophistication in the visual display of information. Try it; you will be as surprised as your audience at the intimate relationship you can generate by excluding the distracting images on the screen. Slide-free discussions after slide-dominated talks are a familiar example of the energy this format can generate.

M.F.M.
D.S.M.

CHAPTER 22

Chairing a Session

H. Troidl and A.S. Wechsler

An invitation to chair a scientific session is an honor that carries substantial responsibility. The honor should not overshadow the important duties that the chairperson must perform. The chairperson must be knowledgeable about the subjects to be discussed during the session to be able to conduct the meeting effectively. He or she must know whether the session is to be a presentation of a collection of scientific papers or will convey a general approach to a specific topic by involving a panel of experts, each of whom will present a prepared part of the program.

When invited, it is particularly helpful to ask who will participate. In general, the personal relationship between the chairperson and the individual speakers, or a personal knowledge of their work, can contribute enormously to the quality of the session. As with any commitment, it is important to ensure before accepting that your schedule will allow you the time necessary to prepare mentally, arrive in advance of the session, conduct the program in an appropriately relaxed fashion, and close without cutting participants short because of a competing commitment of your own if the discussion is heated and goes slightly beyond the allotted time.

A good chairperson will have read the abstracts prior to coming to the meeting. Because it is unlikely that a chairperson will be an expert in every topic of the multiple abstracts that are to be presented (and because he or she frequently has played no role in the choice of those abstracts) the chairperson should, whenever possible, request copies of the abstracts well in advance of the meeting. If you discover that you are unfamiliar with the content of two or three of them, consult your colleagues about their importance and ask for suggestions of pertinent questions to ask in the event that none are forthcoming from the audience. Ask for a gentle critique of the abstract to ensure that the speaker is given the courtesy of active participation by both the chairperson and the audience during the presentation.

It is a good practice for the chairperson to be familiar with the names and appropriate titles of the speakers. Frequently, individuals presenting scientific work are from other countries, and proper pronunciation of their names will not be intuitive. Courtesy dictates that the chairperson speak to colleagues who may be more familiar with pronunciation and be prepared to introduce all speakers by their names, properly pronounced. Young investigators and presenters maybe disconcerted to hear their names mispronounced. Remember, this may be the first opportunity they have had to address a large audience; they may be very proud of being on the program and would be terribly disappointed to hear their names improperly stated at this important moment in their career. When the participants do not have a prefix such as doctor in front of their name, and you are uncertain whether you are introducing a man or a woman, preparation can avoid embarrassment for both the speaker and yourself.

Preparation for chairing a plenary session is more complex when the chairperson is expected to be an integral part of the session. In an important and large session, one strategy that is used is to meet with the presenters either the evening before or an hour before the talk, as schedules allow. If this is impossible, a group telephone conference of 15 or 20 minutes will make a great difference in how smoothly the program runs. The more comfortable speakers are with one another, the greater the likelihood that they will be comfortable discussing each other's concepts and ideas. They will be less likely to take personally opinions that are different from their own, or to waste time establishing their authority and credibility. When speakers are completely unknown to one another, there is the danger of excessive politeness which minimizes frank discussion or, alternatively, antagonism when ideas are challenged by someone whose opinions are not well understood because of inadequate preparation. The premeeting conference provides an opportunity for the chairperson to remind the speakers of their various roles, tasks, and responsibilities, and to indicate that he or she intends, for example, to be very strict about the time guidelines that have been set for each of the speakers. In addition, the chairperson has the opportunity to explain whether questions will be entertained at the end of each talk or will be held until all the speakers have spoken. The chairperson also has the opportunity to fully prepare the speakers for the program in which they are going to participate. The chairperson may even wish to rearrange the order of speakers to provide a format that is more attractive for the audience. After all, the program is being put on for the benefit of those attending, not for those speaking.

The chairperson must be familiar with the work that is to be presented by each of the speakers. He or she should read each abstract, have questions prepared in advance, and, whenever possible, be able to personalize the introduction for each of the speakers by stating their special qualifications in a particular area. This helps the speaker establish rapport with the audience before beginning to present the topic. Chairpersons must decide for themselves how active a role they will play in the discussion. If it seems appropriate, the chairperson may wish to prepare one or two slides simply for the purpose of provoking discussion, but must always remember that he or she is not the principal speaker and is there primarily to facilitate the discussion between the experts and the audience.

Conduct of the Meeting

The chairperson should arrive at the meeting site well in advance of the audience and the other participants on the program. It is the chairperson's personal responsibility to make certain that everything is well organized for the session. This means checking the projection equipment, the systems available for management of questions, the adequacy of microphones in the audience (if attendees are to be given the opportunity to ask questions from the audience), the lighting on the podium, the sound system, the integrity of the pointer that the speakers will use when giving their talk, the visibility of the screen from the vantage point of the speakers and the audience, and such amenities as having water available for speakers.

As the speakers arrive, the chairperson should greet them individually and advise them about the most appropriate place for them to sit. For example, it is convenient for the chairperson to have all of the speakers on the platform for a panel discussion, but this positioning may deprive them of the opportunity to view slides comfortably while others are speaking. When programs include speakers of multiple nationalities, the chairperson should keep in mind that there may be enormous differences in the manner in which meetings are conducted in their native countries, and great differences in the operation of the equipment. Taking a moment to familiarize the speakers with the equipment is always appreciated. Review the rules of the session if a presession conference was not held. At some meetings, there is no common language for the session, and members of the audience will hear simultaneous translations. The chairperson should bring this service to the audience's attention and clarify the procedure for questions.

Introduction of the Speakers

At the exact minute the program is scheduled to begin, it is appropriate for the chairperson to say a few words of greeting to the audience, introduce the general topic, and explain the format. This introduction should be brief, should not take away from the material that is going to be presented by the speakers, and should serve primarily to stimulate the interest of the audience in what they are about to hear. At scientific sessions where the abstracts to be presented may vary greatly, it is not necessary to provide an overview.

Once the program has begun, each speaker has an allotted amount of time; the chairperson has the responsibility for the entire program. No speaker should be allowed to talk longer than agreed upon. Many systems have a warning light when there are only 2 minutes left, and a final light indicating that there is only 1 minute remaining. If the speaker continues beyond the allotted time, the chairperson should have no hesitation in helping to terminate the talk. This can be accomplished by rising and going over to the speaker's platform, making it clear that you intend to introduce the next person. While a novice chairperson may think this behavior rude, it is unfair to the later speakers in the program to have their time usurped by an inconsiderate early participant.

Questions and Discussion

After the papers are presented, there is usually an opportunity for questions and discussion. Whenever possible, discussion should be initiated from the audience because it gives the members of the audience the opportunity to feel included in the program. Once again, the purpose of the program is to fulfill the needs of the audience and the people on the platform. In the event that there are no questions from the audience, those prepared by the chairperson become extremely important. No paper should be presented without a question asked of the presenter. A young speaker (who has spent a lot of time preparing for the program) may be "crushed" by the apparent lack of interest in his work. After a gentle question from the chairperson, multiple questions often spring up from audience members who may have been somewhat shy about being the first to ask a question.

Some of the greatest challenges to a chairperson occur during discussions. It is the one part of the program for which the chairperson can never be completely prepared. Discussion must be kept on a high scientific plane and never allowed to become personal. No one from the audience should be given the opportunity to monopolize the discussion, nor given the opportunity to present a second, unselected paper. The chairperson must gently remind members of the audience that they are to ask a question, should give them some rough guidelines about how long they may speak, and must not be afraid to interrupt someone who is abusing the privilege of the floor. It is a difficult task, but failure to do so may result in great disruption of the program. Frequently, the chairperson may note members of the audience whom he believes are experts in the field. A meeting is always made more interesting when the chairperson asks someone who is an acknowledged expert for a spontaneous opinion on difficult subject matter or for a perspective viewpoint. In the absence of audience discussion, the chairperson may wish to continue with one or two well-directed questions.

In the case of plenary sessions, the chairperson should try to provoke discussion among the members of the panel by calling on them to discuss specific issues. This reinforces the importance of being aware of the particular expertise of each of the members in the program. The chairperson must be careful not to overly express his or her own opinions but rather be willing to serve as the provocateur, the coordinator, and, on occasion, as a referee.

Chairing a session that has provided lively discussion with a good exchange of ideas is an extremely satisfying experience. While it is true that most of the credit should go to the quality and preparation of the speakers, it is frequently the special effort of the chairperson that has made good speakers coalesce their concepts into an excellent program. When the whole is better than the sum of its parts, the synergy is not an accident, and the chairperson can feel proud of a job well done.

Commentary

Like a successful operation, a good scientific session depends on careful advanced preparation, skillful execution, and the ability to think on your feet when unexpected issues arise and require changes in tactics. Professors Troidl and Wechsler's comments can be profitably read by those who appear on scientific panels, meeting planners, and those of us who sit in the audience enjoying the trials, errors, and triumphs of the moderator.

B.M.

CHAPTER 23

Organizing Meetings, Panels, Seminars, and Consensus Conferences

M.F. McKneally, B. McPeek, D.S. Mulder, W.O. Spitzer, and H. Troidl

Just as they communicate ideas by writing and lecturing, surgeons conceptualize, plan, and organize scientific meetings throughout their careers. Planning and organizing a meeting, especially a new one without an established format, is a major challenge that requires a systematic approach as well as scientific creativity.

Why Are We Meeting?

When you are called upon to plan a meeting, panel, or conference, maintain a clear vision of the *purpose of the meeting* as you choose the venue, program, size, and time of the session, and the relationship of your meeting to others whose rationale and content might otherwise be overlapped or duplicated.

Meetings of large surgical organizations like the American College of Surgeons or the German Surgical Society have several purposes that are simultaneously achieved.

1. They provide a *forum for the presentation of new clinical and scientific information.*
2. They *update the education of practicing surgeons* through postgraduate courses in clinical care and through formal and informal peer interaction.

3. They provide an opportunity for the membership to *inform the leadership* of their views and for the *leaders to present policy recommendations and reports* to the members.

The answer to the question Why, the rationale for the meeting, has an important influence on the choice of a final product to be derived from the meeting. Progression toward this goal should be part of the planning of the meeting and will influence its structure significantly. For example, a meeting to establish an organization will put more emphasis on a final banquet and the establishment of a bylaws committee. A meeting intended to document the state of the art in a field emphasizes the production of a publication based on the material presented and will expend resources for recording and editing the discussions. A meeting called to move an idea forward may terminate in a press conference.

Meetings designed primarily for postgraduate education in North America must be planned to meet continuing medical education (CME) requirements as dictated by a sponsoring university. The accrediting agency will require the proposed program, faculty, length of meeting, budget, and pre- and postsession evaluation formats. To ensure that registrants receive appropriate CME credit, which may be required annually by provincial or state licensing bodies, this planning process must be completed well in advance.

How to Do It

Organizing a meeting is a pleasant and interesting diversion for surgeons and their staff. However, as the complexity and size of the meeting increases, and the day-to-day pressures of clinical and research activities continue unabated, the resources required to ensure a successful meeting may be depleted. Professional organizations are available to assist with scientific meetings of every size, just as they are available to assist with social and business functions. Large organizations of 500 members or more may retain a professional business manager to plan and organize meetings at the direction of the executive council. The experience and skill of the organizer in dealing with international guest lists, arranging visas, accommodating audiovisual requirements and translation systems, and supervising program preparation, publicity, and social functions, far outweigh the additional cost to the organization. Professional management companies minimize confusion over submission of abstracts, preparation of manuscripts, and deadlines in preparing for publication in a journal. The professional management group adds continuity and stability to the organization and to the planning for any meeting. Professional management companies are experienced in negotiating for facilities and supplies for the meetings. Their involvement in the budgeting process and their ability to identify sources of revenue is very helpful.

International meetings present special problems and opportunities. They are more difficult and costly to organize because of differences in language and travel distances, but they contribute to the shrinkage of the world in terms of dissemination of surgical knowledge. An international meeting may be designed to fulfill any of the functions of meetings described above. International meetings entail certain specific considerations, such as jet lag or time zone changes, that should be factored into the scheduling of international speakers. Language problems should be anticipated in the development of panels. A clear policy must be delineated from the outset regarding the choice of language for the meeting. Arrangements for international meetings may be complicated by poor communication. Time zone changes, local holiday schedules, and imperfect distribution systems for information demand a much greater lead time. Telefax and telex are useful, as are international couriers and even diplomatic pouches, when the mail and the telephone will not do the job. Electronic mail (E-mail) and the Internet are rapidly opening up communication across time zones and national boundaries, facilitating international meetings. These advances can be used by planning committees for posting, advertising, registration, abstract submission, program publication, and access to presented papers. The Cardiothoracic Surgery Network web site (www.ctsnet.org) provides worldwide communication in that surgical specialty.

Some common features of the organization of a surgical meeting include the *organizing committee*, which should meet well in advance to plan the topics, speakers, chairpersons of sessions and panels, location, time, and size and length of the meeting. The objective or rationale for the meeting provides the guidelines for the decisions of the organizing committee.

A meeting that is primarily directed at the collection and dissemination of new scientific knowledge usually requires a request for abstracts. Plan enough lead time for the abstracts to be submitted and screened by a *program committee*, which will ultimately determine the final program for the meeting. Many scientific meetings request that each speaker produce a paper for publication to be delivered to the recorder at the time of presentation. This document must meet the publication requirements of the sponsoring journal or publisher of the symposium. It is imperative that a decision regarding manuscript preparation be made and communicated well in advance. Attempts to record oral presentations and turn them into a permanent record of the meeting are notoriously difficult.

Meetings developed to promote a specific idea or new surgical concept often include investigators with a special interest in the concept or technique, who have a leadership role and interesting data to present. Other investigators with a more traditional or different approach are invited to present an opposing viewpoint. This may take the form of sequential short presentations followed by discussion, chaired by a carefully chosen moderator. Small group discussions carefully spaced between formal presentations enhance discussion and allow for the definition of a position paper based on the available data. Publications of the proceedings of these meetings may well require recording of discussions as positions evolve during the course of the meeting. It is important that an editorial committee take on the responsibility of collating and editing the manuscript and subsequent discussion.

Business Meetings

Surgical organizations generally hold a business meeting in conjunction with their scientific meetings. These should provide a well-organized opportunity for introduction of new members and committee reports, as well as allowing direct communication between the leadership and the members. Committee reports and controversial agenda items should be well prepared. To avoid lengthy floor discussion, major decisions such as changes in bylaws or policies are sometimes presented in writing at a preliminary meeting at the onset of the congress.

Where to Meet

The location of the meeting and the associated social program enhance free exchange of ideas. A degree of isolation in a resort setting increases attendance at the scientific sessions and facilitates informal discussion in a relaxing atmosphere. The degree of isolation, however, should not preclude relatively easy access for busy surgeons. The overall length of the meeting should be realistic, as should the length of the scientific session. Group discussions lasting longer than an hour usually become nonproductive. A change in format or a diversion from the topic at hand will increase overall productivity.

Paying for the Meeting

Careful thought must be given to the financing of any meeting, particularly an international meeting. Professional organizers are helpful in developing and strengthening funding. The meetings associated with a scientific organization are usually supported by the membership through annual dues or the levy of an attendance fee. This may include the cost of all social functions, or it can be designed to cover the cost of the entire meeting, minimizing the subsidy required by the organization. Surgical meetings designed to promote a concept or develop a consensus usually require the support of a surgical organization, hospital, or university. In many cases, the funding can be augmented by obtaining support from the many companies represented in the surgical-industrial complex. To be certain that the sponsors' expectations for publicity or endorsement are not unrealistic or unmet, specific guidelines must be established at the outset and administered uniformly.

Format

The format of the meeting varies with its purpose. Small breakfast sessions, fireside chats, or meet-the-professor sessions give participants informal access to leaders in the field. Motion pictures provide a venue for exchange of technical information in a relaxing format. Fun is important, and opportunities to swim, hike, and participate together in sports or other physical activities enhance the attractiveness of a meeting.

The social program should be interesting, diverting, and appropriate to the interests of the participants, their spouses, and guests. Educational programs about the interesting features of the setting for the meeting provide common and stimulating diversion, which can increase the energy and enthusiasm of the scientific portion of the meeting. Many successful scientific meetings are carefully programmed to allow substantial periods for relaxation and social activity, which increase absorption and reflection on the scientific material presented. A dense program of continuous scientific activity reduces creativity and responsiveness of the participants.

Panels

Panel discussions have been particularly popular and successful in the United States for many years, and they are now widely used in most other countries as well. There are two common formats. One is the combined half-hour panel discussion as a joint question-and-answer period following several individual formal presentations. The other format is a true panel discussion, in which the panelists take their places on the platform at the outset. The moderator offers brief introductory remarks, and each panelist speaks for not more than 5 to 8 minutes on a particular aspect of the main theme. An open discussion follows to illuminate what the speakers have said. Panel discussions are informative in an authoritative and emphatic way because of the participation of several experts who are able to offer well-based opinions on any issue that may be raised. Properly handled by the moderator, such a group can provide a lively and entertaining exposition of the subject under consideration.

For variety, the moderator may pick a controversial clinical problem and have each of the speakers present their views on the optimal management in a short, formal, illustrative talk. The moderator then presents a clinical case to the panel. The results of key investigative studies are progressively revealed when they are requested by a member of the panel or prompted by a question from the audience. Surgeons with opposing views are asked to defend their positions in relation to the particular problem. This leads to a stimulating discussion in which the audience can participate by written or spoken questions.

Panels are popular with audiences because of their informality and variety, and because they offer the opportunity to hear and contrast different points of view. Listeners particularly enjoy the opportunity to participate in the interchange of ideas through questions or comments. This aspect of a panel discussion, though sometimes technically difficult or inconvenient for the moderator and the panel, is an important one and is well worth the effort required to make it successful.

The success and productivity of a panel depends on the expertise, tact, and wisdom of the chair, the specialized knowledge and communication skills of the participants, and the care and thought put into the planning and organization of the panel.

The Choice of Speakers

The best speakers for a panel may differ somewhat from those who would be ideal to address a congress because the panel requires a greater degree of spontaneity and interactive skill.

Panelists should represent fairly both sides of any controversial issue. The ideal panelist is an accepted authority who is expert at expounding his ideas and engaging in debate. At international meetings, panels can be very challenging. If a common language is chosen, it is usually English. Many doctors whose native language is not English have a good command of the language during a prepared talk, but few are up to a brisk, hard-hitting panel discussion that is not in their mother tongue. It is particularly difficult to transmit humor across the language barrier because it so often depends on subtle nuances. As a consequence, panel discussions in English with multinational participants tend to be rather humorless, in sharp contrast to the spirit that pervades a first-class discussion in which an element of humor is an important, if not indispensable, ingredient. The use of simultaneous translation at international meetings, despite the immense skill displayed by experienced interpreters in translating complex ideas extemporaneously, inevitably slows and occasionally confuses the process of discussion. It also tends to suppress attempts to enliven the proceedings.

The person responsible for the selection of participants should be certain to include with their invitation the names of all other panelists, the anticipated composition of the audience, a clear statement about the duration of the presentation, specific questions regarding required visual aids, a request for a current curriculum vitae to assist in introductions, an indication of the method of reimbursement of travel and expenses, and whether there will be an honorarium.

The Moderator

The key to opening a successful panel discussion, the moderator should be a good speaker whose knowledge and credibility in the field allow firm and positive intervention, reasonable discipline, and the maintenance of an agreed timetable and agenda. A good moderator has a sound overall knowledge of the subject, but need not be familiar with its more abstruse aspects. A moderator who is well known as a strong protagonist of certain controversial beliefs must allow and encourage the expression of contrary views, controlling the assertion of their personal convictions. Biased moderators are like defense or prosecution lawyers who are elevated to a judgeship. To be effective, they must assume an impartial attitude appropriate to the higher office. When planning a meeting, it is useful to know the personality and style of the candidates for moderator, based on previous performance in similar situations. Some individuals have rightly earned reputations as superb moderators and are widely sought after for this role.

A good moderator brings out the strong points of each member of the panel by skillful questioning. This is best done in an atmosphere of cordiality and good humor. A moderator who knows the panelists well can foster such an atmosphere. At the close of a panel, it is useful to have a closing statement from the moderator, which can be developed from notes taken during the course of the discussion.

At the end of a panel discussion, the speakers and audience should feel that the moderator has exercised firm control, maintained a reasonably objective stance, and given all the members of the panel a fair opportunity to express their views. This will not happen as a matter of luck or even of considerable skill, if exercised only during the meeting. To ensure success, the moderator will need to get in touch with the speakers before the meeting to define the limits of their discussion very clearly and to obtain outlines of what they intend to say.

Every attempt should be made to start and finish at the appointed hour. Mechanical timers are helpful in controlling brief presentations. Time discipline can be maintained with tricks such as gavel pounding, placing a samurai sword, a water pistol, or a rose on the table in front of the moderator (leaving the intended use of such objects to each speaker's imagination), or announcing that a trap door will open or the lights and microphones will go off at the end of the assigned time. If an inconsiderate speaker fails to observe the time requirements, the moderator should walk to the podium and gently take the microphone to share the problem of time pressure with the speaker and the audience. The moderator may then invite the speaker to continue the discussion during a subsequent part of the program which may never materialize.

Prediscussion Planning. The moderator is responsible for making certain that the topic to be discussed is well covered. The success of the panel depends on the moderator's explicit instruction to the panelists to be sure that the main theme is covered without overlap. *A carefully written mandate to individual speakers from the moderator well in advance of the panel discussion is the only effective method of preventing duplication and ensuring adequate coverage of the chosen topic.*

Briefing. Most successful moderators hold a preliminary meeting with their panelists the day or the morning before the discussion is to take place. If you have been chosen to act as a moderator, use this occasion to explain your thoughts on how the discussion should be conducted, and briefly review the presentation of each speaker. Some rather surprising things may be learned at such meetings. For example, a speaker who has been instructed to present an 8-minute summary of his subject may announce that he has carefully budgeted 30 minutes of formal discussion with 60 slides. The preliminary meeting is the time to clarify what will happen in the conduct of the panel. Refine general strategy; change the order of talks, if necessary, to make them more effective, and deal with technical problems to ensure that the formal presentations go smoothly.

The panel members can decide who is best equipped to handle particular questions, and panelists can be prepared for preselected questions to lay the groundwork for a lively debate. Occasionally, it is impossible to arrange a preliminary meeting of this kind, and the moderator may have to rely on the second-best arrangement, which is a telephone conference. The third choice is correspondence; this is usually the least satisfactory. Use whatever means are required, but do not omit the preliminary meeting.

Questions

The classic method of securing audience participation is to invite written questions. Cards are distributed to the people in the audience so that they can write down their questions during the formal presentation. Preprinted question cards should indicate to whom the question is directed and the name and address of each individual raising a question. The question cards are collected by assistants who stroll the aisles. There is often a break for coffee between the portion of the symposium allocated to the presentation of papers and the subsequent period assigned to the panel discussion. This convenient interval is available to look through the questions before the discussion begins. If there is not a break, time pressure makes the sorting of questions difficult. An assistant and some planned questions will help you through this difficult period. It is always best to have two people available for sorting questions. If the moderator is sorting while asking questions, the panel discussion may get out of control.

For foreign guests, very clear questions prepared in advance may avert the problems inherent in their participation in panels when there is a language problem. Know the communication skills of your panelists and prepare them for the questions they will be asked. There are some very interesting and pertinent questions that should be asked about the topic under discussion. Even if you intend to collect questions from the audience on question cards, it is perfectly reasonable to have a prepared set of questions that will focus the discussion, and to forewarn your individual panelists. This reduces spontaneity only slightly and helps the panelists compose their thoughts about some questions. You can enliven boring sessions by altering the age or setting of the clinical problem presented by the audience. The discussion can be controlled effectively by grouping submitted questions into topic areas that fall within the expertise of particular panelists. If you make up three questions for each speaker from your own knowledge of the topic and choose three additional questions from those submitted by the audience, an orderly and interesting discussion can be anticipated.

The alternate way of obtaining questions from the audience is to allow them to use microphones strategically placed about the conference room. This provides spontaneous and direct contact with the audience, but it suffers from several disadvantages. Some people are inhibited by the equipment itself. Floor microphones sometimes have technical problems. The most serious problem is that the microphone takes control of the discussion away from the moderator. Floor microphones should be monitored, and a technician should be on duty to activate and deactivate a microphone on the command of the moderator. Turning off the microphone is an effective way to deal with audience members who present lengthy statements or arguments instead of questions. If discussion from the floor is to be recorded for transcription, the moderator must assure that the discussant's name and city are clearly stated.

The use of an interactive audience response system allows listeners to display a "pedagogic vote" on what they think is the best answer to a question, particularly about patient management. Although they are expensive, these systems can add vitality and fun to meetings; they may clarify the extent to which new ideas and techniques have diffused into current practice among the participants.

Seminars

Seminars are usually small group presentations in which the seminar leader serves as a facilitator, eliciting participation of the audience. Skillful direction of a seminar is a fine teaching art; the keynotes are informality and participation. The purpose of the seminar and the general rules for its conduct should be clearly stated. Since an enthusiastic audience may use up all the available time, it is important to announce the subheadings of the seminar clearly through an outline on the blackboard or a transparency; this allows the discussion to progress through the full range of the topics scheduled for review.

Seminars may serve to expose students to the thinking of the seminar leader or visiting professor. Case presentations or research project presentations by the students provide an excellent format for accomplishing this purpose. Slides tend to reduce the spontaneity and creativity of seminars; they should be used sparingly.

Consensus Conferences

A consensus conference is a formalized way of seeking advice. It may be called by a policy maker, such as the minister of health, or science and technology. The convening authority seeks the advice of the conference members to deal with unresolved scientific, medical, or social problems when a summary of the current state of scientific knowledge in the field is required for the development of a new course of action. The policy recommendations may relate to treatment of patients or to assignment of resources to fund research. Consensus conferences almost always attempt to reach an agreement among experts as to exactly what is known about the specified topic, what issues are settled, and what issues are still open to debate. It usually tries to focus the attention of the convening authority on areas of potentially fruitful research.

Participation in a consensus conference is almost invariably by invitation. The sponsor wants advice that cannot be successfully assailed or discredited. Members of consensus conferences are sought from a wide spectrum of scientific backgrounds, and representation of minorities, political groups, and partisans is emphasized. The attempt to ensure that the whole process will be perceived as thorough, complete, inclusive, and honestly executed may lead to an inconclusive, bland position paper that displeases no one. Beware of this.

Consensus conferences have proven to be useful for translating evidence from research studies into professional policy. Consensus conferences should emphasize scientific evidence and attempt to minimize the impact of the unsupported personal opinions of panel members, no matter how senior or prestigious they may be. The National Institutes of Health in the United States have used consensus conferences to integrate considered opinions of recognized experts in many controversial areas.

If you are asked to chair such a conference, be fair, but take a position. Seek the support of a very skillful, informed scientific secretary to take notes during the deliberations and to write a clear account of what has happened, so that the report of the discussion will reflect the true consensus faithfully. *It is extremely difficult to chair a meeting effectively and take notes at the same time.* With a scientific secretary it will be easier for you to develop a report that avoids introducing your own biases more heavily than is warranted.

Conclusion

Maintain a clear vision of the purpose of your meeting.

The location, social program, and format influence the scientific productivity of a meeting.

Publication of the proceedings and presentations from a meeting requires more lead time and much more forethought.

Professional management provides continuity, stability, and knowledge.

Successful panels require explicit mandates to the speakers, and careful briefing.

The ideal panelist is an engaging, spirited debater.

Humor is an important, if not indispensable, ingredient of panel discussions.

Question periods are inconvenient but very engaging for the listener.

Consensus conferences guide policy through carefully balanced summaries of the current state of knowledge.

Fairness and representativeness may lead to bland, inconclusive consensus. Be fair, but take a position.

The keynotes for successful seminars are informality and audience participation.

Checklist for Organizing a Meeting

Develop a time table: Call for abstracts and establish a program deadline

Develop a budget and seek sponsorship

Assess adequacy of site: Consider conference rooms, banquet facilities, hotels, transportation

Reserve adequate space for scientific or industrial exhibits

Select hotels

Develop a promotional schedule and consider advertising

Travel arrangements: Appoint an experienced travel agency

Social program: Final banquet, spouse tours; appoint an experienced agency

Scientific program: Publication of abstracts, recorder at meeting, CME certification

Audiovisual requirements: Microphones, projection (slides and video), translation, professional projectionists

Appointment of guest speakers: Honoraria, plaques

Press conference

Administrative: Staff for registration, CME credits

Recognition: Certificates for participants, gifts for support staff and special guests

Acknowledgments. The authors are grateful to Mr. William T. Maloney of Professional Relations and Research Institute, Inc., 13 Elm Street, Manchester, MA 01944, for helpful advice and review of the manuscript.

Additional Reading

Hoaglin DC, Light RJ, McPeek B, Mosteller F, Stoto MA. Data for Decisions. Cambridge, MA: Abt Books, 1982.

McPeek B. Consensus conferences: seeking advice. Theor Surg 1989;3:169–170.

Neugebauer E, Troidl H. Meran Conference on Pain after Surgery and Trauma. A Consensus Conference of Various Clinical Disciplines and Basic Research, 10–14 May 1988 in Meran, South Tyrol, Italy. Theor Surg 1989;3:220–224.

Professional Meeting Management, 2nd edn. Birmingham, AL: Professional Convention Management Association, 1990.

Commentary

One of the first recorded consensus conferences was held in 1348 in Paris. Its summary statement went something like this:

> We the faculty of the University of Paris at the Sorbonne, after careful discussion and thoughtful consideration, solemnly declare that in a region of India, near the sea, the stars which struggle against the sun and the fire in the sky caused the water of the sea to vaporize. The cloud of vapor darkens the sun. After 28 days of intense struggle the water evaporated, the fish died, and the vapors formed a miasma, covering Arabia, Crete, Macedonia, Hungary, Albania. When this miasma comes to France and Sardinia, there will be many deaths. No one can save the inhabitants, unless they follow the special rules declared from this consensus conference.[1]

Their recommendations emphasized staying indoors, or at least under cover to avoid contracting the plague from the miasma in the air or the rain that fell from it. The consensus view on the etiologic agent seems to be that the monsoon in India caused the plague in Europe.

The European Society for Endoscopic Surgery used the consensus conference as a way to summarize current knowledge of laparoscopic procedures.[2,3] This was an exception to the rule that most large surgical societies, conscious of the impact of their endorsement and their vulnerability to lawsuits, avoid the issue of systematic evaluation for new surgical technologies. "The Cologne method" was developed to meet the need for an accurate statement about the state of the art of endoscopic surgery.

1. One year before the conference, the topic was chosen, based on the availability of preliminary data in the literature and a real need for a focused opinion. There was no general agreement about the new technology and its place in clinical surgery, and there was some concern about potential harms related to the treatment.

2. The literature was reviewed and scored using strict criteria for scoring of evidence (unconfounded randomized trials ranked highest, anecdotal experience and case reports ranked lowest).

3. A panel of experts and nonexperts was chosen. Nonexperts were viewed as important because of their lack of bias toward the new technology. Experts were chosen on the basis of their scientific reputation, influence, and published work, and considerations of geographic representation. All of the panelists were queried with a survey asking them to define the questions that should be addressed by the conference, emphasizing the clinical relevance of the question. Through an iterative process, the question list was modified to assure that the most

important answers would be developed by the conference.

4. The selected literature was then circulated to all members of the panel. (It is important to note that panelists were not informed of who the other panel members were, in order to prevent interaction and premature coagulation of views, leading to bias.) Written opinions based on their own experience and their evaluation of the literature were sought from the panel. The answers and the grades of evidence were correlated at the conference center in Cologne for presentation at a subsequent meeting.

5. Panelists were asked to come two days before the general meeting of the consensus conference and meet each other for the first time, to begin the consensus process. They received a summary of the results of the survey and had a face-to-face discussion on every question. Conclusions were drawn, and dissenting opinions recorded, including the reasoning behind the opinion. The organizers and the panel then presented these conclusions and their reason-

ing to the general endoscopic meetings in Cologne and in Madrid. Audience responses to the views of the panel were factored into the report. Following review of all of this material, a preliminary document was published.

Although this was a very open process, it excluded some important stakeholders; for example, it lacked the viewpoints of patients, representatives of government, or insurers.

M.F.M.
H.T.

1. Schipperges H. Die Kranken im Mittelalter. München: Beck Verlag, 1990, p. 40.
2. Neugebauer E, Troidl H, Kum CK, Eypasch E, Miserez M, Paul A. The EAES Consensus Development Conferences on laparoscopic cholecystectomy, appendectomy, and hernia repair. Surg Endosc 1995;9:550–563.
3. Neugebauer E, Troidl H. Consensus methods as tools to assess medical technologies. Surg Endosc 1995;9:481–482. Editorial.

CHAPTER 24

Speaking at International Meetings: Surviving on the Road

A. Fingerhut and J. Perisat

As medical societies and meetings multiply, surgeons are strongly and repeatedly solicited to travel to give a talk, participate in a scientific conference or meeting, or meet with a group of other physicians to elaborate on specific issues. When this means taking an airplane, traversing different time and weather zones, eating different food, sleeping in strange places and conditions, and meeting many new people, "battle fatigue" can take its toll. In this chapter, we endeavor to advise the traveling surgeon how to survive when on the road.

When you are invited as a speaker or when you have been chosen to present a paper in a foreign country, remember the following rules:

- You are a *guest*, and usually a well-taken-care-of guest. But as a guest, you must remain in your place, be polite, and be respectful of local customs, traditions, and protocols. Although being polite is usually self-evident in all countries, special attention must be paid to the tone of your voice, especially in public places, the way you give reverence to highly placed officials, elders, and women (for men), and the way you drive a car, dress, and pay for services (bills and tips).
- You are a *representative* of your country, your city, your hospital, in that order of decreasing importance. What you say, either in your talk or as a comment from the floor, will often be interpreted as being the policy of your country.

Specify, when you talk, that what you say represents the results of (personal) study, the results of a national school of thought, or a national study or trend.
- You are a foreigner in a country where the culture and language are not yours. Be aware of the problems that language barriers can create. Misunderstandings may be very poorly accepted and will taint your own (and your country's) reputation.

Preparation

The Invitation

Either your free paper has been selected, or you have been invited to give a talk on a specific topic. In the first case, you can skip the rest of this section and go directly to the "Travel Plans" section.

Once the invitation has been received, it is polite and correct to respond as quickly as possible. This can be done directly by telephone when you receive the invitation via a telephone call, or by telephone or fax if the invitation comes by mail, but you should *always confirm your participation in writing*. A telephone call has the advantage of enabling the two parties to converse and make sure that there are no misunderstandings. Begin to prepare (see checklist 1 in Box 24-1). About one month before the meeting, give the person who is inviting you another telephone call to confirm that you are coming and to learn of any changes (see checklist 2 in Box 24-1).

The person who invites you is not always the one who takes care of other matters, so it is important to know who takes care of what. Will registration be paid for directly by the host or should the speaker pay for it and then be reimbursed? Should the speaker make his or her own travel plans, or will the host take care of this with a local travel agency? If the host makes the arrangements, it should be clear whether the plane tickets are first or economy class. Putting everything in writing will avoid later confusion.

Travel Plans

Plan your trip well in advance. Fares are cheaper if you reserve your tickets well ahead of the date of departure and stay over a Saturday night. You might want to take advantage of your trip to a far-off destination to visit with friends or visit another destination. If your traveling expenses are covered by the organizing committee or by your host, sometimes the tickets are economy but the speaker can pay the difference to fly first or business class. On other occasions, the hosts reimburse first or business class, but the speaker is free to bring his spouse along if both go economy class. Along more sordid lines, beware of invitations without written confirmation, because reimbursement can be a problem later on. Strange as it may seem, this happens in one's own country more often than in foreign countries! Be prepared to give the *original* ticket stub to the local organizers for reimbursement.

Preparation of Luggage

Remember that your overall luggage weight is theoretically limited to 20 kg. This is especially adhered to when traveling economy and on some airlines. One way to avoid being overweight is to put the heavy articles (books, full bottles as gifts, for instance) in your hand luggage. The inconvenience is that you have to carry it. Do not put anything in the checked luggage that is essential to your talk (slides, videos); if your slides or other

materials are lost or delayed in arrival, you may have to give your talk without them.

Suits and dress shirts may get very wrinkled during the trip, because valises get squashed and are often mishandled. Special attention must be paid to the way you pack them. Separate packaging for shirts and suits, or wrapping these in commercially available cellophane or plastic bags (placed in the valise) is recommended. Carry-on suit holders are very convenient, but they usually do not allow you much room to include anything else.

Clothes

Preparing one's garments and paraphernalia for travel takes a little time. There are shirts, trousers, suits, blouses, dresses, and skirts made out of "wrinkle-free" or "crease-free" material. They do not wrinkle or crease in your traveling cases, and most are also "drip-dry," which means that these clothes can be washed when on the road, hung up in the bathroom, and worn only a few hours later without ironing. The only problem is that they are not available or easily found in all countries. Most department stores, especially in North America and Hong Kong, have them.

Look carefully at the program and your personal invitations before leaving to make sure that you have the proper attire for every event. Many countries (especially the United States) have dinners where formal dress ("black tie") means wearing a tuxedo, dinner or smoking jacket, or a long dress or gown. Ask your host about the dress requirements for social events. If you don't own formal attire, you can often rent it.

Take into account the local climate. In hot, humid climates you might need to change shirts several times a day. Don't forget special attire such as a swimming suit, sunglasses, sandals, and so forth. Check on weather conditions in the country where you are going just before leaving. In this way, you will not forget that extra sweater or raincoat that you planned on leaving home. Boots and other specific attire can be planned accordingly.

Travel light. Count the number of days you will be away and the number of events for which you have to be "presentable." This means that you take enough clothes for the number of days you are away, or wash some in your room, or send them

---

Box 24-1. Travel Checklists

Checklist 1: Between the moment you
receive the invitation and at
least 1 month before the
meeting

1. Check if you need a visa. Make certain your passport has not/will not expire.
2. Call your travel agent to make travel arrangements.
3. Start research on your talk; either get out the old slides or start to make new ones. Think of an original idea specific to your host.
4. Get acquainted (through the guide) with the area and the country you are about to visit.
5. Make sure you have told your host how you are registering and how you are traveling.

Checklist 2: Less than 1 month before the
meeting

1. Check if the visa is ready. Locate your passport.
2. Check if your travel plans correspond with last-minute changes in meetings outside of the program. Check if travel plans include other (noncongress) meetings as well as pre- or postmeeting tours.
3. Review your slides before leaving home. Start rehearsing.
4. Have you bought (or thought about) the gift for your host?
5. Plan your valises according to the nature and length of your stay.
6. Ask your bank if it is better to change money before you leave, or to change your own currency in the country where you are going. Ask if it is best to bring along your own currency or dollars (cash or travelers' checks).
7. Ask your host what the weather is usually like. (Do you need an overcoat, umbrella, scarf, boots, bathing suit?)
8. Inform your host of your travel plans (airline, flight number, exact time of arrival and departure). Ask your host how to get from the airport to the hotel (maybe this way he or she will arrange for someone to pick you up).

Checklist 3: Last minute

1. Make sure you have your tickets, passport, and visa.
2. Ask your host what the weather is like.
3. Make sure your valise is complete but light. (Don't forget changes according to last-minute weather report modifications.)
4. Check your foreign currency.

---

to a laundry. You may, according to the country to which you travel, take advantage of your trip to purchase new attire. Cotton is especially inexpensive in the United States, wool is inexpensive in Australia, and silk a good buy in Asia.

Gifts

Bring a gift to the person who invites you (and/or to his or her spouse). Especially welcome are specialty gifts from your home country, perhaps bought duty-free upon departure. Try to remember what you brought along the last time so that gifts are not duplicated. The gift should be offered either directly to your hosts if you are staying with them, or when they pick you up at the airport, or else when you arrive at the dinner or reception they will inevitably give.

Vaccinations and Chemoprotection

Check with the embassy of the country you are traveling to in order to know what vaccinations if any are mandatory and what advice may be given for malaria chemoprevention. Make sure that you are correctly vaccinated for tetanus, poliomyelitis, and diphtheria. Vaccination for hepatitis A and typhoid is recommended only if you are going to rural countries with known risks.

Malaria is probably the widest spread parasitic disease in the world, and frequent flyers like you are as susceptible as any other tourist. The risks vary, and chemoprotection differs accordingly. Seek information at the local embassy, because the endemic areas differ from one country to another, and from one region of a given country to another. Chemoresistance varies according to the species prevalent in the country or area you are traveling to, and progress in drugs is continually accelerating. The following points might help in prevention. *Anopheles* mosquitoes usually bite at dawn or during the night. One single bite is enough! The risk of mosquito bites increases after the rainy season for 6 weeks. When in infested countries, use the protection offered locally (screens) and restrict going out at night, but if you do go out, wear long clothing, do not leave lights on and doors or windows open. Commercial repellents and insecticides are available worldwide and in most airports.

Chemoprotection is a must, but it differs from one country to another. In case of fever, nausea, vomiting, or unusual fatigue during your stay or the two months following your return, a high index of suspicion should be the rule. See a specialist immediately.

The Talk

Be sure it is clear in what language you will speak. Ask about the audience; if the members of the audience do not speak the official language, it is often advisable to have someone translate your slides into the local language and do a double projection (same slides at each show). Are they general surgeons or specialists? Are they academics or in private practice? You may have to modify your talk accordingly (see checklist 1 in Box 24-1).

In a long talk, it is appropriate to begin with a kind word to your host, your audience, your host country, or, ideally, all three. Avoid implying that where you come from seems better. A highly appreciated introduction might include a few words of history, a mention of local customs as they influenced your talk or venue, or, in some cases, just a few words in the local language if you can manage it. Specific introductions, however, require research and a little more preparation. Do your homework in advance.

WHEN THINGS GO WRONG

Do not blame your host.
Do not blame yourself.
Just go on as though you had not noticed and do your best.

Videos

Meeting organizers will usually specify the type and format of video that can be shown. If you do not have this information, you must ask beforehand, or you may not be able to show your film. Some projectors will convert formats. Within Europe, in some countries, your color PAL version, although VHS, will come out in black and white only. If the correct projectors are not available, it

is often possible to have your photography department do the necessary conversion. Just as a reminder, in Europe, most videos are PAL-SECAM, whereas in North America the videos are U-matic.

Always travel with two complete sets of your slides and two complete manuscripts of your talk. Carry a copy of your talk and a set of the slides carefully packed in some hand luggage you never let out of your sight. You don't want the airline to send your slides to Boston and you to Bombay.

Slides

Sizes

The size of slides is usually standard. However, be sure that the thickness of the plastic frame is standard. In some countries, thick (usually metal-reinforced) plastic is used and will not fit into most slide projectors. Beware of paper (fragile) frames that do not always work in some settings and are easily mishandled. Several commercially available software programs make excellent quality slides. Do not go overboard, however.

Double Projection

Don't count on double projections unless agreed to or specified in advance. Rehearsal is of utmost importance before trying your luck in this domain. Nothing is more annoying to the audience or frustrating to the speaker than to have mismatched slides and then have to say "forward on the right," and "backward on the left," which usually turns out to be the wrong way around anyway. Do not plan on any specific maneuvers when the operator does not speak or understand any of the languages you know. This will invariably lead to disaster.

Generalities

Never put your slides (or videos) in checked luggage. Always carry them with you on the plane. If your luggage is lost or delayed, you will still be able to give your talk. Number your slides and place a mark (sticker or arrows) to show a specific direction (usually the top), so that if they fall out of the bin when you are not around, the slide projector operator can put them back in order. Arrive at the meeting in advance. It is *very important* to show up ahead of time in order to place your slides in the bin yourself and preview them. Most meetings have a slide projection room for this. In some settings, you may be asked to give a talk, but the organizers have no slide projector. Ask before hand. Also, plan to come in advance to the room in which you will be speaking. This will familiarize you with the general atmosphere and help you get a sense of the size of your potential audience. You will also be able to learn how the spotter works and whether the microphone will be placed around your neck or if you have to turn your head to speak into it (this also concerns how well you need to see your slides to give your talk). Consider bringing your own laser pointer and extra batteries from home. Podiums now often have buttons and switches that you, the speaker, will be required to use to advance (or reverse) your own slides. Try the system out in advance so you will not to lose time during your talk by asking for the "next slide." Often, the slide operator, although he or she can usually do so, will *not* help you out.

Be aware that old or thick slides might not work in the locally available equipment. Sometimes, the slide projector or video will break down or fail to work as expected. Be prepared to continue your talk without your visual aids. Rehearsal and good notes are essential for this.

Timing

Be sure you know how long you are expected to speak. You must not go over the time limit.

---

1. Take a big breath before you start to talk.
2. Speak slowly and loudly.
3. Enunciate clearly.
4. Be confident in yourself.
5. Keep an eye on the time.

Time limits of talks are very important. A time limit for your talk is usually determined when the program is planned and published, but last-minute modifications are always possible. Some speakers may be absent, some parts of the program may have been canceled, or, in some countries, speakers may be added to the list at the last moment. This means that when you plan your talk, there should be room either to lengthen or shorten it. Notwithstanding last-minute changes, staying within your allotted time is a mark of excellence. This takes experience and diligence in the preparation of your talk. For the beginner, rehearsal is essential. Time may be lost fiddling with the pointer (you should have checked it out before) or in asking to advance the slides when you are supposed to do that yourself.

Travel

While the risks when traveling in one's own country or even continent are small, what about the risks when traveling to other countries? Problems are related mainly to jet lag, diseases prevalent in the country being visited (or the common "Turista"), differences in local organization or logistics, differences in electricity, working hours, and extramedical life. Tens of millions of people travel to and from Europe, North America, and Asia every year. The main points of interest to the frequent traveler (aside from a free mileage card) are vaccination, alimentation, chemoprevention, and what to bring along when traveling. Circumstances that have their own importance include pregnancy, seropositivity, and chronic disease.

On the positive side, traveling to foreign countries and cities is a time for leisure and sightseeing. This entails visiting local sites, going to the "inside" of cities, or taking a swim in a local river, lake, or sea. To make the best of your trip, a minimum of information must be known beforehand. Travel guides are usually time-consuming, and your spouse might be the ideal person to take care of this. Some pharmaceutical companies publish "pocket survival guides" available for specific meetings (American College of Surgeons).

When you are invited to visit another city, enjoy the trip, but remember that *your first responsibility is to your hosts.* Make sure they will be pleased you came and will want to ask you back. Give them good value for their effort and generosity.

Jet Lag

Probably the most prevalent and annoying of travel problems, jet lag is due to disturbances in the circadian rhythm of the human being. Human circadian rhythms depend on several factors such as weather and temperature, alternation of day (light) and night (darkness), eating times, and social contacts. Rapid trans- and/or intercontinental travel in high-speed airplanes does not allow the body to adapt to the environmental changes, and invariably the traveler will experience fatigue, sleep disorders (somnolence, insomnia, early awaking), decrease in appetite, and decreased physical and mental capacities.

Traveling from east to west (the day or night prolonged) is generally better tolerated than the contrary (from west to east, with the day or night shortened). As a rule, the symptoms take 1 day per 2 time zones to disappear. Suggestions to shorten these delays include adapting to local time customs (eating and sleeping) as quickly as possible. When traveling from east to west, one should try to stay awake as long as possible and adapt eating and sleeping to the local time, even if still traveling. When traveling from west to east on an overnight flight (North America to Europe, for instance), taking a sleeping pill as soon as you board the flight (which means you should sleep through the meal and video!) usually will allow you to survive the next day and be alert on the following. It may be necessary to regulate one's sleep with sleeping pills for one or several days in the foreign country. Melatonin is now available over the counter in some countries. It acts essentially like a sleeping pill and helps regulate the circadian cycle quicker than just hanging on. Instructions for use are given with the drug.

In warm or humid countries, there may be a long break in the afternoon while everyone waits for the heat to cool down. Most people take advantage of this for their siesta. But this means that the evening and nightlife will be longer. Try to get into rhythm with the local customs or you will increase your fatigue.

Diarrhea

"Turista" is also called "Kaboulite," "Montezuma's revenge," or other names. More than one-third of voyagers will experience a syndrome of benign acute diarrhea that ordinarily does not last more than a few days. The risk of contracting "Turista" depends essentially on the country to which one travels. R. Steffen has distinguished three categories of risk, calculated for a traveler coming from an industrialized country and for a trip of at least one week:

- Low risk (8% of travelers): USA, Canada, northern Europe, central Europe, Australia, New Zealand
- Medium risk (8–20% of travelers): Japan, Korea, South Africa, Israel, Caribbean islands, the northern shore of the Mediterranean Sea.
- High risk (>20% of travelers): the southern shore of the Mediterranean Sea, developing countries in Africa, Asia, and Latin America.

Usually these bouts of diarrhea are due to bacteria, sometimes to viruses. Rarely, the cause is parasites. When the symptoms are slight (nonetheless occasionally embarrassing), no specific treatment is necessary. The first thing to do is to compensate for fluid loss. Symptomatic treatment includes medication to reduce the frequency of bowel movements and relieve symptoms such as fever, abdominal pain, and cramps. When symptoms are more severe, antibiotics or even parenteral rehydration may be necessary. The following guidelines can be given to prevent "Turista" in a large majority of cases. Be careful of what you eat (no fruit) and drink (only bottled fluid) in the high-risk countries and, in most instances, you will not get sick. Preventive antibiotics are not recommended. They can be more dangerous than efficient, but in some specific cases (a very important meeting in a high-risk place combined with a very short—less than 48 hours—stay), they might be justified.

Other Medical Risks

Contaminated needles are an obvious source of disease transmission. Not only are the "unnecessary" intravenous or intramuscular injections and use of drugs a danger, but contaminated needles are also a danger in the case of tattooing, acupuncture, and piercing of earlobes. Even razor blades can be a danger. When on a trip, accept an intravenous or intramuscular injection only when the oral route or suppositories are not feasible. When traveling to distant Third World countries, and for a trip of long duration, bring along a few sterile IV and IM needles as well as sterile syringes. The fact that you are a doctor doesn't give you any privileges, but if the needles and syringes are neatly arranged in a first aid kit or with other medications, there should not be any real problems going through customs.

Avoid *blood transfusions* in Third World countries where the blood is rarely tested for HIV or other foreign substances. Accidents serious enough to require blood transfusions are fortunately rare. In the future, blood substitutes should be commercialized, and it will be possible to bring adequate quantities along. Make your blood group obvious in your identification papers.

Altitude

Several large cities or attractions in the world are not at sea level. Altitude sickness may occur in anyone, even when the person is used to going to high altitudes. Altitude sickness is rare under 3,000 m. Traveling directly to cities such as Cusco, Peru, and La Paz, Bolivia, for instance, will bring you to altitudes as high as 3,360 and 3,631 m, respectively. The altitudes of some "high" cities are as follows: Mexico City, 2,216 m; Quito, 2,890 m; some parts of Darjeeling, 3,365 m; Lhasa, 3,684 m; the Lincoln observatory (Colorado), 4,332 m; the Aiguille de Midi observatory (Chamonix, France), 3,806 m.

Remember that pulmonary and/or cerebral edema can begin at altitudes as low as 3,000 m, especially when traveling from sea level. Beware of headache even when the onset precedes your arrival in high altitude. Headache, nausea, cough, and inordinate difficulty in respiration or breathlessness should be adequate and sufficient warnings. *Rapid descent* is essential, whenever possible, *before* taking the time to consult health care providers at the nearest medical facilities.

Pocket Survival Guides

Travel guides are available in most bookstores for practically any country in the world, even the most remote. Most organizers will inform you of the essentials in the first announcement. Take the time to browse through the guides sufficiently in advance. If traveling for the first time to your destination, and this information is missing, do not hesitate to contact your travel agent.

Dining Out

Most countries and cities have their special restaurants and food. To take best advantage of these, it is best to consult the guides. Most appreciated are invitations to dine with your hosts. It is courteous and well-bred to be informed concerning the specialties of the host country and to be prepared to eat "strange" and "different" food and to drink different-tasting beverages, some of which might not be agreeable. Be aware that your hosts may be offended if you refuse or manifest dislike of their specialties.

Points of Interest

The major points of interest of the country or city you visit are best discerned from the travel guides or from people or friends who have already traveled to the country in question. Museums are very popular and a unique occasion when traveling to certain parts of the world. Tours are usually ample and well organized by your host. Often, however, it is interesting to arrive one or more days before to tour the city or country by yourself or with friends. This is better than touring after the meeting, for several reasons. First, it is always interesting to learn about the country you are visiting as well as learn about its customs. You will communicate better with your hosts and the local people. You will feel more at ease, especially if giving the talk in a language that is not your mother tongue. Second, it also will allow you to get over the jet lag before giving your talk. Getting over the tiredness of travel will enable you to talk with bravo.

Commentary

Visiting other hospitals and other cities exposes us to new ideas; the thoughtful questions of others advance our own work. We feel honored when others want to hear us, especially when the invitation comes from another country. International meetings provide more opportunity for discussion from a global perspective than do domestic meetings, but extra effort is required to exploit the advantages gained from international exchange. It is difficult for all of us to reach out across language barriers for these rewards. You are indeed fortunate if the occasion allows you to present your thoughts in your native language, or if the language of presentation is one you have made the effort to learn. Remember to speak slowly and enunciate more clearly than you might do at home. Avoid the use of slang, colloquialisms, or technical jargon. Try to put your thoughts in straightforward, simple language. Remember that nonnative speakers will have to work especially hard to follow your words. If the language used at the meeting is one you do not speak well, you must give even more careful thought to the words you select to express scientific ideas. The greatest disadvantage of international meetings is the language barrier. There is a real possibility that adequate discussion of your paper may not be possible due either to your own language disabilities or to those of the audience. There is the possibility that errors will arise in the audience's understanding of your presentation as a result of misinterpretation, so you must think carefully about answers to questions and perhaps prepare scripted answers or discussion slides in advance to answer questions you can anticipate will be asked. As a speaker, give yourself every advantage.

The usage of titles varies between countries; for example, surgeons in England are addressed as "Mister," and professors in Europe—and particularly in Germany—are addressed as "Professor," whereas in America they are addressed as "Doctor."

B.M.

SECTION IV

Design and Methods

CHAPTER 25

Turning Clinical Problems into Research Studies

B. McPeek, H. Troidl, and M.F. McKneally

The experimenter who does not know what he is looking for will not understand what he finds.
—Claude Bernard

Turning a question or a problem into a research question is a special skill that allows investigators to "link facts to reason, and create the opportunity to advance knowledge," as Bernard explains in his fascinating book *An Introduction to the Study of Experimental Medicine.*[1] The design of a research study depends on clear formulation of a researchable question, for example, "Will aprotinin reduce perioperative blood loss?" rather than "What will happen if we give aprotinin?" or "What drugs might reduce blood loss?" Postoperative bleeding is the problem; the research question links the antifibrinolytic effect of aprotinin to established reasoning about fibrinolytic effects of surgery. Available methods and their cost, convenience, reliability, and appropriateness influence the decisions about study design. A controlled experiment in the surgical laboratory using an animal model, a controlled clinical trial in humans, an observational review of case experience, or a survey of a practitioner's experience might all lead to an increase in generalizeable knowledge about the problem of postoperative bleeding (see Figure 25-1).

Selecting the Right Methods: Experiments

Questions about cause and effect are best answered through experiments. Some questions in surgery, particularly mechanistic ones, are best answered by experiments conducted in the laboratory. Many practical questions in clinical surgery are best answered by experimentation outside the laboratory. Spitzer and Horowitz define (chapter 28) an experimental design as one in which a group of subjects (patients, mice, or test samples) is exposed to an intervention, and one or more control groups are not exposed to the intervention or treatment of interest. The essential characteristic of an experiment is assignment of the intervention by the investigator to the exposed group, and assignment of the comparison intervention, such as placebo or best accepted current therapy, to the control group.

1. The essential characteristic of an experiment is assignment of treatments under the control of the investigator.
2. The assignment of subjects to the control and experimental groups is done by systematic prespecified methods presumed to guarantee the assembly of two comparable groups.

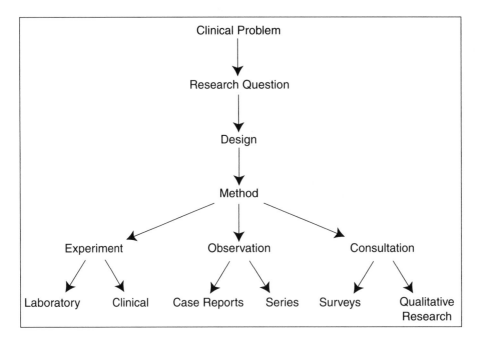

Figure 25-1. A variety of research methods for addressing clinical problems.

Clinical Experiments

In a clinical experiment or controlled trial, the investigator imposes two or more different treatments on selected groups of individuals to see how well each treatment achieves a prestated goal. *The strength of a controlled experiment lies largely in the strength of the control.* We place our greatest faith in the results of a controlled trial where the allocation to treatment groups of subjects drawn from a single population is done by a secure random method—where every member of the population has the same chance to be allocated to each group. Only a truly random allocation will insure that the groups are similar, provided the samples are large enough. When nonrandom methods are used to allocate subjects to treatment groups, our confidence that the two samples are matched is lessened. The randomized controlled trial is the gold standard for evidence of a treatment's effectiveness, and for answering questions about cause and effect. A nonrandomized, concurrent controlled trial is our second choice. A special case of controlled trials uses a crossover design, in which each patient is his own control: treatment A is offered in January–February, and the same patient gets treatment B in March–April, and so forth. This

is feasible only if the treatment effects are short-lived, as with the therapeutic effect of an antibiotic, not an appendectomy.

Matched pairs represent another special case. Here we select a treated patient and then try to locate another patient who is similar but has received another treatment. The reliability of this method depends on the accuracy of the match; it is difficult to explain convincingly to readers.

Weakly controlled trials provide less secure evidence. Historical control groups drawn from another time (for example, patients treated in 1987 compared with those treated in 1997), or from another place (for example, patients from Boston serving as the control group for patients treated in Cologne) rarely provide convincing comparisons, except in the unusual case in which there is a *well-known* course of events and no question about the accuracy of diagnosis. For example, since rabies patients with neurologic signs almost always die, a series of six patients treated by a new method that yielded, say, a 50% survival rate would be most compelling, even if no control group other than historical records was offered.

Solomon and McLeod of Toronto[2] made a computerized search of all clinical studies published in a single year. They compiled a careful sample of treatment evaluation questions involving comparisons of a surgical procedure with another procedure, a medical treatment, or a nonsurgical intervention. They defined problems precluding a randomized control trial and evaluated the questions asked in their sample to determine whether a controlled trial could have been performed. If it could not have been, the predominant reasons precluding a trial of these surgical problems were recorded, and they included such reasons as uncommon condition, patient preference, and lack of equipoise in the surgical community. They found that about 40% of treatment evaluation problems *could have been* answered by a randomized controlled trial in an ideal clinical research setting, but only 7% of published articles comprised randomized controlled trials.

Since Solomon and McLeod found that controlled trials could have been performed for only 40% of the treatment questions they surveyed, 60% of these surgical issues required methods other than randomized controlled trials. Simpler, easier to accomplish, nonexperimental strategies do provide information about what happens after a treatment is given.[3] We sometimes describe them as being "almost as good," but their weaker designs lack the strength of inference one can provide with a controlled trial. The carefully executed controlled trial continues to supply our best evidence of cause and effect and our best evidence of the effectiveness of diagnostic and therapeutic maneuvers. It should be used whenever ethically and practically feasible. But for many questions the controlled trial is simply not feasible. If resources of patients, investigators, and money were unlimited, more therapeutic innovations might be assessed by randomized trials. In the real world, we must prioritize our efforts and make the best use of our resources. Our patients need informed treatment decisions today, and the best feasible alternative strategies. Generally speaking, the more an alternative strategy appears similar to an experiment or controlled trial, the more confidence we will have in its results.

Cohort Comparison Studies

If one cannot do an experiment, a cohort comparison study is the next strongest strategy. Cohort studies are follow-up studies. We select a group of people, for example, patients suffering from cholecystitis. Those patients treated by laparoscopic cholecystectomy are compared to patients treated by open cholecystectomy. We follow each group through time and observe what happens. How well do they do? Are their symptoms relieved? Are there any negative events? What are the costs and the benefits of each treatment arm? We have less confidence in cohort comparison studies, in which the investigator does not assign treatments but simply identifies patients at the time treatments are offered and follows them forward in time to record and to compare their outcomes. The danger here is that, because treatment was not assigned by the investigator in a way that assures comparability, we cannot be certain that the patients offered laparoscopic cholecystectomy did not differ in some important respect from the patients offered open cholecystectomy. Perhaps one group was sicker, younger, or better nourished.

Case-Control or Case-Referent Studies

The next strongest method or strategy for answering a treatment comparison question is probably the case-control or case-referent study. Here we look at a group of patients who have a specified outcome, such as incontinence following low anterior resection for carcinoma of the middle third of the rectum. We identify these patients and then search the records of the hospital and the surgeons to collect data, retrospectively, on how the patients were treated. How did their sphincter function before operation? Was the operation in one group more or less extensive than that in the other? Were special steps taken to preserve the nerve supply? Case-control methods are often the *only* feasible way to study rare diseases. One of the disadvantages is that one must be satisfied with the information in the available records, which may lack accuracy and completeness (e.g., testing for sphincter function was not done before the operation, or the test was unrecorded or lost.)

In a cohort study, both the treatment cohort and the control cohort are identified at or before the time the treatment is given. This often allows detailed record-keeeping measures to be established specifically for the study. In a case-controlled study, the information is collated at the end, after the endpoint is known, and one goes back in time to seek information from the routine records about what happened to the patient. We call such records "management records," because they were collected in the course of the institution's ordinary routine or business, not specially for a research study. Often, management records will work nicely for a research purpose. They are usually inexpensive to use because someone else ordered and paid for their collection, but you have to take what is available; sometimes the records contain no information on a particular item crucial to the research question, such as continence in the example above.

A Series without a Control Group

A weaker method is the series with no control or comparison group. It simply reports on the outcome of a group of patients treated in a specific way. How did a patient get into the series? Does the series contain all such patients treated that way, or only the patients of Dr. Famous? Were only healthy patients offered the treatment? Perhaps only the sickest patients were offered the new treatment, or perhaps they alone were excluded from the series. Published reports are often vague or silent about these issues. We have more confidence in an uncontrolled series if it is consecutive and includes all patients with the problem who were treated over a period of time at a specific clinic or center, rather than a selected group of younger or more healthy patients.

Isolated Case Reports

We learn much from case reports. Isolated case reports often serve as our first warnings that a complication can follow a specific treatment.[4] They serve to alert us to potential complications that have actually occurred. They give us no information about the frequency with which we might expect to encounter such cases in the future, because we do not know the number of patients who had the treatment but did not suffer the complication.

Table 25-1 gives a rough idea of the hierarchy of reliability of the information derived from each of the various strategies described.

Surveys, Censuses, and Management Records

Another approach to learning what is going on in the world around us, besides observation and experiment, is to ask people for information. In sample surveys we seek answers from a sample of, for example, 10% of German hospitals, or 1 in every 35 English surgeons. In the last 50 years we have learned how to perform surveys that give reliable results. Sample surveys can work well, depending on three factors: (1) How frequently do we encounter the outcome of interest? (2) How was the sample drawn? A sample seeking information about surgical practice drawn only from professors of surgery may not reflect what happens in small-town private practice. (3) What was the response rate? A response rate of 75% might be adequate for some questions or samples, but too low for others. If a question seeks information about a rare occurrence, a sample survey may well miss it; a complete census might be needed to ask the question of everyone. When thinking about a sample survey, one of the questions to ask yourself is, Would a census answer the question? If a census would not, then no sample survey will, regardless of the resources available. (A census may be thought of as a sample in which the proportion included reaches 1.0.)

Instead of a special survey, we sometimes tap into information already gathered, perhaps by the government and published as an official statistic, perhaps from the hospital's billing department or pharmacy. The trouble with gathering information from "management records" is that the information at hand may not be adequate to answer all the questions of interest.

Modeling

Sometimes we have questions about the effectiveness of treatment that, for practical or ethical reasons, cannot be resolved by experimental methods. A fire chief who wants to study different methods of extinguishing fires cannot conduct an

Table 25-1.   Hierarchy of reliability of research methods for ascertaining diagnostic or treatment effectiveness.

Research Method (Arranged in descending order of level of reliability)

True experiments (Investigator controls both allocation to groups and determination of treatment)

    Randomized concurrent controlled trial including crossover design with random order of treatment

    Historical controls only in special case of *certain* diagnosis and *known* course of events (see text)

    Randomized concurrent controlled trial with weakly-randomized assignment or systematic assignment (odd/even, alternate appearance, etc.), including crossover design with systematic order of treatment

    Nonrandomized concurrent controlled trial

    Short-interval sequential trials within same institution or service

    Longer-interval sequential trials within same institution or service

    Controls from separate institutions or services with documented attention to coordination

    Controls from separate institutions or services with poor or no attention to coordination

Nonexperimental methods

    Cohort comparison studies

    Historical controls (not in special case)

    Nonexperimental case control or case referent studies

    Series of cases (all comers to a center over a time interval)

    Large series of cases (consecutive)

    Small series of cases (consecutive)

    Large series of cases

    Small series of cases

    Isolated case reports with documentation of active surveillance

    Isolated case reports (volunteer)

    Case report

experiment in which the houses in a neighborhood are randomly allocated into two groups, the houses are set afire, and then the houses in group A are treated with one fire-fighting method and those in group B are treated with another. A wise fire chief might erect model houses for the experiment. Full-size houses are expensive so you might use very small models of houses and carefully record the progress of the fire with motion picture cameras and laboratory equipment. Engineers might abstract the problem further by developing a mathematical model to use in place of the physical model. Animal models and physical models are widely used in surgical research, and the development of computers has made mathematical modeling an increasingly popular way of conducting experiments. Virtual reality techniques are narrowing the difference between mathematical and physical models.

Seeking Advice

Sometimes we seek information about a problem that we understand or can describe so poorly that we cannot pose the right questions let alone do any serious modeling. In these circumstances we turn to friends whose advice we have relied on in the past; we seek our teachers and others who have special knowledge or experience in relevant fields. Governments, health ministries, and scientific societies often develop specialized ways of seeking advice through the use of advisors or consensus conferences; these are particularly useful because questions or opinions offered by one advisor may stimulate fresh thought from another. Face-to-face meetings are sometimes subject to unwarranted influence from the eminent, the powerful, the rhetorically skillful, or simply the persistently noisy. It is for this reason that techniques like the Delphi technique were developed. A special case of seeking advice can be thought of as seeking advice from yourself, or introspection. Introspection as a technique of medical decision making has received much interest in the last few years from serious, thoughtful workers.

What Will Happen in the Future?

What training must we offer today to prepare sufficient surgeons, anesthetists, nurses, and technicians for practice 20 years from now? What will the needs of developing countries be? Questions that seek information about future occurrences generally involve looking at the past (particularly the recent past) and the present, and attempting to project trends into the future. Looking into the future involves methods of forecasting using special analytic techniques. Specific statistical methods such as regression are frequently used for projections. The development of computers has enabled us to take into account a great deal of information when trying to predict the future. Gradually we seem to improve at forecasting, but, as Yogi Berra has said in his translation of the old Chinese proverb, *Prediction is difficult, especially about the future.*

References

1. Bernard C. An Introduction to the Study of Experimental Medicine. Greene HC, trans. New York: Macmillan, 1927.
2. Solomon MJ, McLeod RS. Should we be performing more randomized controlled trials evaluating surgical operations? Surgery 1995;118:459–467.
3. Hu X, Wright JG, McLeod RS, Lossing A, Walters BC. Observational studies as alternatives to randomized clinical trials in surgical clinical research. Surgery 1996;119:473–475.
4. Paul A, Troidl H, Peters S, Stuttman R. Fatal intestinal ischaemia following laparoscopic cholecystectomy. Br J Surg 1994;81:1207–1208.

CHAPTER 26

Clinical Trials

M.F. McKneally, B. McPeek, F. Mosteller, and E.A.M. Neugebauer

Nothing improves the performance of an innovation more than the lack of controls.[1]

Introduction

Surgery is constantly changing, and some of the changes are dramatic advances instantly recognizable for their benefit to patients. William T.G. Morton's administration of ether anesthesia to John Collins Warren's patient on October 14, 1846, required no confirmation. Warren's immediate and definitive conclusion—"Gentlemen, this is no humbug!"—was soon accepted throughout the world. A similar example is the introduction of antibiotics into clinical practice in the 1940s.

Most highly effective innovations such as Semmelweiss's hand washing and Lister's antisepsis are introduced against resistance and adopted only after a prolonged period of sometimes rancorous dispute. Surgeons have a strong tradition of conservative practice. Their skepticism about new methods, and their tendency to revere the techniques they have come to rely upon are part of an important tradition that helps make surgery safe. Solid experience with a new method must be developed before arguments to change proven and trusted procedures are accepted. It took a good 20 years for Lister's work to be widely adopted.

In contrast, sometimes ineffective but intuitively appealing innovations (such as gastric freezing to eliminate acid-secreting cells, or external carotid to internal carotid artery bypass to increase cerebral blood flow beyond a critically stenotic vessel) have gained more rapid and widespread implementation because of their intuitive appeal to the medical and lay public. After substantial investment in equipment and specialized training, these popular remedies were proven ineffective in credible, definitive field trials.

More often, we simply do not know whether an innovative treatment is better than what we are now doing, or better than providing only encouragement and sympathy. We can think, compute, theorize, observe, or guess, but the answers to such questions, even approximate and uncertain answers, must finally be found by studying treatments in a controlled, practical tryout under field conditions. Our language reflects how well we know this: the proof of the pudding is in the eating. This chapter is about the practical evaluation of innovations in the field, using controlled trials to compare alternative treatments.

Controlled Clinical Trials

In a controlled trial, the investigator imposes two (or more) different treatments on selected groups of individuals to see how well each treatment achieves a prestated goal. The results are usually also reviewed for effects not included in the original plan.

The Logic of Trials

A simplified version of the rationale of basing inferences on a comparative trial assumes the following:

1. Initially, the individuals in each group receiving one treatment are similar to the individuals in the groups receiving the other treatment(s).
2. The difference in the treatments is the only factor affecting the outcomes in the different groups.
3. The individuals in the treated groups react to the treatments in the same way as the rest of the population would react.

We then conclude that because the only difference lies in the treatment, it must be the treatment that caused any differences in observed outcome, and because the individuals in the trial react like the rest of the population, applying the treatment to other members of the population will produce the same effect as it did on the individuals in the trial.

Strength of a Trial

Many simpler strategies provide information about what happens after a treatment is given; each is sometimes used to say something about the effectiveness of a treatment. They all lack the strength of a controlled trial because their designs are inherently weaker. They are frequently described as being "almost as good as" or "closely approaching," but it is never suggested that their weaker designs offer the strength of inference one can provide with a controlled trial. For this reason, the carefully executed controlled trial continues to supply our best evidence of cause and effect, and our best evidence of the effectiveness of diagnostic and therapeutic maneuvers.

The confidence we have in the results of a controlled trial lies, in large measure, in the strength of the control. Were the groups of individuals that received the different treatments truly initially similar? We are most likely to be convinced of this if the

groups were selected from the same population and divided or allocated into groups by a reliably unbiased method.

The most convincing of such methods is randomization using a table of random numbers, giving each individual an equal chance to be assigned to each of the groups. Although "randomization" based on throwing dice, tossing coins, or drawing cards can seem to be reliable, it may have serious weaknesses. Such methods are more easily interfered with and cannot be checked if questions about them arise later.

Odd or even birthdays, patient identification numbers, or alternate arrival in the clinic are not proper bases for random allocation. They are systematic allocation procedures. They may appear to be unbiased, but such procedures have the weakness of tipping the patient assignment in advance so that someone who knows the procedure, perhaps a referring physician or clinic secretary, can allow personal prejudice to bias allocation by pushing forward or holding back otherwise eligible patients.

The use of concurrent control groups from the same population lends strength to our belief in the initial similarity of the treatment and control groups, but such confidence would quickly run down the drain if we thought the selection had been done in a biased fashion, resulting in sicker, younger, or wealthier patients being assigned in greater number to one group or the other.

Weaker Controls

Sometimes a controlled trial is designed to use nonconcurrent treatment groups. For example, treatment 1 may be applied to everyone in January and February, and then treatment 2 is applied to everyone in March and April. This strategy, at least, selects group members from the same population in the same institution, but we wonder what other changes may have occurred. Did the surgeons on the service change at the time the treatment change occurred? Were there more or fewer nurses in March than in January? The possibility for such differences increases if the groups are separated more widely in time. A design that compares one treatment given in the 1980s with another treatment administered in the 1990s raises real questions. Have our diagnostic criteria remained stable over time? Have other treatments been introduced, or other changes occurred in the patients or their environment?

Occasionally, a controlled trial in which the treatment group comes from one institution and the control group from another is attempted. It is always difficult to assure ourselves, let alone those who will later read the published reports of such a trial, that the treatment groups were indeed initially similar and that the only difference lies in the treatments being compared.

Sometimes trials attempt to draw a comparison group from patients previously reported in the literature. It is usually very difficult for such "control" groups to be convincing, except perhaps in the special case of a known course of events with literature that is quite clear. For example, if a specific cancer is invariably fatal, and its diagnosis is clear, we may have confidence in historical controls from the literature if the new treatment results in, for example, a 25% survival rate.

Poorly Controlled Trials

What happens when poorly controlled trials are carried out? Physicians, especially uncritical physicians, may begin to believe the results of sloppy trials, especially when repeatedly poorly controlled trials arrive at the same conclusion: the innovative therapy is a winner. As Hugo Muench has taught us, nothing improves the performance of an innovation more than lack of controls.[1]

Performing a poor trial has serious long-run drawbacks. First, the results of a weak trial may foreclose—for a long period—the possibility of a good evaluation by a strong trial. Second, a weak trial may leave a well-established yet ineffective therapy in place for years to come. The losses associated with applying ineffective or less effective therapies to large populations soon outweigh 1000-fold the costs of careful trials.

History of Trials

The background, history, and evolution of randomized clinical trials has been presented in a clear and readable form by Alan Pollock in his chapter "The Historical Evolution of Clinical Research (chapter 6). This history brings us up to the era of the randomized trial of streptomycin for treatment of tuberculosis in the 1940s. Subsequently, Professor John Goligher, a highly respected clinical surgeon and teacher from Leeds, startled the surgical world 40 years ago by assigning patients to surgical treatments for duodenal ulcer disease using randomization.[2] His leadership made surgeons realize that they could legitimately tell their patients that there is a state of uncertainty, of "clinical equipose"[3] (see also chapter 60), which is *a legitimate difference of opinion among respected members of the clinical community about the relative merits* of a given surgical procedure. This uncharacteristic, counterintuitive statement of uncertainty about the comparative value of operative procedures (or anything else!) violates the paternalistic, authoritarian image of the surgeon so cherished by the populace and the surgical community. Because of the magnitude of their interventions, surgeons are widely expected to be fully informed and confident about their decision making ("sometimes wrong, but never in doubt"). Goligher destroyed this caricature, to the lasting benefit of surgical science. Nevertheless, many practitioners and many institutions, particularly those who see themselves dependent on a referral practice, prefer to maintain the illusion that they are always fully confident and always correct in their choice of the best available treatment. This public position has kept several prominent clinical units from entering patients in randomized trials.

Goligher's courageous leadership taught surgeons that randomized trials are valuable instruments and that good surgeons perform them. His studies clarified the role of vagotomy and drainage procedures, and choice of postgastrectomy reconstructions. Goligher's most important contribution, in our view, was the lasting credibility he gave to the concept of randomized trials as an important element of surgical practice.

Random Does Not Mean Haphazard

By a randomized controlled trial, we mean *a planned experiment to assess the effectiveness of treatments by comparing the outcomes in subjects drawn from the same population and allocated to two or more treatment groups by a random method.* Randomization of a large enough group of patients provides the theoretical basis for assuming that the treatment groups were initially comparable in terms of both known and unknown confounding factors. In using the term *random* we do not mean haphazard or unplanned, but a deliberate choice based on probabilities. We want each possible patient, treatment, and sample to have the same probability of being chosen for a particular treatment or for the control group. Balancing the probabilities lends strength to analyses based on statistical methods, protects against conscious or unconscious bias, and reduces the influence of potent confounding factors. The most convincing method of randomization uses a table of random numbers, to give each individual an equal chance of assignment to any treatment group.

Errors

Statisticians often speak of type I and type II errors, usually in the context of testing whether a new treatment differs from a standard or, more generally, whether differences might reasonably be thought to be negligible. In confirmatory statistical analysis, exemplified by significance tests, we may well ask at what rate per experiment we will falsely claim that a difference exists even when the two therapies are equal in effect. Such a false claim is called a type I error. This rate is associated with the significance level of the test, often chosen to be 0.05. When the observed difference falls beyond the 0.05 level, we say the result is significant, while admitting that we are risking a 5% frequency of a type I error.

Failing to recognize a difference when one is present is called a type II error. Given the method of testing for the difference and the significance level chosen, say 0.05, then what is the probability that we will fail to recognize a true difference, that is, make a type II error? This probability depends, of course, on the size of the true difference—larger differences are not as likely to be missed in our sample as smaller ones.

For a given significance level, we can control the rate of type II errors for a given difference in performance of the tests by adjusting the sample sizes. The rates of type I and type II errors we will

accept are important considerations in designing investigations. Ideally, we would have no error of either kind, but to assure this requires infinite sample sizes.

To put a small touch of reality back into the discussion, no one believes that two different therapies have *exactly* the same performance rates, but we might feel they were so close that we couldn't afford to measure their difference, or that very small differences were negligible from a clinical point of view. Thus, a declaration of no significant difference does not promise zero differences.

Trials That Convince

Over the past generation in medicine and surgery, we have come to agree that, when well executed, a randomized controlled trial provides the strongest evidence available for evaluating the relative effectiveness of the interventions tested.

We know how to conduct clinical trials that provide strong information about the relative effectiveness of two or more therapies. *Most controversies with clinical trials arise from investigators' desire to modify or avoid some requirement of the classical randomized controlled trial design.* They worry that it will be difficult to get enough patients, that some will think randomization is unfair, or may wish to substitute historical experience for a control group or avoid some other requirement or strengthening feature. In some situations, requirements can be relaxed with little or no harm to the trial, but often what seems acceptable to some investigators will not satisfy later readers of the trials' reports.

The randomized controlled trial and its analysis have been developed to protect investigators from untoward influences including their own biases that might invalidate the data and the conclusions to be drawn. If we could be sure that a particular biasing influence does not threaten the study at hand, we might not need to take advantage of the aspect of the trial that protects against that influence. For example, if you knew that all experimental units were the same and there was no variation from one unit to another, you would not have to randomize.

What if the investigators' assumptions about

the trial are not shared by readers? The trial loses its ability to convince; readers will criticize the design and conduct of the trial. The trial will fail, even if it gives an answer that is ultimately accepted as being right, because its failure to convince other clinicians means it will fail to affect clinical practice.

Strengthening Features

Some of the strengthening features of randomized controlled trials include the following:

Use of a prespecified explicit question
Clearly defined conditions for admission to the trial
Defined therapies
Entrance of patients into the trial prior to allocation to treatment groups
Blindness to treatment (by patient, experimenter, and evaluator, if feasible)
Systematic evaluation and follow-up of both treatment and control groups
Adequate sample size (for power to discriminate when treatments differ in their performance)
Appropriate statistical analyses of outcomes and side effects
Careful, complete reporting

To provide the strengthening features of the randomized controlled design, careful planning is necessary before starting a trial. The study protocol must fulfill scientific, ethical, and organizational requirements, so that the trial can be conducted efficiently. The protocol should be developed before the beginning of subject enrollment and should remain essentially unchanged throughout the study. The key elements of a study protocol are outlined in Table 26-1.

When Should a Randomized Trial Be Undertaken?

Although generally regarded as the definitive instrument in clinical research, the randomized clinical trial is nevertheless "a last resort for the evaluation of medical interventions" because "it is slow, ponderous, expensive, and often stifling of scientific imagination and creative changes in ongoing protocols" in Baillar's view.[4]

Table 26-1.   The key elements of a study protocol for a prospective controlled randomized trial.

1. Background and description of the clinical problem
2. Clearly defined question(s) or hypotheses
3. Reasons for the need to perform the designed study
4. Description of the type of the study
5. Definition of the study population
   Inclusion criteria
   Exclusion criteria (escape and dropout)
6. Definition and description of intervention and control group
7. Type and execution of the randomization
8. Reason for and execution of blinding
9. Sample size estimates
10. Data of the study
    Definition of basic data of patients
    Definition of endpoints of the study
    Data collection, quality assurance, and quality-control
    Data analysis (tests of hypotheses, descriptive statistics)
    Data protection
11. Ethical considerations (informed consent)
12. Description and schedule for a single patient (logistics)
13. Organizational structure of the study
14. References
15. Forms and data handling for a single patient

Reprinted with permission for Neugebauer E, Rothmund M, Lorenz W. Kunstruct Strukture und Praxis Perspectives Klinische Studies. Chirurg 60:203–213 1989, Springer-Verlag Heidelberg. FRG.

In a humorous, thoughtful essay entitled "The demise of the randomized controlled trial," Herman[5] has advanced the argument that randomized trials are no longer practical or feasible based on their unwieldiness, inconclusiveness, and expense. Despite his sobering arguments, randomized trials remain one of the most powerful and reliable tools of scientific medicine and surgery. Because it is expensive and cumbersome, a randomized trial should be undertaken only when Sacket's six criteria are fulfilled[6] (see Table 26-2). It seems reasonable to require randomized trials before marginal improvements are introduced, if the putative improvement will add to the cost of medical care. When improvements reduce cost, their introduction may not require a trial unless there is a possibility of harm or reduction of an established benefit, for example, when the frequency of an established screening test for cancer is reduced. Established treatments that have troublesome side effects warrant systematic testing, particularly those treatments established by custom rather than by evidence. The progressive reduction in the use of radical mastectomy for early stage breast cancer is a clear example. Alternative accepted treatments for the same problem (e.g., radiation vs. laryngectomy for early stage laryngeal cancer) merit randomized comparison.

Trials are difficult and time-consuming, and they require a genuine commitment on the part of the investigators and their associates—a commitment of enthusiasm, energy, and discipline, as well as resources in terms of time and money. Most trials ought to require a relatively large number of cases, and the investigators must assure an adequate number of patients in a relatively short period of time. *Trials that take many years to complete run the risk of being overtaken by new developments in diagnosis or therapy that make them difficult to finish or irrelevant.* Most research teams find the discipline of a trial irksome, and the required enthusiasm and energy difficult to maintain over long periods.

Sometimes the collaboration of a number of institutions across the world is required. Some problems, particularly those involving truly rare conditions, simply cannot be studied by clinical trials, even large multicentered ones. Many other problems will be judged of insufficient importance to warrant the effort.

Deciding to Start a Trial

The first requirement for a trial is that the physicians and surgeons who participate be honestly uncertain of the comparative merits of the treatments they propose to compare. At the same time, they must have a proper skepticism about the state of their real knowledge, not confusing mere prejudice with knowledge. Even careful and thoughtful people frequently have been found to be much too confident of what they think they know.[7]

The potential investigators must believe that the treatments may differ in outcome, and these

Table 26-2. Sacket's six prerequisites for a successful clinical trial.

1. The trial needs to be done.
2. The question posed is both appropriate and unambiguous.
3. The trial architecture is valid.
4. The inclusion/exclusion criteria strike a balance between efficiency and generalizability.
5. The trial protocol is feasible.
6. The trial administration is effective.

differences may be clinically important. There are too many important problems in medicine and surgery to expend resources on issues we do not expect to matter. Finally, a trial's planners must believe that a trial is feasible with the resources of patients, enthusiasm, personnel, and money that can be made available.

Once you have weighed the benefits and burdens of performing a randomized trial, carefully considered the problems described by Baillar, and accepted the conclusion that the question is worth the effort and can't be solved by any less expensive method, visit your statistical consultant.

The statistical consultation process should begin at the design phase and continue throughout the trial. Biostatisticians prefer to be significant and practical contributors to clinical trials from the outset, rather than posttrial analysts of accumulated data. The two-way street of statistical consultation in clinical research is well described by Lincoln Moses in Baillar and Mosteller's useful book *Medical Uses of Statistics.*[8] (Moses's chapter is reprinted in this textbook as chapter 39).

Structure of a Prospective, Controlled Randomized Trial: The Study Protocol

When the decision to run a trial has emerged, trial planners, including the statisticians, meet to develop a study protocol. The study protocol provides detailed specification of the trial procedure.

Protocol development is the most critical step in turning the research plan into a practical, productive, workable action guide that will provide useful data and excellent patient care. As you are developing the protocol, walk through it step by step with nurses, physicians, data managers, patients, and laboratory personnel who will be affected by it. The team approach will provide commonsense solutions and improvements that might not occur to investigators working alone. If you seek early consultation with the research ethics board, you can facilitate review and minimize delay in approval. Institutional review boards send 80% of protocols back for revisions, many of which could be anticipated during the development phase.

The study protocol is a working document, used by data managers and staff to conduct the trial efficiently. The key elements of a study protocol have been outlined by Neugebauer and his colleagues (Table 26-1). This very useful checklist is helpful for preparing a presentation to a granting agency or research ethics board. Working through it with your study team step-by-step will minimize unexpected problems. A simplified form of the protocol and the permission form is greatly appreciated by staff, patients, and families, who are confused and put off by the excessive detail and legalistic language that has progressively infiltrated and congealed in research documents. If team members who are responsible for the day-to-day conduct of the protocol write the simplified forms, they will have a clearer understanding of the research mission and greater facility in communicating it.

What Is the Clinical Problem?

A description of the background and the clinical problem explains why the trial is needed and how it builds on the experience gained from previous research.[9] What kind of improvement would be important? The statistician can help you prove that an improvement has been demonstrated with "highly significant" probability; the clinician must define an *important* difference, one that has meaning and value in patients' lives.

What Is the Question?

Although a trial may have several purposes, we explicitly define a principal question in advance.

This question serves to guide planning of the whole study. The principal question should be the one the investigators are most interested in answering and is the question on which the sample size of the study is based. We frame the principal question in the form of a testable hypothesis.[10]

Problems of Multiplicity

If a number of questions are investigated, a statistical problem arises. If we look at a large enough number of questions in a single investigation, inevitably some of them will display an unusual outcome. If we compare a number of treatments, even if they are truly equivalent, sampling variation alone would make some of them look better than others. Similarly, when individual institutions are compared in a cooperative multiinstitutional therapeutic trial, even if they are equivalent in excellence, sampling variation will make some look much better than others.

One way of asking many relevant questions and causing problems of multiplicity is to use multiple endpoints. For example, in a controlled trial of coronary bypass surgery, are we preventing death, first myocardial infarctions, second myocardial infarctions, or angina? All these may be legitimate endpoints, but usually one is fundamental and the others are side interests. If that is true, explicitly naming the primary endpoint in advance strengthens statistical appraisal and clarifies suitable experimental design. Analysis becomes more complicated when there are two or more endpoints because larger samples are required to maintain the power required to detect differences.

We may well want to look at additional questions and analyses that suggest themselves in various ways after the data analysis has begun. This is information we are not anxious to throw away, but it may be quite difficult to know how much value we should place on the answers we get. With a statistical test chosen on the basis of a peek at the data, it is hard to say what the properties of the test are because every set of data has unusual features. Thus, it may be difficult to say whether a rare event has occurred if a test of significance is chosen from a large number of possibly related tests. These problems are not unique to randomized controlled trials; they can occur with equal or greater impact in any statistical study.

Why a Further Study?

After the primary question has been framed, we review and analyze the published literature on the issue. Several approaches to systematically reviewing previous work are outlined in chapter 38. As a result of the literature analysis, we formulate a convincing statement of the need for the suggested trial on the primary question. The statement may contain a list of the relevant references.

Type of Trial

The type of trial is determined by the kind of principal question posed. Schwartz and Lellouch[11] distinguish two different kinds of questions that trials frequently ask.[12] The first kind asks for scientific demonstration of efficacy or superiority: Will operation A produce better results than operation B? This is sometimes called an *explanatory* trial, or an *efficacy* trial; it seeks to compare the effects of treatments with close control under ideal or restricted circumstances.

The explanatory or efficacy trial seeks to determine whether the treatment can work under the best circumstances. Such a trial might restrict its admission of patients to those most likely to respond well, and it may call for elaborate monitoring, regulation of treatment, or more frequent follow-up.

The second kind of question deals with *pragmatic* management or clinical effectiveness under wider conditions more nearly like ordinary clinical practice. The *pragmatic* or *effectiveness* trial, sometimes called a management trial, asks the question, Can this procedure or treatment be generalized easily to practice?

A pragmatic or effectiveness trial is likely to accept a wider spectrum of patients, perhaps treated by a varied group of surgeons or practitioners. Its treatments usually strive to replicate clinical practice to obtain a better estimate of the overall usefulness of a therapeutic maneuver in widespread use.

Who Are the Patients?

A trial's protocol must specify the conditions for admission to the trial, that is, which patients or subjects are eligible for admission. The inclusion/exclusion criteria must be clearly defined.

Later readers of published reports will almost always want to assess whether the findings of a trial can be generalized to another patient group or applied to individual patients seen in their own practices. Such extrapolation requires specific information about who the subjects of a trial were and how they were selected. Published reports that lack this information make generalizing a trial's findings to groups other than the subjects themselves very difficult.

What Are the Treatments?

Each therapy must be clearly defined. We ought to know what will be done, how it will be done, and by whom.

Allocation to Treatment Groups

Patients must be entered into the trial before the choice of therapy is made. Determination of admission to a study after treatment assignment is known may bias subject selection. Those in the know may push forward or hold back potential subjects, as a result of conscious or unconscious prejudice about treatment assignment. Assignments based on birthdays, odd or even chart numbers, or alternate arrival often tip the assignment in advance and allow bias to creep in.

Assignment of treatments using published random number tables reduces bias in clinical trials. Frequently, known prognostic factors are used to stratify patients prior to randomization. This can help to achieve balance among treatment groups—at least with respect to known factors. The exact procedure used should be specified so that readers can be assured that the randomization was reliable. The time of randomization and the chosen procedure must be explained and described in detail.

Blindness

Studies should be blinded to the extent possible. Ideally, the patient, the physician giving the treatment, and the person doing the evaluation should not know which treatment is given. Some degrees of blindness may not be feasible, especially in surgical trials (consider a trial of amputation vs. medical treatment), but blindness is an important strengthening feature and should be used whenever possible. For example, histological slides, X rays, or laboratory tests can be read by a physician blinded to the patients' treatment allocation.

The protocol should state which parts of the study are blinded and should describe how to assure that the blinding conditions are met.

Power and Sample Size

The probability of detecting an event of given size in a comparative study is called the "power." The larger the sample size and the larger the size of the treatment effect, the greater is the power. Power also depends on study design, the statistical techniques of analysis, and the significance level, chosen by the investigators. Smaller significance levels give smaller power.

It is important to concentrate on sample size because it is, at least, partially under the control of the investigator. One way to think about power is that it quantifies the probability of detecting a substantial improvement and also the probability of missing one—the probability of a type II error.

A fundamental question that must be faced by investigators planning a clinical trial is how many patients are needed? Beginning investigators will want to seek the advice of a statistician experienced in clinical trial design. There are various published formulas and tables for determining the number of patients necessary to meet the trial's principal objectives, but seemingly minor changes in trial design may make a given formula or table inapplicable. For example, sample size and power calculations can differ depending on the question being asked and on whether the outcome measure is dichotomous (e.g., success or failure) or a quantitative measurement. Standard textbooks[9,13] ordinarily devote one or more large chapters to sample size and power determinations.

How large is the usual treatment group in a clinical trial? Zelen drew a systematic sample of clinical trials reported in the journal *Cancer* and concluded that the usual size is about 50.[14] Mosteller and associates[15] examined 285 samples from randomized clinical trials in three areas of cancer. The median sample size was 9 for studies of multiple myeloma and chronic myelocytic leukemia, 7 for studies of gastrointestinal cancer, and 25 per treatment group for randomized trials of breast cancer. In all these distributions, sample sizes larger than 200 were rare. Only 7% of the samples exceeded 200. Small trials have very low power. Why is power important? Weak trials, trials with very low power, can fail to detect even big improvements in performance.

Freiman et al.[16] document the risk of missing substantial improvements when a trial's power is low. They investigated 71 clinical trials that reported no statistically significant difference between the therapies. They looked at the 90% confidence intervals to see whether substantial improvement might have been missed because of the breadth of the intervals. These intervals contained potential 25% improvements in 57 comparisons and potential 50% improvement in 34 comparisons. The designs were so weak that they left open the possibility that such sizable improvements would be missed.

Emerson et al. found that only 5% of published reports of surgical trials disclose the trial's power to detect treatment differences.[17] This suggests that investigators as well as editors, referees, and readers fail to appreciate the importance that discussions of power should hold for readers.

Data of the Study

Baseline Assessment

To describe study subjects accurately, baseline data should reflect the condition of the subjects before the start of the intervention. The protocol defines the appropriate baseline measures and their assessment. In general, they consist of socioeconomic and demographic characteristics, and medical data with attention to known risk or prognosis factors. Published baseline data allow readers to evaluate whether the study groups were really comparable before intervention started (randomization, except in truly large trials with many hundreds of patients in each group, does not guarantee balance between comparison groups). Imbalance in important characteristics can yield misleading results.

Beside comparability, baseline assessment offers opportunities for stratification and subgrouping. Stratification can be done at the time of allocation to treatment or during analysis.[18] The definition of subgroups normally relies on baseline data, not data measured after intervention. Subgroup analysis in most cases serves only to generate new hypotheses for subsequent testing.

Inclusion/Exclusion Criteria and Study Endpoints

A key element in study documentation is the assessment of the inclusion/exclusion criteria and study endpoints. Study endpoints are response variables measured during the course of the trial that answer the questions of the study (see chapter 35). The methods for measurement must be described in detail. If a number of methods are available, the protocol should state the reasons for the choice of a particular method (e.g., practicability, reliability, validity).

Data Collection, Quality Assurance, and Control

To have data collected as completely as possible, develop a data-handling form for each patient. All data should be clearly defined in terms of how, when, and by whom they are to be collected. To minimize observer variation and to increase the quality of the data, a training course for standardization of the assessment of response variables may be necessary.

Analysis of the Data

Variation among individual patients, physicians, and institutions, and other sources of variability outside the investigator's control usually require statistical inference to evaluate the outcome of a clinical trial. In terms of statistical tests of significance, we gain control much more readily by prespecified analyses of the significance level of the investigation than by postspecified analyses. If we know what questions we want to ask, we can specify the statistics to be used, choose the significance level we feel would be appropriate and convincing to others, and discuss other properties of the statistical test—all in advance.

The protocol should specify the statistical methods to be used and how they are to be applied (see chapter 37).

Data Protection

The increasing use of electronic data processing raises problems of data security. Investigators must devise methods (e.g., passwords, separate data files for baseline data, response variables, and hard copies in secure places) to ensure data protection.

Ethical Considerations

The ethical issues surrounding randomized trials are substantial and sometimes daunting. The investigator must maintain clinical equipoise as a stable state of suspended judgment regarding the unequivocally proven relative advantage of each of the treatments compared. This state is uncharacteristic of surgeons and challenges the Hippocratic beneficence typical of our role when issues are in doubt. Ethical considerations including those related to informed consent and the selection of patients for randomized trial are well discussed by Lebacqz[19] and by Roy in chapter 60.

Investigators have a duty to protect subjects from harm or from deprivation of beneficial treatment should one arm of the trial prove unequivocally superior. This is best done through a monitoring committee comprising statistical and medical experts who are distanced from the point of clinical care. A particularly good example of the termination of a trial based on proven benefit of one of the arms is well described and graphically illustrated in the report of the Multicenter Automatic Defibrillator Implantation Trial (see especially Figure 1).[20]

Schedule for a Single Patient (Logistics)

Before creating data-handling forms for a single patient, trace the path of an individual patient coming through the study. Consider special arrangements and personal relationships as well as specific organizational structures within the institution. After completing the protocol, the investigator then develops data forms for each patient.

Organization for the Trial

The organization should be as straightforward as possible and should avoid overlapping tasks. A simple team consists of the leader of the study, who is closely connected with the study secretary. The study secretary is responsible for collecting the data from physicians and nurses at each patient's bedside. Depending on the type of study, a data monitoring committee may be necessary. Commonly, an advisory group provides professional expertise on special parts of the protocol. All members of the team must keep abreast of the study's progress and work well together.

Collaborative Trials

Most clinical trials, like most biomedical research, have their genesis as individual, investigator-initiated ideas that come from individual scholars or small groups of interested collaborators. Many clinical trials are rather small for what they seek to do; that is, they have relatively few patients in each treatment arm of the trial. Small trials usually have low power, and a low-powered trial will reliably identify only large differences between treatment arms.

One solution is to organize a multiinstitutional collaborative trial. Joining groups of investigators together to work on a trial can increase power by enlarging treatment groups and accelerating the rate of recruitment, but it also brings its own problems.

Multicentered collaborative trials require special care in their planning and execution (see chapter 27). There are problems in assuring that the patients and treatment in Toronto are the same as in Boston or Berlin, and special efforts must be made to maintain investigator enthusiasm, accurate recording of events, and all the myriad issues that cause problems even in trials in single institutions. We have now had a good bit of experience at such large enterprises. A number of groups are set up to function as coordinating centers and advisers for such trials, but multicentered trials are usually very expensive to organize and conduct.

Over the past few decades, groups of investigators have joined together to coordinate long-term programs of treatment evaluations by randomized clinical trials.

These government-funded, collaborative research groups represent one of the most important scientific resources of North American medicine and surgery. These groups have developed long-term mechanisms for data collection, review, and analysis by a relatively constant group of collaborators. They incorporate statistical and design consultation at the outset of each project from statisticians who have a well-developed sense of the history and problems of the group and its particular strengths and aptitudes. Through surveillance of the basic science literature, the members are able to recognize new treatments appropriate for evaluation using their cooperative group. Much of their success comes from the fact that their organization takes advantage of continuing experience. They mount clinical trials that build on the results of the trials just completed. Their organization permits a targeted, systematic approach to the evaluation of treatment in their areas of interest. Continued development and growth of this system is likely to prove advantageous for surgery in the future.

Current Status: Evaluation in Surgery

Although surgeons are often criticized, frequently unjustly, for the quality of their evaluations of both standard and innovative surgical treatments, the record shows that clinical trials in surgery are being done frequently and, on the whole, well.[21] Surgical leaders around the world are concerned with good clinical evaluation and research, are actively pursuing both, are gaining increasing support from practicing surgeons, and merit our support and applause for their efforts.

A significant advance in public appreciation of randomized trials in surgery was gained through the publicity associated with the trials of limited surgery for breast cancer. Further public education and systematic education of surgeons in the value and proper conduct of randomized trials will facilitate their application.

References

1. Bearman JE, Loewenson RB, Gullen WH. Muench's Postulates, Laws, and Corollaries, or Biometricians' Views on Clinical Studies. (Biometrics Note 4) Bethesda, MD: Office of Biometry and Epidemiology, National Eye Institute, National Institutes of Health, 1974.

2. Goligher JC, Pulvertaft CN, Watkinson G. Controlled trial of vagotomy and gastro-enterostomy, vagotomy, and antrectomy, and subtotal gastrectomy in elective treatment of duodenal ulcer: interim report. Br Med J 1964;1:455–460.

3. Freedman B. Equipoise and the ethics of clinical research. New Engl J Med 1987;317:141–145.

4. Baillar JC III. Introduction. In: Shapiro SH, Lewis TA, eds. Clinical Trials, Issues, and Approaches. New York: Marcel Dekker, 1983, p. 1.

5. Herman J. The demise of the randomized controlled trial. J Clin Epidemiol 1995;48:985–988.

6. Sacket DL. On some prerequisites for a successful clinical trial. In: Shapiro SH, Louis TA, eds. Clinical Trials. New York: Marcel Dekker, 1983, p 65.

7. Gilbert JP, McPeek B, Mosteller F. Statistics and ethics in surgery and anesthesia. Science 1977; 198:684–689.

8. Moses LE, Louis TA. Statistical consultation in clinical research: a two-way street. In: Baillar JC, Mosteller F, eds. Medical Uses of Statistics, 2nd edn. Boston: NEJM Books, 1992, pp. 349–356.

9. Pocock S. Clinical Trials—A Practical Approach. New York: Wiley, 1983.

10. Friedman LM, Furberg CD, De Metz DL. Fundamentals of Clinical Trials, 2nd edn. Littleton, MA: Littleton Publishing Co., 1985:1–307.

11. Schwartz D, Lellouch J. Explanatory and pragmatic attitudes in clinical trials. J Chronic Dis 1967;20:637–648.

12. MacRae KD. Pragmatic versus explanatory trials. Int J Technol Assess Health Care 1989;5:333–339.

13. Meinert CL. Clinical Trials—Design, Conduct, and Analysis. New York: Oxford University, 1986.

14. Zelen M, Gehan E, Glibwell O. Biostatistics in cancer research. In: Hoogstralen B, ed. Importance of Cooperative Groups. New York: Mason, 1980, pp. 291–312.

15. Mosteller F, Gilbert JP, McPeek B. Reporting standards and research strategies for controlled trials. Controlled Clin Trials 1980;1:37–58.

16. Freiman JA, Chalmers TC, Smith H. The importance of beta, the type II error, and sample size in the design and interpretation of the randomized controlled trial. New Engl J Med 1978;290:690–694.

17. Emerson JD, McPeek B, Mosteller F. Reporting clinical trials in general surgical journals. Surgery 1984;85:572–579.

18. Shapiro S, Louis A, eds. Clinical Trials: Issues and Approaches. New York: Dekker, 1982.

19. Lebacqz K. Ethical aspects of clinical trials. In: Shapiro SH, Lewis TA, eds. Clinical Trials, Issues, and Approaches. New York: Marcel Dekker, 1983, pp. 81–98.

20. Moss AJ, Hall WJ, Cannom DS, Daubert JP, Higgins SL, Klein H, Levine JH, Saksena S, Waldo AL, Wilber D, Brown MW, Heo M. Improved survival with an implanted defibrillator in patients with coronary disease at high risk for ventricular arrhythmia. New Engl J Med 1996;335:1933–1940.

21. Schwartz D, Flamant R, Lellouch J. Clinical Trials. New York: Academic, 1980.

Additional Reading

A variety of textbooks and journal articles are now available to guide those undertaking or evaluating a trial. An especially readable book, *Clinical Trials: Issues and Approaches,* edited by Stanley Shapiro and Thomas A. Louis,[18] deals with the controversies, design, analysis, and methodology of clinical trials. This will be appreciated by both novices and experts.

While there is general agreement about the conduct of a randomized clinical trial and about what constitutes a good trial, the field is by no means static. Many thoughtful, innovative ideas appear each year. The official journal of the Society for Clinical Trials, *Controlled Clinical Trials,* began publication in 1980 and deals with all aspects of clinical trials.

Emerson JD, McPeek B, Mosteller F. Reporting clinical trials in general surgical journals. Surgery 1984;85:572–579.

Freiman JA, Chalmers TC, Smith H. The importance of beta, the type II error, and sample size in the design and interpretation of the randomized controlled trial. New Engl J Med 1978;290:690–694.

Gilbert JP, McPeek B, Mosteller F. Statistics and ethics in surgery and anesthesia. Science 1977;198:684–689.

Meinert CL. Clinical Trials—Design, Conduct, and Analysis. New York: Oxford University, 1986.

Mosteller F, Gilbert JP, McPeek B. Reporting standards and research strategies for controlled trials. Controlled Clin Trials 1980;1:37–58.

Pocock S. Clinical Trials—A Practical Approach. Chichester, NY: Wiley, 1983.

Schwartz D, Flamant R, Lellouch J. Clinical Trials. New York: Academic, 1980.

Shapiro S, Louis TA, eds. Clinical Trials: Issues and Approaches. New York: Dekker, 1982.

Commentary

Innovative treatments seem obvious candidates for controlled trials, but they rarely enter practice in this way. The research ethics board may not learn about laparoscopic cholecystectomy until one of its members undergoes the procedure. Singer, Siegler, and Lantos, et al.[1] have developed a practical and useful technique for conducting a trial of innovative treatment. They recommend a formal sequence of steps to insure that new technology is evaluated in a timely way under defined conditions. First, the novel procedure is published in the medical literature; this public statement commits the workers to give a follow-up when their clinical observations on a defined number of patients become available. Second, a working paper is submitted to the hospital or clinic where the procedure will be conducted. This summarizes and explains the research plan. Third, after a defined number of patients have been exposed to the new treatment (for example, after 20 living related donor liver transplants), a follow-up publication is submitted to share the experience, regardless of the success or failure of the program.

M.F.M.

1. Singer PA, Siegler M, Lantos JD, Emond JC, Whitington PF, Thistlethwaite R, Broelsch CE. The ethical assessment of innovative therapies: liver transplantation using living donors. Theor Med 1990;11:87–94.

CHAPTER 27

Multicenter Collaborative Clinical Trials

R.G. Pollock, C.M. Balch, and E.C. Holmes

The controlled clinical trial is the most rigorous method we have to evaluate and compare alternative treatments. During the past three decades, controlled trials have almost replaced historical reviews or extensive personal experience as the basis for choosing treatment strategies.

Multicenter clinical trials have played a major role in advancing surgical knowledge and treatment approaches over a range of diseases (e.g., antrectomy vs. highly selective vagotomy for duodenal ulcer, duodenal ulcer surgery vs. acid inhibitor treatment, coronary or carotid surgery vs. medical treatment, cyclosporin in organ transplantation, etc.). Such studies have been performed by groups of clinicians banding together, for a single study or a series of clinical protocols, through such formal cooperative group mechanisms as the National Surgical Adjuvant Breast and Bowel Project (NSABP), the Trauma Cooperative Group, the Veterans Administration Cooperative Group, the World Health Organization Melanoma Group, and the large National Cancer Institute–sponsored cooperative groups such as the Southwest Oncology Group (SWOG), the Eastern Cooperative Oncology Group (ECOG), and the Cancer and Leukemia Group B (CALGB).

We will describe some basic principles and organizational structures that we consider to be necessary to ensure high quality, reproducible results in multicenter studies. Although many of the ex-amples arise from extensive experience with cancer cooperative groups, the principles also apply broadly to other surgical disease.

Types of Trial

Phases of Trials

Clinical investigations of a new treatment are usually classified according to three sequential stages: phases I, II, and III.

Phase I. Trials in the first phase cover the introduction of a new treatment concept or drug. Examples are new chemotherapies that usually involve a small number of patients and which are tested primarily for safety and complications. When the studies focus on drugs, dose-limiting toxicities are sought by beginning with a low dose and increasing it until toxic levels are reached. Demonstration of a therapeutic gain is not necessarily a goal in this phase.

Phase II. Phase II trials are conducted as single-arm studies involving a limited number of patients treated consecutively within each disease category. The aim is to establish some degree of treatment efficacy. The phase II trial also provides an opportunity to define the effect of a new treatment on already-established subsequent treatments. For example, a phase II trial could determine the effects of preoperative chemotherapy or radiotherapy on a subsequent surgical resection (e.g., the difficulty of the surgical procedure, wound-healing problems, etc.). If responses are seen, the feasibility of a phase III trial is explored to see if the benefits can be extended and clarified.

Phase III. In the third phase, the new treatment or drug is compared to known, effective, standard treatments in a prospective, randomized fashion. The new therapy or drug may be evaluated by itself or in combination with other standard treatments as a new combined modality. Phase III trials require large numbers of patients and frequently have to employ the multicenter collaborative group mechanism.

Sometimes, clinical investigators stop at phase II without sufficiently proving that the new treatment is effective. The converse is also true; phase III trials have been started before optimization of the treatment approach and minimization of any associated morbidity. Many clinical research endeavors should take the form of a logical series of different investigations over time.

Randomized Controlled Clinical Trials

The most exacting and widely accepted design for clinical trials is the randomized controlled trial. Participating patients are assigned to treatments by random selection rather than by any conscious decision, to ensure the formation of a control group that differs from the treatment group only in the treatment being studied—and in no other respect. Even though randomized trials can lead to important information of lasting value, *a poorly designed or inappropriately analyzed randomized trial can lead to just as much confusion and conflict* as the biases in nonrandomized studies with historical controls.

Without careful evaluation and confirmation by phase III trials, expensive or dangerous treatments can be widely applied with little chance for benefit. The immediate acceptance of postoperative radiation therapy for breast cancer in the years following World War II is a good example. Improvement in equipment had made safe and effective radiation therapy available, and it was widely assumed that supplementing the then standard operation of radical mastectomy with radiation would improve the rates of control and cure. This assumption went unquestioned for a long time, and radiation, although unproven as an adjunctive therapy, became standard treatment throughout North America. By the late 1960s, the biology of cancer was better understood, and randomized controlled clinical trials to evaluate the postoperative use of radiotherapy were finally undertaken. The eventual result[1,2] was discontinuance of routine adjunctive radiation and a consequent reduction in morbidity and costs, without impairment of survival.

Evaluation of a widely established therapy is often difficult because the need for a "no treatment" control arm suggests the withholding of a putatively useful treatment. The evaluation of a new therapy is preferably made before its use becomes widely established, so that it can be compared to "standard therapy." The difficulty in entering patients in a trial in which treatment is determined by random selection has prompted a long search by investigators for other methods of choosing control groups, but a better method than randomization has yet to be found.

Historical Control Trials

Historical controls remain a popular alternative to randomized controls. This approach uses a selected group of patients treated in the past as a control for a group currently receiving a new treatment; the patients can be matched for such factors as age, sex, and extent of disease. Although this method sounds useful, it has many limitations, including the following:

1. Criteria for patient selection are difficult to define.
2. Investigators may be more selective than past physicians in choosing patients for a new treatment.
3. Changes occur in the natural history of the disease.
4. Changes occur in the pathological definitions or staging of the disease.
5. Changes occur in patient referral patterns.
6. Recorded data may be of inferior quality.
7. Criteria for response may be difficult to ascertain consistently in the records.

8. Improvements in patient care may improve new treatments.

Nonrandomized trials with concurrent controls also introduce bias that may cause incorrect interpretation of the results. Nevertheless, because some types of nonrandomized study provide important information needed for the better design of randomized clinical trials, they do have their place in the sequential scheme of research. For example, a retrospective review of 294 melanoma patients treated at the University of Alabama at Birmingham[3] led directly to the design (including stratification criteria) for a multicenter randomized clinical trial involving various surgical treatment options.[4]

There is clear evidence that uncontrolled studies are much more likely than controlled trials to lead to falsely enthusiastic recommendations for a treatment.[5,6] A study by Gilbert and colleagues[7] showed that only 50% of the surgical innovations tested by randomized clinical trials were associated with significant improvements, even though all of them tested treatments already shown to be efficacious by historical or noncontrolled comparisons.

Advantages and Disadvantages of Multicenter Trials

Advantages

Consider a multicenter trial under six conditions, outlined as follows:

1. *When a large number of patients is required.* Many types of clinical questions can be addressed only in clinical trials involving a large sample size. For example, in a 10-year period, the NSABP entered 10,000 patients into randomized clinical trials to assess the comparative value of using one, two, or three drugs and multimodality combinations of chemotherapy and hormonal therapy. Without the resources of a large collaborative group, it would have been exceedingly difficult to allocate a smaller number of patients to so many drug choices and combinations. The collaborative group mechanisms usually already have in place the expensive and labor-intensive infrastructure needed to conduct a large trial. It is difficult if not impossible for a single institution or small group to marshal the needed resources to conduct a large trial. Using large collaborative groups to generate data can be highly cost-effective by preventing the duplication of resource expenditures that would be required if several small groups were funded that were trying to consider the same question. The collaborative group mechanism has enabled us to gain much more knowledge of the biology of breast cancer than we could have obtained within a single institution.

2. *When rapid accrual of patients is needed.* If it takes too long to recruit the required number of patients, other findings or treatment advances can make a study obsolete before it is completed. A recent NSABP trial (adjuvant colon carcinoma NSABP-C03) entered 830 patients and closed to patient accrual within a 16-month period.

3. *When studying rare events.* Multiinstitutional protocols make it possible to study uncommon diseases or specific subgroups of patients rarely seen at tertiary medical centers. Studies of surgical and adjuvant therapy for childhood cancers (e.g., rhabdomyosarcoma and Wilms' tumor) were feasible only with a series of national trials. The Intergroup Melanoma Surgical Trial made it possible to study a specific subgroup of melanoma patients with intermediate tumor thickness to ascertain the optimal surgical management of the primary melanoma and the regional lymph nodes.[4] This protocol has accrued more than 700 patients treated at more than 200 institutions; it could not have been conducted in any single institution.

4. *When more precisely defined subject groups are needed.* Large numbers of patients for each protocol make it possible to stratify for important patient characteristics. In an NSABP protocol for evaluating the efficacy of adding tamoxifen to the standard two-drug regimen, estrogen receptors (ER) and progesterone receptors (PR) were measured and recorded for all patients. A good response to tamoxifen was seen in patients with high ER and PR levels and in older age groups. In subsequent studies, pretreat-

ment determinations of ER and PR levels were used as the basis for assigning patients to different treatment groups to explore research questions related to differences in ER status.

If studies like those just described were attempted with only 150 patients in each arm, much of the needed information could not be obtained. Splitting trial participants into groups that are large enough to be meaningful may require a total of 2,000 patients. Since a busy urban hospital may average only about 100 new cases of primary breast cancer each year, it is impractical to attempt a study requiring 2,000 cases without some form of multicenter collaboration.

5. *When improved generalizability is important.* Many collaborative groups comprise a combination of university, large urban, and smaller community hospitals that affords access to a more representative mix of patients than would be found in any one type of institution. As a result, their findings are more readily generalizable to broad clinical practice. The necessity of having all participating hospitals comply with such special protocol requirements as immunochemical staining or high-energy radiotherapeutic treatments may, however, exclude some institutions that wish to be involved. Such obstacles can often be surmounted by making referral arrangements within the group.

6. *When rapid technology transfer is needed.* Involving community clinicians in routine clinical trial group meetings is an excellent way to promote the rapid transfer of ideas, techniques, and knowledge. Discussing new protocols and hypotheses, participating in clinical research, and using good clinical trial methodology are valuable learning experiences that lead to better clinical care for participating patients.

Disadvantages

Multicenter trials are both expensive and complex.

First, the cost of supporting a trial group's central operations, travel to group meetings, and research personnel within member institutions usually ranges from $1,500 to $3,000 (US) per

patient entered. The National Cancer Institute in the United States spends more than $60 million per year to support multiinstitutional clinical trials. Allocations of funds for these clinical research studies are approved through an extensive and rigorous peer review process.

Moreover, as the number of investigators participating in a study increases, there must be a parallel increase in quality control efforts to minimize variability among patients, treatments, assessment, investigators, and institutions. This is only a relative disadvantage, however, because the results are generally more representative, and achievable only by a diverse group of institutions and physicians.

The Organization and Management of Multicenter Clinical Trials

The best time to build a collaborative group is during the design phase of a trial. Early in the planning stage, all the possible participants should be invited to a meeting to consider a clearly stated study question accompanied by relevant background material and the rationale for the proposed study. The enclosed concept paper should not be longer than three pages.

If you are participating in the organization of a multicenter trial, give consideration to establishing the following committees, if they are in accord with the scope of the project and the planned duration of the group.

A *protocol committee* is a suitable way to create the actual trial. Circulate the concept paper to interested people who have experience in the subject area to be studied and ask them to discuss the pros and cons of various aspects of the proposed protocol.

Writing the protocol is one of the most important components of a study. The protocol serves two purposes. The first is to describe the scientific design, which is always built best around a biological hypothesis; if it is, your results are more likely to be publishable—whatever answer you obtain. The second purpose is to create an operations manual that will enable all the participating investigators to perform in a uniform, systematic way. A basic outline of a clinical research protocol and a list of data forms to be generated are provided in Tables 27-1 and 27-2, respectively. Some examples of the issues and questions that should be addressed in the development of a protocol are as follows:

1. The surgery or other intervention to be performed must be defined. (A standard version of the operation is necessary. Any variations considered important or unimportant must be specified.)
2. What are the inclusion/exclusion criteria?
3. What preliminary studies need to be performed before a patient is entered (e.g., kidney function tests if a renal-toxic drug is involved)?
4. What special procedures need to be performed on the surgical specimen or the patient (e.g., receptor or immunofluorescent studies)?
5. What pathology controls will be performed?
6. What follow-up intervals will be used, and what observations will be made and recorded?
7. What records are to be kept?

A *study chairperson* (or cochairpersons) should be designated for each protocol. This person (or persons) has responsibility for the ongoing conduct of the study. He or she can respond on an ad hoc basis to unanticipated questions about patient eligibility for entry, or about the conduct of the study. The chairperson assumes responsibility for ensuring that data reports come in on time, that eligibility requirements are met, and that no deviation occurs.

Table 27-1. Basic outline for a clinical research protocol.

1. Objectives
2. Background and rationale
3. Criteria for patient selection
4. Surgical guidelines
5. Pathology guidelines and procedures
6. Studies to be done
7. Randomization procedure
8. Reporting procedures and follow-up
9. Patient evaluation criteria
10. Quality control and evaluation
11. Statistical requirements
12. Forms and records to be submitted
13. Patient consent
14. Bibliography

A *principal investigator* should be identified at each participating institution. The principal investigator has overall responsibility for the conduct of the studies and the maintenance of the institution's level and quality of activity. He or she is the focal point for disseminating information about progress or changes in ongoing studies, and the institution's representative in the collaborating group, especially for the administrative and organizational aspects of the study.

A *surgical monitoring committee* is necessary for any surgical clinical investigation. The surgical operation should be clearly defined, and a description of how it is to be performed should be provided in the protocol. The anatomic limits of the dissection, and the anatomic structures to be preserved or removed should be clearly specified. For example, in NSABP colon studies, each type of segmental colon resection is clearly described, the vasculature to be divided is identified, and the scope of the operative report is specified and compared to the check-off data form to ensure that the surgical requirements are being met. Similarly, the Intergroup Melanoma Committee developed surgical guidelines and check-off forms for lymph node dissections at each anatomic site.

A *pathology monitoring committee* is required to formulate guidelines for examining all surgical specimens, delineating criteria for the diagnostic and prognostic features of the pathology, and developing forms for reporting pathology results in a standardized fashion. Many pathological features are difficult to quantify because they require personal interpretation (e.g., histological grading). A pathology reference center is the best way to ensure standard diagnoses. A data form should be created to prompt the pathologist to provide answers to all relevant questions and ensure good data control.

A *radiotherapy monitoring committee* should be created whenever radiotherapy is employed. If the effects of radiotherapy are being tested in a protocol, very careful attention to the planning and monitoring of the treatment is mandatory. All the collaborating institutions should have their radiation therapy units calibrated, their methodology standardized, and their dose calculations reviewed centrally. Complications and toxicity should be monitored and recorded on data forms designed for the purpose.

Table 27-2. Data forms that might be necessary for a multicenter clinical trial.

Form	Function
On-study form	All vital information about the patient and the diagnosis. When a patient enters the study, the names and addresses of three relatives, who will know the patient's whereabouts in the event he or she moves, should always be obtained. This information can be invaluable after several years of follow-up when a patient suddenly relocates without leaving a forwarding address.
Progress forms	For recording data about the patient status during the conduct of the study, including such study parameters as drug dose received, toxicities encountered, and the status of the patient (e.g., free of relapses or site of relapse).
Follow-up forms	May include results of physical exam and laboratory and X-ray results.
Off-study form	Completed when a patient goes off study because of one of the following quality control reasons; intercurrent illness (e.g., a second type of serious cancer), or death from unrelated cause (e.g., auto accident).
Surgery checklist	Created for reviewing operative reports; can be a part of the protocol documentation and should be filled out by the operating surgeon following each operation. A second data form, for such complications as an anastomotic leak or a seroma, should also be created so that a good statistical analysis can be performed at a later date.

A *drug monitoring committee* is needed to control adherence to the protocol, monitor for drug toxicities, and develop specific criteria and schedules for adjusting drug doses for defined levels of toxicity. A data form should be designed for easy supervision of any departure from the stipulated schedules or doses and for recording toxicities and unanticipated problems.

All these monitoring committees have a double function. One is to ensure conformity to the protocol and the recording and evaluation of any deviations; the other is to monitor and document toxicity and alert investigators to serious problems requiring changes in the protocol when a patient's safety is concerned.

An *executive committee* should be created to make decisions and to oversee the continued functioning of the collaborating groups and their protocols. Ideally, this committee should comprise the principal investigators at each participating institution and representatives from the various monitoring committees. The committee should have guidelines for the probation and suspension of any individuals or institutions failing to participate or violating protocol guidelines. Because inadequate performance by an individual or an institution will sometimes make it necessary to invoke one of these unpleasant actions, appropriate

rules and regulations should be agreed on prospectively, when the group is organized, to facilitate the handling of problems if the need arises. The existence of the monitoring process and rules for dropping a center may help to prevent its occurrence.

Decisions to close or abort a study or any portion of it should follow guidelines laid down in the protocol. The monitoring process, maintained by the executive committee, should provide information on when to close or abandon one arm of a study that is jeopardizing an otherwise good program. For example, in some aggressive chemotherapy programs, unexpected life-threatening toxicities may occur; careful monitoring and evaluation will allow the study to be closed before too many patients are exposed to danger.

Group Meetings

Information dissemination increases in importance as the group grows and gains experience. Annual or semiannual group meetings with a backup system of mailings and updates is one way to keep group communications current. Group meetings provide opportunities to disseminate information on the status of various studies, discuss any problems, explain any changes or clarifications in the conduct of the study, and keep participants abreast of what has been learned. Results will not be published until accrual targets are met, but toxicities can be discussed, and findings and correlations in ancillary areas can be presented. Group meetings also provide a forum for the exchange of information between participants and are an ideal way to stimulate and maintain interest in the study.

Headquarters

One institution should act as the headquarters from which a full-time director and data manager(s) will supervise the day-to-day conduct of the trial. The infrastructure support includes a strong statistical center that may or may not be located adjacent to the trial headquarters. Nurse practitioners and data managers are needed on site at each institution that is participating in the multicenter trial. The operations office at trial headquarters is responsible for monitoring the studies, providing the principal investigators with the data, and providing periodic reports to the entire group. Visits by an audit committee to the participating institution are necessary to monitor the quality of the data, resolve any possible misunderstandings, and proactively identify areas of confusion that might otherwise not come to light until much later when it may no longer be possible to make necessary early or midcourse corrections.

Authorship

If a publication committee does not exist, a clear decision about who will be responsible for writing the report should be made at the outset. This ensures the completion of this task and helps in the assignment of appropriate credits for authorship and participation in the study. A committee can also help to choose the journal for publication or the scientific meeting at which the report will be presented.

Ethics

It is imperative that a clinical trial follow ethical guidelines. A carefully written consent form, counseling about the trial's investigational nature, and full disclosure of its risks and uncertainties are inherent ethical components of any clinical trial. In North America the law requires the creation of review boards composed of scientists not involved in the project, physicians who are not necessarily investigators, and representatives of the nonmedical community, such as lawyers and members of the clergy. The board's role is to determine whether the proposed research is scientifically and ethically appropriate, and whether provision has been made to ensure that patients will receive adequate information about the choices presented to them. It is important that investigators cooperate with review boards to assure the proper conduct of the trial.

Finances

Each participating institution needs money to maintain one or more secretarial data managers and to cover travel expenses for group meetings. The headquarters for a large project will need data managers, supervisors, biostatisticians, computer experts, and adequate computer resources. In addition, large studies may require salaries for investigators. Even though the total outlay of funds for the entire apparatus may be large, a demonstration of the usefulness of some treatments, and the desirability of abandoning others that are not will result in reductions in morbidity and health care costs.

Statistical and Data Management

A *quality control data management program* should be instituted at the group headquarters. It is one thing to specify the data to be collected, the forms to be used, and the records to be kept, but another to ensure that they are accurate, complete, and punctual. Some form of audit will be needed to ensure that the data collected are correct. This is usually best done by a spot check method in which the original hospital charts of randomly selected patients and certain predetermined data (e.g., the accuracy of eligibility criteria and the consistency of drug administration) are examined. Pharmacology logs should also be examined and nursing notes correlated to make sure that the chemotherapy was given according to the protocol, and that the dose actually given corresponded with what was reported on the data forms.

The *biostatistician* is an important and integral member of the collaborative clinical research team. The biostatistician must participate at the study design and protocol planning stages, at the inception of the trial, and also throughout the data accrual, analysis, and presentation phases. In the attempt to answer too many questions, principal investigators will frequently create protocols that are too complicated, have too many arms, or create a study in which no valid results can be obtained. The biostatistician can help the research group avoid initiating a trial that will never give meaningful statistical information, thereby helping to prevent a great deal of wasted effort and resources. Since many phase III trials are blinded to the investigators, the biostatistician is critical for monitoring the study and determining that undue negative effects are not occurring or that a positive effect is not so overwhelming that the trial should be closed.

A *data manager* should be appointed for each institution accruing cases and will be responsible for maintaining and submitting accurately completed data forms on schedule. The data manager becomes involved with each patient at the time of consideration for entry into the protocol—to verify eligibility, perform the randomization, contact trial headquarters to register the patient, and transmit the treatment assignment to the investigator. The data manager immediately assembles a dossier containing the required study forms, and eventually keeps a parallel protocol chart for each patient containing all the paperwork required by the protocol. A copy of every document sent to headquarters should be kept in the patient's protocol chart so that verification can be easily done on a moment's notice.

The data manager is also responsible for scheduling return visits for treatment or follow-up and for maintaining records on long-term scheduling. As patient numbers increase, it is very important to maintain complete follow-up and to ensure that no patient is lost to the process.

Data manager seminars at group meetings are an invaluable way of exchanging information and teaching the newer members of the organization the techniques of data management.

As the number of patients being followed increases, difficulties in tracking and scheduling can occur. The Institutes at McGill University have designed a computer-aided scheduling system, the McGill Protocol System, which contains master or template schedules for each protocol. Patients can be matched to a specific treatment program, and a schedule can be generated at any time to show the data manager which patients are due for which treatments or tests in which time period. As dividends, patients can be given copies of their schedules for the next time frame, and each participating laboratory can have advance lists of all the patients it will have to schedule in the coming weeks. This kind of system minimizes mistakes and assures the flow of good quality data.

Quality Control Criteria and Monitoring

Considerable effort must be devoted to establishing quality control guidelines for each adjuvant therapy protocol. Quality control review mechanisms must be established within each member institution and centrally at the operations or statistics office. In oncology protocols, for example, quality control measures are used to monitor drug dose schedules (including adjustments for toxicity), radiation therapy (including dosimetry and port planning), and surgery (to ensure the surgical procedure was conducted according to written guidelines).

Surgical guidelines must be written for each adjuvant therapy protocol to describe the minimum amount of surgical dissection required for different anatomical settings. The melanoma surgical protocol specified that a parotid dissection was essential for patients with metastatic melanoma from a primary site in the anterior scalp, temple, or face. Precise definitions of regional node dissections were described for cervical, axillary, and inguinal lymphadenectomies.

In NSABP protocol B-06, the segmental mastectomy operation was new to most surgeons in North America, and early experience revealed unanticipated problems in its performance with respect to tumor control and cosmetic outcome. Several NSABP investigators who had extensive experience with the operation proposed solutions that were discussed and refined in workshops of participating surgeons. The workshop concept was so successful that it was continued over the 8-year period of accrual to the protocol, to ensure that surgeons joining later did not have to learn the operation by repeating the same initial errors.

Pathology guidelines must also be defined. For example, all lymph nodes must be examined, and the pathologist must report the total number of nodes examined and the number that contained metastases. A minimum number of nodes must be examined to maintain quality control; in our studies, it was 5 for superficial inguinal dissections, 10 for axillary dissections, and 20 for cervical dissections. Outside pathology slides had to be reviewed by a pathologist at the member institution or by the pathology committee of the entire group.

A surgeon at each member institution should review the operative note and pathology report and sign the on-study form certifying that the minimum surgical guidelines were adhered to before the patient was randomized into the protocol. The operative record and pathology report are forwarded to the statistics office for central review by the surgical investigator assigned to each adjuvant therapy protocol.

Communicating the Results of Multicenter Trials

After the clinical trial has been closed to patient accrual, the investigators must decide when to analyze the results, how to interpret them, and when to publish.

It is important to "let the data speak for themselves" and not overinterpret results, especially before the information on follow-up has become sufficiently mature. Because there is a natural tendency for others to overinterpret, distort, or amplify the results, it is vitally important that the authors frame their interpretations of the results carefully and realistically; premature publication and overinterpretation of results still in a state of flux must be avoided.

Even large randomized clinical trials may not yield absolute conclusions; but the results and the interpretation of data may increase the level of confidence that the treatment under study should be adopted as standard treatment in defined subsets of patients, at least. It is important to publish the results, even when they are negative.

The following questions or issues should be addressed when investigators are deciding when to publish and what to say:

1. Is the follow-up of the patients long enough to permit the drawing of valid conclusions?
2. In studies with survival endpoints, especially oncology studies, is the difference in relapse-free survivals great enough to permit a definite prediction that they will also translate into significant differences in overall survival rate?
3. In patient studies with very large sample size, small differences may be statistically significant, but the investigators will have to ask whether these statistically significant differences are also clinically significant—especially in settings where toxicity, cost, or morbidity might be involved.
4. Are the patients entered into the trial representative of the entire universe of similarly staged patients?
5. Are there any subsets of patients in which different results occurred? Caution must be exercised in interpreting results in subsets of patients defined by criteria not used in the original design of the trial.
6. Are the results internally consistent using different statistical approaches, and consistent with existing knowledge of the biology of the disease under study?

The Future of Clinical Trials in the Managed Care Era

As we move toward the millennium, finances to support health care (at least in the United States) are undergoing a fundamental reorganization. Standard indemnity insurance in support of traditional fee for service is being rapidly replaced by managed care contractual arrangements. This transformation has been fueled by the private sector where there is a perception that the imperatives of economic competitiveness will not sustain a continued 13% of gross national product expenditure on health care. This emerging reality has created a milieu in which cost-competitive pressures on health care delivery are having a major negative impact on biomedical research support in American academic health care centers. Historically, in academic health centers upwards of $850 million have annually been extracted from generated clinical revenues and then used to cross-subsidize research and educational missions, including clinical research. Costs of health care delivery must be cut for academic health centers to compete in the managed care environment; yet any decline in clinical revenue margins may derail cross-subsidization strategies.

Additional detrimental factors are also emerging in this "brave new world" of health care economics. Medical schools have come under increasing pressure to train generalists at the expense of specialty training support, including the surgical specialties. This decreasing specialist physician workforce may result in fewer fellowship training positions, thereby further decreasing the pool of investigators capable of asking "cutting edge" clinical research questions. Alterations such as these could ultimately result in a shrinking faculty pool that has the capacity to design, initiate, and conclude clinical trials as well as mentor new clinical researchers.

Finances in the pharmaceutical industry may also negatively impact clinical research support. Low-overhead mail delivery pharmaceutical suppliers are frequently mandated in lieu of retail outlets as providers for specific managed care contractors. As competitive pressure from these suppliers increases, a traditional source of industrial pharmaceutical financial support for clinical research may also become threatened.

An additional concern arises from the obligation that many academic health care centers have incurred to serve as a safety net for uninsured or underinsured patients. Recent data from the Association of American Medical Colleges suggests that the 287 university academic health care centers, although only 6% of all hospitals, generate 26% of all gross medical revenues, absorb 28% of all medical debt, and deliver 50% of all charity care in the United States.[8]

The increasingly competitive local medical market place will impose further difficulties on the clinical research enterprise. In a capitated environment it is not clear if voluntary enrollees will sign up at academic health care centers instead of more geographically convenient and amenity-rich nonuniversity community facilities, thereby potentially removing themselves from access to clinical trials while simultaneously further eroding academic center clinical revenue streams.

The above emerging forces are of concern to all who are involved in the clinical research endeavor. Managed care entities are presumably aware that clinical research is critical for medical progress and ultimately cost-effective health care. However, most are apparently not interested in paying for research or experimental treatments that do not lead to near-term savings or that place them at a competitive disadvantage vis-á-vis other managed care organizations. There is usually a considerable difference in the time frame in which a new treatment is conceived, tested, and proven effective versus the emergence of proof that the new treatment is medically necessary for certain patients. This time-denominated tension between trial eligibility and trial-derived proof of medical necessity has resulted in patients being denied authorization by managed care organizations to participate in clinical trials. This has led to several highly publicized and expensive legal confrontations that have ultimately forced managed care groups to authorize patient trial enrollment. Proposed alternatives to insurers' varying reimbursement policies include an all-payer research fund, a tax on all managed care companies to support research, and the establishment of public-private partnerships to forge incentives for providers, payers, and patients to participate in clinical trials.

In this rapidly shifting environment it is clear that new medical center coping strategies will need to be developed if clinical trials research is to thrive. The recent molecular insights into a wide variety of surgical diseases, coupled with potential therapeutic benefits as the Human Genome Project is completed over the next several years, offers unparalleled opportunity to advance health care. As such, we may be, in reality, entering a golden era for clinical trials to rapidly define these new molecularly driven standards of health care. In a generalized era of government cost containment, it is unlikely that there will be sweeping legislative relief of the difficult financial scenario now confronting academic health centers, as described above. Some centers may choose to discontinue support for expensive clinical research programs. Indeed, some institutions may not be able to respond to and overcome these difficult economic realities, and fall by the wayside.

In the face of these challenges, many academic health centers are responding by internal financial reengineering while simultaneously pursuing strategies that will expand external patient population pools. This approach will require new partnerships with other institutions and professional entities to secure the patient base needed to support clinical research programs. One strategy calls for creation of hub-and-spoke networks of academic tertiary care centers linked with community-based care organizations that also incorporate private foundations, pharmaceutical companies, and emerging biotechnology firms. Such networks are now being rapidly assembled in many locales on a regional basis. These efforts may require new cooperative and collaborative efforts involving several formerly competitive medical schools or other hub centers to secure the patients needed for meaningful clinical trials. These approaches may also lead to diversification of funding to include extramural peer-reviewed sources, clinically derived funds, and industrial and foundation sources that will most likely be directed toward those patient care clinical research networks that are optimally poised for patient accrual. Reconfiguring the academic health center hub clinical research infrastructure to make it accessible and accountable throughout the network will be required as part of this overall new creative strategy.

This process of reengineering the clinical research enterprise will be built on new and highly sophisticated informatics hardware, software, and personnel to link the network components together. Many academic health centers are engaged in such information access reorganizations as a needed first step to determine true costs in pathways of care required to successfully compete for managed care contracts. The intensity of a given institutional commitment to developing and initiating "cutting edge" informatics may be considered by funding agencies as a litmus test of the ability to construct an effective patient care clinical research network.

In an era of scarce resources, it will be necessary to develop guidelines for the overall quality of clinical trials. This latter issue will be determined by the importance of the question being asked, the quality of care being delivered, as well as the traditional clinical trial outcome parameters. Cost issues and patient satisfaction criteria will almost certainly be entered into future clinical trial guideline assessments, and may themselves become the focus of future health care research and clinical trial initiatives that seek to define a more rational delivery of health care. Such new health care delivery research programs will require new faculty and research facilities, perhaps at the expense of other programs that have not stood up as well to the passage of time. The future clinical research mission, while most likely having a different emphasis from current programs, will still ultimately focus on improving the quality of patient care. The only limitations to our participation in these exciting new developments will be self-imposed: inability to seek new pathways through collaboration, or not imagining broadly enough to encompass new opportunities in clinical care. The studies cited in this chapter clearly show that these constraints have not fettered surgeons in the past. There is every reason to expect that surgeons will develop equally imaginative solutions for the future.

Conclusion

If you are considering a multicenter clinical trial, all the points discussed in this chapter should be taken into account, although some will be more important in some studies than in others. In practical terms, you should always design the ideal study and then make the compromises necessary for feasibility. Setting down rules and guidelines at the beginning is the best way to proceed, but unrealistic rigidity can be self-defeating. All rules or compromises should be considered in the light of how to anticipate and prevent adverse criticism about the conduct of the study or its outcome. The objective is to do good clinical science and contribute to meaningful progress.

The randomized controlled clinical trial is the most reliable and useful investigative tool in clinical medicine. Despite its imperfections, it produces the most credible and generalizable results and has justifiably become—and is likely to remain—the mainstay of clinical research. It is doubtful that any clinical research program can be developed without a good understanding of how randomized controlled trials are designed and implemented. A collaborative multicenter randomized controlled trial is expensive, but the return on investment is worthwhile if the question it seeks to answer is clinically and socially important.

Acknowledgments. We would like to acknowledge the invaluable assistance of Carol MacKinnon and David Bradley of The Advisory Board Company, Washington, D.C., for their invaluable help in completing the chapter section about the future of clinical trials in the managed care era.

References

1. Butcher HR, Seaman WB, Eckert C, Saltzstein S. An assessment of radical mastectomy and postoperative irradiation therapy in the treatment of mammary cancer. Cancer 1964;17:480–485.
2. Paterson R, Russel MH. Clinical trials in malignant disease: III. Breast cancer: evaluation of postoperative radiotherapy. J Fac Radiol 1959;10:175–180.
3. Balch CM, Murad TM, Soong S-J, Ingalls AL, Halpern NB, Maddox WA. A multifactorial analysis of melanoma: prognostic histopathological features comparing Clark's and Breslow's staging methods. Ann Surg 1978;188:732–742.
4. Balch CM. The role of elective lymph node dissection in melanoma: rationale, results, and controversies. J Clin Oncol 1988;6:163–172.
5. Chalmers TC, Block JB, Lee S. Controlled studies in clinical cancer research. New Engl J Med 1972;287:75–78.
6. Moertel CG. Improving the efficiency of clinical trials: a medical perspective. Stat Med 1984;3:455–468.
7. Gilbert JP, McPeek B, Mosteller F. Statistics and ethics in surgery and anesthesia. Science 1977;198:684–689.
8. Richardson WC. The appropriate scale of the health sciences enterprise. Daedalus 1993;122:179–195.

CHAPTER 28

Selected Nonexperimental Methods: An Orientation

W.O. Spitzer and S.M. Horwitz

Clinical investigators and members of interdisciplinary research teams may often find that they must employ nonexperimental strategies characteristically used by epidemiologists and biostatisticians, particularly when randomized controlled trials (RCTs) are not ethically or practically feasible. These designs are used less frequently than controlled trials in surgical and anesthesia research. This chapter is intended as an orientation for those who seek meaningful and knowledgeable partnership in clinical and epidemiologic research. The bibliography will assist those who wish to pursue an in-depth understanding of the strategies presented here.

Uncontrolled case studies and case series have been mentioned in this textbook. Such efforts are indispensable precursors to good clinical and epidemiological research. However, the role of such work should be restricted to *hypothesis generation,* except when findings are dramatic. The discovery that penicillin could cure hitherto consistently incurable disorders was so striking that controlled studies and inferential statistics became unnecessary. Such dramatic advances in any field of medicine are, however, the exception rather than the rule. Characteristically, advances in clinical science are small, and progress is incremental. Improvements can be so subtle that the changes must be demonstrated carefully with the best attainable rigor of design and the highest sophistication of

appropriate statistics. Admissible rules of scientific logic must be followed.

One of the key rules is that research questions or hypotheses are tested only after they have been set forth in advance, not through fishing expeditions in existing data or even data-dredging of information we may have gathered ourselves. It is important to generate hypotheses, but it is essential to test them following an explicit protocol written and evaluated according to principles that assess the extent to which the results support a causal association.

Association Is Not Necessarily Causation

All clinicians must constantly remind themselves that association does not mean causation. Ordinarily, we can develop truly convincing evidence for causation only through experimental approaches. The strongest and most reliable evidence for cause and effect is the randomized controlled trial. Without evidence from such trials, the determination of whether an association is a causal one becomes more problematic. Sir Austin Bradford Hill suggests the consideration of nine features in looking at associations between factors and outcomes when the evidence is derived from nonexperimental methods. If many of these features are present, we are more secure in postulating causation.

Hill put the *strength of the association* first on the list. If the exposed population shows the outcome variable in a very marked degree, we are much more comfortable in inferring causation. High odds or risk ratios mean a strong association. Of course, we are sometimes misled. A very strong association between two factors may be just that, a strong association and not cause and effect.

Next on Hill's list of features to be considered in attributing causation is *consistency* of the observed association. The connection between smoking and lung cancer has been repeatedly observed by different workers in different countries within quite different populations over many years. Hill places great weight on similar results reached from studies with quite different designs. He finds this much more convincing than similar results from a collection of similarly designed studies. We know in medicine and surgery that very weakly designed studies all pointing in the same direction have led us to assume causation when, in fact, the consistency of association was merely the repetition of a mistake.

Hill's third characteristic is the *specificity of the association.* If the association is unusual, if it is limited to specifically exposed persons who develop unusual outcomes, this is a strong argument in favor of causation. The peculiar form of deformity in newborns produced by exposure of pregnant women to thalidomide, and the association between acquired immune deficiency syndrome and very rare Kaposi sarcomas are examples of this characteristic.

The fourth factor Hill considers is the *temporal relationship of the observed association.* An inference of causation is severely undermined when the effect appears before the cause. In the epidemics of Minamata disease seen in several parts of the world a few years ago, the emission of organic mercury toxic wastes preceded the great increase of reported cases of the neurological disorder.

As a fifth factor, Hill looks for an association that reveals a *dose-response curve or a biological gradient.* For example, those who smoke more cigarettes have higher death rates from smoking than both nonsmokers and those who smoke but a few cigarettes. A reverse gradient, such as a decreasing incidence of cancer of the lung among former smokers, is particularly persuasive.

The sixth feature Hill looks for is *biological plausibility.* If the association seems to make no sense at all, as in a relationship between the number of Presbyterian ministers in Scotland and the increasing population of Chicago, Hill suggests that we should be cautious in inferring causation. However, as we learn more and more about biology, associations that once made no sense become biologically plausible. When Professor Oliver Wendell Holmes of the Harvard Medical School drew attention, in 1847, to the association between the hand-washing habits of obstetrical surgeons and the incidence of puerperal fever among the mothers they attended, no one paid much attention because people could see no biological plausibility in the association. Twenty years later, after the work of Pasteur and Lister, the association acquired biological plausibility.

Hill's seventh factor is *coherence of the evidence.* Hill says that a cause and effect interpretation of an association should not seriously conflict with the generally known facts of the natural history and biology of the disease studied. Hill points out that the association of lung cancer and cigarette smoking is coherent with the increase in smoking among men that took place between 1910 and 1920, and the later increase among women. The isolation of carcinogenic factors from cigarette smoke and the histopathologic evidence of irritation of the airway epithelium of heavy smokers lend further evidence of coherence.

For his eighth factor, Hill asks if the *trends are reversible.* When the government withdrew the suspect pharmaceutical from the market, did reported cases of phocomelia fall? When smokers stop using cigarettes, do the rates at which they develop lung cancer fall? We call this evidence of reversibility.

Finally, as a ninth factor, Hill suggests we look for *analogies.* After having discovered a drug effect of thalidomide on fetuses, we are readier to accept somewhat similar evidence that another drug might cause fetal defects.

None of the nine factors brings indisputable evidence for or against a cause-and-effect hypothesis. Nevertheless, they do, with greater or lesser strength, suggest instances when an association may be one of causation.

For causation we prefer to have the evidence of a soundly conceived and well-executed experiment—one that employs the strengthening factors of random allocation to treatment, and appropriate varieties of blindness on the part of the experimenter, the patient, the evaluator of the outcome, and, perhaps, the statistician who analyzes the data. The employment of strengthening factors such as random allocation and blindness is no more an aspersion on the honesty of experimenters than requiring rubber gloves is a comment on the personal hygiene of surgeons.

Ascribing causation is serious business. The best advice about drawing conclusions on cause and effect from nonexperimental designs is to invoke Bradford Hill's criteria judiciously and to interpret the relationships carefully.

Experimental versus Nonexperimental Designs

An experimental design is one in which one group of eligible subjects or patients exposed to an intervention or a maneuver is compared to one or more control groups comparable to the intervention groups in all respects, save for the intervention or maneuver of interest. *The first essential characteristic of an experiment is that the intervention or the maneuver is assigned by the investigator to the exposed group and that the comparison interventions or maneuvers (e.g., placebo or the best-accepted current therapy) are also assigned by the investigator to the control group or control groups.* To express it another way, the *assignment of the maneuvers is under the control of the investigator.*

The second essential characteristic of an experiment is that assignment of subjects to the control and experimental groups be done by systematic, prespecified means presumed to guarantee the assembly of two absolutely comparable groups, except for the effects of the maneuver of interest. Generally, an investigator chooses to assign subjects to the intervention and control groups randomly, assuming that, with a large sample size, random assignment will evenly distribute unmeasured potential risk factors. However, experimental and control group assignment may be done in a systematic fashion by other preselected means such as alternate assignment rules (e.g., odd-even hospital file numbers).

In our current understanding of clinical science, the experiment that is an RCT is the "gold standard" of research. In their chapter on clinical research, Walters and Sackett discuss the advantages of the randomized and controlled approach for the assessment of effectiveness.[1] Yet no matter how well designed, these RCTs are not without problems due to human error, human folly, and chance. RCTs are difficult to carry out, must often sacrifice internal validity for generalizability, and evaluate clinical maneuvers only under optimal circumstances, as opposed to conditions approximating usual clinical care.

Designs belonging to a group in which random assignment of subjects is not possible (although investigator control over the assignment of the clinical maneuver is maintained) are called *sub-experimental* (a term used by Walters and Sackett) or *quasi-experimental* (a term borrowed from the social sciences). These designs can employ one group or multiple groups. In the one-group design, the comparison of interest is the outcome variable before and after the application of the intervention. Consider all eligible drivers in the state of Victoria, Australia, as a group; for the intervention of interest, take the introduction of compulsory use of seatbelts while driving. Given that it is possible to determine the number of injuries entailing death or physical injury to drivers and passengers per 100,000 persons "exposed to automobile transport," you could conduct a "before-and-after study." You could determine the number of injuries in the exposed citizens of that state, within certain age groups, for the full year prior to the new law. With the same determinations for one full year after the law came into effect, you could see whether there was any difference in rates. If the change (presumably a drop) is truly dramatic, you may not need comparison cohorts or concurrent experimental trials of any kind.

When before-and-after studies must be done, the design is strengthened by having several sequential measurements before the event or "independent variable" of interest, and several measures after. In the seatbelt example, suppose you had taken measures for odd-numbered years for a decade *before* the introduction of the law, and suppose further that the rates of identically classified and measured injuries were stable. If you made the same ascertainments for odd years for a decade *after* the introduction of the new law, and there was a stable, *sustained* new lower level, your conclusions about the relationship between the new law and the prevention of accidents and death would be greatly strengthened. If you are doing before-and-after studies, seek every opportunity to have at least two before measures and two after measures. A "step down" or "step up" of the measurement in the dependent variables coinciding with the "treatment" or exposure to the independent variable is a much stronger set of data on which to base conclusions on association.

If a "before-and-after" study does not give convincing evidence of change, you should be very cautious in interpreting the results, even if you have several before-and-after determinations. Other factors (confounders or effect modifiers) could have been operating at the same time. The price of gasoline might have changed, driving habits might have altered, or other laws setting lower speed limits might have affected the rate of accidents. It then becomes important to attempt additional before-and-after studies, historically or concurrently, in other jurisdictions (multiple group comparisons). The replications can be helpful in elucidating the confounding or effect-modifying impact of unrelated factors.

Designs that incorporate neither random allocation nor investigator assignment of the maneuver of interest are called observational or nonexperimental designs, even if two or more groups of study patients are compared. The balance of this chapter will introduce you to the major types of nonexperimental design, but our discussion of them will not be exhaustive. Many variations of these basic designs exist, and our brief orientation provides only a basic road map for this territory of research methodology. We have organized our discussion of nonexperimental designs according to the Canadian Task Force on the Periodic Health Examination[2] hierarchy of evidence: cohorts, case-control studies, cross-sectional research, and ecologic studies. Uncontrolled case studies and case reports will not be considered further.

Before detailing specific designs, we need to introduce a number of concepts that are important to keep in mind when digesting methodologic material. The first is the purpose of the study to be undertaken. Are we simply describing the state of affairs (i.e., *descriptive* study) or are we generating information about the relationship of particular factors to a disease (i.e., an *analytic* study)? We generally undertake descriptive studies when we know little about the determinants of disease or its natural history. Descriptive studies provide us with basic information about the disease or condition of interest and help us generate specific hypotheses about possible etiologic agents.

The second issue is the direction of the study design with respect to the potentially related factor and the outcome of interest. Are we observing a group of individuals at a defined point in time, gathering detailed information on the etiologic agents of interest, and following these individuals *forward* in time, concurrently, to determine disease status? Or, are we assembling a group of individuals with the disease of interest, a second group of individuals without the target disease, and pursuing the information backward with *backward* logic? Finally, are we measuring both etiologic agents and disease at the *same* point in time (cross-sectional)?

Another issue to consider is the unit of observation. Are we measuring our targeted features in individuals, in small groups (e.g., a family), or in larger groups (e.g., countries)? In most medical and surgical studies, the individual is the unit of observation. Further details for subsections of these observational designs can be found in chapters 7, 26, 27, 31, and 37.

Cohorts

The Latin word *cohort* was a Roman military term. It referred to a group of soldiers of a certain category. It could have been 100 or 500 infantrymen, 500 cavalry warriors, and so on. The first and most important use of "cohort" in clinical and epidemiologic research is to designate a number of persons (patients or healthy individuals) who share common attributes considered to be relevant to the research questions at issue. It could be 500 persons, 20–49 years old, experiencing a first incidence of low back pain, who have no clinically objective signs of neurological deficit. The cohort could be 10,000 diabetics 50–79 years old, eligible for inclusion by definite criteria and unaffected by peripheral vascular complications. It could be 25 1-week survivors of liver transplants, aged 13–60 months.

Sometimes the only intervention or maneuver of interest in studying a cohort is the passage of time. Thus, for the diabetics unaffected by peripheral vascular complications, one might wish to discover how many complications affect that *population* of diabetics over a 5-year period, stratified by age in half-decades. Or, a new drug to delay or prevent peripheral vascular complications may have been introduced into the market. A study might then determine the rate of development of such complications in a cohort of persons prone to peripheral vascular disorders and using the drug.

For any cohort, it is important to decide in advance what the dependent variable or the target outcome will be. The outcome events become the numerators for rates (such as incidence) calculated in cohort studies. For survivors of liver transplants, the dependent variable or target outcome might be death. For a cohort of patients with osteosarcoma, it might be length of disability-free survival. For a cohort of women with indwelling urinary catheters, it might be new infections in the postoperative period. The fundamental characteristic of the cohort is that the study subjects are identified and delineated by explicit criteria *before* the declared target outcome or dependent variable of interest is manifest among the same subjects. Cohorts are denominators for target outcomes. The target outcomes or dependent variables are the numerators. *In cohort studies, the denominators are always identified and delineated before the dependent variables are observed.* That is why cohort studies are sometimes called follow-up studies.

Cohorts may be followed in time as a single group without making any comparisons with any other group. Such work is referred to as descriptive. Figure 28-1 diagrams the basic structure of a classical cohort design. Notice that the direction of the study is forward, and the unit of analysis is the individual.

Table 28-1 shows the data layout for the analysis of a cohort. Individuals' exposure status is on the left-hand side, and follow-up disease status is

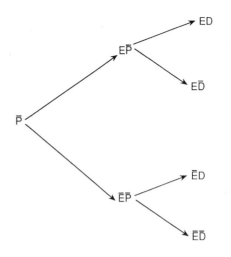

$\bar{P}$ = study population of interest, usually some group of individuals without the disease of interest, some proportion of whom will become exposed to the agent of interest.

E = exposed, $\bar{E}$ = not exposed

D = diseased, $\bar{D}$ = not diseased

Figure 28-1.   A cohort study.

across the top of the table. To determine whether those exposed to the putative agent of interest—for instance, amount of caffeinated beverages consumed daily by a cohort of 40- to 60-year-old men and women, who develop the targeted outcome (gallbladder disease)—we use the ratio of those diseased among caffeine consumers $[a/(a + b)]$ divided by the ratio of those diseased among the nonconsumers $[c/(c + d)]$. The resulting measure, the *relative risk* or *risk ratio*, gives us an idea of the association of caffeinated beverages with gallbladder disease. If this ratio is greater than 1, we usually say that the putative agent is associated with an increased risk of disease. If the ratio is less than 1, we say it is associated with a decreased risk of disease, or it is a protective factor. In his chapter on clinical biostatistics, Kramer presents additional analytic methods appropriate for use with categorical outcome measures.[3]

Sometimes it is possible to compare two or more cohorts and follow them simultaneously. For instance, it may be possible to assemble 20,000 men who became exposed to occupationally related radiation in nuclear plants starting in 1971, and continue to be exposed, and follow them to

Table 28-1. Data layout for a prospective cohort study.

		Disease status		
		D	D	Totals
	E	a	b	$a + b$
Exposure status	$\overline{E}$	c	d	$c + d$
	Totals	$a + c$	$b + d$	$(a + b) +$ $(c + d)$

Disease among exposed a $(a + b)$

Disease among unexposed $= c/(c + d)$

Relative risk $= \dfrac{a/(a + b)}{c/(c + d)}$

determine the total number of new cancers detected through 1995. This could be done at the same time as one follows another 20,000 men in other energy-related industries that are similar in most respects to nuclear power generating plants, except for the exposure to measured levels of radiation in the workplace. This second cohort of 20,000 men assembled in 1971 would also be followed through 1995. Note why this is not an experimental design. The investigator did not assign the men to be or not to be exposed to radiation, or to be or not to be in one type of industry or another. *The men self-selected their own jobs.* However, it can and should be established that the two self-selected cohorts are sufficiently comparable to follow them forward in time and compare the rate of development of new cancers between the two groups. With two or more groups, we have a cohort comparison study. It is worth emphasizing that all 40,000 men, the 20,000 exposed and the 20,000 not exposed, were free of the target outcome of interest (cancer) *at the time the cohort was assembled in 1971.*

One of the main disadvantages of cohort studies is that they generally require a very large number of subjects in the denominator so that meaningful numerators can emerge as dependent variables. That is not true in certain clinically oriented studies (e.g., liver transplant studies, where the outcomes of interest are not rare). The precision of the answers depends greatly on the size of the numerator. Also, cohort studies sometimes require long follow-up with all the consequent problems of logistics, the most important one being losses to follow-up.

One frequently used strategy in cohort studies, which gets around the disadvantage of many years of waiting to ascertain outcomes in cohorts assembled according to exposure criteria, is to do a historical cohort. An investigator studying cancers among cohorts of workers assembled in 1971, in conventional and nuclear plants, could have started the work in 1986. The pursuit of the data is *still forward* from 1971 to 1995, but the investigator has gone backward in time for 15 of the 25 years. The method is partly historical and partly concurrent.

If the investigator had fielded this work in 1995, following the workers from 1971 through 1995, the entire project would have been a historical cohort study. We emphasize, however, that a historical cohort, even when implemented historically, is *prospective* in common terminology, because the pursuit of the data is forward. Other cohort studies that we designate concurrent also pursue the data forward, but from the present to the future. Conventionally, they are also classified as prospective, but this use of the term prospective to qualify cohort studies is ambiguous and confusing. It is also not useful as a qualifier of randomized controlled trials. RCTs are always prospective.

Case-Referent or Case-Control Studies

The distinct feature of the case-referent or case-control study, as it is commonly called, is that the two groups compared, the group of *cases* and the *subjects from the referent group* (i.e., controls), are identified with reference to the presence or absence of the target outcome of interest, usually incident cases of disease. Characteristically, you obtain information on outcomes and exposure at the same time. You then determine, in each of the two groups of patients compared, how frequently a prior exposure of interest occurred.

You might, for instance, take 400 neonates with meningomyelocele from among a group of university childrens' hospitals and compare them to a second reference group of 400 very young children, matched by age, who were referred to the same hospitals for management of severe trauma.

The question of your project is whether exposure of the mother to a particular garden herbicide during pregnancy might be associated with development of meningomyelocele. You would interview the mothers of both groups of children to determine the proportion of exposure of each group during the corresponding pregnancies. Suppose that 32% of the mothers of children with meningomyelocele report being exposed to the chemical herbicide, and only 8% of the mothers of children with multiple trauma report such exposure. You would conclude that mothers of children with meningomyelocele are 4 times more likely to have been exposed to the herbicide. Using these data to calculate an odds ratio, as the exposure ratio in the cases (32/68) divided the exposure ratio in the controls (8/92), you would say that the exposed mothers are approximately 5 times more likely to bear children with meningomyelocele.

Figure 28-2 shows the structure for a case-

referent or case-control study. Notice that the cases and referents or controls are selected from two different populations and that the direction of the study is backward. Subjects are selected on the outcome of interest (disease or condition under study versus no disease), and the information on etiologic exposures is collected retrospectively. Table 28-2 shows the data layout for a case-referent study.

Continuing our caffeinated beverages example, we would gather cases of disease of interest—for instance, cancer of the pancreas—and compare them to a group of patients entering area hospitals for elective surgery with respect to the exposed factor of interest, caffeinated beverages. We would then compare the proportion of those exposed among the cases $[a/(a + c)]$ to the proportion of those exposed among the controls $[b/(b + d)]$. The resulting measure, the odds ratio, gives us a sense of the degree of caffeinated beverage exposure among the cases compared to the referent group. Again, when the odds ratio is more than 1, or unity, we associate an increased risk of dis-

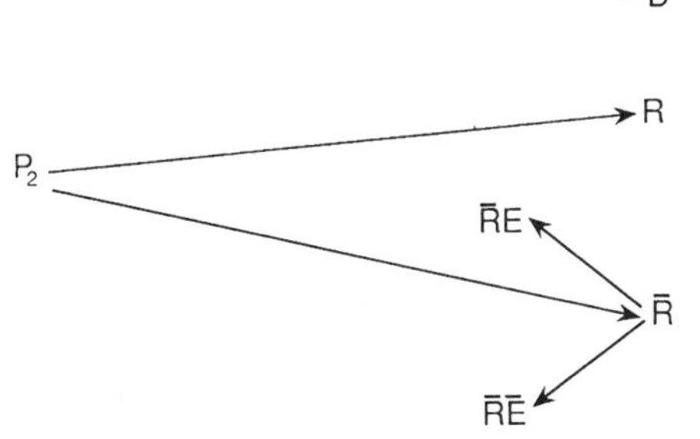

Figure 28-2. The case-referent/case-control study.

D = individuals diagnosed with the disease of interest

P_1 = source population for individuals with disease

$\bar{R}$ = individuals without the disease of interest

P_2 = source population for individuals without the disease of interest

E = exposed, $\bar{E}$ = not exposed

Hypothetically, P_1 = P_2

Table 28-2. Data layout for a case-referent/case-control study

		Cases	Referents or controls
Exposure status	E	a	b
	$\bar{E}$	c	d
		$a + c$	$b + d$

Exposure among the cases = $a/(a + c)$

Exposure among the referents = $b/(b + d)$

Odds ratio = $\dfrac{a/(a + c)}{b/(b + d)} \div \dfrac{c/(a + c)}{d/(b + d)}$ or $\dfrac{ad}{bc}$

ease with exposure. When the disease under study is rare, as is usually the case when we use a case-referent design, the odds ratio comes close to the value of the risk ratio or the relative risk.

In case-referent research, if you obtain odds ratios that are high, such as 6 or 11 or 20 (meaning that a target outcome is 6 or 11 or 20 times more likely to occur in the presence of a suspected risk factor as compared to the absence of the risk factor), you have evidence of *association* between the target outcome and the risk factor, and the strength of the association, as reflected in the high odds ratios, *would strongly suggest but does not prove causality* of the risk factor with respect to the target outcome. Findings from case-referent studies can seldom be taken as conclusive evidence of cause, no matter how high the odds ratios. Moreover, odds ratios from case-referent studies are weak, often only in the order of 1.3, 1.8, or about 2. In such cases (assuming that statistical significance has been attained), the evidence of association can be invoked to draw causal inferences only at great peril. The previously discussed specific ground rules about diagnosing causality from association should be invoked when evaluating evidence from case-referent studies.

In recent years, Miettinen[4] developed the theory underlying case-referent studies that permitted substantial advances in the understanding of this strategy. He introduced the concept of *study base* as the hypothetical conceptual denominator of relevance for these types of studies. Clinicians participating with methodologists in case-referent studies should make a serious attempt to master both the theory and the logistical challenges of the case-referent approach. The theoretical and practical difficulties can be formidable despite the advantages of smaller sample sizes and much shorter study periods.

The key disadvantages to the case-referent method are vulnerability to bias[5] and the difficulty in judicious choice of reference groups for comparison. The advantages include smaller numbers of patients and shorter follow-up. In the case of a rare disease, the case-referent method is often the only feasible way of evaluating association between a risk factor and a clinical outcome.

Cross-Sectional Designs

Cross-sectional designs are those in which denominators are delineated at the same time as the numerator events are measured. You might enumerate all victims of motorcycle accidents within a particular city of 500,000 persons and designate them as the denominator of interest; for the target outcome in the numerator, you might measure the extent of their resulting physical disabilities. This outcome will be established *at the same time* as the eligible study subjects are included in the denominator.

Figure 28-3 shows the structure of a cross-sectional study. The absence of lines indicating the passage of time shows that data on exposure status and the outcome of interest were collected at the same time. Unlike the case-referent study, in which exposure and outcome are also gathered

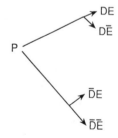

P = population from which individuals under study were sampled

D = disease; $\bar{D}$ = not diseased

E = exposed; $\bar{E}$ = not exposed

Figure 28-3. The cross-sectional study.

at the same time, all individuals under study come from the same source population. If we did a cross-sectional study on the effects of caffeinated beverages, focusing on minor gastric disorders, we would choose a sample of individuals from a population of interest (e.g., community A) and interview them on their use of caffeinated beverages and their symptoms of gastric upset. The unit of analysis is the individual and the study is nondirectional.

Table 28-3 shows the data layout for a cross-sectional study. The comparison of interest is the ratio of the rate of disease among those with exposure to caffeinated beverages *(a/b)* divided by the rate of disease among those without caffeinated beverage exposure *(c/d)*. An elevated risk ratio or relative risk would suggest, but not prove, some association.

A more rigorous approach is a cross-sectional study that makes comparisons among groups of people. You might study all motorcycle victims in one city of 500,000 and compare them with motorcycle victims in another city of 500,000 in a neighboring state. The difference is that the use of helmets is not mandatory in the first city, but is in the second. You could make a quantitative assessment of the extent of disability among the victims in both cities, using a new "disability index" (where 0 is "death," and 100 is "freedom from disability"). Suppose you measure an average "disability index" of 68 points in city A and 48 points in city B. You would tend to conclude that city B is better off than city A and impute the benefit to the law on helmet use.

This example was chosen to show the pitfalls cross-sectional designs can harbor and to illustrate how cohort studies are superior, when feasible, because they are not as vulnerable to biases and misinterpretation. Community A could actually be better off than community B by virtue of having had lower mortality; community B may have had higher mortality with less disability among the surviving victims. If you had started with a cohort approach that identified all motorcycle *riders* in both communities before introduction of the law and followed both groups forward from a time close to the introduction of the new law in city B, there would be no confusion between survival and residual disability.

Budgetary limitations, unavailability of data, lack of time, or ethical constraints may often preclude a cohort study, however, and all we can do is a cross-sectional study. Remember that when your data emerge from cross-sectional studies only, you can reach only tentative conclusions that a particular exposure factor or a particular intervention is *associated* with a particular target outcome or dependent variable.

Cross-sectional designs do not provide reliable information on the temporal relation between suspected causal factors and the health outcomes of interest. Only cohort studies and controlled studies give such information.

Ecologic Studies

Ecologic studies, also called heterodemic, aggregate, or descriptive studies, use the group as the basic unit of analysis. Groups are commonly defined according to geographic, geopolitical, or time criteria. Although ecologic studies often use mortality data as the outcome of interest, they may use any commonly collected types of data such as rates of hospitalization for various conditions, numbers of cases of reported infectious diseases, or numbers of births. Beginning with Durkheim's analysis of the relation between the number of suicides in European countries and the proportions of Protestants in the regions under study, ecologic studies have been used to show relationships on the group rather than the individual level. Wennberg and Gettelsohn's study showing

Table 28-3.   Data layout for a cross-sectional study

		Disease status		
		D	$\bar{D}$	Totals
Exposure status	E	a	b	a + b
	$\bar{E}$	c	d	c + d
	Totals	a + c	b + d	(a + b) + (c + d)

Disease among exposed = $a/(a + b)$

Disease among unexposed = $c/(c + d)$

Prevalence odds ratio = $\dfrac{a/b}{c/d}$ or $\dfrac{ad}{bc}$

the relation between rates of surgical procedures and the numbers of physicians performing surgery is a more recently published example of this type of analysis.[6]

Figure 28-4 shows the basic structure of an ecologic study in which the joint distribution of exposure and disease is not known. We gather information on exposure or disease only, the information commonly found in the marginals of a standard data layout table (Table 28-4). In our illustrative study of caffeinated beverages, we might be interested in the relation between caffeinated beverage consumption and bleeding ulcers. An ecologic study might look at the association of caffeinated beverage sales with hospitalizations for bleeding ulcers in two demographically similar regions that differ in their use of caffeinated beverages. If such an association were found, it might encourage the interested investigator to pursue the possible causal relationship further.

Ecologic studies warrant much caution. They are attractive because they use existing data and require less time and money, but they may be subject to a phenomenon known as the "ecologic fallacy." The data available in an ecologic study consist of the information portrayed in the marginals of a standard data layout table. If the grouping of the individuals studied distorts the effect of interest, *or* if certain factors related to the group affect the occurrence of the outcome of interest, an ecologic study will lead us to the wrong conclusion about the relationship under investigation. If we found a relationship in the caffeinated beverages study, we would have no way of determining whether the individuals who were hospitalized with bleeding ulcers were actually drinking caffeinated beverages.

Conclusion

The three broad purposes of clinical and epidemiologic investigation are (1) *describing what is,* (2) *predicting what could happen* in the future, and (3) *establishing cause and effect* in etiologic and therapeutic investigation.

The experiment is by far the strongest evidence that can be invoked to differentiate causality from association. It is the gold standard of clinical, epidemiologic, and health care research that should be used whenever ethically and practically feasible. In the history of medicine, nonexperimental studies have rarely led to firm conclusions about cause and effect.

If one cannot do an experiment, a series of nonexperimental strategies can be considered. To establish a causal significance from an association, the hierarchy of rigor of evidence gives highest weight to the cohort comparison study. The next levels, in order of descending rigor, are the well-designed case-referent study, the cross-sectional study, and, finally, the ecologic association study. Only when striking findings show major changes should case studies be invoked to establish cause-and-effect relationships. Generally, unless it is an experiment, no single study should be used as conclusive evidence about any one question.

It is important to create a profile of several nonexperimental studies. If most of them tend to point in the same direction, especially if they were planned and designed by different investigators in

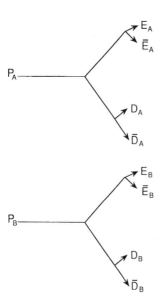

P_A, P_B geopolitical units under study

E = exposed; $\bar{E}$ = not exposed

D = diseased; $\bar{D}$ = not diseased

Figure 28-4. The ecological study.

Table 28-4.   Data layout for an ecologic study

Population$_j$	Disease status		
	Diseased	Not diseased	
Exposure status			
Exposed	–	–	$a_i + b_i$
Not exposed	–	–	$c_i + d_i$
	$a_i + c_i$	$b_i + d_i$	N_i

Population$_i$	Disease status		
	Diseased	Not diseased	
Exposure status			
Exposed	–	–	$a_j + b_j$
Not exposed	–	–	$c_j + d_j$
	$a_j + c_j$	$b_j + d_j$	N_j

Comparison: $\dfrac{a_i + b_i}{N_i} > \dfrac{a_j + b_j}{N_j}$ and $\dfrac{a_i + c_i}{N_i} > \dfrac{a_j + c_j}{N_j}$

different countries at different times, with complementary designs in different kinds of patients, causality may become a tenable verdict. Other important rules about the scientific admissibility of evidence were summarized earlier in this chapter in Bradford Hill's criteria.

Prediction of the future depends, in part, on how faithfully interventions—assessed through experimental, subexperimental, and nonexperimental methods—reflect current and future realities. There must be an adequate sense of all the circumstances surrounding an intervention, such as competing medical treatments, the milieu in which health service organizations operate in a particular country, and the conformity between the characteristics described and studied in a particular project and the basic nature of the population for which predictions are being made.

Mathematical modeling, based in part on empirical evidence gathered through experimental and nonexperimental studies, can play an important role in predicting the future. Although this chapter has not dealt with such modeling, nor has it presented laboratory simulation in detail, a balanced overview of selected strategies requires that they be at least mentioned.

Some investigators scorn the use of anything less than the gold standard of randomized controlled double-blind trials in clinical and epidemiologic research. While we believe that the highest feasible level of rigor in design should always be attempted, we also feel that it is usually better to have some data rather than none. When legitimate real-world constraints do not permit randomized controlled trials, every other avenue to new knowledge should be followed as far and as carefully as possible.

The substantial compromises in strategy that must be made in nonexperimental research require the exercise of even more care in the choice of all patients or study subjects, in the validity and reliability of data gathering, and in the selection of the best possible statistical techniques, than is required in experimental trials.

References

1. Walters BC, Sackett DL. Why clinical research? In: Troidl H, Spitzer WO, McPeek B, Mulder DS, McKneally MF, Wechsler AS, Balch CM, eds. Principles and Practice of Research: Strategies for Surgical Investigators, 2nd edn. New York: Springer-Verlag, 1991, pp. 231–248.

2. The Canadian Task Force on the Periodic Health Examination. 1989 update. Can Med Assoc J 1989; 141:209–216.

3. Kramer MS. Clinical biostatistics. In: Troidl H, Spitzer WO, McPeek B, Mulder DS, McKneally MF, Wechsler AS, Balch CM, eds. Principles and Practice of Research: Strategies for Surgical Investigators, 2nd edn. New York: Springer-Verlag, 1991, pp. 126–143.

4. Miettinen OS. Theoretical Epidemiology: Principles of Occurrence Research in Medicine. New York: Wiley, 1985.

5. Ibrahim M, Spitzer WO. The case-control study: consensus and controversy. J Chronic Dis 1979;32: 1–190.

6. Wennberg J, Gettelsohn A. Small area variations in health care delivery. Science 1972;182:1102–1108.

Additional Reading

Bradford Hill A. Principles of Medical Statistics, 9th edn. New York: Oxford University, 1971, ch. 24.

Campbell DT, Stanley JC. Experimental and Quasi-Experimental Designs for Research. Skokie, IL: Rand McNally, 1963.

Cook TD, Campbell DT. Quasi-Experimentation. Skokie, IL: Rand McNally, 1979.

Feinstein AR. Clinical Epidemiology: The Architecture of Clinical Research. Philadelphia: Saunders, 1985.

Fletcher RH, Fletcher SW, Wagner EH. Clinical Epidemiology: The Essentials. Baltimore: Williams & Wilkins, 1982.

Friedman GD. Primer of Epidemiology, 2nd edn. New York: McGraw-Hill, 1980.

Kelsey JL, Thompson WD, Evans AS. Methods in Observational Epidemiology. New York: Oxford University, 1986.

Kleinbaum DG, Kupper LL, Morgenstern H. Epidemiologic Research. Belmont, CA: Lifetime Learning Publications, 1982.

Lilienfeld AM, Lilienfeld DE. Foundations of Epidemiology, 2nd edn. Oxford: Oxford University, 1980.

Sackett DL, Haynes RB, Tugwell P. Clinical Epidemiology: A Basic Science for Clinical Medicine. Boston: Little, Brown, 1985.

Schlesselman JJ. Case-Control Studies. Oxford: Oxford University, 1982.

Swinscow, TDV. Statistics at Square One. London: British Medical Association, 1976.

CHAPTER 29

Qualitative Research

D.K. Martin and M.F. McKneally

Introduction

Qualitative research is an interdisciplinary, interpretive field of inquiry. The qualitative researcher uses predominantly nonstatistical analytic procedures to generate information from data gathered from field observations, structured interviews, focus groups, case studies, document analyses, and other sources that describe routine and problematic moments and meanings in individual lives.[1]

The antecedents of the discipline have existed for as long as curious people have asked analytic questions about social phenomena, but social scientists within the last century have developed qualitative research into a rigorous, systematic way of exploring social phenomena in context. The goal of qualitative research is to understand the meaning of social phenomena in their natural settings, particularly for the people and institutions involved. Qualitative researchers ask questions such as, "Why is this happening?" or "Why is the prevalence of gunshot wounds (or tonsillectomies) so high in this population?" They do not count the number of events, or test defined hypotheses about them. Their inquiries and analyses may generate hypotheses for subsequent testing by quantitative methods described throughout this book.

A Brief Background to Qualitative Research

Qualitative research is often contrasted with quantitative research which, as its name suggests, is concerned with quantifying or counting phenomena under various conditions, and testing defined hypotheses about causality or relatedness, based on numerical data. Quantitative research seeks generalizability and controls intervening or confounding variables through careful constraints. Qualitative research is concerned with understanding the unique characteristics of the phenomena under study, and less concerned with generalizing to other contexts. Qualitative researchers admit the influence of all naturally intervening variables and, rather than controlling or eliminating them, attempt to understand their confounding influence. Qualitative researchers accept that research interventions and, indeed, researchers may influence the phenomenon under study. A qualitative researcher will include the effects of the intervention as "data" to be examined and will also be honest and transparent about personal biases that inevitably shape research interests, questions, data collection, analysis, interpretation, writing, and the dissemination of results.

Qualitative researchers of the early 1900s (Malinowski and Margaret Mead are well-known examples) studied foreign "others," attempted to write "objective" reports of their findings, and were concerned with the reliability and validity of their interpretations. They were committed to objectivism, monumentalism (creating museumlike representations of the culture studied), and timelessness.[2] From the 1950s through the 1970s, qualitative researchers of the "modern era" focused more on subjective reality. This new version of qualitative research, characterized by a more realistic, forgiving, eclectic view, maintains that reality can never be fully understood, only approximated. More recently, qualitative researchers of the "postmodern" school seek to include emotionality, responsibility, an ethic of caring, multivoiced text, and a dialogue with subjects, often with political overtones, in their analyses.

Today, we recognize that an investigator's perspective is always filtered by language, profession, gender, class, and ethnicity, among other influences. Moreover, we recognize that research participants are often unable to provide full explanations of themselves, and that researchers, who are people with their own experiences and influences, may never completely understand the participants. One result of this evolution of the research model is that today's researcher no longer feels compelled to impersonate the aloof, objective "other," but can now be free to be more of an activist, utilizing a wide range of interconnected interpretive methods.

Like an intuitively gifted detective, the qualitative researcher can pursue a line of evidence systematically and analytically, without the constraints of quantitative research that require all questions to be prespecified before the data are gathered and examined. By carefully combining the techniques of qualitative and quantitative research, observations can be developed into descriptions, explanations, and theories that can then be tested.

The following example illustrates the strength of qualitative research. Rich and Stone interviewed 18 African-American men between 18 and 25 years old who were recovering in an urban Boston hospital after being shot or stabbed.[3] Their qualitative approach enabled the authors to elucidate important details of the interpersonal and societal influences that contributed to violent injury of young urban males. The authors introduce a recurring theme: the phenomenon of "being a sucker"—one who is not tough, who does not have the courage to fight back, even if he will be wounded or killed. The wounded men were proving to their peers that they do not run or back down from violence; by standing up against potential injury they avoided being consigned to an unacceptably subordinate social class of victims. "Standing up for what's yours" prevents robbery and extreme victimization; failure to respond violently to a challenge is more dangerous in their context than striking back. This concept is known to street workers but, until now, has been absent from the trauma research literature, despite the large number of published books and articles on penetrating injury. It took an in-depth qualitative study to examine this segment of surgical practice, expose the "why's" and "how's," and explore interventions that may help reduce its prevalence.

An issue in surgery that is ripe for qualitative research is the dramatic differences in the incidence of certain surgical operations between small geopolitical units. These variations are generally discussed in a speculative analysis of possible causation. This is an ideal target for the application of qualitative research methods because these methods investigate problems systematically to answer questions such as, "Why do the doctors in this region perform so many tonsillectomies, prostatectomies, or coronary bypasses?" Speculation can be replaced by direct quotation from practitioners and patients, and this information can be enhanced through observation of practice behavior.

Six Practical Tips for Rigorous Qualitative Research

These six tips will orient you to qualitative research techniques and help you to ensure that your studies are scientifically rigorous and your findings are meaningful.

1. Ask the Right Question

All research begins with a question; before you begin, critically question your question. The research method should be determined by the question—too often the reverse is true. Because many investigators are steeped in a particular methodological tradition, the questions they can address are predetermined, and as a result the knowledge gained is one-dimensional. Table 29-1 shows how different research questions can shape the research approach.

The quantitative research questions in Table 29-1 can be answered by relatively simple measurements involving questionnaires or a chart review, and comparisons can be made with *t*-tests. The qualitative research questions in Table 29-1 can be answered only by exploring the perspectives of the people involved and the institutions that shape their environment. In the first example, you could observe what surgeons do, analyze the decisions they make about time management, and ask them about rewards, frustrations, and priorities in their work. In the second example, you could listen to elderly patients as they describe their postsurgical experience.

Qualitative research may be used to develop basic descriptive knowledge, clarify quantitative findings, develop research instruments, evaluate programs, guide practice, develop theory, and influence policy.[4] The purpose of your research will influence your research approach. Table 29-2 provides examples of research questions along with corresponding strategies, other disciplines where one might look for research partners, and potential data sources.

2. Interdisciplinarity Is Key

Here it may be helpful to distinguish between multidisciplinary and interdisciplinary research. In multidisciplinary research, researchers from different disciplines work in parallel or in sequence to address a common problem. In interdisciplinary research, researchers from different disciplines work jointly to address a common problem.[13] Strive for interdisciplinarity. Find others from different disciplines who share an interest in your topic. Scholars in sociology, anthropology, nursing, education, social work, philosophy, theology, bioethics, and other disciplines will bring with them not only different research methods but different perspectives on what knowledge is important and why. You will find that they speak a different language than you do, and a certain amount of humility, to listen and learn, is required.

3. Plan the Appropriate Setting

Some settings are easy to access, others require the cultivation of key contacts and lengthy negotiations. It is relatively easy to mail a questionnaire to a surgeon; it is more difficult to book time with a surgeon for an interview. If you want to observe communication in the operating room, you may need to negotiate for the consent of hospital administrators and the participating surgeons, nurses, and managers; if you want to tape- or video-record the interactions, additional consent is required. The key here is to not only get *permission,* but to get *cooperation.* Your research participants must be (1) comfortable with participating, (2) comfortable with you, and (3) willing to allow you to enter into their world. This is the difference between "getting in" and "getting close." To do high quality research you need to get close.

A cautionary word: it is *extremely* difficult to conduct qualitative research where you work. The roles of investigator and employee often conflict, as do the roles of investigator and colleague. Either get someone else to conduct your research or,

Table 29-1.   Quantitative and qualitative research questions.

Quantitative research question	Qualitative research question
How many hours per week do surgeons spend operating versus examining patients in the ICU?	What tasks do surgeons consider important and what keeps them from doing what they think is important?
How quickly does range of motion improve after total hip replacement?	What do elderly patients find limiting or frustrating about total hip replacement?

Table 29-2.   Research questions and corresponding strategies.

Research questions	Research strategy	Other disciplines	Data sources
What does it mean? Why is it meaningful?	Phenomenology[5,6]	Philosophy	Interviews, written anecdotes
What is it (system, institution) like? What are they (people, group) like? (description)	Ethnography[7,8]	Anthropology	Interviews, observations
What is happening? How is it happening? (processes)	Grounded theory[9,10]	Sociology	Interviews, observations
How do those people communicate? What are they communicating?	Discourse analysis[11,12]	Semiotics	Interviews, dialogues, document analysis

preferably, conduct your research in a setting with which you have no formal affiliation. Even then, negotiate openly with all participants. Make sure roles and assumptions are openly discussed ahead of time and agreed to by all parties. Surprises usually mean problems.

4. Prepare, Prepare, Prepare!

Qualitative research reflects the skills of the researcher as much or more than the reliability or validity of the research techniques. Table 29-3 provides a list of skills that are well developed in a good qualitative researcher.

5. Analyze as You Go

Analysis commences when you first think about the study and continues while you (1) write the proposal; (2) negotiate access (the process of negotiation for access can provide some of the most significant insights into institutional structures and the people who work there); (3) collect data (you should constantly ask yourself, "What am I seeing/hearing?" "What does it mean?" "What am I missing?"); (4) read about the topic and have discussions with colleagues (outside sources of information often impact the way in which you interpret data); and (5) write up the research.

Analysis is a process that involves both inductive and deductive thinking. Concepts and ideas will emerge from the data if you are perceptive. Simultaneously, you should be sensitive to data

that address your theoretical premises. Early in the data analysis your thinking will be mostly inductive, later it will be mostly deductive, but your analysis should always include both approaches.

6. Alter Your Data Collection Based on Your Ongoing Analysis

This is one of the great strengths of qualitative methods. If you analyze the data as you collect it you can see what is coming in, where the interesting leads are, what is missing, what is challenging, and what is unproductive. Alter your techniques or your questions as you go, according to your unfolding analysis. Go back and ask different questions of the same people. Ask new questions if the old ones are unproductive—don't keep asking the same questions if they aren't working. If your original questions have turned up unexpected and interesting data, pursue the interesting data. If you are stumped and you need a fresh perspective, ask for help—use your interdisciplinary team.

Collect data slowly; your analysis should keep pace with your data collection, and future data collection may change dramatically, based on the analysis. If you are conducting interviews, space them apart, especially the early ones. Another cautionary word: transcribing recordings is the most tedious and demanding (and boring) of research tasks. *Arrange ahead of time* for a competent transcriber who can keep pace with your interview schedule. If you are collecting observational data,

Table 29-3.   Skills of the qualitative researcher.

Skill	Description
Theoretical sensitivity	Know your field and the relevant published studies and how they shape your questions and interpretation. Know, ahead of time, what you are doing.
Social sensitivity	Investigators must have good interaction skills and must be trustworthy. Informants will provide rich important information only to someone who can be trusted to listen, observe, understand, and use information appropriately. Maintain the highest standards of confidentiality and communicate those standards to all involved.
Rigour	Be meticulous in documenting and justifying your research decisions, your actions, and the results. Have others on your team who are ready to examine, critique, and even challenge your strategies, analysis, and interpretations. Be prepared to listen to them and learn—be humble and flexible.
Reflexivity	Perhaps the most difficult skill to develop for those who are new to qualitative methods is critical thinking. You must make a conscious effort to step back, critically analyze what is happening, and think abstractly.
Theoretical sampling	Select research subjects who are going to help you answer the research question or who can inform you about a particular phenomenon or experience. Sample different subjects according to the perspectives they bring. Seek variety—rigour demands different views of the same phenomenon. Just as you cannot see all the facets of a diamond until you look at it from different sides, so too you cannot expect to understand a phenomenon until you understand the perspectives of all those involved.
Conceptual saturation	Sample until you are finished—numbers are of secondary importance. In the context of sampling, "adequacy" refers to amount and kind of data, not participants. Ask yourself, "What do I need to know?" and then search until you have all you need. If you are not convinced you have all the perspectives that are available, seek out more situations to observe, more people to interview, and/or more documents to examine. When you find yourself seeing and hearing the same things all the time, you are probably finished. Stop when the concepts you are exploring are saturated and no new data is coming in. Before you leave the setting, take stock of what you are finding and then search for confirming *and* disconfirming evidence.
Member check	Write down your observations and interpretations, then let your participants read them and comment on their accuracy and appropriateness. This will help your results and conclusions to be robust and meaningful.

schedule time to write up field notes and analyze them. Remember: *analysis always takes more time than you think.*

Qualitative Research Resources

Qualitative research is being pursued in many medical specialties. Medical anthropology and medical history, which primarily use qualitative methods, are large and ever-growing subspecialties. Funding agencies (for example, the Social Sciences and Humanities Research Council of Canada) often fund multimethod and interdisci-

plinary research projects focusing on areas in medicine.

For examples of qualitative scholarship, we recommend the journal *Qualitative Health Research.* For a particularly innovative study in surgery you might review "She Won't Be Dancing Much Anyway: A Study of Surgeons, Surgical Nurses, and Elderly Patients" by Fisher and Peterson.[14] There are many examples of excellent qualitative studies on topics in medicine and medical care in journals[15–21] and books.[22–26] There are articles that can help you critically evaluate both published articles and your own work.[27–28] Finally, we recommend Denzin and Lincoln's *Handbook of Qualitative Re-*

search[1] as a thorough, scholarly, and highly readable text. Their introductory chapter "Entering the Field of Qualitative Research"[2] is an excellent summary for surgeons who may wish to become better acquainted with the history, scope, and methods of this interesting approach.

References

1. Denzin NK, Lincoln YS. Handbook of Qualitative Research. Thousand Oaks: Sage Publications, 1994.
2. Denzin NK, Lincoln YS. "Entering the field of Qualitative Research." In: NK Denzin and YS Lincoln, eds. Handbook of Qualitative Research. Thousand Oaks: Sage Publications, 1994, p. 7.
3. Rich JA, Stone DA. The experience of violent injury for young African-American men: the meaning of being a "sucker." J Gen Intern Med 1996; 11:77–82.
4. Strauss A, Corbin J. Basics of Qualitative Research: Grounded Theory Procedures and Techniques. Newbury Park: Sage, 1990, p. 20–21.
5. van Manen M. "Practicing phenomenological writing. Phenomenol Pedag 1984;2:36–69.
6. van Manen M. Researching the lived experience. London: University of Western Ontario, 1990.
7. Hammersley M, Atkinson P. Ethnography: Principles in Practice. London: Tavistock, 1983.
8. Spradley JP. The Ethnographic Interview. New York: Holt, Rinehart & Winston, 1979.
9. Glaser B, Strauss A. The Discovery of Grounded Theory. Chicago: Aldine, 1967.
10. Strauss A, Corbin J. Basics of Qualitative Research: Grounded Theory Procedures and Techniques. Newbury Park: Sage, 1990.
11. Denzin NK. "Symbolic interactionism and ethnomethodology." In: J Douglas, ed. Understanding everyday life. Chicago: Aldine, 1970, pp. 261–286.
12. Denzin NK. Interpretive Interactionism. Newbury Park: Sage, 1989.
13. Rosenfeld PL. The potential transdisciplinary research for sustaining and extending linkages between health and social sciences. Soc Sci Med 1992;11:1342–1357.
14. Fisher BJ, Peterson C. She won't be dancing much anyway: a study of surgeons, surgical nurses, and elderly patients. Qual Health Res 1993;3(2): 20–30.
15. Ventres W, Nichter M, Reed R, Frankel R. Limitation of medical care: an ethnographic analysis. J Clin Ethics 1993;4(2):134–145.
16. Hunt LM. Practicing oncology in provincial Mexico: a narrative analysis. Soc Sci Med 1994;38(6): 843–853.
17. Schwartzberg SS. Vitality and growth in HIV-infected gay men. Soc Sci Med 1994;38(4):593–602.
18. Cecil R. "I wouldn't have minded a wee one running about": miscarriage and the family. Soc Sci Med 1994;38(10):1415–1422.
19. Corbin J. Women's perceptions and management of a pregnancy complicated by chronic illness. Health Care Women Int 1987;84:317–337.
20. Fujimura J. Constructing doable problems in cancer research: articulating alignment. Social Studies of Science 1987;17:257–293.
21. Irby DM. How attending physicians make instructional decisions when conducting teaching rounds. Acad Med 1992;67:630–638.
22. Broadhead R. Private Lives and Professional Identity of Medical Students. New Brunswick, NJ: Transaction Books, 1983.
23. Fagerhaugh S, Strauss A, Suzcek B, Wiener C. Hazards in Hospital Care. San Francisco: Jossey-Bass, 1987.
24. Glaser B, Strauss A. Time for Dying. Chicago: Aldine, 1968.
25. Schneider J, Conrad P. Having Epilepsy: The Experience and Control of Illness. Philadelphia, PA: Temple University, 1983.
26. Brody H. The Healer's Power. New Haven: Yale University, 1992.
27. Elder NC, Miller WL. Reading and evaluating qualitative research studies. J Fam Pract 1995;41 (3):279–285.
28. Cobb AK, Hagemaster JN. Ten criteria for evaluating qualitative research proposals. J Nurs Educ 1987;26(4):138–143.

Commentary

I was introduced to qualitative research by Doug Martin when he was a graduate student in bioethics. During his open but probing interviews with patients who had undergone a major surgical procedure, the patients introduced the surprising information that they had *not* wanted to participate in the formal process of informed consent as it is widely taught, practiced, and defined in textbooks of medicine, law, and bioethics. They wanted a doctor they trusted to make decisions for them. They had a different and much more positive view of their lives than we expected, even when cancer recurred. This information clarified the puzzling and unexpected findings of Roder et al.,[1] whose quantitative analysis of quality of life revealed higher scores in postesophagectomy cancer patients than in patients who are well. We are pursuing this theme in a variety of surgical interventions; we would not have found the theme if we had used the usual objective, structured approach to clinical research I have used throughout 30 years of surgical practice. I believe qualitative methods offer an important complement to more familiar, more quantitative, and more limiting research approaches.

M.F.M.

1. Roder JD, Herschback P, Sellschopp A, Siewert JR. Quality-of-life assessment following oesophagectomy. (Meran Consensus Conference on Quality-of-Life Assessment in Surgery) Theor Surg 1991;6(4):206–210.

Commentary

This chapter gives structure to an aspect of investigation that is unconsciously practiced by physicians everyday. Books about "surgical intuition" explain the thinking processes of surgeons as they analyze components of an illness and translate their formulations into action plans. Many of the questions asked in the course of evaluating a patient or a problem are not quantitative, but they provide the careful interviewer with important information. As I read this chapter I was immediately tempted to look at each of the examples quoted and say to myself, "I could quantitate that." In discussions with Dr. McKneally, it became clear that qualitative research should not be viewed simply as an alternative to quantitative research, but rather as a complementary tool. Interaction between the two approaches can bring us closer to understanding. There are times when quantitative analysis of data stills fails to yield root causes of differences in approaches. These differences may ultimately be identified as cultural, environmental, or based in an ethic that is simply not expressed easily as a numerical difference with a p-value. We could subsequently quantify how many people in a given region might possess that given quality or hold that particular viewpoint, but we would need the qualitative inquiry first to discover the basis for the research question or hypothesis we would refute using quantitative methods. Observational studies may ultimately lead to the development of quantitative scales that allow studies of larger numbers of subjects with more responses. Certainly, many of the quality of life survey instruments were made possible by an initial process that defined the importance of various life qualities in specific populations. Some aspects may never be accurately quantified, such as the intensity of maternal love or the level of fidelity and concern of a doctor for a patient. These qualities may lose their inherent meaning in the process of quantitation. This chapter introduces us to a method of inquiry that focuses on quality rather than quantity, and illustrates its utility as a scientific approach.

A.S.W.

CHAPTER 30

Estimating Risk and Prognosis

S.A. Marion and M.T. Schechter

Risk and Prognosis: The Concepts

An understanding of the natural history of treated and untreated disease is essential to the physician, is an area of utmost concern to patients, and is the basis of most decisions about management. The clinician faces numerous questions about the risk of certain events and the natural history of various disease states. Given a patient of a certain age and sex, what is the probability that symptomatic coronary heart disease will develop in the next 5 years? Given such a patient, together with the results of certain diagnostic maneuvers, what is the probability that significant coronary heart disease is already present? Given a set of characteristics of a coronary bypass surgery candidate, what is the probability that he or she will survive at least 5 years after surgery?

Much scientific research is a quest to better characterize or estimate the probabilities that particular events will occur.[1] Rational clinical decision making requires sound estimates of the probability of various possible events occurring along each available therapeutic path.

The questions posed in the opening paragraph illustrate certain points about the concept of probability. The first is that, to be useful in clinical practice, the probability should refer to very specific circumstances—the more specific the better. Plan-

ners estimating the demand for coronary care beds might find it interesting to consider the probability that a person selected at random from their country's adult population will develop clinically significant coronary heart disease in the next 5 years, but this probability would be of little value to a clinician. The patient seeking consultation has certain known characteristics such as age, sex, and a medical history that will affect the probability of an outcome, sometimes profoundly. In clinical practice, what is desired is a probability estimate that is specific to a given set of circumstances.

The second point about probability is specificity of outcome. To define a probability, one must clearly state exactly which events are to be counted. A relatively easy outcome to measure is death: its correct definition may be disputable, but the fact seldom is. But even here, specificity is required regarding the time period involved. Everyone dies eventually; to provide useful information, an estimate of the probability of death must refer to a specified time interval, such as the next 5 years. For other outcomes, there is the additional problem of arriving at a precise and useful definition of the event itself. The probability of developing coronary heart disease will be different depending on how its presence or absence is defined. Minimal evidence, as defined by small abnormalities on coronary angiogram versus a 50% occlusion, will result in a higher probability. The definition chosen needs to be precise and clinically relevant.

The same examples also illustrate three different clinical purposes for which estimates of probability are useful: risk assessment, diagnosis, and prognosis. Given individual circumstances of age, sex, life style, occupation, and so forth, *risk assessment* considers the probability that an apparently healthy person will develop certain disease states within specified intervals of future time. Given individual circumstances, together with the results of diagnostic maneuvers and tests, *diagnosis* considers the probability that an individual currently has a specified disease. Given similar individual circumstances (age, sex, etc.) and a specified disease state, *prognosis* addresses the question of the probability of important clinical events in the future. Diagnosis is discussed in chapter 31; assessment of risk and prognosis is the focus of this chapter.

The characteristics, called *factors*, that appear to affect risk and prognosis fall into three groups: modifiable determinants, nonmodifiable determinants, and markers. Determinants of risk and prognosis are the factors that are causally related to the outcome or event of interest. Serum cholesterol is believed to be causally related to risk of subsequent coronary artery disease and is therefore called a determinant. Serum cholesterol, smoking, and blood pressure are modifiable determinants of coronary heart disease risk, whereas age and family history are nonmodifiable determinants. Markers are associated with increased or decreased risk, or better or worse prognosis, but are not causally related. The association seen in North America between alcohol consumption and increased risk of lung cancer is believed to be due not to alcohol being a cause of lung cancer, but to the strong association between alcohol consumption and cigarette smoking. Individuals who consume more alcohol tend, on average, to smoke more cigarettes; modifying their alcohol consumption without changing their smoking behavior would not change their risk of lung cancer. Accordingly, alcohol is a marker of risk, not a determinant.

Why Study Risk and Prognosis?

We study risk and prognosis to obtain estimates of the probability of occurrence of important health-related events. A patient with coronary artery disease may need to choose between medical management and coronary bypass surgery. The probability of survival for various time periods, for each option, is a factor that should enter into the decision. If the probabilities are uniformly better with one strategy, and other factors such as pain are similar, the rational choice is the alternative with the higher probability of survival.

Life is rarely so simple; the survival may be better with medical management over the short term (weeks to months) but better with surgical management over the longer term; the side effects may be quite different and difficult to compare. Decision analysis is a formal method for weighing all the options and choosing the one of greatest benefit, but the details of the calculations are beyond the scope of this chapter. The crucial point is that the probabilities of such important events as death or recurrence of disease are fundamental to making informed decisions in the context of formal decision analysis and in routine clinical practice. The example that we have chosen relates to prognosis, but the principle is equally valid in risk assessment.

Measures of Risk and Prognosis

Suppose we are following a homogeneous population, that is, a population in which the major determinants of the outcome of interest are virtually the same for all its members (for a particular outcome, over time). The outcome of interest, generally called the *critical event*, might be recurrence of breast cancer, myocardial infarction, postoperative pulmonary embolism, or death. Probabilities are estimated by taking the observed *proportion* of the population that experiences the critical event.

For example, consider a sample of 2,000 patients for whom the critical event is deep vein thrombosis (DVT) in the postoperative period after total hip replacement. Half were treated with prophylactic heparin; half were not. Table 30-1 presents the hypothetical results from such a study. The columns labeled "Events" show the number of critical events on each successive day in the untreated and treated groups, respectively. Because 16 patients in the untreated group developed DVT *on day 5*, our estimate of the single-

Table 30-1. Hypothetical data regarding occurrences of deep vein thrombosis in the first 21 days following hip surgery in 1,000 patients treated with heparin and 1,000 patients not treated.

Day	Untreated				Treated				Relative rate (rate ratio)
	Events	Prob. (%)	N	Rate (%)	Events	Prob. (%)	N	Rate (%)	
1	1	0.1	1,000	0.10	1	0.1	1,000	0.10	1.00
2	7	0.7	999	0.70	1	0.1	999	0.10	0.14
3	9	0.9	992	0.91	3	0.3	998	0.30	0.33
4	7	0.7	983	0.71	6	0.6	995	0.60	0.85
5	16	1.6	976	1.64	2	0.2	989	0.20	0.12
6	19	1.9	960	1.98	7	0.7	987	0.71	0.36
7	22	2.2	941	2.34	3	0.3	980	0.31	0.13
8	16	1.6	919	1.74	5	0.5	977	0.51	0.29
9	13	1.3	903	1.44	2	0.2	972	0.21	0.14
10	11	1.1	890	1.24	3	0.3	970	0.31	0.25
11	13	1.3	879	1.48	3	0.3	967	0.31	0.21
12	10	1.0	866	1.15	4	0.4	964	0.41	0.36
13	3	0.3	856	0.35	1	0.1	960	0.10	0.30
14	6	0.6	853	0.70	0	0.0	959	0.00	0.00
15	7	0.7	847	0.83	2	0.2	959	0.21	0.25
16	3	0.3	840	0.36	2	0.2	957	0.21	0.59
17	2	0.2	837	0.24	0	0.0	955	0.00	0.00
18	4	0.4	835	0.48	2	0.2	955	0.21	0.44
19	1	0.1	831	0.12	0	0.0	953	0.00	0.00
20	1	0.1	830	0.12	0	0.0	953	0.00	0.00
21	1	0.1	829	0.12	0	0.0	953	0.00	0.00

day probability is 16/1,000 (i.e., 0.016, or 1.6%). These daily probabilities have been plotted as a histogram in Figure 30-1. Because 40 patients in the untreated group developed DVT *by day 5*, our estimate of the cumulative probability at day 5 is 40/1,000 (i.e., 0.040, or 4.0%). These cumulative probabilities have been plotted in Figure 30-2.

Even with the large hypothetical sample of 2,000 individuals, the estimated daily probabilities exhibit considerable fluctuation (Fig. 30-1). The cumulative probabilities are more stable, and it is often preferable to present the data in this form. The complement of the cumulative probability (1—the cumulative probability) plotted over time, called the *survival curve*, is a commonly presented summary of the data. It represents the probability of reaching a given point in time without experiencing the critical event.

An important distinction should be made concerning the probability of events. The probability, faced at the outset by all persons in the untreated group, of suffering a critical event precisely on day 12 (10/1,000, or 1.0%) is not quite the same as that faced on day 12 by those who begin day 12 without having developed a DVT. To calculate the latter probability, we remove from the denominator individuals who developed a DVT on days 1 through 11 and obtain a probability of 10/866, or 1.2%. In epidemiology this is called a *rate*—a special kind of proportion calculated by including in the denominator only people who are truly at risk at the beginning of the interval in question. Since the rate also depends on the length of the time interval, it is customary to recognize this explicitly by expressing the rate in units as follows:

(number of critical events) per (number of persons at risk) per (unit of time)

or

(number of events) per (person-unit of time at risk) [In our example, the denominator would be person-days at risk.]

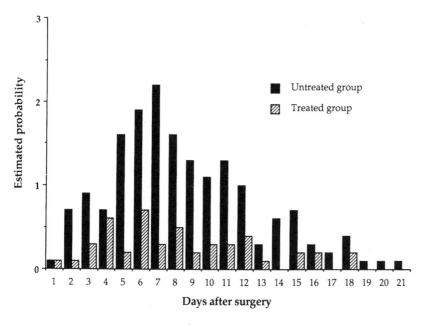

Figure 30-1.   The daily probability of developing deep vein thrombosis in the postoperative period in treated vs. untreated groups.

The rate is a more accurate measure of risk than the proportion, considered previously. However, there is an unfortunate confusion in terminology. To some, "risk" corresponds to the cumulative probability plotted in Figure 30-2. When there is a possibility of confusion, the unambiguous term *hazard* is used. It is the probability of an individual experiencing an event in a specified time interval, given that the event has not already occurred to that individual before the start of the interval. The hazard for an interval is estimated by calculating the observed rate for that interval. In keeping with common usage, we will use *risk* both for the cumulative probability and for the hazard.

The next step is to compare risk or prognosis in the treated and untreated groups, but *remember that the data are hypothetical* and are presented solely to illustrate the concepts under discussion. From inspection of the data, it seems clear that the risk of DVT is reduced with heparin prophylaxis. This is most apparent in the cumulative risk estimates, which illustrates their usefulness in this type of comparison. How do we quantify the difference in prognosis in the two populations? How do we rule out the possibility that the observed difference is simply due to chance?

The simplest approach is to look at the final results of the whole 3-week period of follow-up (i.e., the risk of DVT with heparin is 47/1,000, or 4.7%; without heparin, 172/1,000, or 17.2%). We then calculate the ratio of the two risk estimates—4.7/17.2 or 0.27, which is called the *relative risk*. This means the risk with heparin is only 0.27 of the risk without it; or, inversely, the risk without heparin is 1/0.27 or 3.7 times higher than with it. To rule out the possibility that the observed difference might have arisen by chance, we use the methods described by Kramer.[2] To compare the two proportions, we construct the corresponding 2×2 table, and calculate a χ^2 statistic and a *p*-value. In this instance, $\chi^2 = 82$, and $p < 0.001$ (i.e., there is less than 1 chance in 1,000 that a relative risk of the observed magnitude would occur by chance).

The relative risk has become the most commonly used measure for comparing two risks, but others are available. One is *excess risk,* which is the arithmetic difference between the two risks. In our example, the excess risk in those not given heparin, compared to those receiving it, is 17.2% − 4.7% = 12.5%. This may be interpreted as the net risk of DVT attributable to fail-

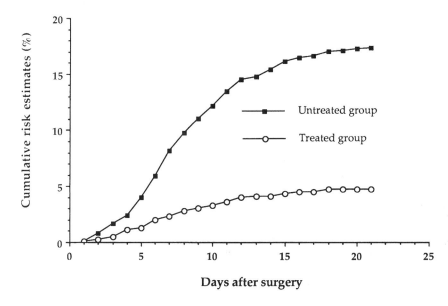

Figure 30-2.   The cumulative risk estimate of developing deep vein thrombosis in the postoperative period in treated vs. untreated groups.

ure to treat with heparin. The excess risk is sometimes called the *attributable risk,* but this term is used for several related quantities and is best avoided. Another measure is the *attributable proportion exposed,* which is the excess risk divided by the risk in the higher risk group. It is interpreted as the proportion or fraction of the risk that is avoidable by treatment, or attributable to nontreatment. In our example, it is 12.5%/17.2% = 72.7%; that is, about 73% of the risk could be avoided by treatment with heparin. The attributable proportion exposed is sometimes also called the attributable risk.

Using the relative risk for the whole follow-up period as the summary measure to compare prognosis in the two groups is problematic in that the calculation is based only on the final cumulative counts of events and ignores everything that happened in between. It focuses on the cumulative probability, but rates are better measures of risk. Another approach is to calculate the *relative rate* or *rate ratio,* the ratio of the rates for the two groups for each successive time interval (one day, in our example). These rate ratios are plotted in Figure 30-3. Because the number of events entering into the calculations for each time interval is quite small, rate ratios exhibit considerable in-

stability, as shown in the figure. This can be circumvented by assuming that, aside from random fluctuation, there is really a constant underlying value known as the *summary relative rate.* This premise about a constant underlying relative rate is a viable assumption under many circumstances and is called the *proportional hazards* assumption. It allows one to summarize the relative rates over time with a single number, the summary relative rate.

Calculation of the summary relative rate from the individual time interval data will not be detailed here. One approach to it, the Mantel-Haenszel technique, produces a summary relative rate and a χ^2 test of whether it is significantly different, statistically, from 1. For our data on DVT, the summary relative hazard is 0.25, and the corresponding χ^2 is 80 (again, $p < 0.001$). A summary relative hazard of 0.25 suggests that, on average, the heparin group experienced a risk of DVT about 25% of that of the nonheparin group. In this instance, the summary relative rate of 0.25 and the relative risk of 0.27 (i.e., the ratio of the cumulative risks) are almost identical. This will generally be true if the cumulative risk over the whole follow-up period is fairly small; in our example, it is 17.2% in the higher risk group. If the

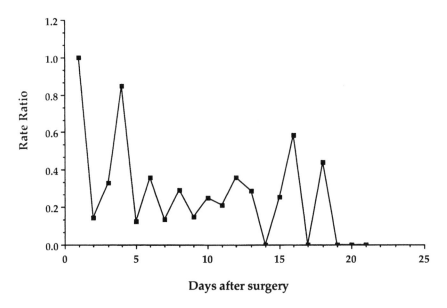

Figure 30-3.   The rate ratio of developing deep vein thrombosis in the post-operative period in treated vs. untreated groups.

cumulative risk over the follow-up period is large, say 50%, the two methods will usually produce quite different estimates, with the cumulative probability method producing estimates that are biased toward 1.

Incomplete follow-up is an important issue in studies that involve monitoring participants over time. Participants may withdraw, become inaccessible by moving away, or cease to be at risk for the critical event because of death or some other intercurrent event. In many studies, recruitment is staggered over time, and participants may be at various uncompleted stages of follow-up when the study terminates. Any individual who does not undergo the critical event and is not followed for the maximal period is said to be *censored*. Censoring, for one or another of the reasons above, may affect a considerable fraction of the study participants. Because simply dropping them from the analysis would waste a great deal of useful data, the method of Kaplan and Meier and actuarial life table methods have been developed for estimating survival curves from incomplete data.

The essential approach in such methods is the inclusion of all individuals followed for any length of time up to the point of being censored; after that, they are no longer considered to be at risk,

and this fact is reflected in the rate calculation. In the DVT example, suppose that on the 10th day, 10 subjects in the untreated group developed DVT, another 3 died of cardiac arrest, and 2 others were transferred to another facility and lost to follow-up. All 15 would be considered to be no longer at risk for DVT after day 10 and would be removed from the rate calculations beyond that point.

In using these techniques of survival analysis, we must make the assumption that loss to follow-up occurs at random or, at least, is not confounded with the relationship of primary interest (e.g., the relationship between deep vein thrombosis and heparin therapy in our example). For further discussion, consult monographs on survival analysis.[3]

Method of Analysis

Under measures of risk and prognosis, we discussed methods of analysis in the somewhat idealized circumstances of comparing two homogeneous groups followed over time, where the proportional hazards assumption is valid. We now turn to more realistic situations in which the sample being followed is heterogeneous with respect to such important prognostic variables as age and sex—the situation of greatest interest to clinicians, who naturally wish to tailor their risk and prognosis statements to the circumstances of an individual patient.

One method is to divide the sample into homogeneous subgroups and carry out a separate analysis for each. The problem with this approach is that, unless the original sample is very large, the subsamples become so small that meaningful conclusions cannot be drawn, and random fluctuation will completely obscure the effects of interest. Nevertheless, when the sample is large enough, separate analysis of each subgroup is a viable approach and has the advantage of not relying on any assumptions about the relationship among the subgroups.

When the total sample is not large enough to support separate subgroup analyses, a regression model can be used. This type of analysis, in contrast to independent analysis of each subgroup, depends on making an assumption that the way in which risk or prognosis varies across subgroups can be described by fairly simple mathematical equations. Suppose the subgroups of interest are defined by age. We might assume that the logarithm of the risk is directly proportional to the age, at least over the range of ages that are of practical importance in a particular context. Such an assumption allows the experience of individuals with different ages to be combined in one analysis.

Now suppose that in our hypothetical DVT study the treated and untreated groups were not similar with respect to age, and that age is a determinant of risk of DVT. A straightforward comparison of the risk of DVT between the groups would not be fair if it did not take account of age differences. Two regression models are presented, one corresponding to the cumulative risk approach, and the other to the rate approach.

If the focus is on cumulative risk, logistic regression is the appropriate model. It takes the form

$$\log\left(\frac{p}{1-p}\right) = b_0$$
$$+ b_1 \times (age - age_0) + b_2 \times (rx)$$

where p is the cumulative risk (or probability) of DVT over the whole follow-up period; "age" is the

age in years; age_0 is a constant reference age, such as the mean age of all subjects; and rx is 1 for those on heparin and 0 for those not on heparin. The coefficients b_0, b_1, and b_2 are unknown quantities (parameters), that are estimated from the actual follow-up data. The detailed method of estimating the parameters from the data will not be addressed here except to say that the method most commonly used is called the *maximum likelihood* method and is available in a variety of statistical software packages. The primary interest in this model is the estimated value of b_2. It turns out that $\exp(b_2)$, the exponential of b_2, is an estimate of the relative risk of DVT in those treated with heparin compared to those not treated. By including the term "$b_1 \times (age - age_0)$" in the model, we have managed to compensate for the age differences in the sample. The estimate of the relative risk obtained is, in a sense, an average over all age groups and is said to be adjusted for age. It should be noted that the equation above explicitly assumes a linear relationship between age and the quantity $\log\left(\frac{p}{1-p}\right)$, called the *logit* of the risk. Although this is unlikely to be exactly true, it may be approximately true in the range of ages in the sample. Using this equation to calculate the risk for a new individual is acceptable, if his or her age falls in the same range. The equation should not be used to extrapolate to ages outside the range represented in the sample data.

If the focus is on rates, the appropriate regression model is called *Cox regression*. The model takes the form

$$\log(\theta) = b_1 \times (age - age_0) + b_2 \times (rx)$$

where θ is the summary relative rate (hazard) for an individual, compared to someone of reference age not on heparin treatment. The similarity to the logistic equation is evident. There is no b_0 term, but, otherwise, the coefficients have a similar interpretation. Again, $\exp(b_2)$ is the summary relative rate adjusted for the differences in age. There is an explicit assumption that the logarithm of the relative rate varies linearly with age, and, as above, this is often a reasonable assumption for the range of ages in the sample. There is also an assumption that the relative rate is constant over time—the same "proportional hazards" assumption mentioned when the summary relative rate was defined earlier. Cox regression is also able to cope with censored data.

There are many sophisticated refinements of the logistic regression and Cox regression models, including incorporation of additional terms to allow adjustment for individual characteristics such as sex or socioeconomic status, possible interactions among factors, and (in the Cox model) variation of the relative hazard over time.

Methodological Issues

Knowing what will likely happen to our patients with given conditions or after certain operative procedures is fundamental to sound clinical decision making, but we must depend on observations from past studies to guide us now, and we must hope that the estimates of what will happen are valid *and* applicable to our own patients.

Earlier we discussed some fundamental concepts associated with the natural history of disease and presented methods of calculating various measures of risk. We now turn to methodological issues associated with studies of prognosis, basing our discussion on the framework used in chapter 7, "Appraising New Information": Why, Who and When, What, How, and How Many.

Why? Clarifying the Purpose

Whenever you are assessing a natural history study, begin with an evaluation of the investigator's stated purpose. Studies that state hypotheses in advance are more reliable than studies that pursue hypotheses after the fact; and studies investigating a single prespecified endpoint are more credible than studies investigating many outcomes, as dictated by the data. In a natural history study, if you follow a group of people and assess them for a multitude of outcomes, there is a strong probability that one or more of the outcomes will be statistically high (or low) by chance. This is analogous to the conduct of multiple comparisons between the treatment and control groups in clinical trials. In the context of natural history studies, it might be termed the *multiple-outcomes problem*.

Studies that test hypotheses after the fact are more likely to use retrospective methods. Be extra vigilant when a prognosis study is conducted retrospectively, that is, when historical data are used to assess outcomes in a population. Such studies can be carried out retrospectively in a valid fashion, but they are made much more difficult by the many pitfalls confronted when groups of patients are assembled retrospectively for follow-up studies.

Who and When? Assembling the Cohort

Ideally, the way to study prognosis is to assemble a group of individuals who share common features and observe what happens to them over time; such a group is usually called a *cohort* (chapter 28). Assembling an appropriate cohort is undoubtedly the most critical step in this type of research. Failure to negotiate this step successfully can doom the study to producing hopelessly biased results that will be useless or, even worse, seriously misleading.

"Who" and "when" remind you of the need to consider the precise nature of the cohort being studied. Who, exactly, is being investigated? When, in the natural history of their condition, have they been sampled? The general principle is that you should assemble a cohort consisting of a *representative* spectrum of people with the condition in question who are at a *homogeneous* and *early* point in its natural history.

The representativeness of the cohort will ultimately determine how generalizable the results will be. The important factors affecting representativeness include the type of patients in the catchment area of the study, the nature of the settings in which the patients are sampled (e.g., primary, secondary, or tertiary), and the mechanisms of presentation or referral that bring the patients into the sampling frame. If, in a study of outcomes in ulcerative colitis, a cohort is assembled by reviewing charts and collecting all people admitted to a given hospital with a diagnosis of ulcerative colitis during a specified period, several sampling biases could be at work to make the cohort nonrepresentative. First, only cases severe enough to require hospital admission are being sampled; individuals with milder disease, managed within their communities, are not adequately represented in the cohort. This biases the results toward worse outcomes. Second, the hospital's referral pattern could play a role: a tertiary care center may admit only the most difficult or intractable cases—another bias toward poor outcomes (unless the study's intent is to examine the natural history of ulcerative colitis in hospitalized tertiary care patients).

The simple way to avoid any bias is to set the sampling frame to target the patient population the study intends to investigate. If the aim is to study the entire spectrum of patients with a given condition, one might sample newly diagnosed patients with the condition at all primary care settings, emergency rooms, and hospitals in a given catchment area. If the intention is to study only hospitalized patients, the sample can be restricted to all hospitals in the catchment area.

How the sample is constructed may seem esoteric to some, who may also consider it an unlikely source of appreciable empirical differences. The importance of the sampling frame has been vividly demonstrated, however, in studies investigating whether children with febrile seizures have an increased risk of recurrent nonfebrile seizures in later life. Ellenberg and Nelson[4] (1980) showed that studies in which children were sampled from hospital clinics and tertiary referral units provided estimates of recurrence ranging as high as 76.9%, whereas all studies that sampled children through primary care settings and in the general population found recurrence rates consistently under 5%.

The cohort of persons under study *must* be homogeneous with respect to where they are in the natural history of their illness. The need for uniformity can best be appreciated by considering what would arise in its absence. What meaning could be derived from the 5-year mortality rate observed in a group of patients who have had bowel cancer for as little as 1 or 2 years, or as long as 15 or 20 years? To whom could such a mortality rate be validly generalized? On the other hand, the 5-year mortality rate observed in a group of people, whose diagnoses of bowel cancer had all been made within the prior year, could be reasonably applied to anyone at the same stage of the illness. To repeat, homogeneity gives the measurement of time internal consistency within the cohort and makes the cohort's experience generalizable to others at the same point in the natural history of a disease. Without such uniformity, the observed incidence rates are not reliable and are simply a function of the relative proportions of the various stages of illness that happen to fall within the cohort in question.

It is equally important that all persons in the cohort be observed onward from an early point in the natural history of the illness. There are two reasons for this. First, early observation allows for a characterization of the entire natural history of the illness. Second, and more importantly, it avoids potential biases associated with assembling cohorts at later points in time.

Consider a study of the subsequent rate of stroke in patients with hypertension. Suppose all patients currently under treatment for hypertension at a few primary care clinics and who have not had stroke are identified and followed forward in time. This sample includes patients who have been treated for hypertension for many years and are still under treatment. This is known as a prevalent cohort, because it includes prevalent cases (i.e., all existing cases at a particular point in time). To fully appreciate the potential biases, consider those not captured in this sample. First, the sample will tend to exclude the patients who were at highest risk and had a stroke soon after developing hypertension. As a consequence, the sample will overrepresent "survivors" who may be more "stroke-resistant"; the study would then underestimate the true risk of stroke. It will also tend to exclude those with very mild hypertension that responded to diet, weight loss, and/or exercise (i.e., essentially, the hypertension was cured by the time of the sampling). Thus, the sample will overrepresent persons with more severe hypertension who require long-term treatment and will lead to an overestimation of the risk of stroke. Both examples illustrate what might be termed *migration bias*.

Migration bias occurs when cohorts are assembled later in the natural history of a disease, because doing so raises the possibility that some members have migrated from the cohort as a result of early ill effects or early cure. Although we might argue that these effects work in opposite directions and might cancel each other, it would depend on the relative weights of the two forms of migration. Using an incident cohort of individuals assembled at an early and uniform point in the natural history of an illness is much preferable to relying on good fortune.

There are usually several points in the natural history of a disease from which to choose an inception point for a cohort. For studying the natural history of an illness, two obvious inception points are the time of onset of symptoms and the time of first diagnosis; each has advantages and disadvantages. Time of onset of symptoms is more closely related to the true biologic onset of the illness, but it may not be reliably documented and cannot be truly validated. Establishing the inception point for a person with ulcerative colitis may be impossible: How can we tell whether an episode of abdominal pain and diarrhea 5 years prior to diagnosis was truly the first episode of the illness or simply a transient infectious gastroenteritis? In contrast, time of first diagnosis is usually well documented on medical charts and accompanied by confirmatory diagnostic evidence, but diagnosis may be separated from the biologic and clinical onset of the illness by varying amounts of time attributable to delays in seeking medical help, or to differences in access to diagnostic facilities.

To study prognosis following a particular surgical procedure, the time of operation is an obvious choice for the inception point of a cohort. The sampling required to obtain such a cohort *must* be carried out in a way that ensures that all persons undergoing the procedure are represented; any form of sampling at a later postoperative point would be subject to bias because those with perioperative or early postoperative events could be missed. It may surprise you to learn that the time of surgery is not necessarily the best inception point for a prognosis study of a surgical intervention. Consider a study of prognosis in cardiac transplantation patients. If we were to assemble a cohort of patients at the time of surgery, only those who survived long enough for a donor to be found would be captured; those with very severe disease who died waiting for a donor would be missed. If we wish to study the policy of attempting to perform a transplant rather than the surgery itself, outcomes during the preoperative waiting period ought to be included and attributed to the policy of attempting to perform a transplant. A preferable inception point might, therefore, be the point at which the patient is deemed eligible for transplant and is entered on the waiting list. Although not perfect, this inception point is much

more uniform than the date of surgery, which is influenced by the availability of donors and applicable only to those who survive to undergo the procedure. Use of this inception point converts the study into an investigation of the natural history of what might be termed *transplant-eligible end-stage cardiac disease*.

Sometimes, it is possible to choose an inception point that is too early in the natural history of the disease. Consider a study of prognosis in women with breast cancer. For convenience, it is tempting to assemble a cohort of all women detected as having breast cancer at an initial visit to a mammography screening program. Although the results of such a study will be generalizable to all women with similarly detected cancers, they will not be applicable to the vast majority of women whose cancers are detected clinically in the community.

The fundamental goal of screening is to enhance the benefit of therapy by implementing it at an earlier stage in the natural history. Even if screening had no beneficial effect on outcome, however, the experience of the screen-detected cohort will not be generalizable to community-detected populations. First, earlier detection will automatically lengthen survival following detection, but this longer survival accrues to the length of time patients carry the diagnosis, not to their life spans—an effect known as *lead-time bias*." Second, a more subtle effect stems from the fact that the cancers that are most amenable to detection at an initial screening visit have the longest detectable phase prior to clinical detection and tend to be the slowest growing. Accordingly, the prognosis for women detected as having breast cancer at an initial screening visit will appear to be more favorable than for women diagnosed in the community because slower growing, less fulminant cancers will have been overrepresented in our cohort sample. This effect is known as *length bias*. An inception point that is too early—as would occur with screen detection—may yield results that are not generalizable to the illness as it is customarily diagnosed.

What? Defining the Endpoints

The "what" criterion reminds the reader to consider precisely what endpoint is being studied.

Outcomes *must* be so clearly defined that the reader of a report will know exactly what was being measured and what must be measured to reproduce the study. This principle applies no less to a study of prognosis than to any other type of biomedical investigation. Even when the outcome is as unambiguous as death, there may be problems if the analysis depends on distinguishing differences in its etiology (e.g., cardiovascular vs. cerebrovascular); death certificates are notoriously unreliable for such purposes. The need for clear criteria is even more marked when the endpoint is less incontrovertible than death. A study of prognosis following femoral-popliteal bypass grafting that uses loss of graft patency as its endpoint will need a precise definition of this outcome.

How? Monitoring for the Endpoints

Once a clear definition of the endpoint has been identified, you should consider how occurrences of the endpoint were monitored. In general, surveillance for the endpoint of interest in a natural history study should be carried out in a uniform fashion and performed, when possible, by individuals who are blind to the prior history or relevant risk factors in the study.

When surveillance is not carried out in a uniform fashion, surveillance bias (so-called) is possible. Consider a prognosis study following a particular operative procedure in which a cohort of patients is assembled and monitored. In the perioperative period, patients are classified as being high and low in risk on the basis of a profile of associated risk factors; high-risk patients are subsequently followed at a specialized clinic. Clinically, it is an excellent idea to provide specialized follow-up for the high-risk patients, but it will likely bias the results in terms of prognosis; the high-risk individuals will likely receive closer scrutiny, more frequent evaluation, and earlier and more frequent diagnostic tests.

The net effect of this differential intensity in follow-up is that events may be uncovered more frequently, or, at the least, endpoints may be detected earlier in the closely followed group. In either case, the incidence of later endpoint events may be artifactually elevated as a result of this surveillance bias. Even in the absence of a specialized

clinic, if those who are conducting the follow-up are aware of the risk status, it may influence them to scrutinize the high-risk persons more carefully for the outcome (i.e, a diagnostic suspicion bias). Similarly, when ambiguous events occur or uncertain diagnostic test results are present, knowledge of the prior status may influence interpretation of the diagnostic test or categorization of the event (i.e., an expectation bias). All these effects can be minimized if (1) the follow-up is conducted in a uniform fashion that simulates routine clinical follow-up in intensity, and (2) interpretations are made by individuals who are blind to the particular risk status of patients.

How Many? Completeness of Follow-up and Methods of Analysis

The final criterion, "how many," alerts you to some of the quantitative issues surrounding natural history studies. How many of the subjects were followed completely and how many were lost to follow-up are crucial questions. We have already discussed the methods of analysis that are applicable when there is incomplete follow-up; the data on any individuals who are lost to follow-up at the time of their last known status are usually "censored," that is, the subjects are not considered to be at risk beyond that point. Although this assumption helps to provide more precise estimates of the incidence of outcome events and maximizes use of the information gained in the study, the estimates will be unbiased only if similar subsequent courses are experienced by those who were lost to follow-up and those who were followed completely. Our knowledge of prognosis in persons who volunteer for studies and in those who comply with study protocols suggests that this is unlikely to be true.

There are several strategies for dealing with this problem. If the proportion of persons lost to follow-up is small, a bias that will seriously distort the estimates is unlikely; if it is not, you can try to gauge how different the persons lost to follow-up are from those who were not lost. If you have baseline demographic information and data on prognostic factors, and you can show that they are similar for those followed and those lost, you have some circumstantial evidence that the bias may not be very severe.

Another strategy is to explore the boundaries of the potential bias by assuming the best and worst possible outcomes in those who were lost—sometimes referred to as best- and worst-case scenarios, respectively. Suppose that, in a 10-year follow-up study of mortality in persons subjected to a particular surgical procedure, approximately 20% of the cohort was lost prior to completion of the study; whether they lived or died beyond the last point of contact with them is not known. Conventional methods of survival analysis, which censor such persons at the last point of contact, provide unbiased estimates *if* these persons have a subsequent mortality experience similar to that of those who were followed completely. Now consider the two possible extremes. The worst-case assumption is that every person who was lost to follow-up died just after the point of last contact; survival analysis using this assumption will provide a maximum estimate of mortality for the cohort in the worst-case scenario. The other extreme is to assume that every person lost to follow-up survived the entire study period; survival analysis using this assumption will provide a minimum estimate of mortality in the best-case scenario. The truth will likely be somewhere in between.

If the extremes lie in a particular direction, they may help to strengthen your conclusion. If the observed mortality in the 10-year mortality study following the surgery remains low, even in the worst-case scenario, you can remain relatively confident it is low despite the incomplete follow-up. Conversely, if the observed mortality remains high, even in the best-case scenario, you can remain confident in the conclusion that mortality is high.

In studies of prognosis in which analytic comparisons are being made, you should ensure that issues of statistical significance are addressed satisfactorily. Suppose a study reports the 5-year survival probabilities of a certain class of heart disease patients are 50% and 60% with medical management and surgical management, respectively. Because these are estimates from a finite data set, they are subject to random error. Could such an observed difference in prognosis easily arise by chance alone, or is there a real difference? The statistical methods provide a *p*-value that may be interpreted as the chance that a difference of the observed magnitude could have arisen by chance

alone (i.e., the "null" hypothesis of no true difference). Confidence intervals around probabilities should be provided to permit an appreciation of the range of values compatible with the data.

When a prognosis study reports a statistically significant difference in outcomes between two cohorts, the canny reader will immediately question whether it is clinically significant. Clinically trivial differences in the probabilities of critical events can be statistically significant when large cohorts are involved. Conversely, when a study finds no statistically significant difference in the probability of certain outcomes between cohorts, the reader should immediately ask whether the cohorts were large enough to provide adequate power for important differences to have been detected. When a difference in prognosis is found, it may have arisen because of other differences between the two groups. Inequalities in socioeconomic status or in severity of disease are almost certain to be present if random allocation to the two groups was not used. Statistical methods are available to allow the prognosis associated with the method of management to be separated from, or adjusted for, other differences between two groups, if the other factors influencing risk or prognosis are known and have been accurately measured. Nevertheless, the possibility remains that an unrecognized factor is present, or a recognized factor is being poorly measured ("misclassified"). The only convincing way to deal with this possibility is to perform a randomized controlled trial in which the random allocation is expected to apportion unrecognized factors about equally between the two groups.

Conclusion

Evaluation of risk and prognosis involves estimating the probability of future events, given present circumstances. Risk assessment refers specifically to the probability of future disease or injury in apparently healthy individuals; prognosis refers to the probability of future health-related events in individuals who already have a disease or injury. The term *risk* is also generally used in both contexts. To estimate risk in simple situations, proportions and rates are used. To compare risk between two groups, relative risk and the summary relative rate are available. A useful graphic technique is to present a survival curve for the study sample, or a set of survival curves for different subgroups. Statistical hypothesis testing can be carried out using the ordinary χ^2 test for a 2×2 table, or the more sophisticated Mantel-Haenzel summary χ^2 statistic.

For more complex situations in which the populations being compared are not homogeneous, logistic regression and Cox regression are used. Censoring (loss to follow-up) is a commonly encountered complication. The survival curve can be estimated in this situation by the Kaplan-Meier method, and the summary relative rate, adjusted for confounding factors, by Cox regression.

A methodological framework has been provided for assessing the quality of an article reporting a study of prognosis (or for planning such a study). "Why" reminds the reader to begin, *always,* with an evaluation of the investigator's stated purpose. In general, studies that state hypotheses in advance are more reliable than studies that pursue hypotheses after the fact, and studies that investigate a single prespecified endpoint are more credible than studies that investigate many outcomes, as dictated by the data. "Who" and "when" remind the reader that, in a natural history study, it is crucial to consider the precise nature of the cohort being studied. Who, exactly, is being investigated, and when in the natural history have these subjects been sampled? The general principle is that the researcher ought to assemble a *representative* spectrum of people with a particular condition who are at a *homogeneous* and *early* point in its natural history. Failure to construct such an inception or incident cohort can bias a study beyond repair.

"What" reminds the reader to consider precisely what endpoint is being studied. The primary outcomes must be clearly defined so that the reader will know exactly what is being measured. The "how" criterion pertains to how occurrences of the endpoint were monitored. Surveillance for the endpoint of interest in a natural history study should be carried out in a uniform fashion and performed, whenever possible, by individuals who are blind to the prior history or relevant risk factors in the study. Failure to perform uniform and blinded surveillance should alert the reader to the possibilities of surveillance bias, diagnostic suspicion bias, and expectation bias.

The final criterion, "how many," is meant to alert the reader to some of the quantitative issues surrounding natural history studies. How many subjects were lost to follow-up and how they were handled in the analysis are crucial questions. Techniques of survival analysis can utilize censored observations, but losses to follow-up are assumed to have similar subsequent experiences. Best- and worst-case scenarios can be used to explore the boundaries of any possible bias. Like studies of therapeutic interventions, prognosis studies should explore the statistical significance of important differences, should assess whether statistically significant differences are clinically meaningful, and, in the case of negative hypothesis tests, should document adequate power to have detected important differences if they were present.

References

1. Knaus WA. The science of prediction and its implications for clinicians today. Theor Surg 1988;3: 93–101.
2. Kramer MS. Clinical biostatistics. In: Troidl H, Spitzer WO, McPeek B, Mulder DS, McKneally MF, Wechsler AS, Balch CM, eds. Principles and Practice of Research: Strategies for Surgical Investigators, 2nd edn. New York: Springer-Verlag, 1991, pp. 126–143.
3. Lee ET. Statistical Methods for Survival Data Analysis. New York: Wiley, 1992.
4. Ellenberg JH. Nelson KB. Sample selection and the natural history of disease: studies of febrile seizures. JAMA 1980;243:1337–1340.

Additional Reading

Beslow NE, Day NE. Statistical Methods in Cancer Research, vol. 2. The Design and Analysis of Cohort Studies. Lyons, France: International Agency for Research on Cancer, 1982.

Buck N, Devlin HB, Lunn JN. Report of a confidential inquiry into perioperative deaths. The Nuffield Provincial Hospitals Trust/Kings Fund, 1988.

Cooper JB, Newbower RS, Long CD, McPeek B: Preventable anesthesia mishaps: a study of human factors. Anesthesiology 1978;49:399.

Ellenberg JH, Nelson KB. Sample selection and the natural history of disease: studies of febrile seizures. JAMA 1980;243:1337–1340.

Kleinbaum DG, Kupper LL, Morgenstern H. Epidemiologic Research: Principles and Quantitative Methods. Belmont, CA: Lifetime Publications, 1982.

Knaus WA. The science of prediction and its implications for clinicians today. Theo Surg 1988;3:93–101.

Kramer MS. Clinical Epidemiology and Biostatistics. Berlin: Springer-Verlag, 1988.

Lee ET. Statistical Methods for Survival Data Analysis. New York: Wiley, 1992.

Lunn JN, Devlin HB. Lessons from the confidential enquiry into perioperative deaths in three NHS regions. Lancet 1987;2(8572):1384–1386.

McPeek B, Gasko M, Mosteller F. Measuring outcome from anesthesia and operation. Theor Surg 1986;1: 2–9.

Rothman KJ. Modern Epidemiology. Boston: Little, Brown, 1986.

Sackett DL, Haynes RB, Tugwell P. Clinical Epidemiology: A Basic Science for Clinical Medicine. Boston: Little, Brown, 1985.

CHAPTER 31

Sensitivity, Specificity, and Predictive Value

M.T. Schechter

Yerushalmy's pioneering work[1] on observer variability in the interpretation of chest roentgenograms initiated a still-expanding interest in the evaluation of the diagnostic process. He introduced the terms *sensitivity* and *specificity* as measures of the validity of diagnostic tests, and an entire methodology including the concept of *predictive value* has developed in response to the geometric growth in and reliance on diagnostic testing in clinical practice.

Diagnostic Test Validity

Clinicians use diagnostic tests to ascertain whether a disease is present. For example, you can use a gallium scan to test for the presence or absence of an intraabdominal abscess, or mammography to help you determine whether a palpable lump is malignant.

The disease state that a diagnostic test is meant to detect is sometimes referred to as the *target disease*. The *validity* of a diagnostic test refers simply to its ability to register an abnormal result for patients in whom the target disease is present, and a normal result for patients in whom the target disease is absent. An ideal diagnostic test would exhibit both these behaviors; that is, it would register abnormal results only for patients who have the target disease, and normal results only for patients who are free of the target disease. Such a diagnostic test would be perfect in the sense that its results would be perfectly predictive of absence or presence of the target disease. Unfortunately, most diagnostic tests do not perform this well, and a number of concepts and techniques have been developed to gauge just how satisfactorily a given diagnostic test performs.

To judge how well a test performs in detecting a target disease in certain patients, we need some way of determining the truth about the disease's presence or absence in the same patients. To judge the capabilities of the gallium scan in diagnosing intraabdominal abscess, we need to know whether such abscesses are present in a group of patients so that we can compare this information with the results obtained by means of the gallium scan. We could use the findings of laparotomy and subsequent pathological confirmation of an abscess as the determinant of the true target disease state. Similarly, we could use the results of laparotomy as the determinant for the presence of intraperitoneal injury, to assess the performance of peritoneal lavage as a diagnostic maneuver. To assess mammography as a means of detecting malignant breast tumors, we could use pathological examination of the tumor as our determinant. The method used to confirm the presence or absence of the target disease in such determinations is known as the *gold standard*; it should be the best clinical standard currently available.

When surgical exploration and pathological confirmation are part of the usual clinical management, they are obvious choices as gold standards; when they are not, other standards must be used. To determine the validity of newer scanning techniques as diagnostic tests for deep vein thrombosis (DVT), the best clinical standard currently available is venography. Consequently, the results of this radiological procedure are usually used as the gold standard for the presence or absence of DVT. Similarly, to check the validity of such tests as radionuclide scans in the detection of coronary artery stenoses, where surgical confirmation is available only in the relatively small number of patients who come to bypass surgery, coronary angiography is often used as the gold standard.

Figure 31-1 sets out the structure of a diagnostic test assessment in general terms. In essence, we merely compare the diagnostic test result (abnormal vs. normal) with the gold standard result for the target disease (present vs. absent). By convention, the test result is set out in the rows of a 2×2 table, while the gold standard result is displayed in the columns. Adoption of this arbitrary convention will help you to recall some of the definitions we will come to later.

The upper left-hand cell displays the number of patients who have the disease, according to the gold standard, and also have positive test results; that is, the test correctly identifies them as having the target disease. Such patients are called *true positives* (TP). The lower right-hand cell displays the number of patients who do not have the disease and have negative test results, the *true negatives* (TN). Taken together, the true positives and true negatives constitute all the patients in whom the diagnostic test is correct. The greater the proportion of patients found in these two groups, the more accurate the diagnostic test.

The patients who fall into the two remaining cells give rise to whatever uncertainty there is. The number in the upper right-hand cell represents the patients who do not have the disease but who have erroneously positive test results. These patients are called *false positives* (FP). The costs of this type of error are the unnecessary further investigations and treatments that might be undertaken, and the effects of falsely labeling the patient. The number in the lower left-hand cell represents the patients who have the disease, but erroneously negative test results, *false negatives* (FN). The costs of this type of error are the morbidity and mortality associated with lack of im-

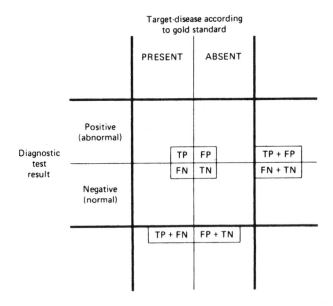

Figure 31-1.

mediate treatment. We have completed the table by adding the rows and columns: TP + FN, FP + TN, TP + FP, FN + TN.

Sensitivity is defined as the proportion of those with the disease who have a positive test result. This is sometimes shortened to "positivity in disease." Sensitivity is a measure of how well the test performs at detecting the disease when it is present. It can be calculated from the first column of the table by the formula

$$\text{sensitivity} = \frac{\text{TP}}{\text{TP} + \text{FN}}$$

Specificity is defined as the proportion of those who do not have the disease who have negative test results—sometimes referred to as "negativity in health." Specificity is a measure of how well the test performs at registering negative results when the target disease is absent. It can be computed from the second column of the table by the formula

$$\text{specificity} = \frac{\text{TN}}{\text{FP} + \text{TN}}$$

If you prefer the terminology of conditional probabilities, *sensitivity* is the conditional probability of a positive test given the presence of disease, and *specificity* is the conditional probability of a negative test given the absence of disease. These latter definitions are included only because you may encounter them in the literature.

To illustrate these concepts, we will use a well-known example from the recent history of medicine, namely, the evaluation of prostatic acid phosphatase (PAP) for the detection of prostatic cancer, adapted from Foti and colleagues.[2] Although PAP has been superceded by other tests, most notably prostatic-specific antigen, the events surrounding the evaluation and dissemination of the prostatic acid phosphatase test remain an excellent example with which to illustrate the concepts in this chapter.

Foti and his colleagues used 113 patients with prostatic carcinoma, confirmed by the gold standard of surgical biopsy, and 217 individuals free of prostatic cancer. The latter group consisted of normal individuals and patients with benign prostatic hyperplasia, previous prostatectomy, gastrointestinal disorders, or nonprostatic cancer. Sera from the 330 individuals were assessed by the assay for the presence of PAP, and each specimen was characterized as positive (abnormal) or negative (normal). The results were compared with the true prostatic cancer status of the 330 individuals to produce Figure 31-2.

In the 113 patients with prostatic carcinoma, the PAP test was positive in 79, for *a sensitivity* of 79/113 or 0.70. A *sensitivity* of 0.70 or 70% prompts the inference that, given 100 patients with prostatic carcinoma, the test will detect approximately 70 of them and miss about 30. The latter figure, derived by subtracting the *sensitivity*, in percent, from 100, is known as the *false negative rate*.

In the 217 patients who did not have prostatic carcinoma, the test was negative in 204, that is, a *specificity* of 204/217 or 0.94. A *specificity* of 0.94 or 94% suggests that, given 100 patients without prostatic carcinoma, the test will be negative in about 94 of them and falsely positive in the remaining 6. The last figure, obtained by subtracting the specificity, in percent, from 100, is known as the *false positive rate*.

Sensitivity and *specificity* are measures of a diagnostic test's validity; the higher these values are, the better the test is at detecting the presence and absence of disease, respectively. The higher the sensitivity, the lower the false negative rate; that is, the lower the chances are of missing the target disease when it is present. The higher the specificity, the lower the false-positive result when the target disease is absent. The PAP test, with a sensitivity of 70% and a specificity of 94%, exemplifies high specificity with only moderate sensitivity.

Diagnostic Test Utility (Usefulness)

To calculate sensitivity and specificity, you *must* know the true presence or absence of the target disease. This was illustrated earlier by the 113 patients in whom biopsy had already established the actual presence of prostatic carcinoma. In many clinical situations, we do not know whether the target disease is present or absent. If the results of a gold standard were available, there would be no need for another diagnostic test.

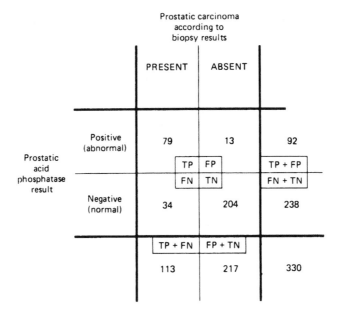

Figure 31-2.

In clinical practice, we are often confronted by additional problems when the presence of the target disease is uncertain. First, given that a patient has a positive test result, we need to know what the probability is that the target disease is present, that is, the *positive predictive value* (PPV) of the test. The PPV reflects how certain we may be about the presence of the target disease in patients with a positive test result. Similarly, for patients with negative test results, we need to know the probability that the target disease is absent, which is the *negative predictive value* (NPV). The higher the PPV, the better the test is at "ruling in" the disease when the test result is positive; the higher the NPV, the better the test is at "ruling out" the disease when the test result is negative. Whereas sensitivity and specificity measure the test's intrinsic abilities to detect the presence and absence of the target disease, respectively, the predictive values measure the test's utility in clinical practice.

Consider a typical patient drawn at random from the entire group of 330 individuals in the study by Foti and his colleagues (Figure 31-2). Suppose we do not know whether the individual has prostatic carcinoma, as would be true in clinical practice, and we are going to rely on the PAP assay for the answers. Since 113 of the 330 indi-

viduals in the study have prostatic carcinoma, we know there is a probability of 113/330 or 34.2% that our randomly chosen individual has the disease. This measure of the proportion of diseased patients within the total population is known as the *prevalence* and is calculated using the formula

$$\text{prevalence} = \frac{\text{TP} + \text{FN}}{\text{TP} + \text{FN} + \text{FP} + \text{TN}}$$

The numerator (TP + FN) is the total number of individuals with the disease (i.e., the sum of the cells in the left-hand column of Figure 31-2); the denominator is the total number of participants (i.e., the sum of all four cells in Figure 31-2). Since there is a 34.2% chance that our typical patient, drawn at random from the sample, has prostatic cancer prior to undergoing the PAP test, the prevalence is also referred to as the *pretest probability* or *pretest likelihood* of the disease.

Let us now see how well the PAP test performs at predicting the presence or absence of disease in our typical patient, by supposing that his test result is positive. Since there are 92 patients with positive test results, of whom 79 actually have prostatic cancer, there is a 79/92 or 85.9% chance that our patient has prostatic carcinoma, given a positive test. This is the PPV for this population (Figure 31-2), that is,

$$PPV = \frac{TP}{TP + FP}$$

Since the PPV represents the probability of a patient having a given disease when the test result is positive, it is also referred to as the *posttest probability of a positive test* (PTL +). In this case, the PPV (or PTL +) is substantially higher (85.9%) than the pretest probability of 34.2%, and the test has performed very well at "ruling in" prostatic carcinoma by markedly increasing the probability of the presence of the disease when the test is positive.

Now, suppose the PAP result in our randomly chosen individual is negative. Since there are 238 patients with negative test results, of whom 204 do not have the disease, there is a 204/238 or 85.7% chance that our subject is free of prostatic carcinoma given a negative test. This is the negative predictive value (NPV) for this population (Figure 31-2), that is,

$$NPV = \frac{TN}{FN + TN}$$

This NPV of 85.7% represents the probability of not having the disease when the PAP result is negative. If there is an 85.7% chance of not having the disease, there is a 14.3% chance of having it; subtracting the NPV from 100 gives the probability of having the disease even when the test is negative, which is the *posttest probability of a negative result.* As you might anticipate, the probability of having the disease after a negative test (14.3%) is lower than the pretest probability of disease (34.2%). Consequently, the negative test result has contributed to "ruling out" prostatic carcinoma by decreasing the probability of the disease from 34.2% to 14.3%.

You may have noticed an asymmetry. The "positive predictive value" (PPV) and the "posttest probability of a positive test" (PTL +) are synonymous, but the "negative predictive value" (NVP) and the "posttest probability of a negative test" (PTL −) are not. The NPV refers to the probability of the disease being absent in those with a negative result, while the PTL − refers to the probability of the disease being present in

those with a negative result. Although the two quantities are not the same, they are strictly related, since they sum to 100%, and one can be easily derived from the other.

The results of the PAP test in this particular population can be depicted by a diagnostic tree diagram (Figure 31-3). Such representations are very useful in clinical decisions analysis, the science of structuring clinical decisions. The patient enters the test at the left of the diagram with a pretest probability of prostatic carcinoma of 34.2%. If the test is positive, this probability rises to the posttest probability of a positive test (85.9%); if the test is negative, this probability falls to the posttest probability of a negative test (14.3%). The test appears, therefore, to provide some potentially useful information in this population. For patients with positive results, the probability of disease is sufficiently high (85.9%) to warrant biopsy and possible surgical exploration; but if the results are negative, the probability of disease is sufficiently low (14.3%) that such patients may be followed, or given another noninvasive test, if one is available.

On the basis of the sensitivity and specificity results of Foti and his colleagues, many concluded that the PAP radioimmunoassay could serve as an effective screening test for the early detection of prostatic cancer. In an editorial accompanying the report of Foti et al., Gittes stated, "The grim finding has been that, overall, 90% of cases are first detected when they have already metastasized. The clear implication of the accompanying report is that mass screening on the basis of a blood test

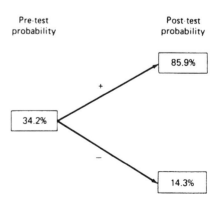

Figure 31-3.

alone can reverse this gloomy experience."[3] The popular press reported that a new blood test promised to do for prostatic cancer what the Papanicolaou smear had accomplished for cancer of the cervix.

The *utility* of a test refers to its usefulness and its ability to affect patient care positively in a specific clinical situation. It can be judged only in relation to a *particular* clinical situation; a relatively good sensitivity and specificity do not suffice to establish the clinical utility of a given test in *any* situation. Although sensitivity and specificity measure intrinsic qualities of a test's validity and may be assumed to remain relatively stable in different clinical situations, the predictive values and posttest probabilities can change drastically. Since the predictive values and posttest probabilities depend very heavily on the pretest probability (prevalence), changes in prevalence can lead to marked changes in the predictive values and the clinical utility of a test. In other words, to adequately assess a diagnostic test for a specific clinical purpose, you must analyze it in relation to that particular purpose.

The original analysis of the PAP assay was carried out in a population of patients in whom the prevalence of prostatic cancer was 34.2%—hardly representative of the usual screening situation. Three years after the report of Foti et al., Watson and Tang presented their analysis of the PAP test as a screening test for prostatic cancer.[4] On the basis of national data for the United States for 1964, these authors assumed that the prevalence of prostatic carcinoma among white American men was 35 cases per 100,000. They then used the PAP test's established sensitivity and specificity of 70% and 94%, respectively, to calculate its predictive values in the screening situation.

To make these calculations, you begin by putting the hypothetical population of 100,000 as the total at the lower right-hand corner of the 2 × 2 table (TP + FP + FN + TN) (Figure 31-4A). Since there are an estimated 35 cases among this hypothetical group, the sum at the bottom of the left-hand column (TP + FN) should read 35. It follows that the sum of the right-hand column (FP + TN) should be 100,000 − 35 = 99,965 (Figure 31-4A). Of the 35 men who have prostatic cancer, the test will be positive in about 70% (sensitivity), that is, approximately 25, and this

quantity can be entered in the TP cell (Figure 31-4B). The remainder, 35 − 25 = 10, can be entered in the FN cell. Similarly, of the 99,965 men without prostatic carcinoma, the test will be negative in about 94% of the men (specificity), that is, approximately 93,967, and this quantity can be entered in the TN cell (Figure 31-4C). The remainder, 99,965 − 93,967 = 5,998, is entered in the FP cell (Figure 31-4C). The table can be completed by simply adding the row totals (Figure 31-5).

We can now calculate the predictive values and posttest probabilities for the screening situation. The PPV (or PTL+) is TP/(TP + FP) or 25/6,023, that is, 0.42%. The NPV is TN/(TN + FN) or 93,967/93,977, that is, 99.99%. Consequently, the posttest probability of a negative test, obtained by subtracting the NPV from 100%, is 0.01%. The probability of prostatic carcinoma prior to the test (the pretest likelihood or prevalence) was set at 35/100,000 or 0.035%.

Figure 31-6 is a diagnostic tree diagram summarizing these results for the screening situation. The average asymptomatic man, who would be screened by such a test, approaches the test at the left of the diagram with a pretest probability of prostatic cancer of 0.035% (35 chances in 100,000). If his test is positive, the probability rises to only 0.42% (1 chance in 240). Even with a positive test result, the chance of having prostatic cancer is still extremely slim, and it would be hard to justify further invasive testing. Obviously, the test is of little clinical help when it is positive in a screening situation.

Moreover, since approximately 6% (6,023/100,000) of all white American men would have positive PAP screening tests, any policy of investigating positives further would involve the needless testing of significant numbers of healthy men. If the test is negative, the probability of disease falls to 0.01% (10/100,000). Although one could argue that the test is useful in the screening situation, since it virtually rules out prostatic carcinoma when it is negative, this decrease in probability is of little benefit because the disease is exceptionally rare in the given population (35/100,000).

Our example illustrates the relation between posttest likelihoods and pretest likelihoods. In the diagnostic analysis carried out by Foti et al., the

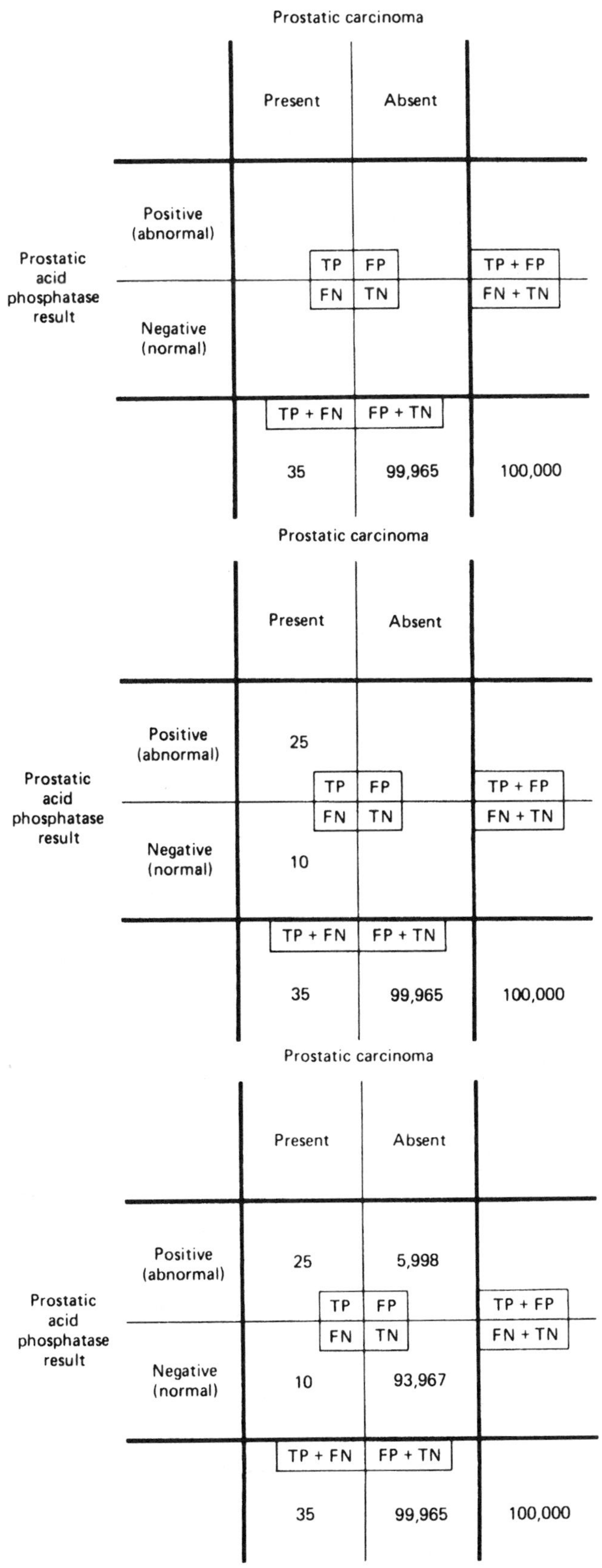
Prostatic carcinoma
Present
Absent
Positive (abnormal)
Negative (normal)
Prostatic acid phosphatase result
TP
FP
FN
TN
TP + FP
FN + TN
TP + FN
FP + TN
35
99,965
100,000
Prostatic carcinoma
Present
Absent
Positive (abnormal)
Negative (normal)
Prostatic acid phosphatase result
25
10
TP
FP
FN
TN
TP + FP
FN + TN
TP + FN
FP + TN
35
99,965
100,000
Prostatic carcinoma
Present
Absent
Positive (abnormal)
Negative (normal)
Prostatic acid phosphatase result
25
5,998
10
93,967
TP
FP
FN
TN
TP + FP
FN + TN
TP + FN
FP + TN
35
99,965
100,000

Figure 31-4.

Prostatic carcinoma

Prostatic acid phosphatase result		Present	Absent	
	Positive (abnormal)	25 TP	5,998 FP	6,023 TP + FP
	Negative (normal)	FN 10	TN 93,967	FN + TN 93,977
		TP + FN 35	FP + TN 99,965	100,000

PPV = TP/(TP + FP) = 25/6,023 = .0042 or 0.42%
NPV = TN/(TN + FN) = 93,967/93,977 = 0.9999 or 99.99%

Figure 31-5.

posttest likelihoods of a positive and negative test were relatively high (85.9% and 14.3%, respectively) because the pretest likelihood was high (34.2%) prior to the test. In the screening analysis carried out by Watson and Tang, the posttest likelihoods of a positive and negative test were extremely low (0.42% and 0.01%, respectively) because the pretest likelihood was very low (0.035%) prior to the test. The pre- and posttest likelihoods can be linked by a mathematical expression known as Bayes' theorem. The following are two of many equivalent expressions for Bayes' theorem:

$$\text{PPV} = \frac{\text{P} \times \text{SENS}}{(\text{P} \times \text{SENS}) + (1 - \text{P}) \times (1 - \text{SPEC})}$$

$$\text{NPV} = \frac{(1 - \text{P}) \times \text{SPEC}}{(1 - \text{P}) \times \text{SPEC} + \text{P} \times (1 - \text{SENS})}$$

where P, SENS, and SPEC represent the pretest probability, sensitivity, and specificity, respectively, in decimal (e.g., 0.80) rather than percent (e.g., 80%) format. The different expressions used for Bayes' theorem have the common feature of portraying the posttest probabilities or predictive values in terms of the pretest probability. They all demonstrate how dependent the former values are on the latter value, and they provide a method for calculating posttest probabilities and predictive values for a given diagnostic test and a given pretest probability. You are encouraged to calculate the predictive values for the PAP test in the screening situation by setting P at 0.00035, SENS at 0.70, and SPEC at 0.94, in the formulas above. You should derive the predictive values that were obtained before, except for possible slight differences due to rounding error. These formulas provide an attractive alternative to the series of calculations and tables we went through earlier, to derive the predictive values and posttest probabilities (Figures. 31-4A–C and 31-5). Bayes' theorem, in whatever form, is a relatively straightforward method of deriving the predictive values and the posttest likelihoods that are central to the consideration of clinical utility. This type of analysis is sometimes referred to as "Bayesian analysis."

The PAP radioimmunoassay illustrates several fundamental things about diagnostic tests:

1. Sensitivity and specificity measure the validity (accuracy) of a diagnostic test. They have no direct bearing on its clinical utility.
2. The clinical utility of a test is best assessed by considering its predictive values and posttest probabilities in a specific clinical situation.

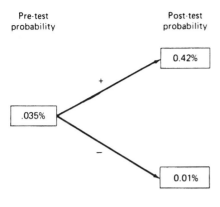

Figure 31-6.

3. Predictive values and posttest probabilities depend very heavily on the pretest probability (prevalence) of disease and, as a consequence, on both the clinical situation and the patient population in which a test is applied. This differs greatly from the popular misconception that test results are definitive (i.e., positive tests imply that patients are diseased and negative tests that they are not) and that the conclusions to be drawn from test results are independent of the patient who is tested.

The Assessment of Diagnostic Tests

New diagnostic tests and technologies are being developed at a constantly increasing rate; we have, for example, the prostatic specific antigen (PSA) test, positron emission tomography (PET), and magnetic resonance imaging (MRI). These new tests and techniques must be evaluated before they enter into widespread clinical use, and the medical literature contains more and more articles about their "assessment."

Guidelines for the Assessment of New Tests or Techniques

The Purpose of the Diagnostic Test

Any proper assessment of a diagnostic test begins with a clear statement of its proposed clinical purpose. The prostatic acid phosphatase radioim-

munoassay test illustrates how a clinical test may perform well in one situation (diagnosis) and fail in another (screening). The proposed clinical function dictates how the assessment should be carried out.

Clinical tests serve five different clinical functions: diagnosis, screening, staging, monitoring, and triage. *Diagnosis* is the "ruling in" or "ruling out" of a disease in a patient in whom the disease is clinically suspected (e.g., coronary angiography for detecting coronary artery disease in a patient with angina). *Screening* refers to the presumptive detection of a given disease in a group of individuals who are asymptomatic for, and not suspected of having, it (e.g., mammography for the presumptive detection of breast cancer in middle-aged women). *Staging* is the use of a clinical test to gauge how far a disease has advanced as a guide to treatment (e.g., mediastinoscopy to determine the resectability of a lung cancer). *Monitoring* is the use of a test to assess and adjust ongoing therapy (e.g., prothrombin times to monitor the effect of anticoagulant therapy). *Triage* refers to the use of a test to determine which patients should receive further invasive testing (e.g., Doppler studies to determine which patients should have cerebral angiography).

Accordingly, you must state the type of patient, the intended clinical setting, and the purpose of a test before you embark on any assessment of it. The importance of these requirements will become more apparent as we continue.

The Spectrum and Number of Patients

When you are choosing the patients who will participate in a diagnostic test assessment, observe the following rule: *the type of patient used in the assessment of a test should replicate the type of patient for whom the test is intended in clinical practice.* Unfortunately, this rule is not always followed. To carry out an assessment, you require a population with the target disease to estimate sensitivity, and a population free of the target disease to estimate specificity. You may be tempted to use an already-identified group with established, florid disease as the diseased group, and a group of normally healthy controls as the nondiseased group. A moment's thought should convince you that such disparate groups would not challenge the clinical test with the wide spectrum of patients you and others will face in normal clinical practice. A test proposed for *diagnosis* should be assessed in a wide range of patients suspected of having the target disease or other diseases often confused with the target disease. A *screening* test should be challenged with asymptomatic individuals like those it will be applied to in clinical practice.

The use of obviously diseased and healthy individuals as cases and controls will spuriously inflate both sensitivity and specificity values, because these individuals will likely have positive and negative tests, respectively. If you start with a statement of the test's proposed function, the proposed type of patient in whom it is to be used, and the proposed setting for its use, you merely need to assemble, consecutively, all the patients matching the specified profile who are seen in the appropriate setting(s) over a sufficient interval of time. The use of consecutive patients minimizes the possibility of introducing bias into the selection of patients and replicates the spectrum of patients the test will be applied to in its eventual clinical use.

If you wish to assess a new diagnostic test for DVT for use when patients first present themselves at the primary care level, consider using every consecutive patient who consults his or her family practitioner, or arrives at a local emergency room with a swollen calf and suspected DVT over a specified interval of time. Such a group will include patients who actually have DVT, in varying degrees of severity, and some who have confusing disorders, such as ruptured Baker's cysts or superficial thrombophlebitis. The performance of the test in such a group of patients will accurately reflect its performance in similar groups in similar primary care settings. If you propose to assess a *screening* test for the early detection of prostatic carcinoma, you should state that the test is proposed for use in elderly men who are both asymptomatic and clinically normal, and then assess it in a large population of such individuals.

Too often, inadequate numbers of patients are used. An investigator may assess a test in 25 diseased individuals, find that 20 of them have positive results, and conclude that the sensitivity is 80%. Although this is technically the best estimate for sensitivity based on the data, the 95% confidence limits around it are very wide (64% to 96%). The investigator should take the conservative approach and use the lower limit (64%) as the estimate of sensitivity, but, more often than not, the sensitivity is simply stated as being 80%. The result is an overestimation of test validity. The only acceptable exception to the use of sufficient numbers of patients to ensure precise estimates occurs when a test for a rare target disease is being assessed, and the number of available patients is inescapably small.

The Gold Standard

The gold standard is the set of criteria used by investigators to determine which patients are truly diseased and which are not. These criteria have a crucial impact on the 2 × 2 table and on the determination of the sensitivity and specificity of a test. Gold standards may be definitive (e.g., histopathological results from biopsy, surgery, or autopsy) or may simply be the results of other diagnostic tests currently accepted as standards for the diagnosis of the target disease in question. In certain situations, the gold standard may be a complex of symptoms, signs, and test results (e.g., the classification systems for the diagnosis of rheumatoid arthritis, systemic lupus erythematosus, and rheumatic fever). In diagnostic test assessments, it is critically important that the gold standard be well defined, repeatable, and accepted as a current clinical standard for the diagnosis of the target disease. Anyone who reads a report on a diagnosis test assessment will want to know how the test will perform at detecting the presence or absence of the target disease in relation to the gold standard. If the gold standard is not well defined or does not represent the current standard for diagnosis of the target disease, the assessment will be of little use because it will not be directly applicable to clinical practice. For example, since autopsy results or surgical findings are not usually available for patients with coronary artery disease (CAD), the results of coronary angiography are widely accepted as the clinical standard for diagnosis. Consequently, if you wish to assess the performance of a new test in the diagnosis of CAD, you might well utilize coronary angiography as your external gold standard for verifying the presence or absence of CAD in each patient; the angiographic criteria you use to establish the presence of CAD should be explicitly stated in your assessment report. Such explicit statements should include such clear, repeatable criteria as "a stenosis of greater than 75% seen on independent review by two cardiologists" and avoid such vagueness as "any abnormality seen on angiography." Describe the exact methods used to carry out the gold standard so that readers can determine whether the gold standard, as used in your study, corresponds with the one in use in their clinical settings.

The Diagnostic Test

An exact detailed description, as prescribed for your gold standard, is equally necessary for the diagnostic test you are assessing; that is, you must describe explicitly your test methodology, the conditions under which the test was performed, and how the patients were prepared. Supply enough detail to enable your readers to perform the diagnostic test exactly as you did in your assessment.

When the test produces a quantitative result (e.g., the concentration of a serum constituent), you should assess its precision. The variability produced by the test technology can be assessed by comparing the results for several samples taken from the same patient at the same time: the intrapatient variability can be assessed by comparing the results for samples taken from the same patient at different times. The sensitivity, specificity, and predictive values should not be calculated at several threshold values (e.g., the value that separates normal from abnormal results). When you choose a single threshold value, your choice should be justified.

If the test produces a qualitative result that requires interpretation (e.g., CT scans must be interpreted by a radiologist), state clear and repeatable interpretation criteria. In addition, assess both the inter- and intraobserver variability in the interpretative component of the test by presenting the same consecutive panel of test results to two or more observers for independent review, and to a single observer for independent review on two or more separate occasions.

Independence

When each patient in your sample has undergone the diagnostic and gold standard tests, the results are compared in a 2 × 2 table (Figure 31-2) to determine the test's validity and utility.

The diagnostic test and the gold standard test *must* be independent. Each patient *must* undergo both tests. The diagnostic test result must not influence the selection of who is to have the gold standard test. The process should be triple-blinded if possible, that is, those who perform the tests, those who interpret them, and those who undergo them (the patients) should be kept "blinded" until both tests have been performed and interpreted. The various individuals who perform, interpret, or undergo the diagnostic test should be unaware of the gold standard results, if possible. Conversely, the various individuals who perform, interpret, or undergo the gold standard test should be unaware of the diagnostic test results, if possible. If this independence is not maintained, expectation bias can occur and can result in a spurious increase in the derived sensitivity, specificity, and predictive values. This is especially true when there is a significant subjective patient component or a significant interpretive component to the diagnostic test.

Assessment of Validity and Utility

When you have produced a 2 × 2 table, derived sensitivity, specificity, and predictive values, and concluded the test is useful, if the values are reasonably high, you may think your job is finished. A proper assessment, however, goes on to consider the predictive values, the posttest probabilities, and their significance in the clinical situation proposed for the test. Since these values depend very heavily on the prevalence of the target disease in your patient sample, as determined by the gold standard, you must assess whether this prevalence is reasonably close to the true prevalence of the same disease in the proposed target population. This will almost certainly be so if you obeyed the principle of using all consecutive patients who are like those for whom the test is intended and who arrived at one or more settings similar to those in which use of the test is envisaged.

If the prevalence in your patient sample is not

a realistic estimate for the target population, re-calculate the predictive values and posttest probabilities on the basis of a more realistic prevalence. You can do this easily by using Bayes' theorem with the new prevalence value (P), and the derived sensitivity (SENS) and specificity (SPEC). Your assessment of clinical utility should center on whether the test provides enough information, on the basis of predictive values and posttest likelihoods, to cause a change in management. The radioimmunoassay test for PAP failed in the screening situation because the posttest likelihoods of a positive and negative test were not sufficiently different from the pretest likelihood (prevalence) to affect any management decisions. A proper assessment, based on a realistic prevalence, could have demonstrated this in the initial analysis before the use of PAP as a screening test had been suggested.

When you assess clinical utility and the impact of the predictive values and posttest likelihood on clinical decisions, you must consider the consequences for false positives and false negatives. If the target disease is frequently fatal and a treatment exists that markedly alters the outcome (e.g., intraabdominal bleeding, subdural hematoma, bacterial meningitis), false negatives are extremely undesirable, and a high sensitivity is required. A high sensitivity value has the effect of markedly reducing the posttest likelihood of a negative test (i.e., the negative predictive value is raised) and provides reasonable certainty that the target disease is absent when the test is negative. If you are screening for a disease that is not immediately fatal if missed, for which no effective treatment is available, and/or for which the costs of labeling and further investigation of positives are high (e.g., cystic fibrosis in newborns), you will want to keep the number of false positives to a minimum, and a high specificity will be required. A high specificity has the effect of markedly increasing the posttest likelihood of a positive test (i.e., the positive predictive value is raised) and provides reasonable certainty that the target disease is present when the test is positive.

In general, the impact of posttest likelihoods and predictive values on clinical decisions cannot be assessed without reference to the subsequent management of and consequences for positives and negatives.

References

1. Yerushalmy J. Statistical problems in assessing methods of medical diagnosis with special reference to x-ray techniques. Public Health Rep 1947;62: 1432–1449.
2. Foti AG, Cooper JF, Hershman H, Malvaez RR. Detection of prostatic cancer by solid-shape radioimmunoassay of serum prostatic acid phosphatase. New Engl J Med 1977;297:1357–1361.
3. Gittes R. Acid phosphatase reappraised. New Engl J Med 1977;297:1398–1399.
4. Watson RA, Tang DB. The predictive value of prostatic acid phosphatase as a screening test for prostatic cancer. New Engl J Med 1980;303:497–499.
5. Bayes T. An essay toward solving a problem in the doctrine of chance. Philos Trans R Soc London 1763;53:370–418.

Additional Reading

Department of Clinical Epidemiology and Biostatistics, McMaster University. How to read a clinical journal. II. To learn about a diagnostic test. Can Med Assoc J 1981;124:703–710.

Department of Clinical Epidemiology and Biostatistics, McMaster University. Interpretation of diagnostic data (six parts). Can Med Assoc J 1983;129: 429–432, 559–564, 587, 705–710, 832–835, 947–954, 1093–1099.

Diagnostic tests. In: Kramer MS, ed. Clinical Epidemiology and Biostatistics. Berlin: Springer-Verlag, 1988, pp. 201–219.

Feinstein AR. On the Sensitivity, Specificity, and Discrimination of Diagnostic Tests in Clinical Biostatistics. St. Louis: CV Mosby, 1977;214–226.

Galen RS, Gambino SR. Beyond Normality: The Predictive Value and Efficiency of Medical Diagnoses. New York: Wiley, 1975.

Griner PF, Mayewski RJ, Mushlin AL, Greenland P. Selection and interpretation of tests and procedures: principles and application. Ann Intern Med 1981; 94:557–592.

Jaeschke R, Guyatt GH, Sackett DL. Users' guides to the medical literature. III. How to use an article about a diagnostic test. A. Are the results of the study valid? The Evidence-Based Medicine Working Group. JAMA 1994;271:389–391.

Jaeschke R, Guyatt GH, Sackett DL. User's guides to the medical literature. III. How to use an article about a diagnostic test. B. What are the results and will they help me in caring for my patients? The Evidence-Based Medicine Working Group. JAMA 1994;271:703–707.

McNeil BJ, Keeler E, Adelstein SJ. Primer on certain elements of medical decision making. New Engl J Med 1975;293:211–215.

Schechter MT, Sheps SB. Diagnostic testing revisited: pathways through uncertainty. Can Med Assoc J 1985;132:755–760.

Sheps SB, Schechter MT. The assessment of diagnostic tests. A survey of current medical research. JAMA 1984;252:2418–2422.

Sox IIC Jr. Probability theory in the use of diagnostic tests. Ann Intern Med 1986;104:60–66.

Vecchio TJ. Predictive value of a single diagnostic test in unselected populations. New Engl J Med 1966; 274:1171–1173.

Weinstein MC, Fineberg HV. Clinical Decision Analysis. Philadelphia: Saunders, 1980.

Commentary

Based on my own personal experience, Schechter's chapter remains one of the most frequently used chapters in this textbook. An experienced methodologist provides us with a concept for measuring the validity of diagnostic tests. It introduces the reader to the terms *sensitivity* and *specificity* and then leads us through the concept of *predictive value*. These terms frequently appear in the literature and require a firm understanding in order to intelligently judge the literature. The concepts of sensitivity and specificity are carefully defined and then well illustrated with a surgical example. We are then guided through the use of negative and positive predictive values and how we can use this information to assess the validity of laboratory or imaging tests. The author carefully points out that, while sensitivity and specificity may measure the validity of a diagnostic test, they may have no direct bearing on its clinical utility. Clinical utility is best assessed by examining the predictive values. There is a very useful list of additional readings at the end of this chapter, including two publications from Sackett and the Evidence-Based Medicine Working Group in the *Journal of the American Medical Association* on the use of diagnostic testing in clinical medicine. This short but practical chapter should be read and understood fully prior to any study examining the role of diagnostic tests.

D.S.M.

CHAPTER 32

Scaling, Scoring, and Staging

M.E. Charlson, N.A. Johanson, and P.G. Williams

The world of scales often appears to be murky, filled with inscrutable jargon and even more incomprehensible analytic techniques. Clinicians planning clinical research must take a common-sense approach to the use of scales or indices. A scale, like a thermometer, is an instrument to measure clinical phenomena; a score is a value on the scale in a given patient. Clinical scales provide a standardized, repeatable measure of a patient's condition or functional status, just as thermometers provide a standardized repeatable measure of temperature.

Scale Anatomy

From the simplest to the most complex, scales have similar structures. Scales consist of one or more elements or questions and their answers. The answers may be either dichotomous, yes/no, or rank-ordered. The simplest scales consist of only one element. Complex scales many contain many elements organized into domains of interest. For example, physical function might be one domain, and psychosocial function another. In assessing a scale, first inspect its constituent parts.

Ranks for an Individual Scale Element or Question

The simplest scale addresses only one question. For example, a scale for rating peripheral edema ranges from $1+$ to $4+$. To use this scale in clinical research, we must clearly define the individual ranks. For example, $1+$ edema might be defined as noticeable only after digital pressure applied for more than 10 seconds. We define each of the other ranks, $2+$ through $4+$, in a way that is both clear and mutually exclusive. In clinical practice, the difference between grades $2+$ and $3+$ may not appear to be critical. However, if you study the response of patients to two different diuretic regimens after a shunt procedure and want to assess peripheral edema as one outcome, you would need to clearly define ranks with no confusion between them. If one observer rates a patient as having $1+$ edema and another rates the same patient as having $3+$ edema, you will not have meaningful results. If $2+$ and $3+$ peripheral edema are truly indistinguishable, the scale should not force an artificial division.

Other problems arise if the ranks are not *mutually exclusive*. For example, one disability status scale[1] has ranks for no, minimal, moderate, and severe disability but uses a separate rank for patients who require a cane or crutches to walk. Clinically, however, the extent of disability and the requirement for assisting devices are separate phenomena. How would one classify a patient who has minimal disability but requires a cane?

The ranking must yield a *clinically sensible, hierarchical order*. The scale should progress in an orderly way from least to most, or best to worst.

Generally, we take hierarchical progression for granted. For example, the TNM staging systems[2] rank local disease as stage I, locally advanced disease as II, regional extension as III, and metastatic disease as IV. It would create confusion if regional extension was I; local disease, II; and metastases, III. In the disability scale cited above, the lack of mutual exclusivity precludes ranking in a defined hierarchical manner. In summary, a scale element or question must assess a single type of qualitative phenomena, have ranking that is clearly defined and mutually exclusive, and be arranged hierarchically.[3]

Scale ranks must encompass a range of responses relevant to the patients being studied; that is, *the scale must have an adequate range* for the patient population. Consider weighing patients. The usual adult scale is not useful for a baby, nor will it be useful for a patient who weighs 350 pounds. The same phenomenon occurs with indices—the index must encompass a range that is relevant to the patients studied. For example, there are a number of scales that measure strenuous physical activity.[4] However, if you used one of these scales to compare patients before and after total hip replacement, you might find that there was no change, since few patients are likely to play basketball or to jog either before or after this operation. Since the activities measured are more than most patients are likely to do, such a scale could not reasonably be expected to change in response to total hip replacement. On the other hand, if you used the Activities of Daily Living (ADL) scale,[5] which measures patients' ability to dress, wash, and generally care for themselves, there also may be little postoperative change, because most patients undergoing hip replacement were at the highest level of that scale before operation. In short, a scale's range in relation to the patients under study must be adequate to permit detection of both improvement and deterioration. If patients are clustered at the top or bottom of the scale before treatment, it may be impossible to detect improvement for those at the top, or deterioration in those at the bottom.[6]

Scale Questions or Elements

While the simplest scales contain only one question or element and are designed to measure only one phenomenon, more complicated scales consist of a number of separate elements or questions that cover different issues. For example, the New York Heart Association classification has four ranks of physical function in relation to angina ranging from no angina on strenuous exertion to angina at rest. In contrast, the Goldman cardiac risk scale for noncardiac surgery patients is a complicated scale that incorporates nine different elements including age, presence of congestive failure, severity of congestive failure, and others.[8] The responses to each element are assigned weighted scores, which are then summed to arrive at a total score for each patient. For example, age greater than 70 years has a weight of 5, and a recent myocardial infarction has a weight of 10.[7] A patient with both would have a total score of 15 and would be assigned to the class 3 risk group. This scale is simpler than some others because it predicts one outcome—cardiac morbidity and mortality in the perioperative period.

Other scales include not only multiple questions or elements, but different domains, such as psychosocial, physical, or emotional function. However, your basic approach to a scale should remain the same, regardless of how complicated it is. You should review the questions and see if they are relevant to what *you* want to measure. You must assess the possible responses to the questions to ensure they are clear and mutually exclusive and decide whether the range is sufficient to assess your patient population. Finally, you must review how the elements are aggregated to see if the combinations are sensible.

What Do You Want the Scale to Do?

A scale may serve three basic functions: prediction, evaluation, or description.[9] Predictive scales divide patients into groups that have prognostic importance over time; many predictive scales are called staging systems. Evaluative scales evaluate change or stability in a population over time, and, particularly, the effect of a therapeutic intervention. Descriptive scales describe and contrast populations at a single point in time; they discriminate between those with and without condition X. The type of scale you need differs substantially depending on how you want to use it.

Predictive Scales

Let us suppose you are conducting a clinical trial to study the effect of two different topical antibiotics on the survival of burn patients. Patients randomized to the two different treatments must, before treatment, have an equal likelihood of survival. If their risk were not equal (e.g., if one group contained a larger proportion of patients with greater than 50% second- and third-degree burns),[9] it would be difficult to tell at the end of the trial whether any differences in survival between the groups were due to the prognostic imbalance or to differences in the efficacy of the therapy. Therefore, you would want to stratify patients prior to randomization according to their likelihood of survival; to help do this, you could use a scale (i.e., the percentage and depth of injury of involved skin) that predicts survival with reasonable accuracy. The importance of predictive scales or staging systems has long been recognized in studies of cancer patients. For example, a breast cancer trial that randomized patients with local disease and those with distant metastases, without stratifying them and balancing them according to stage, would not be clinically sensible because the prognoses of the patients are so different. In fact, randomizing them together might obscure rather than clarify the effects of treatment, because treatment effect could be completely opposite for the two groups. Experience with trials in cancer patients has shown that an effective treatment for patients of one stage may be ineffective for those of another. This underscores the importance of using predictive scales or prognostic staging systems in studies of treatment effectiveness. Apart from oncologic staging systems, predictive indices for survival have been developed for burn patients,[1] trauma patients,[2,10–12] and postoperative ICU patients.[13,14] The scoring system for burns,[1] the abbreviated injury score,[2–5] and scale for ICU patients,[7,14] have been demonstrated to predict patients' survival. A method of classifying comorbid conditions has also been developed for use in longitudinal studies.[6]

However, scales designed for prediction may not serve well to evaluate the effects of therapy. For example, the percent involvement might not be useful in evaluating the response to two different approaches to skin grafts. The Child's classi-fication for cirrhosis,[15] which has clear prognostic importance, might not be helpful in evaluating the response to shunts.

Evaluative Scales

Let us assume that you wish to compare porous ingrowth hip prostheses versus cemented metal implants with respect to long-term patient outcomes, in particular, the patient's physical function. To measure the impact of therapy, you need to assess the patient on at least two occasions: preoperatively and postoperatively. You would want to choose a scale that could measure changes in physical function related to operation. First, the scale should measure phenomena in some way related to physical function and the hip. Second, the scale should show improvement when the patient gets better, and deterioration if the patient worsens. To evaluate the effect of therapy, the patient's preoperative scale rank would be compared with his or her postoperative score. The outcome of interest is a change in an individual patient; the aggregate mean preoperative scores compared to postoperative scores would be of little value, because fundamentally you want to know how many patients improved, or worsened, or stayed the same. Relatively few evaluative scales have been developed specifically for surgical patients. However, some scales that have been developed for other uses may be useful for surgical patients. The Arthritis Impact Measurement Scale (AIMS) is one such example.[16,17]

Descriptive Scales

Both predictive and evaluative scales imply that the status of patients will be observed at two points in time; predictive scales must accurately forecast how the patient will do, and evaluative scales must be able to distinguish patients who have changed clinically from those who have not. Descriptive scales are designed to characterize patients at a single point in time. We use such indices to compare one group of patients with another. The Karnovsky classification of performance status in oncologic studies is an example of a scale that was developed for a descriptive purpose.[18] The American Society of Anesthesiologists' classification of physical status and the New

York Heart Association classification of angina[19] are examples of scales developed primarily for descriptive purposes.[20] Another example of a descriptive scale is the Organ Injury Scaling System for the spleen, liver, and kidney.[21]

Scale Physiology: Reproducibility, Validity, and Responsiveness

Not only are the purposes of the three types of scales distinct, but the design requirements of predictive, evaluative, and descriptive studies and scales differ. The distinctions are crucial, because indices designed for one purpose will not necessarily work for another purpose.

All scales must first be reproducible, that is, they must have minimal intraobserver and interobserver variability. (Translation: the scale gives scores within reasonable range of variation on repeated administrations to the same patient by the same and by different observers.) If reproducibility is poor, the scale will be useless for any purpose. Second, a scale must be a valid measure of what it is supposed to be measuring. The requirements for validity differ according to the scale's purpose. Predictive scales must be useful in predicting outcomes, in other words they must have prognostic validity. Descriptive scales must distinguish between different populations. Evaluative scales must correlate with the results of other methods of assessing outcome; if patients score better, there should be ways of confirming that they are indeed improved. Third, evaluative scales have an additional requirement—responsiveness. If the patient's condition changes, they should change; if the patient does not change, they should not change. We usually do not emphasize responsiveness sufficiently. Let's look at these issues in scale physiology one at a time.

Reproducibility

Reproducibility issues associated with scales are similar to those we encounter every day with the reproducibility of clinical data. Most biologic variables we want to measure are not static, but fluctuate and change. For example, pulse, blood pressure, urine output, and serum sodium constantly change throughout a day. The fluctuations are partly random and partly reflect efforts to maintain homeostasis. The usual range of values through which these variables fluctuate differs for different people. A runner may have a pulse that ranges from 40 to 60 during usual activity, while someone else may have a usual pulse that ranges from 70 to 90. Apart from moment to moment variability, there are often patterns of changes or trends on a daily, monthly, or seasonal basis. These variations also occur in responses to scales. Patients evaluated at the end of a tiring day may rank worse than would have been the case if they had been evaluated that morning.

Scales must have unambiguous questions with enough detail to ensure that the same question will be more likely to receive the same answer. For example, a question about whether a patient has pain on walking will have better reproducibility if specific conditions are considered, such as pain after climbing one flight of stairs.

The circumstances of measurement must be the same. Consider blood pressure. First, the conditions under which we take the measurement are important in minimizing inter- and intraobserver variability. The measurements should be made in the same position, with the same cuff size, applied at the same arm position, using the same deflation rate, and viewing the meniscus in the same way.[22] Second, the sequence of measurement is important. On the second or third measurement, the patient's blood pressure is usually lower than on the first measurement.[23] The results may be different if we scale or score at the end of an exhaustive evaluation, or at the beginning. If the index involves asking the patient to respond to questions, we must use the same wording; varying, or "ad libbing" the questions may adversely affect reproducibility. Furthermore, responses may differ based on whether they are given by the patient, a spouse, or the surgeon. If the scale calls for patient responses, the investigator must not supply the answers. If it is designed to be read to the patient or filled in by the patient, those procedures should be followed. In short, the way we administer indices must be operationally defined with sufficient precision to permit the repetition of subsequent measurements in identical circumstances.

Finally, we must ensure that the patient has *not* changed clinically when the reproducibility of the measurements is being assessed. If you were trying to establish reproducibility of an index designed to measure hip function, it would be foolish to test it before and after hip replacement, because you would expect the patient to change between the assessments. We must establish reproducibility in stable, nonchanging patients.

Even if the circumstances of measurements are standardized and the patient is stable, there may still be differences among different observers or among the reports of one observer on several occasions. One must recognize problems with reproducibility and plan strategies to reduce variability. Contrary to popular belief, observer variability is as much a problem with "hard" data from radiologic and pathologic tests as it is with "soft" data in scales.[24,25] One key question associated with scales is who does the measurement. With clinical scales, particularly for the evaluation of outcomes, the surgeon often is the observer. There may be a natural tendency for surgeons to rate postoperative assessments as improved. Therefore, perhaps one should have someone not involved with the treatment assess the patient. Many studies use "blinded" assessors who are unaware of the patient's treatment.

There are several ways to assess the reproducibility of scales. Without going into detail, most rank-ordered scales should be assessed using a statistic called *kappa*, not percent agreement. Percent agreement does not take into account agreement that occurs by chance alone. If you flip a coin, you will be right 50% of the time whether you call heads or tails. Similarly, when scales are used, some ratings agree simply by chance. The kappa statistic takes this into account and reports the agreement beyond chance.[26]

In summary, assessing reproducibility addresses the following question: Is the scale measurement the same on repeated administrations when the patient has not changed?

Validity

Validity asks whether the scale measures the phenomena it is supposed to measure. The assessment of validity differs according to the purpose of the scale.

This issue is usually fairly straightforward with predictive scales. They are valid if they predict the outcome they are supposed to predict. If patients are classified according to Goldman's cardiac risk class, patients in class I should have lower cardiac morbidity and mortality than those in class IV. Note, however, that none of the predictive scales separate patients perfectly according to outcome. For example, the cardiac risk index score cannot reliably identify two groups of patients; the ones who will die and the ones who will live. Prediction is never perfect.

Does the scale identify a range from those most likely to live to those most likely to die? If you had proposed a new scale to predict the likelihood of postoperative wound dehiscence, you might first evaluate all patients undergoing abdominal surgery to assess their status on your scale. Validation of the scale would require that you show that a larger proportion of patients in the highest risk group in your scale had wound dehiscence than those in the lower risk groups.

With descriptive scales, the question of validity is somewhat circular. Descriptive scales are constructed because there is no standard method of assessing the phenomena you want to measure. Yet, scale measurements at a single point in time should have a reasonable relationship to other related assessments. For example, a patient in New York Heart Association class IV (i.e., angina at rest) should not be able to walk one mile without stopping and should not achieve a maximal treadmill exercise test. The validity of descriptive indices is generally established by their relation to other measures directed at the same qualitative phenomena at the same point in time.

With evaluative scales, the issue of validity is more complex. First, does the scale, on its face value, appear to be qualitatively correct? It is tempting to choose measures that are very precise, but if they do not measure the phenomena you are actually interested in, that precision is useless. For example, if you used pulse rates to measure preoperative anxiety, you would get very precise numbers; however, the pulse rates may or may not relate to anxiety. Second, the scale should measure the phenomena that you believe to be clinically important. For example, a hip score designed to assess patients undergoing total hip replacement that measured only range of motion and did not assess walking ability or pain, would not be very useful because it does not capture the most clinically relevant outcomes. Physicians and patients may place different weights on outcomes. We must consider whether a scale takes into account the issues most important to the patient. For example, most scales include pain, because the extent of pain is extremely important to most patients, despite its "subjectivity."

Responsiveness

A responsive scale shows change when the patient changes, and no change when the patient is stable. The requirement for responsiveness is distinct from those for reproducibility and validity. A scale may be reproducible and valid, but unresponsive to change. For example, the New York Heart Association classification may be reproducible and valid. However, let us say that we want to use it to measure outcome after coronary artery bypass surgery. You assess patient classes preoperatively and postoperatively and find that most patients did not change. Perhaps the gradations in the scale are too gross to measure the change.[27] Consider weighing patients on a vehicle scale that measures only in hundreds of pounds. If you used that device to assess weight loss with dieting, you would be unable to demonstrate that weight loss had occurred. Even if every patient had lost weight, you would be unable to show it because your measurement device was unresponsive to change. To be useful for evaluation of response to treatment, a scale needs responsiveness. Many predictive and descriptive scales have yielded disappointing results because their basic anatomical design is not suited for evaluation.

Many indices have been modeled after scales developed by psychologists to measure personality characteristics and intelligence. Designed to characterize the differences between populations in cross-sectional studies, such scales contained many questions and required 30 minutes or more to administer. Scales that had been shown to be reproducible and valid were then used to evaluate the effect of therapeutic interventions. Often these single-state scales showed no difference before and after treatment, even when everyone agreed that the patient had indeed changed. This occurred because the scales were designed to discriminate between large populations by including many items, many of which would not be expected to change when the patient changed.[28]

This structure impairs a scale's ability to discern change and evaluate response to therapy.[29] For example, when surgical patients were evaluated preoperatively and postoperatively with the Sickness Impact Profile, a widely used descriptive scale,[30] the instrument was able to detect only patients who were worse. It was unable to detect improvement.[31] Recently, this scale has been modified to improve its responsiveness for head-injury patients.[32]

Single-State versus Transition Scales

Most evaluative scales are single-state scales, designed to be administered twice: we use the same scale once before treatment and once after treatment. We attribute any differences in score between the two administrations to treatment effect. Another type of scale is a transition scale. With a transition scale, patients are asked at the second evaluation whether they are better, the same, or worse than they were at the time of the first evaluation. This type of scale mimics the way we, as clinicians, actually assess patients. An example is a scale developed to measure dyspnea.[33] At the baseline administration, we ask the patient to respond to three different elements (level of functional impairment secondary to shortness of breath, magnitude of task resulting in shortness of breath, and magnitude of effort resulting in shortness of breath) and each element receives a rating from 0 (most severe) to 4 (unimpaired). The ratings for each element are added to form a baseline score. On the second administration, the patient is asked how much deterioration or improvement has occurred compared to the baseline state for each element, ranging from -3 to $+3$ level change. We sum the transition ratings on the different elements to arrive at a transition score.

Patient-Specific Indices

To take into account the wide variation in activities of different patients (i.e., questions about grocery shopping or mowing the lawn or playing golf will not be relevant to all patients), patient-specific indices of change have been developed. For example, a patient-specific index of physical function[33] has patients identify one or more physical activities they do frequently and consider to be the most demanding in terms of physical effort. Each patient's response forms the basis for subsequent assessments of change. For example, if a patient says "walking up subway stairs" at the initial evaluation, at the subsequent assessment we ask the patient about whether there has been a change in his ability to walk up subway stairs (i.e., better, the same, or worse; if better, how much better). You can see that this follows the transition-scale model. Patient-specific indices have been developed to measure changes in dyspnea, fatigue, emotional function, and mastery as outcome measures in trials involving patients with congestive heart failure and chronic pulmonary disease.[34] Additionally, the model has been used to develop disease-specific measures of quality of life or function for a number of other conditions, for example, inflammatory bowel disease.[35]

Scale Use

The Clinically Important Difference

What is a clinically important difference in score? All too often, articles report that one group of patients had a mean score that was 2.6 points higher than the other group, but no data are provided to permit the reader to understand what this difference in score actually means. The investigator needs to provide a context so that readers can interpret scores and changes in scores. For example, one study of adult health described a 10-point difference on the physical subscale as being equivalent to the effect of mild, chronic osteoarthritis.[36] We must define the minimal clinically important difference for each single-state scale. Standards for defining clinically important differences have been developed for transition scales.[37]

Quality of Life

The Example of Coronary Artery Bypass Grafts

The issues become more complex when measuring the overall quality of life. Consider the issue of quality of life using the example of coronary artery bypass graft surgery. When many studies

of prognosis after coronary artery bypass graft (CABG) were begun, the work in the area of defining and measuring health status or quality of life was in its infancy. There were only a few scales available for investigators to use, for example, the Karnovsky scale[38] and Katz's ADL scale.[39] Neither scale appeared to be optimal to investigators accustomed to quantitating luminal obstruction or ejection fraction. Furthermore, most patients were too well to have quality of life or function measured by an ADL instrument designed for assessing outcomes in elderly patients and nursing home residents. In the mid-1970s, a series of instruments was developed based on the World Health Organization definition; health status or quality of life was defined operationally by physical, mental, and social function.[40] Most scales developed to assess quality of life included specific measures of physical and psychosocial function, but not mental function.

Why is quality of life important in studies of CABG patients? The Coronary Artery Surgery Study (CASS)[41] and the European cooperative study[42] suggest that patients with left main and triple vessel disease survive longer with surgical rather than medical treatment. Among patients with less extensive disease, survival in the medical and surgical groups was similar. Given the similarity in survival of patients with less extensive disease, the effect of therapy on quality of life (i.e., on physical, mental, and psychosocial function) became the critical question.[43]

The CASS study operationally defined quality of life according to disease-related items (i.e., chest pain, congestive failure, hospitalization, or drug treatment) and activity-related items (i.e., limitations in daily activities, recreational activities, and employment).[41] Surgically treated patients had less chest pain, better exercise tolerance, and fewer limitations in daily activities.[44] In general, after CABG, chest pain decreased significantly, yet the New York Heart Association and Canadian cardiovascular classifications did not change. These scales were insensitive to postoperative improvement.[45] Other studies focused on return to work to assess quality of life after CABG. They found that employment status is not usually altered by CABG[40]; the most optimistic studies report a net gain in employment of only about 10% after CABG.[46–48] For example, patients who were not working before CABG generally did not return to work. Younger patients and those with more education were more likely to return to work postoperatively. In an important but small study that helps to explain these findings, post-CABG patients were asked whether they *wanted* to work[49]; ironically, patients ranked returning to work as least important to their quality of life after CABG. Family relationships, relief of symptoms, and increased physical activity were more important to patients.[50] The emphasis on return to work as a major method of assessing quality of life after CABG is understandable given the pressure to prove that CABG is more effective than medical therapy and that this benefit is worth the additional cost.[51] Demonstrating that patients resumed work would have provided a powerful argument for cost-effectiveness. Other important aspects of quality of life have received less attention than return to work.[52,53] This paradoxical situation arose because of the perceived difficulties in defining and measuring quality of life.

Function and Health Status: Generic Measures

The problems of such indices have been reviewed extensively in other publications.[54–56] There are currently a wide variety of indices available. The Quality of Well-Being scale[57] and the Quality of Life Index[58] require the least time to administer. While some data on responsiveness and the minimal clinically important difference of these scales are available, we need more studies of this important issue. For cardiopulmonary disease[31] and arthritis patients,[16] disease-specific instruments are available. We can now measure quality of life or health status with available instruments that are designed for different patient groups, including both physical and psychosocial function, and have been shown to be reproducible, valid, and responsive to change.

Choosing a Scale, Designing and Testing Your Own

When evaluating a scale for its appropriateness for use in your own research, decide whether it focuses on the elements relevant to the outcomes you are interested in. You may find that there is no scale that directly addresses the issues that con-

cern you. In this case, you may feel that a few additional elements combined with an existing scale would fit your needs or that a minor transformation of an existing scale would be appropriate. Alternatively, you may feel that you have to start from scratch, that there is nothing available that is relevant to your research questions.

You can develop your own scale, based on your own clinical knowledge and experience. For those undertaking such a task, more detailed understanding of the issues is key.[59] Commonsense will enable you to choose questions and responses that cover the various outcomes of interest and are valid at face value. You then need to pilot test your scale to see whether patients understand your questions and to assure that the response ranges are appropriate. You may find that there are redundant elements that can be dropped to yield a briefer instrument. The scale then needs to undergo testing to ensure its reproducibility and validity. If you want to use it to evaluate the effect of therapy, you must make certain that it is responsive. (See also chapters 30 and 31.)

References

1. Hauser SL, Dawson DM, Lehrich JR, Beal MF, Kevy SV, Propper RD, Mills JA, Weiner HL. Intensive immunosuppression in progressive multiple sclerosis. New Engl J Med 1983;308:173–180.
2. International Union Against Cancer (UICC). TNM Classification of Malignant Tumours. Geneva: International Union Against Cancer 1974:51–55.
3. MacKenzie CR, Charlson ME. Standards for the use of ordinal scales in clinical trials. Br Med J 1986;292:40–43.
4. Taylor HL, Jacobs DR, Schucker B, Knudson J, Leon AS, Debacker G. A questionnaire for the assessment of leisure time physical activities. J Chronic Dis 1978;31:741–755.
5. Katz S, Ford AB, Moskowitz RW, Jackson BA, Jaffe MW. Studies of illness in the aged: the index of ADL, a standardized measure of biological and psychosocial function. JAMA 1963;185:914–919.
6. Charlson ME, Pompei P, Ales KL, MacKenzie CR. A new method of classifying prognostic comorbidity in longitudinal studies: development and validation. J Chronic Dis 1987;40:373–383.
7. Goldman L, Caldera DL, Nussbaum SR, South-

wick PS, Krogstad D, Murray B, Burke DS, O'Malley TA, Goroll AH, Caplan CH, Nolan J, Carabello B, Slater EE. Multifactorial index of cardiac risk in noncardiac surgical procedures. New Engl J Med 1977;297:845–850.

8. Kirshner B, Guyatt G. A methodologic framework for assessing health indices. J Chronic Dis 1985;38:27–36.

9. Committee on Medical Aspects of Automobile Safety. Rating the severity of tissue damage. JAMA 1971;215:277–280.

10. Kirkpatrick JR, Youmans RL. Trauma index: an aid in the evaluation of injury victims. J Trauma 1971;11:711–714.

11. Committee on the Medical Aspects of Automotive Safety. Rating the severity of tissue damage: the comprehensive scale. JAMA 1972;220:717–720.

12. Baker SP, O'Neill B, Haddon W, Long WB. The injury severity score: a method for describing patients with multiple injuries and evaluating emergency care. J Trauma 1974;14:187–196.

13. Knaus WA, Wagner DP, Draper EA. Relationship between acute physiologic derangement and risk of death. J Chronic Dis 1985;38:295–300.

14. Knaus WA, Draper EA, Wagner DP, Zimmerman JE. An evaluation of outcome from intensive care in major medical centers. Ann Intern Med 1986; 104:410–418.

15. Conn H, Lindenmuth W, Mayu C, Ramsby GR. Prophylactic portocaval anastomosis. Medicine 1972;51:27–40.

16. Meenan RF, Anderson JJ, Kazis LE, Egger MJ, Altz-Smith M, Samuelson CO, Wilkens RF, Solsky MA, Hayes SP, Blocka KL, Weinstein A, Guttadauria M, Kaplan SB, Klippel J. Outcome assessment in clinical trials: evidence for the sensitivity of a health status measure. Arthritis Rheum 1984;27:1344–1352.

17. Liang H, Larson MG, Cullen KE, Schwartz JA. Comparative measurement efficiency and sensitivity of five health status instruments for arthritis research. Arthritis Rheum 1985;28:542–547.

18. Karnofsky DA, Burchenal JH. The clinical evaluation of chemotherapeutic agents in cancer. In: MacLeod DM, ed. Evaluation of Chemotherapeutic Agents. New York: Columbia University, 1949;191–205.

19. Criteria Committee of the New York Heart Association. Diseases of the Heart and Blood Vessels: Nomenclature and Criteria for Diagnosis, 6th edn. Boston: Little, Brown, 1964:112–113.

20. Dripps RD, Lamont A, Ecknehoff JE. The role of anesthesia in surgical mortality. JAMA 1961;178: 261–266.

21. Moore EE, Shackford SR, Pachter HL, McAninch JW, Browner BD, Champion HR, Flint LM, Gennarelli TA, Malangoni MA, Ramenofsky ML, Trafton PG. Organ injury scaling system: spleen, liver, and kidney. J Trauma 1989;29:1664–1666.

22. Kirkendall WM, Feinleib M, Freis ED, Mark AL. American Heart Association recommendations for human blood pressure determinations by sphygmomanometer. Hypertension 1981;2:509–519A.

23. Armitage P, Fox W, Rose GA, Tinker CM. The variability of measurements of casual blood pressure. II. Survey experience. Clin Sci 1966;30:337–344.

24. Boyd NF, Wolfson C, Moskowitz M, Carlisle T, Petitclerc M, Ferri HA, Fishell E, Gregoire A, Konan M, Longley JD, Simey IS, Miller AB. Observer variation in the interpretation of xeromammograms. J Natl Cancer Inst 1982;68:357–363.

25. Feinstein AR, Gelfman NA, Yesner R. Observer variability in the histopathologic diagnosis of lung cancer. Am Rev Respir Dis 1970;101:671–684.

26. Spitzer RL, Cohen J, Fleiss JL, Endicott J. Quantification of agreement in psychiatric diagnosis: a new approach. Arch Gen Psychiatry 1967;17:83–87.

27. Goldman L, Cook EF, Mitchell N, Flatley M, Sherman H, Cohn PF. Pitfalls in the serial assessment of cardiac functional status. J Chronic Dis 1982;35:763–771.

28. Guyatt G, Walter S, and Norman G. Measuring change over time: assessing the usefulness of evaluative instruments J Chronic Dis 1987;40:171–178.

29. Kirshner B, Guyatt G. A methodologic framework for assessing health indices. J Chronic Dis 1985;38:27–36. A classic article providing a framework for thinking about the use of scales.

30. Bergner M, Bobbitt AS, Carter WB, Gilson BS. The Sickness Impact Profile: development and final revision of a health status measure. Med Care 1981;19:787–805.

31. MacKenzie CR, Charlson ME, DiGioia D, Kelley K. Can the Sickness Impact Profile measure change? An example of scale assessment. J Chronic Dis 1986;39:429–438.

32. Temkin N, McLean A, Dikmen S, Gale J, Bergner M, Almes MJ. Development and evaluation of modifications to the Sickness Impact Profile for head injury. J Clin Epidemiol 1988;41:47–57.

33. Mahler DA, Weinberg DH, Wells CK, Feinstein AR. The measurement of dyspnea: contents, inter-

observer agreement, and physiologic correlates of two new clinical indexes. Chest 1984;85:751–758.

34. Guyatt GH, Berman LB, Townsend M, Taylor DW. Should study subjects see their previous responses? J Chronic Dis 1985;38:1003–1007.

35. Guyatt G, Deyo RA, Charlson ME, Levine MN, Mitchel A. Responsiveness and validity in health status measurement. J Clin Epidemiol 1989; 42: 403–408.

36. Brook RH, Ware JE, Rogers WH, Keeler EB, Davies AR, Donald CA, Goldberg GA, Lohr KN, Masthay PC, Newhouse JP. Does free care improve adult health? Results from a randomized controlled trial. New Engl J Med 1983;309:1426–1433.

37. Jaeschke R, Singer J, Guyatt G. Health status measurement: ascertaining the minimal clinically important difference. Clin Res 1989;37:315A.

38. Karnovsky DA, Abelmann WH, Craver LF, Burchenal JH. The use of nitrogen mustard in the palliative treatment of carcinoma. Cancer 1948;1: 634–656.

39. Katz S, Ford AD, Moskowitz RW, Jackson BA, Jaffe MW. Studies of illness in the aged. JAMA 1963;185:914–919.

40. World Health Organization. The constitution of the World Health Organization. WHO Chron 1947;1:29.

41. CASS Principal Investigators and Their Associates. Myocardial infarction and mortality in the coronary artery surgery study (CASS) randomized trial. New Engl J Med 1984;310:750–758.

42. European Coronary Surgery Study Group. Long term results of prospective randomized study of coronary artery bypass surgery in stable angina pectoris. Lancet 1982;ii:1173–1180.

43. Hampton JR. Coronary artery bypass grafting for the reduction of mortality: an analysis of the trials Br Med J 1984;289:1166–1170.

44. CASS Principal Investigators and Their Associates. Coronary Artery Surgery Study (CASS): a randomized trial of coronary artery bypass surgery quality of life in patients randomly assigned to treatment groups. Circulation 1983;68:951–960.

45. National Institutes of Health Consensus Development Conference Statement. Coronary artery bypass surgery: scientific and clinical aspects New Engl J Med 1981;304:680–684.

46. Niles NW, Vander Salm TJ, Cutler BS. Return to work after coronary artery bypass operation. J Thorac Cardiovasc Surg 1980;79:916–921.

47. Symmes JC, Lenkei SC, Berman ND. Influence of aortocoronary bypass surgery on employment. Can Med J 1978;118:268–270.

48. Gutman MC, Knapp DR, Pollock ML, Schmidt DH, Simon K, Walcott G. Coronary artery bypass patients and work status. Circulation 1982;66 (suppl. III):33–41.

49. LaMendola WF, Pellegrini RV. Quality of life and coronary artery bypass surgery patients. Soc Sci Med 1979;13A:457–461.

50. Flynn MK, Frantz R. Coronary artery bypass surgery: quality of life during early convalescence. Heart Lung 1987;16:159–167.

51. Doubilet R, Weinstein MC, McNeil BJ. Use and misuse of the term "cost effective" in medicine. New Engl J Med 1986;314:253–256.

52. Fletcher AE, Hunt BM, Bulpitt CJ. Evaluation of quality of life in clinical trials of cardiovascular disease. J Chronic Dis 1987;40:557–566.

53. Stanton BA, Jenkins CD, Savageau JA, Thurer RL. Functional benefits following coronary artery bypass graft surgery. Ann Thorac Surg 1984;37: 286–290.

54. Feinstein AR, Josephy BR, Wells CK. Scientific and clinical problems in indexes of functional disability. Ann Intern Med 1986;105:413–420.

55. O'Young J, McPeek B. Quality of life variables in surgical trials. J Chronic Dis 1987;40:513–522. A review of the experience with surgical trials.

56. McDowell I, Newell C. Measuring Health. A Guide to Rating Scales and Questionnaires. New York: Oxford University, 1987. A detailed description and critique of many different health status measures.

57. Kaplan RM, Bush JE, Berry CC. Health status: types of validity and the index of well-being. Health Serv Res 1976;11:478–507.

58. Spitzer WO, Dobson AJ, Hall J, Chesterman E, Levi J, Shepherd R, Battista RN, Catchlove BR. Measuring the quality of life of cancer patients. J Chronic Dis 1981;34:585–597.

59. Feinstein AR. Clinimetrics. New Haven, CT: Yale University, 1987.

Additional Reading

Knaus WA. The science of prediction and its implications for the clinician today. Theor Surg 1988;3:93–101.

Commentary

Measuring Clinical Phenomena: Introductory Comments on Chapters 32, 33, and 34

Martin McKneally's qualitative research colleagues in bioethics suggest that surgeons may be afflicted with "incurable quantomania." These three chapters provide a framework on more effective use of measuring instruments by surgeons. Charlson et al. (chapter 32) provides the theory and definition of scaling, scoring and staging, and this is followed by Eypasch (chapter 33) applying them to everyday surgical problems. Paul and Bouillon (chapter 34) provide the details of developing a "disease-specific" measuring instrument for orthotopic liver transplantation. All three chapters suggest this methodology has limitations and must be a dynamic process that meets the clinical or research question, changing technology, and so forth.

D.S.M.

CHAPTER 33

Surgical Examples of Scoring Systems

E. Eypasch

Are scoring and scaling systems scientific poetry or a clinical necessity? Some current surgical examples will help to answer the question.

In a 60-year-old patient after right hemicolectomy, the Dukes stage is a widely accepted, indispensable descriptive tool for planning further treatment. Adjuvant postoperative chemotherapy is currently the recommended treatment for resected Dukes C colon cancer. This is an example of a well-known staging system, based on pathology of the colon cancer, that now has therapeutic implications.[1]

A 60-year-old woman with resistant symptoms of heartburn and regurgitation needs 24-hour pH monitoring of the distal esophagus to rule out or define gastroesophageal reflux disease. The interpretation of the crude 24-hour esophageal pH profile is a matter of debate. A practical method to distinguish physiological from pathological distal esophageal acid exposure is to use a scoring system that incorporates some criteria of the pH profile, namely, percent time below pH 4 and number and duration of reflux episodes, into a scoring system that discriminates between normal and pathological acid exposure reflux. Such a scoring system is available and well known to gastroenterologists.[2] It can be used to define gastroesophageal reflux disease. This is an example of a necessary, practical scoring system with diagnostic and therapeutic implications that is becoming increasingly accepted as a reference standard, although it has not reached the level of acceptance exemplified by the Dukes classification.

In another example, a 20-year-old woman with right lower quadrant pain and vomiting of one day's duration is likely to have appendicitis or a gynecological infection. After excluding pelvic inflammatory disease, experienced surgeons will diagnose appendicitis based on history, clinical findings, and ultrasound. Though an extensive list of appendicitis scores is available, their clinical application is negligible. The complicated scores have no predictive value and are not widely used.[3]

Definitions

The need to assign numbers to certain phenomena or qualities is a simple necessity that is highly debatable. There is hardly any question that it is necessary to count the number of patients or to measure age by counting the years of life. According to Postman in *Technopoly*,[4] 200 years ago no one had thought of assessing a written work quantitatively, or signifying the intelligence of a person by an actual number. Today intelligence scores or a grade in an essay are well-established numerical tools, and it is acceptable to assign quantitative values to human thoughts. We have accepted that everything has to be counted and measured to make it manageable and "scientific."

However, many phenomena such as individuality, friendship, and sympathy cannot be measured. Nobody would—yet—try to measure love and affection! Nevertheless, scaling, staging, and scoring are mathematical processes used in daily life and clinical practice.

Scales can be very simple or very complex. They can comprise a simple, dichotomous yes/no decision, with a rank order going from smaller to bigger numbers, or a continuous variable going from zero to infinity. A distinction between four ways of using numbers is fundamental in all scaling methods and lies in the mathematical hierarchy. The lowest level is a simple classification grouping individuals or items in different categories such as "female" or "male." In the second type, ordinal numbers are assigned, and these numbers reflect an increasing order of the variable to be measured. The actual value of the numbers and the distance between them do not yet have an intrinsic meaning. In the third type of scale a definite interval between categories is given. This means that in an interval scale, a change of one unit represents a constant change across the whole range of the scale. Temperature is a good example. In the "interval score," differences between scores can be calculated because addition and subtraction of scores are permitted. However, it is not permitted to state how many times greater one score is than the other; this is only allowed in "ratio scales" which include a zero point.

SCALES

Binary
Rank order (small → large)
Continuous ($0 \rightarrow \infty$)
Ratios

Scales and scores reflecting more difficult constructions such as disability, activities of daily life, or quality of life can be a composite of several characteristics. For example, quality of life scales include symptoms, emotions, and physical and social functions.[5,6]

The definition of *staging* implies that a disease has different grades of severity in various patients or that the disease changes over time, either becoming better or worse. The Child classification for liver function is a good example.[7] The structure of a staging system must be reasonable and address the key issues of a question. For instance, local tumor growth (T category), the infiltration of lymph nodes with malignant cells (N category), and distant metastases (M category) reasonably describe the local spread of an epithelial tumor (gastric cancer).[8] However, age, sex, or the central or peripheral location of a tumor might also play an important role in the prognosis and outcome. Furthermore, a staging system should have diagnostic or therapeutic consequences, or define a different outcome or prognosis.[9,10] Staging systems without consequences are "scientific poetry."

The meaning and use of the word *scoring* is twofold. A scoring system is a method to compress clinical information into a mathematical number in order to make a decision. Above a certain reasonably chosen cutoff point, a clinical decision (yes/no or normal/abnormal) is taken. The choice depends on sensitivity and specificity of the scoring system.[11,12] In a given scoring system, the particular value for one patient is also called the score. For instance, a patient may be assigned a particular score on the Glasgow coma scale.

According to de Bono's description of human thinking, the human brain organizes perception from outside into certain patterns.[13] Pattern recognition and comparison to existing patterns is a key process of human thinking. In order to deal with things, the brain lumps them together in groups of similar, previously encountered patterns and is thus able to act on them accordingly. The precise mechanism of this pattern recognition remains largely at an unconscious level. For instance many people know how to run a TV or a video recorder even though they are not aware of the precise mechanism of receiving and producing the TV image. De Bono calls this the "blackbox" mechanism. In other words, the brain simplifies and compresses perceptions and puts them in a blackbox labeled "TV" or "diagnosis of a reflux disease." This process makes communication among individuals possible. This is exactly the purpose of scoring systems: they compress more complex, individual, biological information into a single number or an array of letters or symbols. It has to be kept in mind that this is a modification, compression, and change of the actual basic information, which might lead to a false representation and oversimplification of the original information. This method of information processing abolishes individuality and is reductionistic, neglecting the holistic and individual approach to the patient.[14,15]

Scoring systems can be developed in three different ways: based on clinical plausibility or importance, on statistical grounds, or on a combination of both. Clinical plausibilities are obvious. Albumin, bilirubin, ascites, and neurological function are reasonable variables for the assessment of liver function.[7] Tumor ingrowth, lymph nodes, and distant metastasis are plausible criteria for the evaluation of tumor progression.[8] The methodological approach to developing, evaluating, and using scoring systems is described in chapter 32 by Charlson et al. Practical problems and solutions encountered in the development of a specific quality of life index for liver transplant patients is described in chapter 34 by Paul and Bouillon.

Practical Applications of Scoring Systems

Of the many scores available in the literature, a well-known and widely accepted score can be compared to a successful industry product known by the company name and not the original product itself. For instance a "Kleenex" is a piece of paper used to wipe something. To "Xerox" in American English means to photocopy something. Similarly Apgar, Dukes, Child, Forrest, Breslow, Aitken, NYHA, and APACHE are names so well known for staging or scoring systems that the original purpose no longer needs to be mentioned. Through the course of time these names have become self-explanatory.

Some examples of scoring systems are shown in Table 33-1, classified by their level of acceptance and usage.

Anatomy and Design of Scoring Systems

Some simple criteria must be fulfilled for a scale or scoring system:

1. The system must address a single type of qualitative phenomena, that is, the same variable in different qualities or quantities. It is not possible to count apples and oranges as the same thing on one scale.

2. The scale has to have a clearly defined ranking in a hierarchical order. Stage III should be worse or more severe than stage I, based on reasonable clinical or mathematical criteria that are known and agreed upon.

3. The different stages or categories must be mutually exclusive. A patient with a certain expression of the disease has to be clearly staged as stage II according to a set of criteria. Undefined and uncontrolled overlap of the stages ruins a classification system.

4. A system has to be comprehensive and include all kinds of severities of a disease, from the least harmful to the worst stage, including all kinds of side phenomena. The scale has to be adapted to the area of measurement where it will be applied. To assess knee function in a 35-year-old male individual with moderate leisure sports activities, both the Katz ADL score[24] and the Tegner index for sports activity would be inappropriate.[37] With regard to the ADL index, the patient is too young and too mobile; with regard to the Tegner Index, the sports activity of the patient would not be enough.

5. The complexity and relative weight of different score elements have to be taken into account. A simple score like the Breslow for malignant melanoma assesses only the thickness of a melanoma in millimeters.[38] A more complex score such as the Child classification takes into account multiple facets or descriptors of the disease state: bilirubin, albumin, ascites, neurological symptoms, and nutritional state.[7] Among experienced clinicians, all of these parameters are equally important and representative of liver function. The same probably holds true for the variables of the Glasgow Coma Scale: eye movement, motor activity, and verbal reactions.[18] However things become more complex in a pH score or in an index to assess quality of life.[2,31] Which is more important for the latter: the patient's symptoms, emotional situation, or physical function? What should be measured: a frequent and of-

Table 33-1.   Examples of scoring systems.

Well-known, widely accepted scores	Purpose [Reference]
TNM	Tumor spread and stage [8]
APGAR	Vital function in neonates [16]
Aitken	Fractures in adolescents [17]
Glasgow Coma Scale	Coma [18]
Trauma Score	Injury severity [19]
APACHE Score	Physiological status and age [20]
Child Classification	Liver function [7]
Dukes Classification	Colon cancer stage [21]
Spitzer Index	Quality of life [22]
Nyhus Hernia Classification	Unguinal hernia type [23]
Activity of Daily Life (Katz)	Physical activity [24]
Visick Scale	Symptomatic well-being [25]
Moderately well-known, useful scores	
DeMeester Reflux Score	Esoph. acid exposure [2]
Talley Dyspepsia Score	Dyspepsia [26]
Best-Index for Crohns Disease	Inflammatory activity [27]
Mannheim-Peritonitis Index	Peritonitis [28]
Injury Severity Score	Injury severity [29]
Sickness Impact profile	Sickness and well-being [30]
Gastrointestinal Quality of Life Index	Quality of life [31]
Forrest Classification	Ulcer, bleeding [32]
Published but less well-known scores	
Alvarado Appendicitis Score	Appendicitis [33]
Moore Trauma Score	Pattern of organ injury [34]
Garden Classification	Hip fracture [35]
Cologne Quality of Life Inventory	Quality of life [36]

ten-changing item, or a very rare but very important item? What is more important for esophageal mucosal damage: one long reflux episode or multiple short episodes with a pH less than 4. This brings the problem of weighting into the discussion about the score design. Creating complex or assembled scores representing phenomena such as quality of life, disability, or satisfaction with life requires one to address the issues concerning the inner structure of a score. Again, the weighting can be done based on statistical grounds expressed in certain coefficients, or it can be done based on clinical necessities, experience, and plausibilities as with the Mannheim-Peritonitis Index.[28]

Purpose of a Score: Description, Prediction, and Evaluation

There are three basic characters or design intentions of a scoring system: description, prediction, and evaluation.

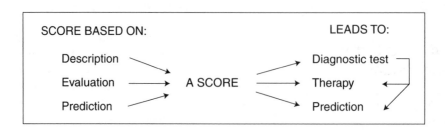

Many scoring systems have been developed for description; their purpose is to group individuals or phenomena according to certain criteria into different categories at one single point in time. This individual with that disease falls into "category IIB." The Karnofsky scale for cancer patients and the Organ Injury Scale by Moore are such static classification systems.[34,39]

The next purpose is to link consequences to the classification system. These consequences can be diagnostic, therapeutic, or prognostic.[9,10] For example, a patient having Forrest Ib ulcer bleeding requires further endoscopies and measurements of central venous pressure as diagnostic actions, and an early elective operation if he or she is old and frail as the therapeutic consequence, followed by a good or bad prognosis. An ideal scoring system is connected to diagnostics, treatment strategies, and outcome/prognosis. The better this link, the greater the usefulness of the system. Scales with no or minimal connection to consequences and outcome are "scientific poetry." Appendicitis scores are such an example.[3]

Descriptive and predictive scoring systems are also indispensable tools for stratifying patients in controlled clinical trials. Without proper stratification based on staging systems, all the "bad" patients might be included in one study arm, while the "good" ones are included in the second arm.

A third and very important purpose of staging or scoring systems is evaluation of change over time. Evaluative systems must be able to measure change or stability over time in a very sensitive way. In many research and daily practice situations, clinicians are interested in change of the patients' condition after treatment. A useful score must be responsive enough to identify this change. The influence of a treatment on a score must be large enough and the score design must be sensitive enough to express the change in a numerical number. Several good examples underline this effect.

The Sickness Impact Profile by Marylin Bergner is a long list of questions describing the sickness of a patient in a very complete and comprehensive way.[30] No dimension of the impact of sickness on life is omitted. If a therapeutic intervention modifies the sickness of the patient, even if it actually improves the patient's condition, only

a handful of items will change, having only a minimal numerical effect on the overall score. Therefore, studies have been published asking whether the Sickness Impact Profile is able to measure change at all.[40] The same effect can be seen with the Cologne Quality of Life Inventory,[36] which is a list of more than 200 questions regarding quality of life. The instrument has been developed by oncological hematologists at the University of Cologne, and again the question is whether an improvement in the quality of life of a patient will be reflected by the overall score of the instrument if only a few items change. On the other hand, there are instruments that are too gross to express the change of a patients' condition. The Spitzer Quality of Life Index is simply too general to measure clinically relevant changes of the patient's situation after esophageal or gastric cancer surgery during the postoperative period. Only when the patient is about to die from progression of the disease can a numerical change of the Spitzer Index be observed (Waterfall effect).[41] In summary, the clinically relevant change or the area of interest must be known, and the scoring system must be appropriately designed to measure change in this area of interest.

Design Criteria

Some additional well-known design criteria for diagnostic tests and scoring systems must be briefly mentioned.

CRITERIA FOR A SCORING SYSTEM

Reproducibility
Validity
Responsiveness

Reproducibility means that the score instrument shows only minimal reasonable variation if it is applied repeatedly in a clinically stable patient. Without adequate reproducibility (statistically expressed as the difference between measurements and their distribution; kappa statistics), a diagnostic test is just a lottery. The aspect of interobserver variation in repeated measurements and other sources of bias have to be addressed.

Validity, the next important criterion, expresses whether the test actually measures what it is supposed to measure. Validity of a new test can be assessed either by comparison to an accepted gold standard of measurement (i.e., comparison of a new laboratory test to an established, exact, but perhaps expensive one), or by constructing a reasonable relation to another known and established criterion. For instance, patients with an increasingly better quality of life should have a parallely increasing grade of physical mobility at home, in the neighborhood, or in the whole city. In a somewhat circular construction, one criterion is compared or linked to another parallel or closely comparable variable. Terms such as *construct validity* and *face validity* express this relation but should be read about in the abundant literature of methodological experts.

The third design criterion is *responsiveness,* which means the ability of an index to pick up clinically relevant changes. This issue has been discussed above in the section on the evaluative purpose of a score.

Transition Scores or Patient-Specific Scores

In transition scores, the patient has to record whether his or her situation is better or worse than during the previous measurement. This approach avoids a clear definition of what is actually measured. The patient simply says "it" is better or worse. Problems arise when measurements are repeated and have to be interpreted, and when comparison between individuals or a group of individuals is intended. The question arises as to whether the better-or-worse information between patients is comparable, or the interindividual difference is too big. Another way of modifying a score is through patient specification or adaptation. For instance, for one patient, reading, relaxing, sleeping, and avoiding any physical exercise can be very important aspects of his or her quality of life. For a second patient, sport activity including competition is of supreme importance for the quality of life. It is difficult to measure quality of life reasonably in both individuals with the same index. This difficulty can be resolved by the adaptation of a scoring system to the patient's needs in order to measure and express whether a medical intervention has improved the quality of life. "Has the cruciate ligament repair in the knee improved your sports activity? Very much—much—a little—not at all—worsened." This example also shows that the spectrum of given answers influences the score result. It makes a big difference whether you offer answers from "very much" to "not at all," or whether you include the negative aspect by offering from "very much" to "worsened considerably." The size of fish (and answers) you catch obviously depends on the size of hole in your fishing net! Again, with these patient-adapted scores you run into the problem of comparison between individuals and groups of patients.[15]

The clinical researcher has to be well aware that the method—a staging system, a score, a laboratory test—influences the result. You only get what you are looking for! Thus the test and its specifications must be well chosen before the measurement is started. No wonder that the planning and setting up of a randomized trial can take years!

Here are some helpful questions to ask when you are faced with choosing an appropriate score. Some classification systems such as Dukes or Child are so well known that their application is mandatory. For less well-known instruments, the following questions should be answered by referring to the original publication and subsequent applications of the score. The more of these questions we can answer in a positive way, the closer we are to an appropriate instrument for the respective study purpose.

1. Is the purpose of the score clearly defined by the authors?
2. How has the score been designed or developed?
3. Is the score a clinical construct based on experience, plausibility, knowledge, or necessities, or is it a mathematical construction with all statistical details and requirements?
4. How much time, detail, and research have the authors invested to create the score?

5. Has the score been validated by an established formal process of validation? By comparison to other scales? By application in other publications?

6. Has the score been validated by other investigators and on study populations other than the original one where it was developed?

7. Has the score been successfully applied by other investigators? Is it widely spread in the literature?

8. Is the score just descriptive or does it have consequences for the diagnostic and therapeutic regimen of the patient, leading to a different outcome and prognosis?

9. Is the score range and design appropriate for the intended research question?

10. Is the calculation of the score clear? What is the numerical quality like? Is the score computerized, easy to handle, and user-friendly? What is the statistical analysis like? How are the results interpreted?

Occasionally, the need may arise to design a new scoring system because you cannot find one in the literature that suits your purpose. Designing your own instrument is not an easy task. It requires time, experience, and support from methodological experts. However, as Feinstein pointed out, clinicians have to do their own basic research and need support from theoretical scientists. Designing an instrument is not a simple task to be accomplished on a Sunday afternoon. The process is described in Paul's chapter in this book (chapter 34). It is time-consuming but worth the effort when a good scoring system is created.

The following helpful hints and questions may make the process easier.

1. Do we really need a new scoring system or is a slight modification and revalidation of an existing instrument a viable option?

2. What is the intended purpose of the new scoring system?

3. Which is the special patient population under consideration? Which group of patients will be assessed?

4. What amount and kind of methodological assistance is needed?

A clear consideration of these questions and adherence to the formal process will help.

Examples of Scores in Clinical Situations

A brief description of staging and scoring systems in different clinical situations underlines the importance of scoring systems to help solve clinical problems and answer important questions.

Gastric cancer. In current surgery for gastric cancer, there is a decline in radical and lymph-node-hunting operations. Recent randomized trials of radical lymphadenectomy have shown an increase in morbidity and mortality with no survival advantage.[42] In the last two decades, no accepted instrument was available to assess quality of life before and after surgery for gastric cancer. In order to select patients for multimodality treatment or withholding of treatment, with respect to progression of disease and with respect to reconstruction of the food passage after gastrectomy, a useful quality of life score became increasingly important. By the Troidl-Kusche score in 1987 and also by the Gastrointestinal Quality of Life Index, it could be shown that patients with a pouch reconstruction after gastrectomy have an improvement in quality of life in the first postoperative year—a period that is of supreme importance because 40–60% of patients die in the first year after surgery.[43]

Knee surgery. One of the most frequent ligament injuries of the knee is anterior cruciate ligament tear. This requires a technically demanding operation that today can be performed by arthroscopy. It takes months to regain appropriate and pain-free knee function. Both subjective (patient self-assessment) and objective (interviewer assessment +/− clinical examination) evaluations have been applied. A practical tool for the assessment of knee function based on subjective evaluation is the Flandry score, which has not been adequately validated, especially not in German. Our group in Cologne has translated and reevaluated the Flandry index. Using this index, the clinical course after anterior cruciate ligament repair and rehabilitation therapy can be depicted in an understandable graphic display that can be easily explained to patients and doctors.[44] In the future this instrument will allow comparison among different treatment options (arthrotomy vs. arthroscopy) for patients.

Liver transplantation. Liver transplantation is one of the most expensive interventions in general surgery. Such procedures can be justified (and paid for in the future) only when they offer a clear survival and quality of life benefit. Quality of life in liver disease has not been well investigated, perhaps in part due to reduced mental capacity of patients with progressive liver failure. Using the recently developed Liver-Quality of Life Index, it was shown that patients after orthotopic liver transplantation clearly have a better quality of life than untreated patients before operation. Such information will be necessary to promote liver transplantation programs.[45]

A quote from McDowell and Newell[46] summarizes the importance and the difficulty of choosing an appropriate instrument:

> Ultimately the selection of a measurement contains an element of art and perhaps even luck; it is often prudent to apply more than one measurement whenever possible. This has the advantage of reinforcing the conclusions of the study when the results from ostensibly similar methods are in agreement, and it also serves to increase our general understanding of the comparability of the measurements we use.

References

1. Moertel CG, Fleming TR, MacDonald JS, Haller DG, Laurie JA, Goodman PJ, Ungerleider JS, Emerson WA, Tormey DC, Glick JM, Veeder MH, Mailliard JA. Levamisol and fluorouracil for adjuvant therapy of resected colon carcinoma. New Engl J Med 1990;322:352–358.
2. Lawrence FJ, DeMeester TR. Development of the 24-hour intraesophageal pH-monitoring composite scoring system. J Clin Gastroenterol 1986;8:52–58.
3. Eypasch E, Felsenstein M, Köhler L, Troidl H. Decision making in acute appendicitis: meta-analysis versus clinical practice. Digestive Surgery 1996;13:309–313.
4. Postman N. Technopoly. New York: Alfred A. Knopf, 1991. German Version: Das Technopol. Frankfurt: Fischer Verlag, 1992, pp. 11–28.
5. Wood-Dauphinee S, Troidl H. Endpoints for clinical studies: conventional and innovative variables. In: Troidl H, Spitzer WO, McPeek B, Mulder DS, McKneally MF, Wechsler AS, Balch CM, eds. Principles and Practice of Research: Strategies for Surgical Investigators. New York: Springer Verlag, 1991, pp. 151–168.
6. Troidl H, Kusche J, Vestweber KH, Eypasch E, Koeppen L, Bouillon B. Quality of life: an important endpoint both in surgical practice and research. J Chron Dis 1987;40:523–528.
7. Child CG, Turcotte JG. Surgery and portal hypertension. In: Child CG, ed. The Liver and Portal Hypertension. Philadelphia: Saunders, 1964, pp. 50–64.
8. International Union against Cancer (UICC). TNM Classification of Malignant Tumours. Geneva: International Union against Cancer, 1975, pp. 51–55.
9. Loop JW, Lusted LB. American college of radiology diagnostic efficacy studies. Am J Roentgenol 1987;131:173–179.
10. Lusted LB. Decision making studies in patient management. New Engl J Med 1971;284:416–424.
11. Bion JE, Aitchison TC, Edlin SA, Ledingham IM. Sickness scoring and response to treatment as predictors of outcome from critical illness. Intensive Care Med 1988;14:167–172.
12. Fletcher RH, Fletcher SW, Wagner EH. Diagnosis. In: Fletcher RH, Fletcher SW, Wagner EM, eds. Clinical Epidemiology: The Essentials. Baltimore: Williams and Wilkins, 1982, pp. 42–75.
13. De Bono E. Thinking Course. BBC Books, 1985.
14. Giebel GD, Troidl H. Möglichkeiten und Grenzen von Scores. Langenbecks Arch Chir 1996;381:59–62.
15. Vollmer G. Wissenschaftstheorie im Einsatz. Stuttgart: Hirzel Verlagsgesellschaft 1993:183–206.
16. Apgar V. Proposal for a new method of evaluation of the newborn infant. Curr Res Anesth 1953;32:260.
17. Aitken AP. The end result of the fractures of the distal radius epiphysis. J Bone Joint Surg 1935;17:302.
18. Teasdale G. Assessment of coma and impaired consciousness: A practical scale (Glasgow Coma Scale). Lancet 1974;II:81–83.
19. Champion HR, Sacco WJ, Carnazzo AJ. Trauma score. Crit Care Med 1981;9:672–676.
20. Knaus WA, Draper EA, Wagner DP, Zimmerman JE. An evaluation of outcome from intensive care

in major medical centers. Ann Intern Med 1986;104:410–418.

21. Dukes CE. The spread of cancer of the rectum. Br J Surg 1930;17:643–648.

22. Spitzer WO, Dobson AJ, Hall J, Chesterman E, Levi J, Shepherd R, Battista RN, Catchlove BR. Measuring the quality of life of cancer patients. J Chron Dis 1981;34:585–597.

23. Nyhus LM, Klein MS, Rogers FB. Current Problems in Surgery: Inguinal Hernia, vol. 28. St. Louis: Mosby Year Book, 1991, pp. 417–419, 436–446.

24. Katz S, Ford AB, Moskowitz RW, Jackson BA, Jaffe MW. Studies of illness in the aged: the index of ADL, a standardized measure of biological and psychosocial function. JAMA 1963;185:914–919.

25. Visick AH. A study of the failures after gastrectomy. Hunterian Lecture. Ann R Coll Surg Engl 1948;3:266.

26. Talley NJ, McNeil D, Piper DW. Discriminant value of dyspeptic symptoms: a study of the clinical presentation of 221 patients with dyspepsia of unknown cause, peptic ulceration, and cholelithiasis. Gut 1987;28:40–46.

27. Best WR, Becktel JM, Singleton JW, Kern F. Development of a Crohn's disease activity index. National cooperative Crohn's disease study. Gastroenterology 1976;70:439–444.

28. Linder MM. Der Mannnheimer Peritonitis-Index. Chirurg 1987;58:84–92.

29. Baker SP, O'Neill B, Haddon W, Long WB. The injury severity score: a method for describing patients with multiple injuries and evaluating emergency care. J Trauma 1974;14:187–196.

30. Bergner M, Bobbitt RA, Carter WB, Gilson BS. The Sickness Impact Profile: development and final revision of a health status measure. Med Care 1981;19:787–805.

31. Eypasch E, Williams JI, Wood-Dauphinee S, Ure BM, Schmülling C, Neugebauer E, Troidl H. The gastrointestinal quality of life index (GIQL), development, validation, and application of a new instrument. Br J Surg 1995;82:216–222.

32. Forrest J, Finlayson N, Shearman D: Endoscopy in gastrointestinal bleeding. Lancet 1974;II:394–397.

33. Alvarado A. A practical scoring system for decision making in acute appendicitis. Ann Emerg Med 1986;15:557–564.

34. Moore EE, Shackford SR, Pachter HL, McAninch JW, Browner BD, Champion HR, Flint CM, Gennarelli TA, Malangoni MA, Ramenofsky ML, Trafton PG. Organ injury scaling system: spleen, liver, kidney. J Trauma 1989;29:1664–1666.

35. Garden RS. Low angle fixation in fractures of the femoral neck. J Bone Joint Surg 1961;43:647 B.

36. Sommer H. Einflußfaktoren der Lebensqualitätsveränderung bei Patienten mit Tumorerkrankung und Therapieerfahrung. (Kölner Lebensqualitätsinventar KLQI). Dissertationsschrift der Medizinischen Fakultät der Universität zu Köln, 1989.

37. Tegner Y, Lysholm: Rating systems in the evaluation of knee ligament injuries. Clin Orthop 1985;198:43–49.

38. Breslow A. Thickness, cross-sectional areas and depth of invasion in the prognosis of cutaneous melanoma. Ann Surg 1970;172:902–908.

39. Karnofsky DA, Burchenal JH. The clinical evaluation of chemotherapeutic agents in cancer. In: MacLeod DM, ed. Evaluation of Chemotherapeutic Agents. New York: Columbia University, 1949, pp. 91–205.

40. Mac Kenzie CR, Charlson ME, DiGioia D, Kelley K. Can the Sickness Impact measure change? An example of scale assessment. J Chron Dis 1986;39:429–438.

41. Stützer JH. Lebensqualität beim Magenkarzinom, Dissertationsschrift an der Medizinischen Fakultät der Universität zu Köln, 1991.

42. Bonenkamp JJ, Songun I, Hermans J, Sasako M, Welvaart K, Plukker JT, van Elk P, Obertop H, Gouma DJ, Taat CW, van Lanschot J, Meyer S, deGraaf PW, von Meyenfeldt MF, Tilanus H, van de Velde CJM. Randomised comparison of morbidity after D1 and D2 dissection for gastric cancer in 996 Dutch patients. Lancet 1995;345:745–748.

43. Troidl H, Kusche J, Vestweber KH, Eypasch E, Maul U. Pouch versus esophagojejunostomy after total gastrectomy: a randomized clinical trial. World J Surg 1987:11:699–712.

44. Höher J, Münster A, Eypasch E, Klein J, Tiling T. Ein neuer Patientenfragebogen mit visueller Analogskala zur quantitativen Erfassung subjektiver Kniebeschwerden. Arthroskopie 1995;8:25–30.

45. Paul A. Outcome nach konservativer und chirurgischer Therapie des akuten und chronischen Leberversagens. Habilitationsschrift an der Medizinischen Fakultät der Universität zu Köln, 1996.

46. McDowell I, Newell C. Measuring Health. A

Guide to Rating Scales and Questionnaires. New York: Oxford University, 1987.

Commentary

An additional criterion for evaluating the usefulness of a scoring system is *sensibility*, "a mixture of ordinary common sense plus a reasonable knowledge of pathophysiology and clinical reality."[1] For example, an index for measuring inflammatory bowel disease that includes questions about headache or that excludes questions about bowel frequency lacks sensibility.[2]

1. Feinstein AR. Clinimetrics. New Haven, CT: Yale University, 1987.
2. Wright JG, McLeod RS, Lossing A, Walters BC, Hu X. Measurement in surgical clinical research. Surgery 1996;119:241–244.

M.F.M.

CHAPTER 34

Developing a Measuring Instrument

A. Paul and B. Bouillon

The traditional outcomes of interest in clinical trials are survival, negative events (complications), failure of treatment, and recurrence of disease.[1] These endpoints are appropriate when the patient's return to normal health and activity can be expected within a relatively short period of time. They have to be altered when we evaluate treatment options that aim to increase general health or overall quality of life. This is especially true when palliative care is applied. In these patients, a return to normal "health" and "activity" cannot be expected (Table 34-1).

Evaluation of established, "objective" outcome parameters is generally accepted; evaluation of "subjective" data such as pain, discomfort, dissatisfaction, and impairment of physical, emotional, and social function (quality of life) is believed to be more difficult or sometimes impossible because of the requirement to correlate treatment effects with the patient's personal perception of health and illness in the context of culture, social norms, roles, and expectations. The measurement of quality of life, an overall measure from the patient's point of view concerning the effects of health-related problems, seems to be important in evaluating the natural history of a disease or a specific medical intervention. Recent advantages in the development of a specific methodology enable us to accurately measure so called "subjective" or "soft" data.[2,3,4]

This chapter focuses on developing accurate "quality of life measurements." The basic principles of the methodology presented here are similar when measuring endpoints such as pain, discomfort, disability, dissatisfaction, fatigue, meaningful life, and so forth. While in many clinical trials the measurement of quality of life is often a vital part in the assessment of a treatment, a measure responding to clinically important interventions is often unavailable. Many investigators are therefore faced with the challenge of constructing an index for a specific condition or even a single trial. In this chapter we will discuss the appropriate methodology in general, illustrated by an example related to liver transplantation.

General versus Disease-Specific Instruments

A great number of non-disease-specific quality of life instruments have been developed for the general population[5-8] that have the advantage of disease-independent comparisons including cost-benefit analysis. Application of these generic instruments may be appropriate, but they are unlikely to detect small differences or even clinically important changes. Therefore, disease-specific instruments for patients with, for example, cancer,[9,10] joint,[11-14] heart,[15] and lung diseases[16] have been developed. Although these instruments,

Table 34-1.   Different types of medical interventions and the importance of health-related quality of life.

Condition	Treatment	Main outcome measure
Acute illness, e.g., appendicitis	Appendectomy	Survival, recovery
Chronic condition, e.g., gallstone disease, ulcerative colitis	Cholecystectomy ileostomy vs. pelvic pouch	Quality of life Quality of life vs. survival
Carcinoma of the prostate	Medical vs. radical prostatectomy	Survival vs. quality of life
"Palliation"	Support, pain relief	Quality of life

once validated, can provide the investigator with most relevant information, they will have a narrow range of applicability (Table 34-2).

Clinical investigators who might have been inexperienced in questionnaire development have responded by creating "ad hoc" measures.[17–19] The results of their measurements are usually difficult to interpret because of failure to address important issues such as clinical relevance, reproducibility, responsiveness, and validity.

Our strategy for developing a questionnaire to measure a disease-specific quality of life is based on previous work and will identify basic principles for constructing instruments to measure changes in individual patients over time; such instruments must be based on what is important to the patients. "Minimal," "elaborated," or "optimal" requirements are presented.[3]

Developing the Questionnaire

The development of a disease specific instrument can be divided into several stages: item selection, reduction of numbers of items, questionnaire format, pretesting, reproducibility, responsiveness, and validity.[3] The stages in the development of a new questionnaire for two models (minimal vs. optimal requirements) are shown in Table 34-3.

Item Selection

Items initially selected must reflect all areas important for patients suffering from the disease and should be derived from how patients, relatives, experts, and associated health care workers estimate how the illness affects their lives. To determine a true frequency of all possible items, a comprehensive series of probes to cover all possible areas of dysfunction must be provided. The nature of these probes will depend on the amount of details the specific research study requires. Ideally, 50–100 patients are necessary to determine all possible areas of dysfunction. To determine the frequency and importance of each item, a further sample of approximately 100 patients is required. This second group of patients is asked via questionnaire whether any of the items are a problem for them, and they are encouraged to rank the importance of each item.

Table 34-2.   Advantages and disadvantages of generic and disease-specific instruments.

Instruments	Comment
Generic instruments (e.g., SF36, Sickness Impact Profile, Nottingham Profile)	Comparison in different diseases and to national norms No specific information Usually less sensitive/responsive Basis for cost-utility analysis
Disease-specific instruments, (e.g., Liver Disease–Specific QL Index, Gastrointestinal QL Index)	Detection of small differences often possible Symptom-related information is usually given No national norms Often less well validated

There are several approaches to determine item importance, each with its own theoretical and practical advantages and disadvantages. Preferably, patients are asked to rate the importance of each item that is a problem for them on a 5-point Likert Scale. Further item selection considers "frequency," "importance," and "expert opinion on completeness." This implies sampling of the complete spectrum of disease severity under consideration (for example, sex, duration of illness, different types of underlying diseases, etc.) and inclusion of patients from all subclasses. The number of patients surveyed at this stage is crucial to obtain a reasonable estimate. To gain a confidence interval of 10%, 100 patients with a frequency of 50% are required. A minimum of at least 50 patients should be included (confidence interval 15%).

Item Reduction

The initial item selection process usually results in more items than can and should be included in the final questionnaire. Important criteria for retaining items at this stage of questionnaire development include the number of patients who listed the item as a problem (item frequency), the importance attached to the items, and the potential responsiveness of the items, that is, the item's ability to detect clinically relevant changes. At this stage, sophisticated analysis such as principal component analysis and factor analysis are helpful and favored by many investigators. Alternatively, a simple and reasonable approach is to modify the frequency of each item by its level of importance. With this rather simplified analysis one can retain the items with the greatest frequency-importance

Table 34-3.   Stages in development of a quality of life measure.

Stage	Maximal requirements	Minimal requirements
Item selection	Literature review Consultation with health care workers Use of existing instruments Semistructured interview with 50 patients	Use of existing instruments Consultation with health care workers
Reduction of no. of items	Questionnaire identifying item frequency and importance Choice of items with highest frequency-importance product or principal-component analysis	Item selection according to presumed importance
Questionnaire format	Choice of response-options scale: 5- to 7-point Likert or Visual Analogue Scale Time specification (2–4 weeks) Availability of previous responses to patients	Choice of response-options scale: 5- to 7-point Likert or Visual Analogue Scale Time specification (2–4 weeks) Availability of previous responses to patients
Pretesting	Analysis of results to ensure that full range of response options is used	None
Sampling for above four stages	Use of random sample of patients to ensure representation of entire range of disease, severity, age, lifestyle, etc.	Use of sample of convenience
Reproducibility and responsiveness	Questionnaire administration to stable patients Administration before and after intervention of known efficacy	No testing before trials
Validity	Use of construct validity Comparison with "a priori" predictions Comparison with a previously validated instrument	Use of face validity

Table modified according to G.H. Guyatt et al. (1986).[3]

product for the final questionnaire. Both approaches to analysis are valuable, and their usage depends on the specific questions to be answered.

The purpose of the questionnaire design is very important. For measurements of changes in individual patients over time, items unlikely to demonstrate changes should not be included. If the intention is to assess an intervention with specific goals, items related to those goals should appear in the final questionnaire. Additionally, core activities that apply to most patients with respect to sex, age, disease severity, and lifestyle (individualized according the study population) should be included in the final questionnaire.[2]

The number of questions remaining after the items have been reduced depends on where the test is administered and, in some instances, on how many other tests and questionnaires the patient will have to complete during the course of the study. In general, we should aim to keep the time required to fill out our questionnaire to less than 20 minutes. The time per question should not exceed 1 minute.

Format of the Questionnaire

Questions must be precise, easy to understand, and specific about the time frame, usually referring to the last 2–4 weeks. Response options refer to the range that patients have in responding to a specific questionnaire item. Only two response options—"yes" or "no"—are always satisfactory. To enhance responsiveness, that is, to detect small changes, a 5–7 point Likert Scale or a Visual Analogue Scale (VAS-Scale) may be more appropriate.[20,21] During a pretesting phase with at least 20 patients, poor wording and inappropriate, embarrassing, or confusing questions are identified and corrected.

Reproducibility and Responsiveness

Reproducibility (reliability and precision) is determined by repeated administration of the same questionnaire to stable patients. Most commonly, reliability is looked for by calculating the variability between subjects versus total variability in response (including between-subject variability and within-subject differences). The resulting statistic is the Pearson's correlation coefficient or,

more precisely, the intraclass correlation coefficient.[22] These correlations also measure how well an instrument is differentiating between subjects. Thus, the ratio of the minimal clinically important differences to the variability in individual stable patients is directly related to the sample size requirements and can be used as an index of the questionnaire's responsiveness.

If the measure of responsiveness changes, the questionnaire is distributed to patients before and after the application of an intervention of known efficacy. Ideally, the questionnaire will not only demonstrate a change or improvement in quality of life, but also a sufficient and large change or improvement relative to the variability shown in stable patients. If therapy is not applied, or therapy will be investigated concerning "known benefit," the serial distribution of the questionnaire to a large group of patients is usually necessary. Then the ratio of variability in patients of the second study group in comparison to those patients of the first study group provides an estimate of the questionnaire's responsiveness.

Validity

An index, test, or questionnaire is considered to be valid if it measures what it is supposed to measure. A simple way to measure validity is to measure "construct validity," that is, does the questionnaire function adequately with respect to quality of life in comparison to other measures? Since evaluative questionnaires primarily measure changes, the correlation between changes in quality of life and other clinically relevant indicative variables has to be examined. Important additional validation derives from a comparison with previously validated health measures. Simple "face validity," although looked upon as being reasonable, (e.g., the index is determined from expert opinions in order to measure quality of life) is often insufficient.

Developing a Quality of Life Index for Liver Transplantation

We have described the theoretical background and generic requirements for the development of an appropriate, meaningful, and reproducible in-

Table 34-4. Results of principal component analysis after VARIMAX rotation of the LDQL Index.

Factor 1 Emotional function		Factor 2 Activities (social and physical function)		Factor 3 Symptoms	
Lack of self-confidence	0.81	Limited in social activities	0.80	Swollen abdomen	0.65
Depressed	0.78	Limited in housework	0.82	Itching	0.59
Loss of control over life	0.75	Dependent on others	0.82	Food restriction	0.66
Frustrated about illness	0.72	Problems in sexual act	0.39	Stomach pain	0.50
Depressed about illness	0.76	Ability to work	0.82	Bone pain	0.32
Nervous about health	0.72	Weakness/loss of strength	0.57	Nausea	0.68
Changes in appearance	0.56	Difficulty to move around	0.76	Headaches	0.63
Changes in mood	0.64	Feeling unwell	0.59	Vision problems	0.64
Thoughts about death	0.61			Dizziness or ringing ears	0.48
				Memory	0.76
				Concentration	0.58

strument. Practical issues and adaptations that might be encountered in the development of such an instrument are illustrated by an example from hepatobiliary surgery. The author recently developed an index to evaluate quality of life in patients before and after liver transplantation, and in patients with chronic liver disease. The underlying clinical problem was that not only long-term survival but also improvements in quality of life have frequently been observed in patients following liver transplantation. In this case, existing major impairments concerning quality of life are contributing factors for (even earlier) liver transplantation, which has traditionally been considered only as a "life-saving" procedure.

Definition of Quality of Life (QL)

Quality of life has been defined as an individual's perception of limitations in relation to personal goals, expectations, standards, and concerns.[23] Following the currently accepted hypothesis, medically relevant QL can be objectively assessed in the subareas of an individual's emotional function, activities (physical and social function, including the level of independence and social relationships), and perception of general health. Furthermore, disease-specific information and symptoms are possibly of direct clinical relevance and affect the patient's QL.[24,25]

Development of the Liver Disease–Specific Quality of Life (LDQL) Index

The liver disease–specific QL instrument was developed according to the standard methods described. Briefly, a total of 82 items that could affect QL in patients with chronic liver disease and after orthotopic liver transplantation (OLT) were selected by a panel of transplant physicians and surgeons, methodologists, specialized health care workers, and selected patients and relatives. The first step of item reduction was achieved through correspondence with other experts and selected patients ($n = 20$). The altered questionnaire (reduced to 55 items) was applied to 49 selected patients and controls, who were chosen to be representative for the future study. This questionnaire was analyzed by calculating frequencies, inter-item correlations, and the ability of each item to differentiate different stages of a disease. It was finally checked for completeness. As a result of this analysis, the questionnaire was reduced to 39 items and was then applied to 78 randomly selected patients. Subsequent frequency-importance analysis resulted in a 5-point Likert Scale–format instrument consisting of 28 specific and 5 general questions that were self-administered and completed within approximately 10 minutes.

Assessment of Quality of Life (QL)

The questionnaire was mailed to an additional 245 available but otherwise randomly selected patients. This group consisted of patients with advanced chronic liver disease (biopsy-proven liver cirrhosis) from a general hepatology practice ($n = 61$), patients currently listed for transplantation ($n = 15$), and patients at three months after successful OLT ($n = 169$). All patients were informed that they were participating in a study assessing QL. The term quality of life was mentioned, but no specific definition of QL was given to the individual patient. Of the 245 patients, 200 completed and returned the questionnaire (response rate 82.8%) and were eligible for further analysis. In addition to the LDQL Index basic demographic data, the staff assessment regarding presence and significance of associated diseases or treatment side effects, and the short form of the SF36, a widely used and well-validated general health measure,[26] were applied to these patients at the same time. The patients' level of education and professional activity were recorded. Additionally, reproducibility (test-retest reliability) was assessed by repeated application (within 2–4 weeks) of the LDQL Index to 34 medically stable patients following OLT.

Data Analysis

The results for every single answer of the newly developed questionnaire, the patients' details, and the SF36 data were entered into a computer-data file. On the 5-point Likert Scale, the answer "never" was coded as "5," and the answer "always" (maximal impairment of QL) as "1." The raw values were then transformed into percentages through multiplication with 100 (raw scale score minus the lowest possible score divided by the possible score range). This allowed for comparisons between different subareas of QL in the

newly developed index, as well as with the results of the SF36. Prior to this analysis, LDQL data had been further processed by factor analysis using the SPSS statistical package (version 4.1). This principal component analysis including varimax rotation identified five different factors with EIGEN values greater than 1. Final analysis was restricted to 3 factors because all symptom-related items loaded on the factors 3–5. Two techniques were used to determine whether a specific item correlated with the scale items: item total correlation (internal consistency) and calculation of Cronbach's alpha.[27] Cronbach's alpha was calculated after $K \times Tii/1 + (K - 1)$ rii (where rii is the inter-item correlation, and K is the number of items). In the different subgroups of patients, the newly developed index was then compared to the results of the SF36, and with the patients' own global ratings of health and quality of life. Sensitivity was evaluated by comparing the impairments of QL with "objective" parameters such as the number and importance of limiting associated diseases and by analyzing whether the newly developed index discriminates among the three different clinical groups of liver disease.

Validation of the Newly Developed Disease-Specific QL Questionnaire

The results of the principal component analysis and internal consistency data of the LDQL questionnaire are given in Table 34-4. The item to own dimension correlation, after correction for overlap, exceeded 0.4 for all except the question about the patients' sexual restrictions and most of the symptom-related questions. Cronbach's alpha exceeded the recommended minimum of 0.8 and

Table 34-5. LDQL-Values in the different subareas of QL and number of limiting associated diseases after OLT.

Areas of QL	Number of limiting diseases;[a]				
	0 ($n = 86$)	1 ($n = 53$)	2 ($n = 36$)	≥3 ($n = 25$)	p-Value
Emotional function	82.4	74.8	69.3	56.0	<0.001
Activity (physical and social function)	80.6	71.2	65.4	50.7	<0.001
Symptoms	82.0	74.7	72.5	66.1	<0.001
General health	68.8	63.0	57.6	45.6	<0.001

[a]Values in percent: 100%, perfect health; 0%, worst health possible.

was 0.92 for the emotional function and activity (social and physical function), and 0.82 for the symptom-related questions. The mean ranges of correlations of variance were 0.45, 0.49, and 0.48, respectively. Ninety-eight percent of cases fell within the 95% confidence interval in all three subareas of QL. The test-retest reliability (reproducibility) in 34 stable patients following transplantation was overall 0.7 and did not reveal any significant differences in the subareas of QL when analyzed separately.

The validity of the newly developed questionnaire was further assessed by checking for sensitivity and by comparing with the SF36 health survey questionnaire. Sensitivity, the proxy that a QL questionnaire measures the currently present medically relevant limitations, was evaluated by comparison with objective medical parameters of the study population. The results of this comparison are shown in Table 34-5. In all subareas of QL, a significant correlation of QL impairment with an increasing number of the patients' limiting associated diseases was found. Furthermore, the newly developed LDQL Index separated the different stages of liver disease more distinctly than the SF36. Detailed information is given in Table 34-6. In all subareas of QL and in the assessment of general health, highly statistically significant differences were detected among the patients with chronic liver disease, those awaiting transplantation, and following successful OLT. There were no significant differences in the subareas of social and emotional function for the SF36.

Quality of Life—Overall Results

As shown in Table 34-6, there are statistically significant improvements in all investigated subareas of QL following OLT. Further subset analysis including age, sex, time from transplantation, number of episodes of rejection, and so forth did not reveal any further significant differences in improvements of QL, when these different subgroups were compared (data not shown). Only patients with primary sclerosing cholangitis (PSC), usually transplanted in the early stage of their disease, achieved significantly higher scores in all areas of QL after OLT (81% versus 72%, mean values for all dimensions of QL, $p < 0.05$). Since no data from a representative cross-section of normal individuals for the newly developed LDQL Index were available, comparisons with normal individuals—corrected for age, sex, and profession (manual workers versus nonmanual workers)—were performed using the SF36 data. The "emotional function" and overall "vitality" of the patients were normal or close to normal following OLT. Minor limitations regarding the symptom "pain" and "general health perception" were still present. The "social" and "physical" functions and the "role limitations related to the physical function" were still impaired when compared to normal individuals.

Using the LDQL Index, there were no statistically significant impairments, but also no improvements of the preexisting symptoms such as bone pain, vision problems, and headaches. Almost all symptoms related to the advanced char-

Table 34-6. Comparison of the LDQL Index within the different subareas of QL.

Disease	Index	Symptoms	Physical	Social	Emotional function	General health
Chronic liver	SF 36	62.7%	67.9%	52.0%	64.6%	44.7%
disease ($n = 42$)	LSLQ	65.9%	65.5%		65.2%	48.7%
Before treatment	SF 36	51.2%	49.6%	54.9%	56.9%	24.7%
($n = 13$)	LSLQ	64.3%	52.4%		64.3%	39.7%
Following Transplant	SF 36	70.5%	67.1%	55.2%	75.9%	62.5%
($n = 145$)	LSLQ	79.7%	75.2%		78.4%	68.3%
p-Value[a]	SF 36	0.01[b]	n.s.	n.s.	0.001[b]	0.001[b]
p-Value[a]	LSLQ	<0.0001	0.0095		0.008	<0.0001

[a]Kruska-Wallis Test, one-tail anova (100%, perfect health; 0%, worst possible health)

[b]for the SF 36 only pain.

acter of their underlying liver disease showed significant improvements.

Conclusion

An "instrument" as discussed in this chapter is a surgical tool to evaluate the most clinically relevant endpoint of a defined intervention, or it functions as a part of the evaluation of the natural history of a disease. From an individual patient's point of view, the quantity and quality of survival—how much fun, happiness, love, and satisfaction one can have and expects to have in the future—is one of the most important endpoints.

Troidl[17] emphasizes that quality of life should be measured in a simple and practical way. The questionnaires applied to patients should be easy to understand and complete within 10–20 minutes and should focus on the most clinically relevant problems.

Applying the methodology described here shows that conversion of quality of life data that is so often believed to be "soft," into reproducible "hard" data is possible. Nonvalidated "ad hoc" questionnaires are not acceptable because no relevant information can be gained by the scientists or clinicians using them. Whenever improvement of quality of life is the indication or part of the intention to treat, the success of the intervention should be checked by means of a reasonably validated QL questionnaire. Validation of such questionnaires is never complete and must therefore be considered an ongoing process. The incompleteness of our methodology must be the motivation for further clinical and experimental research.

References

1. Troidl H. Lebensqualität: Ein relevantes Zielkriterium in der Chirurgie. Chirurg 1989;60:445–449.
2. Guyatt GH, Veldhuyzen Van Zanten SJO, Feeny DH, Patrick DL. Measuring quality of life in clinical trials: a taxonomy and review. CMAJ 1989;140 (June 15):1441–1448.
3. Guyatt GH, Bombardier C, Tugwell PX. Measuring disease-specific quality of life in clinical trials. CMAJ 1986;134 (April 15):889–895.
4. Jaeschke R, Guyatt GH. How to develop and validate a new quality of life instrument. In: B. Spilker, ed. Quality of Life Assessment in Clinical Trials. New York: Raven, 1990, ch. 5, pp. 47–57.
5. Ware JE, Brook RH, Davies-Avery A, et al. Conceptualization and Measurement of Health for Adults in the Health Insurance Study, vol. 1: Model of Health and Methodology, Santa Monica, CA: Rand, 1980.
6. Kaplan RM, Bush JW, Berry CC. Health status: types of validity and the index of well-being. Health Serv Res 1976;11:478–507.
7. Bergner M, Bobbit RA, Carter WB, Gilson BS. The Sickness Impact Profile; development and final revision of a health status measure. Med Care 1981;19:787–805.
8. Parkerson GR Jr, Gehlbach SH, Wagner EH, James SA, Clapp NE, Muhlbaier LH. The Duke-UNC Health Profile: an adult health status instrument for primary care. Med Care 1981;19:806–828.
9. Spitzer WO, Dobson AJ, Hall J, Chesterman E, Levi J, Shepherd R, Battista RN, Catchlove BR. Measuring the quality of life of cancer patients. J Chronic Dis 1981;14:585–597.
10. Preistman TJ, Baum M. Evaluation of quality of life in patients receiving treatment for advanced breast cancer. Lancet 1976;1:899–901.
11. Fries JF, Spitz PW, Young DY. The dimensions of health outcomes: the health assessment questionnaire, disability and pain scales. J Rheumatol 1982;9:789–793.
12. Meenan RF. The AIMS approach to health care measurement: conceptual background and measurement properties. J Rheumatol 1982;9:785–788.
13. Helewa A, Goldsmith CH, Smythe HA. Independent measurement of functional capacity in rheumatoid arthritis. J Rheumatol 1982;9:794–797.
14. Tugwell P, Bombadier C, Buchanan W, et al. The ability of the Mactar disability questionnaire to detect sensitivity to change in rheumatoid arthritis. Clin Res 1983;31:239. Abstract.
15. Goldman L, Hashimoto D, Cook EF. Comparative reproducibility and validity of systems for assessing cardio-vascular functional class: advantages of a new specific activity scale. Circulation 1981;64:1227–1234.
16. Mahler DA, Weinberg DH, Wells CK, et al. Measurement of dyspnea: description of two new indices, interobserver agreement and physiological

correlations. Am Rev Respir Dis 1982;24 (suppl 1):138.

17. Troidl H. Quality of life: definition, conceptualization, and implications—a surgeon's view. Theor Surg 1991;6:138–142.

18. Troidl H. Lebensqualität als entscheidendes Kriterium im Alltag und in der Forschung des Chirurgen. Langenbecks Arch Chir, Suppl II (Kongreßbericht 1989).

19. Wood-Dauphinees S, Troidl H. Assessing quality of life in surgical studies. Theor Surg 1989;4:35–44.

20. Woodward CA, Chambers LW: Guide to Questionnaire Construction and Question Writing. Ottawa: Canadian Public Health Association, 1983.

21. Sudman S, Bradburn NM. Asking Questions: A Practical Guide to Questionnaire Design. San Francisco: Jossey-Bass, 1982.

22. Kramer MS, Feinstein AR. Clinical biostatistics. LIV. The biostatistics of concordance. Clin Pharmacol Ther 1981;29:111–123.

23. WHOQOL Group (Division of Mental Health, World Health Organization). Study protocol for the World Health Organisation project to develop a Quality of Life Assessment Instrument (WHOQOL) Qual Life Res 1993;2:153–159.

24. Fraser SCA. Quality of life measurement in surgical practice. Br J Surg 1993;80:163–169.

25. O'Boyle CA. Assessment of quality of life in surgery. Br J Surg 1992;79:395–398.

26. Ware JE. Standards for validating health measures: definition and content. J Chron Dis 1987;40:473–480.

27. Kline P. A Handbook of Test Construction. London: Methuen, 1986.

CHAPTER 35

How to Choose a Relevant Endpoint

H. Troidl, A.S. Wechsler, and M.F. McKneally

Two well-dressed gentlemen were on their way home from a party, where they had obviously wined and dined too well. One was on his knees systematically examining the sidewalk beneath a streetlight. His friend volunteered helpfully: "I am sure I heard your keys drop back here where it is dark!" The searcher on his knees replied: "I know, but what is the use of looking back there where I can't see, when it is so much easier here in the light?"[1]

The chapter on endpoints in the last edition began with this anecdote, illustrating the classic fallacy of confusing the measurable with the important. We used it to introduce the difference between conventional, easily measurable endpoints (such as mortality), and innovative, less readily quantified endpoints (such as quality of life) in clinical research. This chapter discusses the concept of an endpoint and its decisive significance in clinical and experimental research, illustrated by simple examples. The important methodology for testing their validity is discussed in the chapter by Paul, "How to develop a measuring instrument" (Chapter 34).

"How Are You?"

This ancient and enduringly fundamental question of a doctor to a patient is important before and even more important after a treatment. A question encompasses specific symptoms and the general condition; there is a special nuance hidden in this question—how this particular patient, under the current circumstances and at this particular time, is handling the symptoms and the treatment.[2]

In most cases, symptoms (such as pain, worry, and fear) bring the patient to his doctor. Patient and doctor discuss and carefully consider whether an operation or some other treatment is indicated or not, and decide after the treatment on its success or failure by answering the original question: "how are you?" This scene describes a transaction and a relationship between patient and doctor that has been unchanged for generations. Generally, this is never reflected with the original intensity and significance in the scientific world of congresses, papers, research grants, and protocols.

One example for demonstrating the reality of "seeking for the key in the light of a streetlamp" is the determination of blood sugar in patients with chronic pancreatitis. Every clinician knows that the main indication for surgical intervention in chronic pancreatitis is the patient's unbearable pain. Patient and doctor should pay attention to this "endpoint," because to get rid of pain is the patient's main intention; blood sugar deviations counted in millimoles per liter of plasma are not of interest to the patient.[2]

"How are you?" This simple question with multiple layers of meaning has many possible answers.

This transaction between patient and doctor is often reduced in today's language to "outcome measurement," an essential aspect of clinical research; its significance is just starting to be appreciated and responsibly developed. The endpoint is part of this research— maybe the most important part.

Although "How are you?" is the decisive question according to Feinstein,[3] it is not readily accepted by methodologists, because it is not sufficiently "objective" and "reproducible." Great clinicians have traditionally evaluated their patients according to this question and changed their treatment significantly according to the answers received. John Goligher modified stomach surgery with the "Visik criteria" and brought great benefit to patients, without perfect validation and testing of the criteria according to current methodological standards.[4]

Methodologists have sound reasons for their objections; we have to remember that great clinicians like Billroth realized this more than 100 years ago.

> It is difficult when one's therapeutic management is based on nothing more than the memories of personal experiences, because it is important to realize how fallacious some of these memories can be. . . . What a cautious person calls "sometimes" is "often" or even "always" to the overly enthusiastic, and "seldom" or "never" to the overly sceptic.[5]

Bryan Jennett, a critical and thoughtful neurosurgeon, delivered the theme in a nutshell: "If we would be as interested in outcome measurement as we are in making a diagnosis, most surgical interventions would be changed or even dropped!"[6] How to obtain information on the effectiveness of medical treatment in different local and social circumstances will be one of the most important questions of clinical research in the near future.

Toward a Definition of Outcomes and Endpoints

The English word *outcome* is almost untranslatable to other languages. This short word indicates an effect being experienced and felt by individual patients in individual situations in different periods of life. Since Western science always requires definitions, we now need one. What is fatigue, what is quality of life, what does health or sickness mean? According to Sir Karl Popper, definitions are often senseless or of little use. He demonstrates this with the following sentences: "A human being is a featherless biped" and "A human being is a rational vertebrate."[7]

Nevertheless, definitions are necessary in the real world. We summarize Popper's concept of useful definition in more detail in chapter 1, "Toward a Definition of Surgical Research." Popper feels it is more reasonable to generate a definition from an expandable list of all reasonable, practical characteristics. In this way a definition is always kept open but can be summarized as a hypothesis at any time.

With Popper's cautionary advice in mind, let us look at a possible definition of outcome. Donabedian suggests the following: An outcome is "any change in the actual or future health status of an individual person or society that is related to a previous or ongoing intervention."[8] This definition includes essential components such as the situation of an individual or even of society at one particular time, and the change of this situation over time. However, the most important aspect remains unconsidered, the question "What is meant by health/sickness?" This is a difficult question, we admit, so difficult that it is rarely discussed during congresses or in the literature, not even in daily life or in the education of medical students. This is a peculiar but grave situation.

Henrik Wulff tried to answer this question using two different approaches, singly and in combination, with one or the other dominant.[9] The "mechanical model" uses established biochemical and physiological measuring methods: "Without numbers, there is no science!" The "hermeneutic approach" to health/sickness puts emphasis on the individual's opinion, the explanation of one's situation, and rejection and acceptance of deviations from standard.

The endpoint helps to describe outcome. The right endpoint is the essential prerequisite for obtaining relevant information on outcome. The German word *Zielkriterium* makes this even more clear (*Ziel*, meaning aim, *Kriterium*, meaning criteria). The endpoint is not synonymous with "result," because there may be many results depending on the question (assay) used. Ideally, the endpoint consists of only one variable, but sometimes several are necessary to show the effect more clearly.

The acquisition of information is more critical than methodology and should not be limited by preconceived methodological approaches. If the variable to be used as an endpoint can be objectively measured, it has to be handled methodologically; this is an advantage but not a necessity. An endpoint does not necessarily lose its informational content if it is not reproducible or objectively measurable. Death is also not reproducible.[3] An acute abdomen is rarely measured objectively, even though it is real. Subjective information is still information, even though it is not possible to measure it in centimeters or other units. Vomiting, fatigue, nausea, pain, hate, or love are not unreal or without informational content because they cannot be determined by plasma levels.

The personal, the unique, is essential. Every thoughtful clinician realizes that highly esteemed objective data—obtained for example by X ray and pathology—are not as "hard" as they were thought to be, when looking at them a little closer. On the other hand, "soft data" can be made even harder than "hard data" with appropriate methods.[11]

The arguments of evolutionary epistemology can also be used, such as whether an "objective" observation is objective at all, since observations are always a reproduction, and reproductions are never identical, especially if they were made in different situations.

The relevant endpoint in experiments using animals or small subsystems is as problematic as it is in clinical investigation. Every experiment is a reduction of reality. An experiment as part of methodological research uses manipulation and standardization in an attempt to achieve an outcome.

Irrelevant and Perverted Endpoints

In clinical and experimental research, irrelevant endpoints are sometimes chosen, or the selected endpoint could even be called "perverse." Questions regarding hygiene and surgical infection are often answered via number and kinds of bacteria per cubic meter of air. What is clinically relevant is the infection rate of patients in a hospital and, even more to the point, the effect of the infection on the individual. Nosocomial infection rates—a very sensitive topic that could be seized by the press—include positive urinary tract cultures of unknown clinical relevance. Here the endpoint has become perverted because bacterial counts are used as an inappropriate surrogate for clinical infection—the correct endpoint.

After surgical interventions for chronic pancreatitis, the patient, who is solely interested in getting rid of the pain, will judge the operation as successful if pain has been eliminated, and as unsuccessful if pain remains or gets worse. From the patient's perspective, his or her blood sugar level, although precise, is meaningless.

Oncologists have been aware of inadequate endpoint usage for the past 30 years (Table 35-1).[12] Walter Spitzer, a pioneer in dealing with these problems, stated in the 1986 Sintra symposium on quality of life: "Cure has something to do with surviving, palliation only with quality of life."[13]

In 1971 United States President Nixon called for "a war on cancer." In 1990 J.C. Bailar, a sta-

Table 35-1. Endpoints in oncological research.[12] An example of objective measurement without considering what it means to the patient. From a patient-centered view, this is a *perverted endpoint.*

Complete Response

Complete disappearance of measurable disease for a period of at least 1 month.

Partial Response

A greater than 50% decrease in the sum of the products of the perpendicular diameters of all measurable lesions, which lasts at least 1 month.

Stable Disease

A smaller than 50% decrease of tumor diameter and no tumor diameter increase greater than 25%.

Progression

A greater than 25% tumor diameter increase or the appearance of new metastasis.

tistical expert for the *New England Journal of Medicine*, had to admit: "We have lost the war."[14] Because cancer therapy so rarely achieves cure, and palliation is the reality, the military paradigm for treating cancer with radical interventions is inappropriate. Since this is so, it is hard to justify descriptions of the success of therapy measured by survival rates expressed in months and years.

During surgical congresses, statistical manipulations are more often the topic of discussion than the suffering of patients. Figure 35-1 demonstrates this convincingly. Death is not the worst outcome, dying badly is worse. In 1972 Small and Krause wrote, "What you really want to know, and to show in presenting results, is the quality of patients' lives."[16] As a young surgeon I realized this bitter reality after technically achieving safe pneumonectomy and gastrectomy for cancer therapy. I celebrated surgical success but realized a bad outcome after 3–6 months (see Figure 35-1b). This

was the key issue for starting my interest in patients' well-being as a critical outcome measure. Intense discussion of this issue with Walter Spitzer at a Canadian lake cottage at 4:00 A.M. led to the development of the first edition of this textbook.

Why does the mechanistic approach dominate our thinking? It is based in Western scientific thinking. In contrast with the holistic thinking of the ancients, Cartesian rationalism separated emotions and everything "subjective" from scientific observations. Despite accurate planning, standardization, and reduction, the result is totally dependant on the method and the given question. According to Thomas Kuhn, the paradigm using the same questions and the same methods leads consistently to the same results, even when mistaken, as illustrated by cancer therapy.[17]

Selection of relevant endpoints is essential for the development of scientific theory. It deserves

a.

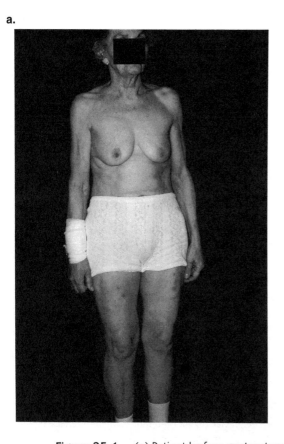

b.

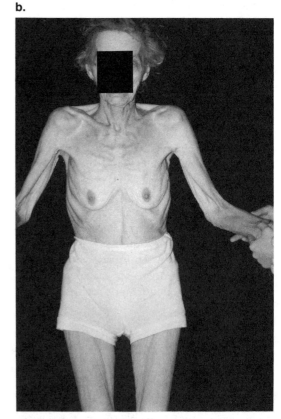

Figure 35-1. (a) Patient before gastrectomy and (b) the same patient 6 months later.

Table 35-2.   The 5 *D*s according to White (1967), showing examples of ranking in different clinical situations.[23]

Clinical situation	Surgical examples	Ranked importance of outcome variables[a]
Impaired quality of life but not life threatening	Hernia Gallstones Lacerated meniscus Peripheral arterial occlusion	Discomfort > Disability > Disease > Dissatisfaction > Death
Impaired quality of life and life threatening; surgery prolongs life but increases morbidity	Stoma for colitis Amputation for vascular disease Transplantation	Discomfort > Disability > Disease > Dissatisfaction > Death
Different therapeutic approaches: similar operative mortality, complications, and survival	Arterial occlusion: bypass vs. profundplasty Stomach cancer: different reconstructions	Discomfort > Disability > Dissatisfaction > Disease > Death
Trade-off between better quality of life and therapeutic risk	Colitis: stoma vs. pelvic pouch Coxarthrosis: conservative vs. endoprothesis	Discomfort > Death > Disability > Dissatisfaction > Disease
Palliation	Esophageal carcinoma Pancreatic carcinoma	Discomfort > Disability > Dissatisfaction > Disease > Death

[a]Read > as "more important than."

to be given the appropriate value in research and methodology. To work in clinical research, common sense is needed. Feinstein stated, "Clinically relevant problems have to be solved by clinicians themselves; methodologists and epidemiologists are useful partners."[18] A scoring system for gastrointestinal disease cannot be designed by someone who has never seen a patient suffering from vomiting.

Some Prerequisites for Relevant Endpoints

Placebo effects. Surgery has a strong placebo effect that varies with the personality, social circumstances, and culture of the surgeon and the patients. It influences animal experiments; when animals receive careful, intensive treatment, their natural history changes.[19]

Motivation. The influence of socioeconomic and cultural aspects are important in clinical research. Returning to work strongly depends on social and economic circumstances.[20] A mother without available help from relatives returns home after cholecystectomy as soon as possible in order to take care of her children. The same is true for an employer who manages the company, quite different from the behavior of an employee who may have financial gain in case of sickness. The influence of motivation in the Third World is outside our comprehension.

Time. It is important to define the time at which an endpoint is assessed. After a knee is operated on, it will function very differently in 1

a.

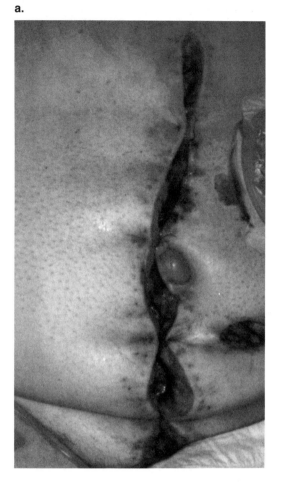

b.

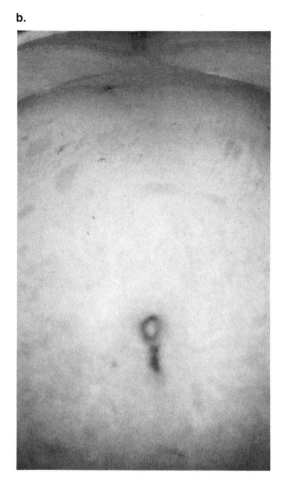

Figure 35-2. Two "midline abdominal wound infections." The dramatic difference from the patient's perspective is not included in the definition of the endpoint.

week as compared with 1 year. Survivors of gastrectomy may present an excellent picture regarding quality of life 1 year later, but probably have been through hell during that year. Appetite is worst in the first 6 weeks after operation but improves after 3 months. Patients not lucky enough to survive the first year after this intervention have no benefit at all.[21]

Social context. A measuring instrument developed according to state-of-the-art methods in clinical research may be easy to process statistically, but less useful than a questionnaire based on the long-term experience of clinical researchers (for example, the Visik classification).[4] Endpoints such as cost-utility, cost-benefit, and cost-

effectiveness may have to be assessed to demonstrate effects in and on society. Because these measurements and inferences are made in complex systems, they may be misleading. The distinguished biologist Rupert Reidel has developed the epistemological position that experiments are reliable when they are done in simple systems such as mathematics and physics; they are far less reliable in complex systems such as human biology and social groups.[22] Inferences from clinical studies, particularly those related to cost, utility, and benefit, may mislead because they focus on the disease, not the individual patient. Clinicians avoid this pitfall in their practice by adjusting the treatment as needed, based on the patient's comorbidity, social situation, and other contextual details. Research protocols restrict this adaptation. Their endpoints should be chosen to insure that they provide clinically relevant information. The clinician will ask, "Does this conclusion apply to my patients, or does it only answer a study question?"

In summary, the final test of relevance of an endpoint is its relationship to the well-being of the individual patient. In choosing endpoints, the doctors should envision themselves as advocates for the patients. The closer the chosen endpoint comes to answering the age-old, elemental question "How are you?" the more appropriate and relevant it will be.

"How to Find a Key in the Darkness"?

An easy way for clinicians to develop their thinking about endpoints is to consider the "5 Ds" approach described by White in 1967.[23] Table 35-2 shows the ranking of the "5 Ds" (death, disease, discomfort, disability, and dissatisfaction) in realistic, clinical situations.

Death. For evaluation of surgical interventions in life-threatening situations, operative mortality is the most definite endpoint. Striking examples are ruptured aorta, transplantation, or multiply in-jured trauma patients. Risk factor adjustments provide better conceptualization of even such a specific endpoint as death. Although complication rates are frequently cited as endpoints, they are of importance only if they are relevant for the sick patient. In Figure 35-2, two examples meeting the definition of "wound infection" are shown. The essential difference in terms of impact on the patient's recovery is clearly evident.

Disease. To determine an endpoint related to disease, the mechanical or hermeneutic approach or a combination of both might be chosen. For example, measurement of blood pressure or the fasting blood sugar would be a relevant mechanistic endpoint appropriate for diseases such as insulinoma or an adenoma of the adrenal gland. In contrast, the impact of an amputation depends much more on the patient's acceptance or refusal of the social implications and context. Some patients participate in the Olympics of the Disabled after limb amputation; others despondently await their old age at home. The nature of a disease (silent carcinoma versus acute and painful appendicitis) and its natural course of ups and downs should be considered in choosing the endpoint for evaluating treatment effects.

Discomfort. Discomfort has been long neglected but is of great importance for the patient. It has become one of the most relevant endpoints in

Table 35-3.   Different endpoints of hernia repair in 1997, including feasibility, economics, and social circumstances.

	Which procedure should you choose?		
		Procedure	
Relevant endpoint	1	2	3
1. Technical difficulty	high	medium	low
2. Overall complication rate	low	medium	low
• seriousness of possible complications	high	low	low
3. Overall rehabilitation	fast	slow	fast
• postoperative comfort	high	medium	high
• return to daily activities and work	fast?	slow	fast
4. Recurrence rate	1%	2%	2%
• formidability of repairing a recurrence	difficult	medium	high
5. Socioeconomic factors			
• charges for operating room, hospital stay, etc.	high	low	medium
• societal costs, notably lost work time	low	medium	low

Modified from Rutkow.[25]

Table 35-4.   A classification as an endpoint (Troidl 1990).

Class I. *Incident-free surgery:*

   no surgical technical problems and no negative outcome for the patient

Class II. *Inconsequential incident:*

   one or more surgical technical problems, but no negative outcome for the patient (intraabdominal stone loss, bleeding)

Class III. *No incident, negative consequence:*

   no surgical technical problems, but one or more negative outcomes for the patient (hematoma, wound infection)

Class IV. *Consequential surgical incident:*

   one or more surgical technical problems with corresponding negative outcomes for the patient (conversion to operation, relaparatomy)

Class V. *Death:*

   in any relation to operation

---

studies of endoscopic surgery. The hypothesis of endoscopic surgery is: "less trauma, more comfort, at equal or better safety."[24] Endpoints for assessing the quality of endoscopic surgery include pain, fatigue, nausea and vomiting, general working ability, daily activity, physical integrity, and cosmesis.

Disability. Equally important is the fourth *D*, disability, to what extent an individual is able to work actively and live independently after treatment. Daily activity is the baseline of this endpoint: to eat independently, bathe, shower, get dressed, go to the toilet. Disability evaluation includes a combination of psychological and physical components such as intellectual competence, being able to read a book, listen to music, or have an interesting conversation.

Dissatisfaction. Dissatisfaction with one's state of health or with medical treatment is a complex and interesting endpoint. Satisfaction does not necessarily correlate with good or improved health. A patient with a serious illness may be more satisfied with his circumstances than someone less severely ill or even fully recovered. Satisfaction or dissatisfaction depends on introspection, acceptance of reality, and balancing expectations with outcome.

Rutkow's evaluation of hernia repair (Table 35-3)[25] considers economic and socioeconomic reality as well as surgical and technical problems. A professional athlete, financially independent,

will choose the method promising quick recovery despite the high cost and the higher risk of needing a repeat operation. For an older, less financially secure person, cost, not time, may be more important.

Endoscopic surgery is formulated on the hypothesis that it yields more comfort and less trauma with equal or better safety when compared with "open" operations. The classification shown in Table 35-4 has been very helpful in our clinic and may lead to a useful method to test this hypothesis.[26] The most important feature of this classification is that the view of the patient has been recognized. The classification ranges from positive to negative, has a differentiated grading, is legally neutral, and is quite practical.

Figure 35-3 illustrates three controlled clinical trials conducted in our department. Their design schema contains some of the patient-centered endpoints discussed above and demonstrates the relevance of an endpoint within the design structure of a trial.

Figure 35-4 illustrates relevant endpoints for three different animal experiments. In the first experiment we tried to determine if helium gas impaired intestinal blood supply less than CO_2, in endoscopic surgery (tested on pigs). The relevant endpoints are the intestinal blood supply and energy changes in the mucosal cells. The second experiment tested whether a liver from a non-heartbeating donor can be used after corresponding

The Clinical Experiment

A. Pelvic Pouch vs Ileostomy after Total Colectomy

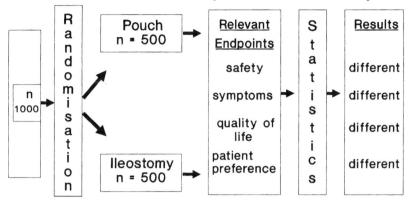

B.
Hunt-Lawrence-Rodino-Pouch vs Oesophagojejunostomy after Total Gastrectomy

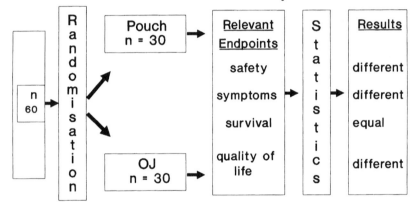

C. Lichtenstein vs Endoscopic Repair of Inguinal Hernia

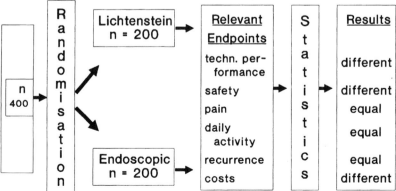

Figure 35-3A–C.   The design of three different controlled clinical trials showing the relevant endpoints within the design.

The Animal Experiment

A.   Helium less danger in haemodynamic

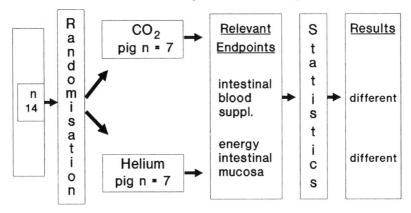

B. O_2-Persufflation vs Cold Ischemia

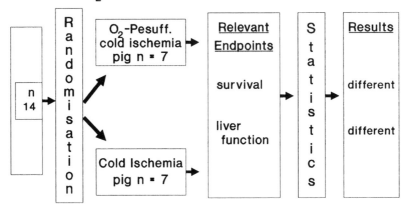

C.   Bacterial translocation reduced by Sucralfat
in hemorrhagic shock

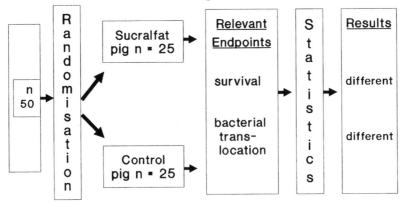

Figure 35-4A–C.   The design of 3 different controlled animal experiments.

Table 35-5.   Selected measures for assessing pain.

Authors	Measure	Dimensions included	Rater	Time	Validity[a]	Reliability[a]	Comments
Huskisson 1974[27]	Visual analogue scale	Intensity	Patient	30 seconds	XXX	XX	Widely used clinically and in research
Melzack 1975[28]	Verbal 5-point rating scale	Intensity	Patient	<1 minute	X	X	May be as useful as entire MPQ[34]
Melzack 1975[28]	McGill Pain Questionnaire	Sensory; affective evaluative	Patient	15–20 minutes	XX	XX	Useful for chronic and acute pain
Melzack 1987[29]	Short-Form McGill Pain Questionnaire	Sensory; affective evaluative	Patient	5–10 minutes	XX	XX	Useful when MPQ takes too long
Pilowski et al. 1983[30]	Illness Behavior Questionnaire	Emotional/ behavioral responses to pain	Patient	15–20 minutes	XX	XX	Used with coronary by-pass patients[35]
Black and Chapman 1976[31]	SAD Index	Somatic, anxiety & depressive response to pain	Physician		X	X	Useful only as a clinical tool
Tursky et al. 1982[32]	Pain perception profile	Intensity; un-pleasantness type	Behavior therapist				Used mainly in research
Zung 1983[33]	Pain and distress scale	Emotional and behavioral responses to pain	Patient	5–10 minutes	XX		Used only with acute pain

[a]X, weak; XX, adequate; XXX, excellent.

Compiled mainly from information contained in McDowell et al.[36]

preparation (O_2 persufflation) for transplantation. Here the appropriate endpoint is survival of the recipient, not just a chemical measurement of liver function. Finally, the third experiment determines whether Sucralfate prevents bacterial translocation and, far more relevant and important, whether it favorably influences survival from hemorrhagic shock.

Symptoms as Relevant Endpoints

Symptoms are important endpoints that may be inadequately assessed if they are fused under too broad an endpoint, such as general well-being.

Failure to probe for a symptom may result in missing a potentially important harbinger of a negative outcome. Alternatively, failure to assess symptoms in a patient "not feeling well" may miss the cause of poor health. Different examiners will be more or less successful in persuading patients to disclose the symptoms.

Symptoms such as anorexia or nausea have to be graded according to their intensity. The problem when looking at isolated symptoms is determining their relationship to well-being in general. Symptoms like dysphagia, nausea, vomiting, loss of appetite, incontinence, impotence, fatigue, and pain may be the relevant endpoints to measure. It is also important to determine how the individual

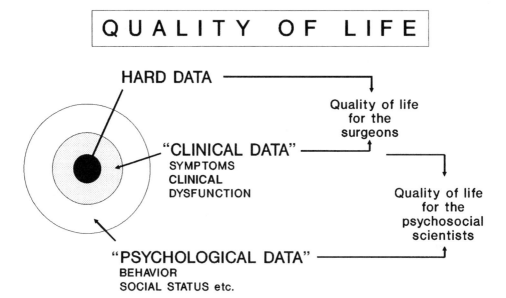

Figure 35-5.   A. Feinstein's drawing modified by H. Troidl approaching the concept of quality of life by combining surgical and psychological aspects.

patient deals with the symptoms and judges his or her own situation.

Symptoms

The intensity of pain and its duration and quality are significant endpoints. Pain is a diagnostic signal, a stressor and at its worst a torment. In many cases pain is the only reason for surgical intervention. Examples of pain as an indication and as an endpoint for successful treatment include biliary colic, pain after herniation of an intervertebral disk, pain of chronic pancreatitis, and so on. Postoperative pain is the endpoint for evaluation of an endoscopic surgical intervention.

Instruments for obtaining detailed information on this endpoint exist:

1. Estimation scales (linear, numeric, verbal)
2. Questionnaires, instruments informing about quality and intensity of pain
3. Dosage of pain killers

Table 35-5 shows several tested instruments for pain measurement.[27-36]

Another important endpoint that has received less attention is the fatigue experienced by patients after surgical interventions. Instruments for determination exist but have not been adequately tested according to the present standards of clinical research. Fatigue has biochemical, physiological, and psychological components. Despite normal muscle function a depressed or fearful patient may still experience fatigue, and muscles impaired by a large incision or by a metabolic disease cannot compensate for fatigue despite a normal or enhanced psychological state.

Physical Functions as an Endpoint

Physical function as an endpoint is generally dominated by the patient's profession, interest, and age. An elderly man may not take up competitive athletic activity after an operation on his knee or hip. Nevertheless, it is important that he be able to carry out his daily activities and interests. A wrist that has not healed in an optimal position after radial fracture may not be a significant problem if it is not painful, but it is a disaster for a musician if the malunion hinders playing his or her musical instrument.

Table 35-6.   Selected health-related quality of life measures.[43–48]

Authors	Dimensions	Response format/rates	Applications	Validity[a]	Reliability[a]	Comments
Spitzer et al. 1981[43]	Daily activities; self care, health; support; outlook	5 items: 0–3 scale/patient, clinician, significant others	Cancer, cardiac transplantation, terminally ill, and ICU patients	XX	XX	Most useful to document net effects of disease and management over time
Padilla et al. 1983[48]	Physical condition, daily activities, personal attitudes	14 items: visual analogue scales/patients	Cancer patients	X	X	Unable to locate usage by other authors
Padilla et al. 1985[48]	Physical, social, physiological well-being; treatment response (surgical)	24 items: visual analogue scale/patient	Colostomy patients	X	X	Unable to locate usage by other authors
Schipper et al. 1984[44]	Daily functioning: symptoms, satisfaction	22 items: 1–7 scale/patient	Cancer patients	XX	XX	Presented on tear sheets to be returned by patients
Priestman & Baum 1976[45]	Physical functioning, physical and physiological symptoms, personal relationships	Variable number of items; visual analogue scale/ patient	Cancer patients	X	X	Extensively used by other investigators
Eypasch et al. 1995[46]	Symptoms, emotions, physical functions, social functions	36 items: 0–3 score points patients	Various benign and malignant GI diseases	XX	XX	Used by other investigators in English and German
Paul et al. 1996[47]	Physical, social, emotional function symptoms; general health	24 items: 5-point Licart scale/ patients	Patients before and after liver transplantation	X	XX	No norms; needs further validation

[a]X, present; XX, strong feature.

Table compiled from information contained in William JI, Wood-Dauphinée S. Assessing quality of life: Measures and utility. In: Quality of Life and Technology Assessment. Mosteller F, Falotico-Tylor J, eds. Washington DC: National Academy Press, 1989; 65–115.[48]

To measure this endpoint, several instruments have been developed. The earliest proposals determined physical fitness with the aid of a scoring system, including push-ups and knee-bends, without considering the patient's age. Physical fitness is an important endpoint for the evaluation of treatment in trauma patients, but it cannot be looked at in isolation. For determining this endpoint in older patients, Sidney Katz developed a "daily activity score" based on six components: bathing, dressing, toileting, transferring, continence, and feeding.[37] The Karnofsky Scale is another pioneer work, developed in 1949, describing physical fitness.[38] This has often been applied in judging physical fitness in carcinoma patients and has an excellent correlation with the well-being and quality of life instruments developed later.

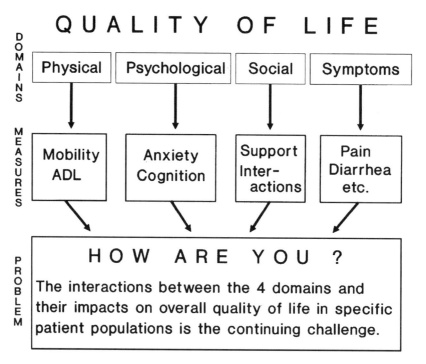

Figure 35-6. The four domains of well-being that may be measured to assess overall quality of life.

Well-Being as an Endpoint

Overall quality of life is the most difficult endpoint to assess. To maintain and improve well-being and quality of life is the ancient approach of medical treatment. For more than 20 years I have followed discussions on the definition, measurement, and feasibility of quality of life assessments.[39–42] My colleagues in the fight for quality of life assessments in the early days were Walter Spitzer, Jack McPeek, Martin McKneally, later Sharon Wood-Dauphinee, Jack Williams, and still later Monika Bullinger, and my present co-workers Ernst Eypasch, Andreas Paul, and Lothar Köhler. Since that time the situation has changed; the topic is now discussed.

The main source of the resistance and skepticism toward quality of life as an endpoint in clinical research lies in our focus on measurability in disease and health. Ignorance, indifference, and preoccupation with the fads and fetishes of measurement have impeded understanding and development of approaches to describe quality of life

with some degree of realism. In 1986 at the Sintra symposium we tried to develop a definition or a reasonable summary of quality of life. Feinstein (see Figure 35-5) summarized the average approach of clinicians and the similarly isolated approach of psychologists, and he thoughtfully and enthusiastically offered "How are you?" as a possible solution.

Pragmatists and methodologically oriented members agreed upon the definition as shown in Figure 35-6 as a possible hypothesis for a suitable definition of quality of life. In general, quality of life is sufficiently described by the domains of physical fitness, psychological aspects, social aspects, and symptoms. Still, the problem of interaction between these domains exists. The individual domains can be determined with acceptable objective methods. A number of good instruments for determination of quality of life have been developed, most of them focused on methodology for present clinical research. A general discussion is ongoing between clinicians and epidemiologists related to an "organ-specific" index;[41] it has the

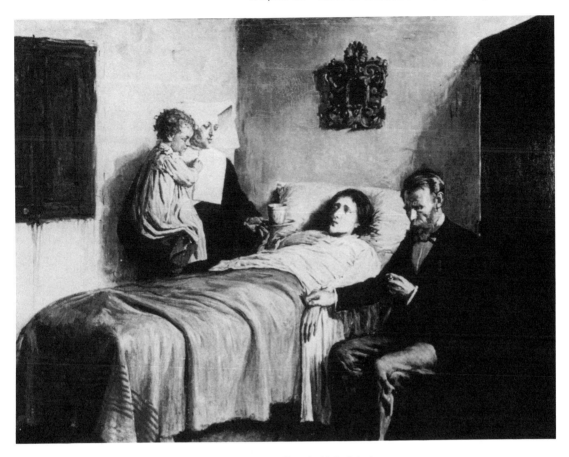

Figure 35-7.   Ciencia Y Caridad.

advantage over global determinations of quality of life of discovering specific symptoms responsible for impaired quality of life that may be treatable. Practicability and sensitivity not only for dying patients, but also for patients in less-advanced stages of disease are important unfilled goals.

Conclusion

We close with the example of organ transplantation. Indications for transplantation of a liver, kidney, lung, heart, or pancreas can be understood more easily if an extremely bad quality of life can be improved. The relevant endpoint in transplantation is often palliation of unacceptable overall quality of life. Quality of life is also the relevant endpoint when treatments offer only small alterations in survival time. Quality of life is a significant endpoint in "trade-offs"; for example, is the

risk of pelvic pouch versus permanent ileostomy worthwhile? Only a quality of life determination can justify the risk of this large, complicated operation for patient and surgeon.

Fortunately, interest in this complex issue is broadening. Newly developed instruments for determining quality of life—not only in carcinomas, but also in diseases of the intestinal organs and transplant surgery—demonstrate this. Table 35-6 shows several important and tested instruments for measuring quality of life.[43–48]

Picasso's painting of "Ciencia y Caridad" (Figure 35-7), which he made at the age of 18, portrays the essence of the medical profession. The nurse with the child stands for "caridad" (care), the physician measuring the pulse represents medical science. After many earlier versions, Picasso evolved this picture dominated by care, with the patient put into the center of the picture. Shouldn't we do the same?

References

1. Wood-Dauphinée S, Troidl H. Endpoints of clinical studies: conventional and innovative variables. In: Troidl H, Spitzer WO, McPeek B, Mulder DS, McKneally MF, eds. Principles and Practice of Research: Strategy for Surgical Investigators, 2nd edn. New York: Springer, 1991, pp. 151–168.
2. Troidl H. Lebensqualität als entscheidendes Kriterium im Alltag und in der Forschung des Chirurgen. Langenbecks Arch Chir Suppl II (Kongreßbericht 1989) 1989;101–107.
3. Feinstein AR. Personal communication, 1986.
4. Goligher JC, Pulvertaft CN, Watkinson G. Controlled trial of vagotomy and antrectomy, and subtotal gastrectomy in elective treatment of duodenal ulcer: interim report. Br Med J 1964;1:455–460.
5. Billroth Th. Über das Lehren und Lernen der Medicinischen Wissenschaften an den Universtäten der Deutschen Nation nebst allgemeinen Bemerkungen über Universitäten. Eine culturhistorische Studie. Wien: Druck und Verlag von Carl Gerold's Sohn, 1876.
6. Jennett B. High Technology Medicine. Benefits and Burdens. Chap.: Technology assessment—a question of information. Oxford: Oxford University, 1986, ch. 9.
7. Popper KR. Personal communication, 1989.
8. Donabedian A. Exploration, in Quality Assessment and Monitoring, vol 3. The Methods and Finding of Quality of Assessment and Monitoring and Illustrated Analysis. Ann Arbor: Health Administration, 1985, pp. 256.
9. Wulff HK, Pedersen StA, Rodenberg R, eds. Philosophy of Medicine: An introduction. Oxford: Blackwell Scientific, 1986.
10. Descartes R. Von der Methode des richtigen Vernunftsgebrauchs und der wissenschaftlichen Forschung. Hamburg: Felix Meixner, 1960.
11. Feinstein AR. Clinical biostatistics. XLI. Hard science, soft data, and the challenges of choosing clinical variables in research. Clin Pharmacol Ther 1977;22:485–498.
12. Miller AB, Hoogstraten B, Staquet M, Winkler A. Reporting results of cancer treatment. Cancer 1981;47:207–214.
13. Spitzer WO. Personal communication, 1986.
14. Bailar JC, Smith EM. Progress against cancer? New Engl J Med 1986;314:1226–1232.
15. Lorenz W. Personal communication, 1996.
16. Small WP, Krause U. An introduction to clinical research. Edinburgh, London: Churchill Livingstone, 1972.
17. Kuhn TS. Die Struktur wissenschaftlicher Revolutionen. Frankfurt: Suhrkamp, 1976.
18. Feinstein AR. Clinimetric perspectives. (The Portugal Conference: Measuring Quality of Life and Functional Status in Clinical and Epidemiological Research). J Chronic Dis 1987;40:635–640.
19. Turner JA, Deyo RA, Loeser JD, Korff MV, Fordyce WE. The importance of placebo effects in pain treatment and research. JAMA 1994;271:1609–1614.
20. Palcedo-Wasicek M, Thirlby RC. Postoperative course after inguinal herniorrhaphy. A case-controlled comparison of patients receiving workers' compensation vs. patients with commercial insurance. Arch Surgeon 1995;30:29–32.
21. Troidl H, Kusche J, Vestweber K-H, Eypsch E, Maul U. Pouch versus oeophagojejunostomy after total gastrectomy. World J Surg 1987;11:699–712.
22. Riedel R. Personal communication, 1996.
23. White KL. Improved medical care statistics and health services system. Public Health Rep 1967;82:847–854.
24. Troidl H. The philosophy of patient-friendly surgery. In: RD Rosin, ed. Minimal Access—Medicine and Surgery. Principles and Techniques. Oxford: Radcliffe Medical, 1993, 10–21.
25. Rutkow IM. Beyond the scalpel. The importance of socioeconomic issues in surgical outcomes: what is a relevant end point? Eur J Surg 1995;161:545–548.
26. Troidl H, Spangenberger W, Dietrich A, Neugebauer E. Laparoskopische cholezystektomie. Erste Erfahrungen und Ergebnisse bei 300 Operationen: eine prospektive Beobachtungsstudie. Chirurg 1991;62:257–265.
27. Huskisson EC. Measurement of pain. Lancet 1974;2:1127–1131.
28. Melzack R. The McGill Pain Questionnaire: major properties and scoring methods. Pain 1975;1:277–299.
29. Melzack R. The Short-Form McGill Questionnaire. Pain 1987;30:191–197.
30. Pilowsky I, Spence ND. Manual for the Illness Behavior Questionnaire (IBQ), 2nd edn. Adelaide, Australia: University of Adelaide, 1983.
31. Black RG, Chapman CR. SAD Index for clinical

assessment of pain. In: Bonica JJ, Albe-Fessard D, eds. Advances in Pain Research and Therapy, vol 1. New York: Raven, 1976:301–305.

32. Tursky B, Jammer LD, Friedman R. The Pain Perception Profile: a psychological approach to the assessment of pain report. Behav Ther 1982;13:376–394.

33. Zung WWK. A self-rating pain and distress scale. Psychosomatics 1983;24:887–894.

34. Finch L, Melzack R. Objective pain measurement: a case for increased clinical usage. Physiother Can 1982;34:343–346.

35. Pilowsky I, Spence ND, Waddy JL. Illness behavior and coronary artery bypass surgery. J Psychosom Res 1979;23:39–44.

36. McDowell I, Newell C. Measuring Health. A Guide to Rating Scales and Questionnaires. New York: Oxford University, 1987, pp. 229–268.

37. Katz S, Ford AB, Moskowitz RW, Jackson BA, Jaffe MW, Cleveland MA. Studies of illness in the aged. The index of ADL: a standardized measure of biological and psychosocial function. JAMA 1963;185:914–919.

38. Karnofsky DA, Burchenal JH. Clinical evaluation of chemotherapeutic agents in cancer. In: Macleod CM, ed. Evaluation of Chemotherapeutic Agents. New York: Columbia University, 1949, pp. 191–205.

39. Troidl H, Menge K-H, Lorenz W, Vestweber K-H, Barth H, Hamelmann H. Quality of life and stomach replacement. In: Herfarth CH, Schlag P, eds. Gastric Cancer. Berlin: Springer, 1979, pp. 312–317.

40. Troidl H, Kusche J. Lebensqualität nach Gastrektomie: Ergebnisse einer randomisierten Studie zum Vergleich Oesophago-Jejunostomie nach Schlatter mit dem Hunt-Laurence-Rodino Pouch. In: Rohde H, Troidl H, eds. Das Magenkarzinom. Methodik klinischer Studien und therapeutischer Ansätze. Stuttgart: Thieme, 1984.

41. Troidl H, Kusche J, Vestweber KH, Eypasch E, Koeppen L, Bouillon B. Quality of life: An important endpoint both in surgical practice and research. J Chron Dis 1987; 40:523–528.

42. Troidl H. Lebensqualität: ein relevantes Zielkriterium in der Chirurgie. Chirurg 1989;60:445–449.

43. Spitzer WO, Dobson AJ, Hall J, Chesterman E, Levi J, Shepherd R, Battista RN, Catchlove BR. Measuring the quality of life of cancer patients. A concise QL-Index of quality of life of cancer patients. A concise QL-Index for use by physicians. J Chronic Dis 1981;34:585–597.

44. Schipper H, Clinch J, McMurray A, Levitt M. Measuring the quality of life of cancer patients. The Functional Living Index-Cancer: development and validation. J Clin Oncol 1984;2:472–483.

45. Priestman TJ, Baum M. Evaluation of quality of life in patients receiving treatment for advanced breast cancer. Lancet 1976;2:899–901.

46. Eypasch E, Williams JI, Wood-Dauphinée S, Ure BM, Schmülling C, Neugebauer E, Troidl H. The Gastrointestinal Quality of Life Index (GIQLI): development, validation and application of a new instrument. Br J Surg 1995;82:216–222.

47. Paul A, Willimas JI, Greig P, Levy GA. Development of a Liver Disease–Specific Quality of Life Index. (In press.)

48. Williams JI, Wood-Dauphinée S. Assessing quality of life: measures and utility. In: Mosteller F, Falotico-Taylor J, eds. Quality of Life and Technology Assessment. Washington, DC: National Academy, 1989, pp. 65–115.

CHAPTER 36

Introductory Biostatistics Texts: Selected Annotated Bibliography

F. Mosteller and B. Rosner

When asked to prepare this bibliography, we selected a few books based upon our personal knowledge. We performed a computer search in the American Statistical Association Institute of Mathematical Statistics Current Index of Statistics to identify reviews of these books and used the reviews to help produce the comments included below. The purpose is to give the potential consumer a quick overview of the contents, orientation, and special features of several texts in biostatistics.

In addition to the full reference, we have indicated the pages of appendices, tables, and other materials.

We indicate the intended audience, where the examples and problem materials come from, the extent of tables, how computing is handled, and special features. This list may be helpful as a starting point for choosing books for a library or for a course of study.

Armitage P, Berry G. *Statistical Methods in Medical Research,* 3rd edn. London: Blackwell Scientific, 1994, pp. 558 + xi + Tables 22 + References 14 + Index 26.

Audience. "This book is intended to be useful both for the medical research worker with no particular mathematical expertise but with the ability to follow straightforward formulae and for the professional statistician interested in medical application" (p. ix). "Statisticians engaged in medical work or interested in medical applications will, we hope, find many points of interest in this review of the subject. In particular, the book may provide a useful framework for the teaching of courses for students trained in medical or biological science. Much of the exposition and many of the examples are based on material used in courses for postgraduate students in the medical sciences" (p. xi).

Chapter titles.

1. The Scope of Statistics
2. Probability
3. Sampling
4. Statistical Inference
5. Regression and Correlation
6. The Planning of Statistical Investigations
7. Comparison of Several Groups
8. Further Experimental Designs
9. Further Analysis of Straight Line Data
10. Multiple Measurements
11. Data Editing
12. Further Analysis of Categorical Data
13. Distribution-Free Methods
14. Survival Analysis
15. Sequential Methods
16. Statistical Methods in Epidemiology
17. Biological Assay
18. Statistical Computation

Examples and problems. Examples are selected almost entirely from real medical research problems, which are a strength of the book. There are no problems, which is a drawback for the purpose of classroom use.

Computing. Computer packages are not explicitly used in the book. Chapter 18 is concerned with statistical computation and summarizes some of the major statistical packages, each in about one paragraph.

Tables. There are ten tables that include the standard tables used in basic statistical inference as well as two special tables concerned with sample size for comparing two proportions, and sample sizes for detecting relative risk in a case control study.

Special features. This book is more comprehensive than most elementary books on biostatistics. It contains some topics that might ordinarily be found in intermediate-level specialty biostatistics books, such as generalized linear models, sequential methods, experimental design, Bayesian methods, and methods for longitudinal data. One of the great strengths of the book is its ability to give the reader an informed glimpse on an introductory level at these more advanced topics, without requiring that the reader be familiar with these specialty areas. Another strength of the book is its fine use of real examples throughout, although the examples are usually presented as excerpts from a study without giving the big picture as to what the study is about. One drawback of the book is that, although little mathematics is used, it is written on a higher level than most other elementary biostatistics books.

Colton T. *Statistics in Medicine.* Boston: Little Brown, 1974, pp. 352 + xii + answers 22 + tables 9 + references 5 + index 12.

Audience. "This book enunciates the principles of statistics for the present or future practicing physician . . . to arm the reader with sufficient statistical expertise so that he can critically evaluate an author's presentation, analysis, and interpretation of data" (p. vii).

Chapter titles.

1. Rationale for Statistics in Medicine

Part I. Fundamentals

2. Descriptive Statistics
3. Probability

Part II. Statistical Inference

4. Inference on Means

5. Inference on Proportions
6. Regression and Correlation*
7. Nonparametric Methods
8. Sequential Analysis
9. Longitudinal Studies and Use of the Life Table

Part III. Statistics in Medical Research

10. Clinical Trials
11. Medical Surveys
12. Fallacies in Numerical Reasoning
13. Critical Reading of the Medical Literature

Examples. Drawn from medical and epidemiological research and practice.

Problem material. Drawn from practical work, about 60 problems composed of 155 parts.

Computing. Not treated.

Tables. Standard statistical tables for the normal, t, χ^2, rank correlation, and a few nonparametric tests.

Special features. Discussion of fallacies.

Daniel WW. *Biostatistics: A Foundation for Analysis in the Health Sciences,* 6th edn. New York: Wiley, 1995, pp. 645 + x + appendices 112 + answers to odd-numbered exercises 18 + index 4.

Audience. "The sixth edition of *Biostatistics: A Foundation for Analysis in the Health Sciences* should appeal to the same audience for which the first five editions were written: advanced undergraduate students, beginning graduate students, and health professionals in need of a reference book on statistical methodology" (p. vii).

Chapter titles.

1. Introduction to Biostatistics
2. Descriptive Statistics
3. Some Basic Probability Concepts
4. Probability Distributions
5. Some Important Sampling Distributions
6. Estimation
7. Hypothesis Testing
8. Analysis of Variance
9. Simple Linear Regression and Correlation
10. Multiple Regression and Correlation

---

*Multiple regression and logistic regression are not treated except for a two-page mathematical discussion about extending simple linear regression.

11. Regression Analysis—Some Additional Techniques
12. The Chi-Square Distribution and the Analysis of Frequencies
13. Nonparametric and Distribution-Free Statistics
14. Vital Statistics

Examples and problems. There are a total of 715 problems. The problems are organized at the end of specific sections as well as in the form of review exercises at the end of a chapter. There are a few problems at the end of many of the chapters that make use of the 20 computer datasets on the data disk that comes with the book. The examples and problems are sometimes from the medical or biological literature and in some cases are fictitious problems. Answers are supplied to the odd-numbered exercises at the end of the book.

Computing. MINITAB output is used through the book. SAS output also appears for the first time in the sixth edition. In addition, an appendix with some MINITAB commands is given at the end of the book. In some cases the author also indicates specific MINITAB commands in the text to carry out particular types of analyses.

Tables. There are 16 tables available, which cover the standard tables used for basic statistical inference. The tables for nonparametric methods are more detailed than one finds in most introductory texts.

Special features. The book spans traditional topics in introductory courses. The book is very strong on nonparametric methods, but somewhat weak on methods used in epidemiologic studies. There is a chapter on vital statistics, which is very brief and does not include some topics of current interest such as the log rank test or the Cox model. The large number of exercises makes the book appealing for classroom use.

Ingelfinger JA, Mosteller F, Thibodeau LA, Ware JH. *Biostatistics in Clinical Medicine,* 3rd edn. New York: McGraw-Hill, 1994, pp. 360 + xxv + additional problems 4 + solutions to odd-numbered problems 14 + tables and charts 30 + index 10.

Audience. "This book prepares physicians to understand probability and statistics and apply them to the care of the individual patient. . . . We em-phasize their use in problems of diagnosis, treatment, and follow-up" (p. xxi).

Chapter titles.

1. Diagnostic Testing: Introduction to Probability
2. Diagnostic Testing: Likelihood and Odds
3. Screening for Breast Cancer. Guidance from Decision Trees
4. Has the Treatment Helped the Patient? Intrasubject and Intersubject Variability
5. Blood Pressure and Hypertension: Distribution and Variability
5A. Ideas of Exploratory Data Analysis: Reanalyzing an Exercise Dataset
6. Assessing Treatment Efficacy by Analyzing Counts
7. What are P Values?
8. What is Chi-Square?
9. Regression: an Overview
9A. More about Regression: A Closer Look at the Regression of Glomular Filtration Rate on Plasma Creatinine
9B. Introduction to Multiple Regression
10. The Management of Stable Angina: Interpreting Life Tables
11. Reading a Report of a Clinical Trial
12. Applying a Clinical Trial
13. Reading a Report of an Epidemiological Study
14. Using Meta-Analysis for Research Synthesis: Pooling Data from Several Studies

Examples and exercises. Almost all examples and exercises are based on data from medical research studies. There are 152 problems composed of 216 parts.

Tables and charts. Tables for the normal, t, binomial, binomial confidence limits, Poisson, F, Poisson confidence limits, χ^2, binomial ($p = 1/2$), and random digits and binomial confidence charts.

Computing. Shows printout from computed regression.

Special features. Each principal chapter contains at least one detailed clinical problem with associated quantitative methods leading to interpretations and solutions. Chapter 14 gives an overview of research synthesis.

Pagano M, Gauvreau K. *Principles of Biostatistics.* Belmont, California: Wadsworth, 1993. pp. 481 + ix + tables 20 + datasets 10 + solutions to selected exercises 8 + index 3.

Audience. "This book was written for students of the health sciences and serves as an introduction to the study of biostatistics—the use of numerical techniques to extract information from data and fact" (p. vii). "Principles of Biostatistics is aimed at the student who wishes to learn modern research methods. It is based on a required course offered at the Harvard School of Public Health. A large number of health professionals in the rest of the Harvard medical area attend as well" (p. vii).

Chapter titles.

1. Introduction
2. Data Presentation
3. Numerical Summary Measures
4. Rates and Standardization
5. Life Tables
6. Probability
7. Theoretical Probability Distributions
8. Sampling Distribution of the Mean
9. Confidence Intervals
10. Hypothesis Testing
11. Comparison of Two Means
12. Analysis of Variance
13. Nonparametric Methods
14. Inference on Proportions
15. Contingency Tables
16. Multiple 2×2 Tables
17. Correlation
18. Simple Linear Regression
19. Multiple Regression
20. Logistic Regression
21. Survival Analysis
22. Sampling Theory

Examples and problems. The author states, "Throughout the text we have used data drawn from published studies to exemplify biostatistical concepts. Not only is real data more meaningful, it is usually more interesting as well. . . . To this end, we have been guided by the backgrounds and interests of our students—mostly public health and clinical research—to choose examples that best illustrate the concepts at hand" (p. viii). There are 113 exercises, some with multiple parts. So-lutions are provided for selected exercises (approximately half).

Computing. There are 12 datasets listed in the appendix, which are also provided on a data disk that accompanies each copy of the book. Most of the datasets contain a few columns of specific variables without any specific context of the studies from which the data is derived. Some of the exercises make use of these datasets. The course that the book is derived from uses Stata, which is the package used to display results of some of the examples in the text, although the datasets can be accessed by any statistical package. No specific guidance is provided on statistical computing techniques.

Tables. There are six tables covering standard tests of significance and nonparametric tests.

Special features. At the end of each chapter is a section on further applications, which provides a few additional examples for discussion.

Rosner B. *Fundamentals of Biostatistics,* 4th edn. Belmont, California: Wadsworth, 1995, pp. 631 + xi + tables 27 + answers to selected problems 5 + flowchart: methods of statistical inference 5 + index 7 + index of applications 4.

Audience: "I have written this introductory-level biostatistics text for upper-level undergraduate or graduate students interested in medicine or other health-related areas" (p. iii). "The material in this book is suitable for either a one- or two-semester course in biostatistics. The material in Chapters 1 through 8 and Chapter 10 is suitable for a one semester course. The instructor may select appropriate material from the other chapters as time permits" (p. iii).

Chapter titles.

1. General Overview
2. Descriptive Statistics
3. Probability
4. Discrete Probability Distributions
5. Continuous Probability Distributions
6. Estimation
7. Hypothesis Testing: One-Sample Inference
8. Hypothesis Testing: Two-Sample Inference
9. Multisample Inference
10. Hypothesis Testing: Categorical Data
11. Regression and Correlation Methods

12. Nonparametric Methods
13. Hypothesis Testing: Person-Time Data

Examples and problems. "Most examples and exercises used in this book are either based on actual articles from the literature or on actual medical research problems that I have encountered during my consulting experience at the Harvard Medical School" (p. iii). "Every new concept is developed systematically through completely worked out examples from current medical research problems" (p. iii). There are a total of 900 problems in the text. An additional 700 problems are available in a study guide that is an ancillary text that students can purchase to supplement the text. Approximately 300 problems are solved in the back of the book. Complete solutions are provided for all problems in the study guide. An Index of Applications provides an index by medical subspeciality of the examples and problems in the text.

Computing. A data disk accompanies the text with 20 datasets that are used for the computer-based problems in the text (of which there are approximately 150). The datasets are available both in ASCII and MINITAB format. In addition, computer output in MINITAB, SAS, and SPSS is provided illustrating the methods throughout the book. However, no specific instructions are given for how to use these packages.

Tables. There are 15 tables in the text, which cover most of the standard distributions used in routine statistical inference. In addition, a few special tables are concerned with exact confidence limits for the binomial and Poisson distribution and tables for outlier detection methods.

Special features. A special feature of the book is the quality and quantity of the examples and problems. The datasets in some cases are based on entire datasets from real studies rather than excerpts from a few selected variables. The scientific questions posed by the datasets have their own substantive interest. There is also a flow-chart of methods of statistical inference that unifies the methods covered through the book. A case study is discussed throughout the book to illustrate different statistical methods. The book can serve both as an introductory text as well as a reference book. Some special topics include power and sample size in many different con-

texts, intraclass correlation coefficient, the cross-over design, analysis of incidence rate data, and outlier detection methods.

Woolson RF. *Statistical Methods for the Analysis of Biomedical Data.* New York: John Wiley & Sons, 1987, pp. 464 + xx + tables 43 + index 5.

Audience. ". . . two audiences in mind. First, the book may fill the needs of medical researchers who would like to reference a book that is more substantial than an introductory biostatistics text. Second, . . . as a text book for an introduction sequence in biostatistics, particularly for majors in biostatistics and statistics. . . . As a text book for a biostatistics program, the book would be suited to those students who are pursuing a master's degree" (p. vii).

Chapter titles.

1. Introduction
2. Descriptive Statistics
3. Basic Probability Concepts
4. Further Aspects of Probability for Statistical Inference: Sampling, Probability Distributions, and Sampling Distributions
5. Confidence Intervals and Hypothesis Testing: General Considerations and Applications
6. Comparison of Two Groups: *t*-Tests and Rank Tests
7. Comparison of Two Groups: Chi-Square and Related Procedures
8. Tests of Independence and Measures of Association for Two Random Variables
9. Least-Squares Regression Methods: Predicting One Variable from Another
10. Comparing More Than Two Groups of Observations: Analysis of Variance for Comparing Groups
11. Comparing More Than Two Groups of Observations: Rank Analysis of Variance for Group Comparisons
12. Comparing More Than Two Groups of Observations: Chi-Square and Related Procedures
13. Special Topics in Analysis of Epidemiological and Clinical Data: Studying Association Between a Disease and a Characteristic

14. Examination and Comparison of Survival Curves

Examples and problems. Many of the examples are drawn from real-life biological or medical data, as are some of the problems. Citations to the original research simplifies follow-up. There are 114 problems, some of which have many parts.

Computing. The author shows tables that might appear as printouts. The regression chapter ends with a paragraph about SAS and BMDP. The analysis of variance chapter closes with more than half of a page devoted to statistical software. Other chapters provide similar brief discussions.

Tables. The appendix provides 16 tables covering random digits, the binomial and Poisson distributions, the usual normal, t, χ^2, F distributions, charts for binomial confidence limits, and tables for various nonparametric methods.

Special features. The parametric tests and the nonparametric tests are presented in parallel.

In addition to the textual description of the various methods, the author provides handy outlines associated with a technique indicating the kind of data, assumptions, and computations, and in hypothesis testing gives the various hypotheses and the decision rules associated with them. Then an associated table gives a worked example following the layout. Additional examples sometimes illustrate several approaches or situations.

Richard G. Cornell alerts us to a notational trap in designating the degrees of freedom for the t distribution. The $(n - 1)$ in the confidence limits $\bar{X} \pm t_{1-\alpha/2}(n - 1)s/\sqrt{n}$ is not a multiplier but indexes the degrees of freedom (p. 121).

Zar JH. *Biostatistical Analysis*, **3rd edn. Upper Saddle River, New Jersey: Prentice Hall, 1996, pp. 662 + x + appendices 205 + answers 11 + references 19 + index 21.**

Audience. "First, it has served as an introductory text book, assuming no prior knowledge of statistics. Secondly, it has functioned as a reference work, covering a sufficient variety of concepts and procedures to satisfy a large portion of the biological disciplines that require statistical analysis, and being consulted long after formal instruction has ended" (p. ix).

Chapter titles.

1. Introduction
2. Populations and Samples
3. Measures of Central Tendency
4. Measures of Dispersion and Variability
5. Probabilities
6. The Normal Distribution
7. One-Sample Hypotheses
8. Two-Sample Hypotheses
9. Paired-Sample Hypotheses
10. Multisample Hypothesis: The Analysis of Variance
11. Multiple Comparisons
12. Two-Factor Analysis of Variance
13. Data Transformations
14. Multiway Factorial Analysis of Variance
15. Nested (Hierarchical) Analysis of Variance
16. Simple Linear Regression
17. Comparing Simple Linear Regression Equations
18. Simple Linear Correlation
19. Multiple Regression and Correlation
20. Polynomial Regression
21. Testing Goodness of Fit
22. Contingency Tables
23. More on Dichotomous Variables
24. Testing for Randomness
25. Circular Distributions: Descriptive Statistics
26. Circular Distributions: Hypothesis Testing

Examples and problems. The author states that the data in the examples and exercises are largely fictional and intended to illustrate statistical, not biological, principles (p. x). There are about 159 exercises composed of 293 parts. The illustrations come from many biological disciplines, not primarily from medicine.

Computing. Occasionally, printouts of computer output are produced for illustration. Appendix A gives advice about the appropriate comparisons for F-ratios and degrees of freedom associated with the analysis of variance.

Tables. Forty-one tables cover the usual tests of significance plus nonparametric tests, including runs and tests associated with data distributed on a circle.

Special features. The author provides many historical remarks about the inventors of statistical techniques. A strength of the book is in its encyclopedic coverage of many topics including some rarely seen in introductory books, such as tests for randomness, extensive handling of analysis of variance, and circular distributions.

Commentary

The editors chose not to include a "primer chapter" on statistics in this edition, but rather asked the dean of American statisticians to guide us through a spectrum of currently available textbooks on statistical methods that might be helpful to the surgical researcher. The reader will find the chapter an insightful critique of existing textbooks on biostatistics that is easy to read. Based on reviews culled from a survey of the American Statistical Association Institute of Mathematical Statistics Current Index of Statistics, this chapter will allow researchers to select a book based on their level of training and needs, and to find out where to go for more information.

My personal favorite of the textbooks evaluated is the book by Ingelfinger, et al., entitled *Biosta-*

tistics in Clinical Medicine. It provides a broad array of well-illustrated information and the basic methodology a surgeon-investigator needs to assess most clinical data. It is reader friendly, and each chapter contains at least one detailed problem illustrating the application of biostatistic methodology.

Professor McPeek, reminding us that the field of biostatistics is a well established, free-standing discipline, makes the point that "a surgeon partially informed in statistical methodology can be almost as dangerous as a statistician attempting an appendectomy after 6 months' exposure to surgical teaching." He counsels working with the statistician as a two-way consultation, as emphasized in Moses's chapter (chapter 39). These chapters, combined with practical surgical examples and advice from Olak and Chiu (chapter 37), will help the reader to become an informed consumer and more effective collaborator in biostatistical methodology.

D.S.M.

CHAPTER 37

A Surgeon's Guide to Biostatistical Inferences: How to Avoid Pitfalls

J. Olak and R.C.-J. Chiu

In this last decade of the twentieth century, surgeons are finding themselves making decisions based on statistical analyses. These analyses appear regularly in professional journals and scientific presentations, but they are also used by governments and insurance companies in the formulation of health care policy documents. Mass media may disseminate this information, often ignoring serious pitfalls associated with the statistical methods used to reach the conclusions published. The consumer generally assumes that the statistical tests used in peer-reviewed journal articles are appropriate. It has been estimated, however, that up to two-thirds of the studies appearing in some of the best medical journals contain statistical errors or unwarranted conclusions.[1,2] In order to critically appraise this information, some understanding of biostatistical methods and their constraints has become essential. Education to enable surgeons to do so is being incorporated into the training of future surgeons and will be a valuable part of the continuing education of practicing surgeons. This chapter is intended to contribute to this effort, building on the information provided in earlier chapters.

In addition to understanding methodological issues and their pitfalls, surgeons need to interpret results in a clinical context. Some experts feel that there has been an unnecessary shift in emphasis from reporting raw data to hypothesis testing, increasing the risk of equating statistical significance with clinical relevance.[3–5] For example, some studies report clinical outcomes using endpoints that are sensitive but of no proven *clinical* significance.[6]

Today the randomized prospective clinical trial is thought to be the gold standard method for the evaluation of the effectiveness of diagnostic or therapeutic interventions. It is felt to provide the best evidence of cause and effect.[7] It is also the most expensive type of trial to conduct.

> **CLUE: Beware of the paper that attempts to establish a cause and effect relationship on the basis of a retrospective or cross-sectional study. This is best established within the context of a randomized clinical trial.[8]**

Trial methodology has evolved substantially since the first randomized prospective clinical trials were published 30 years ago.[9] The strength of this approach lies in the similarity between control and treatment groups, resulting from the random allocation of patients to these groups. Historical observational studies achieve a higher rate of statistical significance than randomized trials. This is usually attributable to the fact that the control groups do more poorly in these studies, and this, in turn, relates to the difficulty in eliminating selection bias whenever random allocation of subjects is not practiced.[10] Unexplained variability among historical groups might account, to some extent, for this phenomenon as well. It is not always possible, however, to perform a randomized clinical trial in order to answer a surgical question. The reasons for this are manifold. For example, the condition under question might be so rare that it would take an unacceptable amount of time to complete a trial. On the other hand, the cost of a trial when weighed against the importance of the question might be prohibitive and thereby preclude its being done. Finally, it might not be considered ethical to withhold therapy from a control group if, for example, the disease of interest is uniformly fatal.

This chapter will discuss comparability of study groups, prognostic stratification, randomization, the issue of sample size, and *p*-values. It will also address the difference between positive and negative trials, as well as the difference between statistical and clinical significance. Statistical comparisons of two treatment strategies are meaningful only when they can detect *clinically* important differences.

This chapter will also address confidence intervals, statistical power, and survival statistics including life-table methods, regression, proportional hazards, correlation, and decision analysis. Meta-analysis will be discussed in a subsequent chapter.

Evaluation of Study Groups

The first paragraph of the results section of a typical journal article usually describes the study groups in terms of demographic characteristics and prognostic factors. This enables the reader to verify whether the groups were sufficiently similar to one another. It is important to establish similarity of study groups, since all tests of statistical significance are predicated on the supposition that the study groups are drawn randomly from the population. Of course, this is strictly true only in properly randomized clinical trials.[7] It does not mean that the results of tests of statistical significance are not otherwise accurate, but rather that they should be interpreted with caution. The *level* of significance reported and the *generalizability* of the result to the population can be affected by the failure to randomly allocate patients to the different treatment arms.

In randomized trials it is not necessary to *prove* that control and treatment groups are similar to one another by testing for statistically significant differences between them. It is considered sufficient to report the absolute number of subjects with each pertinent variable in table form. In nonrandomized trials it is particularly important to check for imbalance between study groups because bias may enter into the selection of a particular patient for one treatment arm as opposed to the other. If an imbalance between groups with respect to a particular variable is apparent, a single test of statistical significance should be performed to determine its potential for impacting on the results.[8] In addition, a look back at how the patients were accrued to the study might illustrate that selection bias could be influencing the results.

If the surgeon suspects that not all eligible patients were offered participation in the study, selection bias may indeed be acting. In a truly randomized study, the authors should indicate not only how many patients were ultimately randomized, but how many otherwise eligible patients did not participate and the reasons for failure to participate. For example, an individual patient may not have been made aware of the study. The surgeon may have felt the patient to be higher risk, lower risk, or otherwise unacceptable for the study, or may have forgotten about the study. The referring doctor might have requested a particular approach for the patient. The reader must judge based upon the information provided whether or not selection bias might be acting and to what extent it may affect the generalizability of the results to patients.

There are three questions that a wary reader should be able to answer to ensure that the data are correctly summarized: (1) Do the numbers add up, that is, are all patients accounted for with regard to each parameter reported? (2) Are the observations counted correctly? Just because multiple observations are made on a treatment group does not mean that the sample size increases. (3) Are the baseline variables similar among control and treatment groups?[8]

Stratification for prognostic variables should be sought because it is much more meaningful when patients are stratified prior to randomization (a priori) in a study rather than performing subgroup analyses at the end. In the former instance, the investigators anticipated a difference in response between subgroups defined by a particular attribute and attempted to ensure that equal numbers of patients with that attribute were randomized to each treatment arm; whereas, in the latter instance, the investigator found a difference in response rates and elected to analyze the data according to subgroups after the fact (a posteriori). For example, in a study of antibiotic prophylaxis in surgical patients, one might anticipate a difference in wound infection rates in diabetics when compared to nondiabetics and stratify for the presence of diabetes *before* randomization to ensure equal numbers of diabetics in each group. Subgroup analysis, on the other hand, can be both informative and potentially misleading.[11] The strength of inference regarding a proposed difference in treatment effect among subgroups is dependent on several factors. If the magnitude of the difference would not impact on clinical decision making, subgroup analysis is not useful. In addition, the performance of separate significance tests on different subgroups increases the likelihood of obtaining a statistically significant difference by chance alone and thus may not provide direct evidence that a prognostic factor affects the observed difference.[12] In this instance, a test for interaction can be performed and is a valid method of assessing the relationship between the variable and treatment response. If the authors anticipated a differential treatment effect, subgroup analysis has more credibility than the post-hoc finding of an effect for which they might be accused of data dredging. The finding of a differential treatment effect in a second separate study adds to its credibility as well. Finally, a differential treatment effect that makes biological sense is even more plausible.[11]

CLUE: Be careful not to overinterpret data that have been subjected to multiple subgroup analyses. Subgroups may be of very different size (n), and the p-values associated with subgroup analysis must be taken within the context of each group's size. Beware of the study whose primary outcome is not statistically significant but reports a series of secondary outcomes, some of which are significant: if you perform enough tests of statistical significance, you increase the likelihood of obtaining a positive result due to chance alone.

Only rarely is the effect of an intervention really confined to one subgroup of patients. Without a positive test for interaction, the factor being assessed is unlikely to profoundly influence the outcome.[12] Stratified randomization can be used to reduce the risk of having any imbalance in prognostic factors.

It is important to ascertain whether or not all patients who entered the study are accounted for in the results section. If the number of dropouts or withdrawals was high overall or disproportionately high in one treatment arm, a significance test should be performed to ascertain whether or not this created inequality between control and treatment groups because this might impact on the validity of the study. For example, in a comparison of two drugs for the treatment of hypertension, one drug might result in a disproportionately high incidence of undesirable side effects, resulting in more patient withdrawals from that treatment arm and thereby create an imbalance between control and treatment groups. It is likewise important to be assured that there were equal numbers of observations made on each subject studied. For example, if a researcher reports on the antihypertensive effect of two drugs 1 hour after their administration, but reports only 20 observations in the control group and 100 observations in the treatment group, the reader should be suspicious of possible reporting bias. Reporting bias could affect either the control or treatment group.[13]

This information is important to the reader. Patients drop out or withdraw from studies for many reasons. For example, they may (1) suffer severe side effects or complications of therapy and withdraw from the study, (2) recover and not want further follow up, (3) die, or (4) move and be unable to complete follow up. In a report addressing prognosis it is especially important to indicate the fate of every patient enrolled in the study and to include each one in the analysis of results. If a study does not account for all of its patients, the impact can sometimes be assessed by recomputing the statistics, assuming that all patients lost to follow-up experienced the least desirable outcome. If the conclusion is unchanged despite this adjustment, then the physician can assume that the results are robust; whereas, if they do change, their clinical relevance must be questioned.

Analysis of Results

p-Values

When p-values began to be incorporated into surgical articles, physicians learned that "$p < 0.05$" meant that the difference in whatever was being compared was statistically significant. What does this really mean?

First of all, most statisticians urge the publication of the actual p-value (e.g., $p = 0.04$ instead of $p < 0.05$) as well as the value of the test statistic from which the p-value is obtained (e.g., t-value for student's t-test, or F-value for analysis of variance (ANOVA)). This will enable a doubting reader to verify the value on his or her own tables. For most studies, two-tailed statistical tables should be used. As stated previously, these are more conservative, and thus statistical significance is harder to achieve. By using two-tailed tables, the investigator is allowing for the possibility of either a positive or negative effect to occur.

When $p = 0.05$, it means that there is a 5% probability that the difference observed between the control group and the treatment group with respect to whatever is being compared has occurred by chance alone. Conversely, it means that there is a 95% probability that the observed difference is really the result of the intervention. p-values imply little, however, about the magnitude of the difference between groups. When $p < 0.0001$, for example, it does not mean that the result is very important, but rather that a large sample size was used. It does mean that chance is an unlikely explanation for the difference observed. In the real world, however, this result might be clinically irrelevant. In any study, the author should specify beforehand what magnitude of treatment effect would be considered clinically meaningful.[1]

Several reasons why a statistically significant difference (e.g., $p = 0.05$) might not translate into a *clinically* relevant difference are outlined below:

1. The population of patients upon whom the intervention was applied might not represent the patients whom you treat. For example, age, race, or coexisting illnesses might be quite different, and this information must be gleaned from the article in order to determine the clinical applicability of the result to patients.

2. The cost of the intervention might be prohibitive for the magnitude of difference in outcome seen, even though the outcome is statistically significant. For example, a new chemotherapeutic regime might prolong life by 4 weeks in women with breast cancer compared to the current regime, but is 4 weeks clinically significant? Do the side effects of this new regime reduce a patient's quality of life for a longer period of time than the presently used regime, thereby reducing the actual 28-day life benefit? Is 28 days a clinically important amount of time for patients suffering from breast cancer? What is the cost of the therapeutic intervention? You must decide if this new treatment regime is practical and feasible within the constraints of your clinical setting.

3. The risk of the intervention might, in your patient population, be considerably greater, so that you would be unwilling to accept even a 5% probability that the observed difference in outcome was due to chance alone. For example, a trial of resection and primary anastomosis in patients with obstructing colonic cancer might come out in favor of this approach over resection, colostomy, and secondary colocolostomy. Your patient population might have a higher percentage of diabetics, patients on steroids, or elderly patients than in the clinical trial and for whom this surgical approach might not result in the same outcome. On the other hand, you may be willing to accept an even higher probability (say 10%) of the difference having occurred by chance alone if the intervention had no associated risk or cost in your patient population.

CLUE: Rely more on the author who reports the exact value of the test statistic he or she calculated, along with its associated p-value.

When a p-value is reported as greater than 0.05, or NS, the clinical relevance of this information is even more difficult to decide. Small differences in treatment effects may be important to the clinician even though not statistically significant. Reporting p = NS deprives the reader of potentially important information, since p = 0.07 as opposed to p = 0.70 may have clinical relevance. A slightly larger sample size in the former instance might result in a statistically significant outcome; whereas, an increase in sample size in the latter instance would be unlikely to change the interpretation of the result. Many readers and researchers wrongly conclude that two treatments or tests are equivalent when a value of $p > 0.05$ is reported.[3] All that can, in fact, be concluded from this result, is that if there is a difference in the groups, the study failed to detect it. Failure to detect a statistically significant difference might not mean that in clinical practice the difference does not exist or is not relevant. There are three possible explanations for this: (1) the number of subjects being compared might be too small, so that the p-value is greater than 0.05 only because the sample size was too small to detect a difference when a difference did exist; (2) the method used to measure treatment effect might be too insensitive to detect a difference when one did exist; or (3) a significant difference might indeed exist, but by chance it was not detected in the study.[14] In a review of 71 "negative trials" that had been published in the *New England Journal of Medicine,* nearly all of the accepted null hypotheses were erroneously interpreted to mean there was no treatment effect, despite some differences as great as 25%. While these differences failed to reach statistical significance, they may have had considerable *clinical* relevance.[1]

Negative Studies and Confidence Intervals

One way to appraise the value of a negative study (one that has not demonstrated a statistically significant difference between control and treatment groups) is to calculate 95% confidence intervals around the observed difference. Confidence intervals reflect a range of values that are plausible for the *population* of patients from which the sample came. They are complementary to p-values, and both should be reported in negative studies. Confidence intervals say something about the size

of the difference observed. If the confidence interval is narrow and contains zero, it supports the notion that the difference observed is really not statistically significant. Most often, confidence intervals are used to aid predictions and comparisons, either of proportions or of time-related events. For example, in my (J.O.) randomized study involving patients undergoing elective thoracotomy, comparing the number of wound infections using one preoperative dose of antibiotic to six perioperative doses, the 95% confidence interval was − 0.008 to + 0.048.[15] This indicated that there was no more than a 4.8% chance that one dose was better than six doses, and no more than a 0.8% chance that six doses were better than one dose. The fact that this interval was both narrow and contained zero indicated that it was unlikely that a clinically significant difference in wound infection rates would result from adoption of one approach over the other. I anticipated that the outcome would be negative, that is, the number of wound infections in the one- and six-dose groups would be similar. Anticipating no difference, I estimated the sample size required by calculating the 95% confidence interval on the difference in proportion of wound infections. Thus, I felt safe in concluding that it was very unlikely that six doses of antibiotic conferred a clinically important benefit upon the patients compared to one dose.[15] Table 37-1 helps to illustrate the relationship between p-values, confidence intervals, and trial size. The values presented are based on the assumption that the true improvement in survival in the treatment group compared to the control groups is 55%, up from 50%.

The exact location and width of the confidence interval suggests a good deal about where the truth lies and the adequacy of the sample size to determine it.[8] Confidence intervals are not appro-

Table 37-1.

Trial size	95% confidence interval	p-value
20	(0.12, 3.79)	0.33
200	(0.47, 1.43)	0.24
2,000	(0.69, 0.98)	0.01
20,000	(0.77, 0.87)	<0.00001

Modified from Parmar MKB (1994).[16]

priate, however, to use with descriptive data (e.g., patient weights), for which means and standard deviations should be used.[17]

The relevance of a negative study depends on how large a difference it could detect if one existed, that is, on its *power*.[18]

> CLUE: In a negative study, look for confidence intervals to help you to determine whether or not the sample size was large enough to detect a difference if one did exist, that is, if the power of the study was adequate.

The width of the interval depends on its standard error and thus on both the sample size and the standard deviation of the sample measurements. A wide interval should alert the reader to the possibility that the sample size was too small, a commonly encountered finding in the literature.[17] Alternatively, though less likely, a wide confidence interval might reflect natural variation. The level of confidence reported (90% vs. 95%) also affects the size of the interval. A 90% confidence interval is always narrower than a 95% confidence interval because the researcher is taking a greater (10%) chance that the truth lies outside the calculated limits. Confidence intervals are probably most valuable in situations where the sample size is neither very small nor very large.[19]

> CLUE: Confidence intervals are a useful way of expressing the range of differences in outcome that can be expected between control and treatment groups. If the interval includes zero, the reader knows that it is entirely possible that the observed difference in outcome may have been due to chance alone. If the interval is narrow, the reader can be reassured that the sample size was sufficient.

Some journals are now moving away from reporting standard errors in favor of confidence intervals, because of the added information contained in the latter statistic.

> CLUE: The same problem can arise with computation of multiple confidence intervals as can arise with the calculation of multiple *p*-values, that is, with every 95% inter-

val reported, there is a 5% chance that the truth lies outside the range.

Power

The power of a study relates to its ability to detect a difference between groups, if one exists. This, in turn, relates to the sample size. Power levels are usually set at 80%. In a negative study, for example, a power level of 80% means that there is an 80% probability that a real difference between control and treatment groups does not exist, that is, that the "negative" conclusion is correct. In other words, the authors are willing to accept a 20% possibility that a "positive" conclusion eluded their detection due to insufficient sample size.

Researchers often design studies in order to determine if one drug, diagnostic test, or operation is better than another. They most often elect to take a 5% chance that a difference, if observed, is due to chance alone. What they do not do often enough, however, is assign a risk of being incorrect in the event that the study fails to yield a significant result. When a trial reports results that are not statistically significant, it cannot necessarily be said that the two drugs or tests studied are equivalent. Without knowledge of the power of the study, interpretation of a statistically nonsignificant result is difficult, if not impossible, to make. In a review of 84 therapeutic trials appearing in six general surgical journals from July 1981 through June 1982, only 5% of authors discussed the power of their study.[20] Reed et al. stated that almost 86% of articles published in six medical journals, and which reported negative results, could have missed small effects, 60% could have missed medium effects, and 40% could have missed large effects.[14] That is, the articles lacked sufficient power to detect differences of these magnitudes. The clinical relevance of a negative study generally depends on how large a difference between groups the study can detect, in other words, on its power.[8] In general, confidence intervals are more useful for interpreting clinical relevance than power calculations, because the latter do not take into account the actual results obtained.

Survival Rates, Life-Table Methods

A properly calculated survival rate is the best single statistical index available for measuring the efficacy, for example, of one cancer therapy compared to another.

In a clinical trial, the mean duration of survival may be calculated for each group being studied. Its meaningfulness is limited by the duration of follow-up. Unless all patients have died when the calculation is made, the reader may not be able to ascertain whether or not prognosis or survival is different between the groups being studied.

Alternatively, a mortality rate may be calculated. This is the percentage of patients dead at the end of the study. This rate also depends upon the duration of the study; if the duration of follow-up is too short, there might not have been enough deaths in either arm to allow the reader to decide on the risks or benefits of the treatment under investigation.

Yet another rate, a survival rate, may be calculated. This is the percentage of patients in each arm of a study who are alive at the end of a specific interval. This rate also wastes potentially valuable information, however, because it does not permit patients who have been followed for shorter intervals to contribute to the rate.

An "adjusted" survival rate reflects the proportion of patients in the group who escaped death from the cause of interest. It ignores those who died from other causes (and hence adjusts the survival rate) and might be appropriate to use when it is ascertained that the death rate in one group from causes unrelated to the disease was disproportionately higher than in the other. Admittedly, this would be unlikely to occur within the context of a randomized trial.

> **CLUE:** Beware of the data from an author who reports an "adjusted" survival rate. Ask yourself what was adjusted for and whether or not the adjustment was appropriate.

A "relative" survival rate reflects the proportion of patients in a group who died compared to the expected rate for a group of people in the general population who are similar with respect to race, sex, age, and period of observation. This method should be used only when information on cause of death is incomplete.

Actuarial or life-table methods, on the other hand, provide a means for using all follow-up information accumulated up to the date of assessment.[21]

Life-table analysis is the method most commonly used to summarize survival data in clinical trials. It is also used when reporting results of longitudinal investigations whose objective is to determine, for example, prognosis or outcome in a study of chronic disease. Its principal advantage over reporting 5-year survival data is that it uses all survival information gathered on patients enrolled in a study including those who have not yet reached the 5-year point. The method is not standardized, however, and it is incumbent upon the authors to describe how they handled their patients. A clearly defined "time equals zero" should be indicated (e.g., date of diagnosis, date of initial treatment, or date of hospital admission). In addition, a clearly defined endpoint should be indicated (e.g., death). To avoid the potential for biased results, authors should attempt to minimize the number of patients lost to follow-up and report how they did so.[21]

Life-table analysis takes into account the fact that patients are enrolled into studies at different points in time, partake in the study for variable amounts of time, and may be either alive, deceased, withdrawn, or lost to follow-up at the end of the study period. Life tables quantitate the proportion of patients alive at the end of various intervals compared to those alive at the beginning of the interval. In general, patients who survive less than a complete interval are most often credited with having survived one-half the interval.

The advantages of using all patients are that (1) if there are only a few cases of a particular disease, all of the potential information is included in the life table; (2) if the mortality rate within the first few years is more substantial and trails off subsequently, patients who contribute for the smaller periods of time provide as much relevant information as those who contribute to the entire life table; (3) survival information is more completely described, and a smaller percentage of patients are considered to have been lost to follow-up; and (4) if subgroup analysis is undertaken, the reliability of the survival rate increases with the use of all available patient information for the same reason as (2) above.

In cancer trials, for example, mortality rates are often higher within the first 2–3 years of surgery, as are recurrence rates (events). However, in a report of 5-year survival or late mortality, which are usually reported as a percentage, a patient who had survived for 3 years would not "count" for anything; whereas, in a life table this patient would contribute to the first 3 years of data tabulated. Reporting 5-year survival data or mortality data as a simple percentage ignores the distribution of patient-events over time, information that is of potential value because it might influence follow-up protocols and so forth.[21] Furthermore, using every patient's survival information reduces the standard error of the survival data.

CLUE: Beware of the study that reports "survival rates" when patient follow-up to the date of assessment is largely incomplete. There might be important information that is not incorporated into the rates, which life-table methods would have included.

All patients who contribute to a life table must be categorized by the closing date of the study as either (1) alive, (2) dead, (3) withdrawn, or (4) lost to follow-up.

Patients who withdraw from a study are generally considered to contribute fully to the life table until the interval immediately preceding the one during which they withdraw. They are considered to have contributed to one-half of the interval during which they withdraw. The author should document the number of patients who withdrew from the study and the reason(s) for their withdrawal in his or her report.

Patients lost to follow-up can be dealt with in a number of ways. The most conservative approach is to consider them to have died as of their last follow-up. This is, however, contrary to fact in most cases. Registry experience with intensive field investigation of lost cases has resulted in the recovery of some patients and indicated that such patients often live for several years beyond the initial date of lost contact.[22] The method most often opted for is to assume that patients lost to follow-up have a survival experience similar to that of the remaining cases. This approach might overestimate survival. Yet another method for dealing with patients lost to follow-up is to omit these patients from the table altogether. Most epidemiologists agree that this discards available and potentially useful information. Whatever method is adopted, the author should state how many patients were lost to follow-up, how their status was ascertained, and how they were handled in the data analysis.

CLUE: Even though patients who are lost to follow-up and those who withdraw from a study are dealt with in the same fashion when generating a life table, it is important to distinguish between the two. If, for example, a large number of patients are lost to follow-up in a particular study, conclusions might be biased as a result.

The study authors may invoke removal for cause. Any patient whose status changes during the period of observation and who no longer meets criteria for inclusion in the table may be removed for cause. Failure to do so may bias results. The reason for removal of all such patients must be stated. For example, in a life table examining the survival of patients undergoing cardiac valve replacement using two different valves, one might argue that considering a study patient who dies during the follow-up period as a result of coronary artery surgery as a death during the study might distort data. There are others who would argue, however, that the likelihood of this event occurring in either group of patients would be expected to be similar. This is the "intention to treat" principle.

Life-table methods also can be used to describe outcome data other than survival. Analysis of nonfatal events by actuarial methods is also appropriate.[21] For example, in a study of two cardiac valves, freedom from reoperation for valve failure can be translated into a curve with patients considered to cease contributing to the curve when they require reoperation.

When interpreting a life table, one should look for the number of data points contributing to the curve at various points along the x-axis. This will give an indication of the number of patients who are contributing to the curve as time from entry into the study increases. If these numbers are not published, less significance should be placed on the curve as it goes further out from time zero. The number of patients contributing to the curve generally decreases with time, making it a less reliable estimate of the truth. When less than 10 persons are contributing to a point on a survival curve, it is generally felt that the curve should be terminated.[23] There has been much debate about the most appropriate method of analyzing life tables, that is, whether the curves should be compared in their entirety or whether comparison at selected points in time is also appropriate.[24] The latter method of analysis is appropriate when clinicians are discussing treatment options with individual patients, though it might not be applicable when generalizing results from the sample studied to the population.

The Kaplan-Meier method of survival analysis is similar to the life-table method. It involves calculation of the proportion of patients surviving to each point in time that a death occurs, instead of survival to some present interval of time.[25] This method generates a stepwise curve, whereas, the life-table method results in a line.

Decision Analysis

Decision analysis is a way of attempting to address a health question when a clinical trial is considered either not feasible or too expensive to conduct considering the importance of the question. It can be used to improve, verify, or support intuitive decision making when a medical problem is rare and thus the question is unanswerable by the usual means. It has become a popular method used by health policy makers and textbook writers. It is a technique based on quantitative reasoning and probabilistic models.[26] It involves the development of strategies and tests the impact of uncertainty on the result of these strategies by varying the estimates (sensitivity analysis).[26] It employs a computer software program that generates a decision tree, branches of which describe various treatment strategies. The risks and benefits of each branch generate subbranches, and the endpoint of each of these has a utility attached. Utility reflects a patient's preference for different

health states and can be estimated using any of several techniques.

In 1990 one of the authors (J.O.) used decision analysis to compare three strategies for the management of the patient undergoing esophagogastrectomy for carcinoma of the distal esophagus or gastric cardia. The question was, "Should all, some, or no patients undergoing esophagogastrectomy with esophagogastrostomy for carcinoma have a drainage procedure performed at the time of initial operation?" The few studies that addressed the question had either included too few patients, had short follow-up times, examined different types of esophageal resection, or included different drainage procedures. The goal of the analysis was to minimize the proportion of patients in whom any complication developed either as a result of gastric outlet obstruction or as a result of the drainage procedure. The decision tree had three branches: (1) drain all patients and accept the risk of a drainage-associated complication, (2) drain no patient and accept the risk of gastric outlet obstruction, and (3) assess each patient's risk of development of gastric outlet obstruction and perform the drainage procedure on those patients felt to be a high risk. All risks were estimated from available published studies. It was determined that all patients should undergo a drainage procedure in a clinical setting when the risk of gastric outlet obstruction is greater than 10%, as long as the drainage procedure is 95% effective. Furthermore, the analysis indicated that if a test were developed to stratify patients into high and low risk groups for the development of gastric outlet obstruction, it would have to have a sensitivity of 80% if its specificity was 100%. The likelihood that a test as good as this could be developed is slight.[15] From a health policy perspective, this finding indicates that it might be unwise to fund research aimed at developing this type of test.

Decision analysis can be applied both to generic clinical problems and to decisions involving individual patients, as in the above example.[27] It is useful, however, only to the extent that it alters clinical behavior, and thus the reader must have a basic understanding of the concepts underlying the development of the analysis to have faith in its results.

Correlation

Correlation can be used as an alternative to hypothesis testing. It describes the strength of the linear relationship or association between two variables. The correlation coefficient ranges from −1 to +1. Correlation is used most often to describe the relationships between risk factors and a disease. A correlation coefficient between −1 and 0 implies an inverse relationship between a factor and a disease (e.g., modest alcohol consumption and coronary artery disease); whereas, a coefficient between 0 and +1 implies that a factor changes in the same direction as the risk of developing a disease (e.g., number of pack-years smoked and the risk of developing carcinoma of the lung).

CLUE: A small correlation between two variables can be due to (1) little linear association between two variables, or (2) large errors in the measurement of the variables.[28]

The type of correlation coefficient calculated in a particular article will depend on the type of data that have been collected. The Pearson Product-Moment r (Pearson r) is used to quantify the strength of a linear relationship between continuous variables (of interval or ratio type) from normally distributed data. The Spearman Rank Order r (Spearman r) is used for data that are either not interval or ratio, not normally distributed, or not linearly related. Correlation quantifies the strength of the relationship between a risk factor and a disease, as well as the direction of the relationship (direct versus inverse). It does not, however, imply causation.[29] To determine whether or not the relationship between two variables is statistically significant, standard hypothesis testing can be performed. The question answered by performance of a test of statistical significance is, "Is 'r' significantly different from 0 because of chance or because the true population correlation coefficient is not 0?"[30]

CLUE: It is generally felt that correlation coefficients should be reported with their corresponding level of significance.[29]

Once again, however, the question of clinical relevance is left to the discretion of the reader.

Regression and Multiple Regression

Correlation actually belongs to a larger class of statistical techniques known as regression.[31] Regression can be used to describe the relationship between two or more variables. It fits a line or curve to paired data points. Its principal use is in describing the relationship between two variables that are nonlinear, or between multiple variables.[30] Regression describes both the strength and magnitude of the relationship between variables. Regression techniques are being used more often in the surgical literature, most often to describe diagnostic and therapeutic predictive models.[31] Assumptions underlying simple linear regression include that (1) the values of the independent (x) variable are set by the investigator, (2) the independent (x) variable should be measured without experimental error, (3) for each independent variable there is a subset of y variables that are normally distributed, (4) the variances of the y variables should be homogeneous, (5) the y variables are distributed linearly, and (6) y values are independent of one another.[32]

Many regression techniques have been described, all of which involve the manipulation of multiple variables simultaneously in order to determine which one(s) best predict the outcome of interest.[31] These techniques include logistic regression, log linear regression, stepwise multiple regression, and discriminant function analysis.

Significance testing for linear regression is conceptually similar to ANOVA. It generates an F ratio for which a p-value can then be found using the appropriate table. Significance testing answers the question, "Is the slope of the regressions line statistically different from zero?"

CLUE: Authors who perform tests of statistical significance on regression data should report the corresponding p- or F-value obtained.

Conclusion

In this chapter, an attempt has been made to review the statistical tests commonly used in surgical studies, pointing out their strengths as well as the pitfalls associated with their use and interpretation.

It is also hoped that this chapter has served to illustrate the difference between statistical and clinical significance.

A heightened understanding of how statistics should be applied to datasets and how the results of statistical testing should be interpreted will improve the quality of surgical studies and reduce the number of studies reporting conclusions that are not supported by the data presented.

References

1. Sheehan TJ. The medical literature: let the reader beware. Arch Intern Med 1980;140:472–474.
2. Gardner MJ, Machin D, Campbell MJ. Use of check lists in assessing the statistical content of medical studies. Br Med J 1986;292:810–812.
3. Mainland D. Mathematics in medicine: statistical ritual in clinical journals. I. Is there a cure? Br Med J 1984;288:841–843.
4. Feinstein AR. XXXVII. Demeaned errors, confidence games, nonplussed minuses, inefficient coefficients, and other statistical disruptions of scientific communication. Clin Pharmacol Ther 1976;20:617–631.
5. Gardner MJ, Altman DG. Confidence intervals rather than p values: estimation rather than hypothesis testing. Br Med J 1986;292:746–792.
6. Chiu RC-J. Cardioplegia: From the bedside to the laboratory and back again. Ann Thorac Surg 1991;52:209–210. Editorial.
7. McPeek B, Mosteller F, McKneally MF, Neugebauer EAM. Experimental methods: clinical trials. In: Troidl H, Spitzer WO, McPeek B, Mulder DS, McKneally MF, Wechsler AS, Balch CM, eds. Principles and Practice of Research: Strategies for Surgical Investigators, 2nd edn. New York: Springer-Verlag, 1991, ch. 14, pp. 114–125.
8. Freiman JA, Chalmers TC, Smith H Jr, Kueler RR. Importance of beta, the type II error, and sample size in the design and interpretation of the randomized control trial. New Engl J Med 1978;299:690–694.
9. Sacks H, Chalmers TC, Smith H Jr. Randomized versus historical controls for clinical trials. Am J Med 1982;72:233–240.
10. Elenbaas JK, Cuddy PG, Elenbaas RM. Evaluating the medical literature. III. Results and discussion. Ann Emerg Med 1983;12:679–686.
11. Oxman AD, Guyatt GH. A consumer's guide to subgroup analyses. Ann Intern Med 1992;116:78–84.
12. Pocock SJ. Further aspects of data analysis. In: Clinical Trials: A Practical Approach. New York: Wiley, 1983, ch. 14, pp. 211–225.
13. Gore SM, Jones IG, Rytter EC. Misuse of statistical methods: critical assessment of articles in BMJ from January to March 1976. Br Med J 1977;1:85–87.
14. Reed JF III, Slaichert W. Statistical proof in inconclusive "negative" trials. Ann Inter Med 1981;141:1307–1310.
15. Olak J, Jeyasingham K, Forrester-Wood CF, Hutter J, al-Zeerah M, Brown E. Randomized trial of one-dose versus six-dose cefazolin prophylaxis in elective general thoracic surgery. Ann Thorac Surg 1991;51:956–958.
16. Parmar MKB. Pitfalls and biases in the reporting and interpretation of the results of clinical trials. Lung Cancer 1994;10(1):S143–150.
17. Morgan PP. Confidence intervals: From statistical significance to clinical significance. CMAJ 1989;141:881–883.
18. Arkin CF, Wachtel MS. How many patients are necessary to assess test performance? JAMA 1990;263:275–278.
19. Simon R. Confidence limits for reporting results of clinical trials. Ann Intern Med 1986;105:429–435.
20. Emerson JD, McPeek B, Mosteller R. Reporting clinical trials in general surgical journals. Surgery 1984;95:572–579.
21. Anderson RP, Bonchek LI, Grunkemeier GL, Lambert LE, Starr A. The analysis and presentation of surgical results by actuarial methods. J Surg Res 1974;16:224–230.
22. Cutler SJ, Ederer F. Maximum utilization of the life-table method in analyzing survival. J Chron Dis 1958;8:699–712.
23. Hess KR. Confidence intervals and survival estimates. J Thorac Cardiovasc Surg 1991;102:456–457. Letter to the editor.
24. Kirklin JW, Blackstone EH, Naftel DC. Confidence intervals and survival estimates. J Thorac Cardiovasc Surg 1991;10:457–459. Reply from the editor.

25. Kaplan EL, Meier P. Non-parametric estimation from incomplete observations. J Am Stat Assoc 1958;53:457–481.

26. Detsky AS, Redelmeier D, Abrams HB. What's wrong with decision analysis? Can the left brain influence the right? J Chron Dis 1987;40:831–836.

27. Pauker SG, Kassirer JP. The threshold approach to clinical decision making. New Engl J Med 1980; 302:1109–1117.

28. Elston RC, Johnson WD. Essentials of Biostatistics. Philadelphia: Davis, 1987.

29. Gaddis ML, Gaddis GM. Introduction to biostatistics. 6. Correlation and regression. Ann Emerg Med 1990;19:1462–1468.

30. Knapp RG: Basic Statistics for Nurses, 2nd edn. New York: John Wiley and Sons, 1985.

31. Gehlbach SH. Interpreting the Medical Literature: Practical Epidemiology for Clinicians, 2nd edn. New York: Macmillan, 1988.

32. Daniel WW. Biostatistics: A Foundation for Analysis in the Health Sciences. New York: John Wiley and Sons, 1974.

Additional Reading

Emerson JD, McPeek B, Mosteller R. Reporting clinical trials in general surgical journals. Surgery 1984;95:572–579. This paper reviews deficiencies in design and analysis found in clinical trials in surgery from six general surgical journals from July 1981 through June 1982. The authors review the information that a reader needs to be made aware of with regard to trial design and analysis so that an evaluation and interpretation of the results can be made.

Freiman JA, Chalmers TC, Smith H Jr, Kueler RR. Importance of beta, the type II error, and sample size in the design and interpretation of the randomized control trial. New Engl J Med 1978;299:690–694. This paper illustrates the importance of having an adequate sample size when designing a clinical trial, and the impact of sample size on the interpretation of results.

Gardner MJ, Altman DG. Confidence intervals rather than *p*-values: estimation rather than hypothesis testing. Br Med J 1986;292:746–792. This paper discusses the limitations of *p*-values and the value of confidence intervals in the reporting of results of clinical studies. Confidence intervals enable the reader to determine whether or not the magnitude of effect seen is of clinical importance.

Commentary

Even when something is demonstrated to be statistically significant, there is still a probability that an erroneous interpretation of the data has been made and that what is observed is simply a chance occurrence. The increased power of computing allows a greater number of tests to be applied to data, including tests of increasing complexity. Although there is no substitute for a trained biostatistician as a collaborator in research projects, Drs. Olak and Chiu provide good advice to help you analyze the literature on your own. They illustrate some of the common and important pitfalls in the use of statistics in a clear, collegial style. Readers are referred to the excellent bibliography provided by Mosteller and Rosner (chapter 36) for a more extensive exploration of this critically important discipline.

A.S.W.

CHAPTER 38

Systematically Reviewing Previous Work

E.A.M. Neugebauer, R. Lefering, B. McPeek, and S. Wood-Dauphinée

Reviewing previously published literature seems time-consuming and boring when compared to performing clinical or laboratory experiments to develop new information in surgery. For this reason, the task of reviewing and summarizing the literature is often delegated to a research assistant or the most junior member of the team.

This is a major error in thinking. The accumulation of evidence is an important goal underlying all scientific inquiry; an individual study is seldom an isolated event, but rather part of a continuum in which each new endeavor builds on preceding work. New findings lose much of their value if they have not integrated the accumulated knowledge, both theoretical and empirical, of earlier reports. When you discover that some of your findings or problems have already been addressed or even published by someone else, you will probably recognize the necessity of a thorough literature review. Performing a review not only avoids errors and saves you time and money, but will enable you to estimate more accurately the significance of your ideas and results. It is even possible to base whole textbooks on meta-analytic principles,[1] using quality criteria to separate valid results from questionable or invalid results.

On a practical level, a thorough critical appraisal of existing literature provides background information for developing a research proposal, a grant application, or a report for publication.

A research review will likely lead to one of four products:

1. It may bring together what is known about a specific research area and lead directly to new work designed to test a specific hypothesis, or add to the knowledge base.
2. It may analyze data from previous studies in a new way, to answer new research questions.
3. It may summarize what is known in an area, appearing in a journal in its own right as a "state-of-the-art" paper. Such a review will not only be of interest to those working in the specific field, but will also be particularly helpful to other specialists who wish to bring themselves up-to-date quickly.
4. It may inform clinical decisions made by individual clinicians about the care of patients, or by chiefs of units about policy matters.

Approaches to Reviewing the Literature

Traditional Reviews

The task of examining and evaluating previous work is frequently done by experts in the specific field who write traditional narrative review articles. Performed carefully, this is a quick way to get an overview of a specific topic. However, one must always be aware that the bias of its author can subtly contaminate a traditional narrative review. The studies used are often selectively chosen in order to support the author's view. Equally able reviewers often disagree about basic issues and occasionally arrive at diametrically opposite conclusions. With little concern for scientific rigor, some reviewers turn to a simple vote count. When some studies show a positive treatment effect, others no effect, and still others a negative effect, the reviewer counts the number supporting each result and selects the majority view. This procedure, also called "box score analysis," or the vote-counting method,[2] ignores the size of the effect found and the strength of the research design. If the number of previous studies is large, the traditional reviewer easily gets lost. Despite the subjectivity, questionable scientific validity, and inefficiency of the traditional narrative approach to reviewing the literature, most scholars in medicine and surgery still use this antiquated procedure. Over the past generation, new methods have been developed. They are increasingly known to clinical scientists and represent significant advances in the methodology of reviewing scientific literature.

Data Analysis

Gene V. Glass[3,4] has written about three levels of data analysis: primary analysis, secondary analysis, and meta-analysis.

Primary Analysis

Primary analysis is the original analysis of data from a research study. This is what most of us think of as research, and articles describing such work form the bulk of medical communications.

Secondary Analysis

Secondary analysis, as described by Glass, is the reanalysis of original data to bring current statistical methods to bear on them or to answer new questions. We can learn much from secondary analysis. Better ways of looking at the data gathered in a project may be suggested after they have been published. For example, a variety of useful secondary analyses of the data collected by the

University Group Diabetes Project (UGDP study) in medicine[5] advanced our understanding of how diabetes should be treated. Similarly, new hypotheses can be tested by the imaginative re-analysis of data already collected for a similar or even an entirely different purpose. Secondary analysis can be particularly useful in dealing with volunteer case reports, where volunteer reporting bias may have produced an effect if the data were collected prospectively.

Meta-Analysis

Like secondary analysis, meta-analysis uses existing data, but it focuses on the quantitative integration of findings across a group of independent studies and provides a more scientific alternative to the traditional narrative method of literature review.

There is no question that meta-analysis is a major advance, but we must remember that it is a comparative observational study with all the strengths and weaknesses of observational studies. We celebrate the fact that we now have a way to review work systematically, but guard against trying to extend it too far.

In thinking about meta-analysis, we lean heavily on three principles. First, *develop a strategy*. Bear in mind that the most effective review strategies and analytic techniques arise from the answers to the specific questions that are leading you to make the review. What do you want from the review? Do you seek a broad exploration of available information on a subject, or do you want to test specific hypotheses? Is an overall answer desirable, or are you interested in identifying interactions between specific treatments, patient populations, or settings, such as hospitals or clinics? Are you interested in the feasibility of implementing a new program locally? If the plan is for an exploratory review, you ask what is known about a particular area of research, a specific disease, a clinical problem, or a treatment, such as an operation or an element of pre- or postoperative care. Your strategy will be to include diverse studies to increase the chance of uncovering interesting findings that may lead to new directions for future research. Unless you know what you are doing at the start, you may finish with a simple recitation of previous findings that does little to advance research, contribute fresh insight, or inform decisions.

The second principle is that *conflicting results must be carefully investigated*. When we find dozens of previous studies, we hope that most of them will agree. If they do, a review is easy, but this rarely happens. Conflicting findings have several potential explanations. There may be substantial differences between operations with the same name. Follow-up care may be quite dissimilar. Perhaps the treatment works poorly for some kinds of patients and well for others, or is effective in certain hands or settings but not in others. These explanations can be uncovered only through the careful study of the narrative reports of patients, treatment descriptions, and details of hospital, clinical, or laboratory procedures. A letter or telephone call to the authors may uncover new postpublication information or insights that clarify the analysis.

The third principle is that *we often need formal, quantitative, analytic methods to identify small effects across studies* that are not apparent through simple inspection of the results of the studies individually.

Beware! Drawing inferences about findings uncovered from exploratory analyses can be risky. Searching among many research studies for factors significantly related to outcome will lead to some false positives—statistically significant relationships due only to chance. If you examine many separate relationships, each at the 0.05 level of significance, you should not be surprised to discover that 1 in 20 is significant due entirely to chance—a finding consistent with probability theory.

If several treatments are compared, sample variation alone may make some look better than others even when they are truly equivalent. Similarly, when institutions are compared for success with an operation, sampling variation will make some look much better than others even if they are equal in excellence. For example, in the United States National Halothane Study[6] 34 institutions were compared for standardized surgical mortality rates, and they appeared to differ, initially, by a factor of 24; after allowance was made for sampling variation, the ratio between the highest and lowest was only 3:1.

One way to prevent a review from *over-capitalizing on chance* is to break the data into parts. Half of the studies can be used to generate hypotheses about effective treatments or to predict treatment success; the other half can be used to test the hypotheses so generated. If the entire set of studies has some systematic bias, this procedure cannot eliminate it. Regardless of how you perform the review, your inferences will be only as valid as the underlying studies.

If your review is aimed at testing a previously established hypothesis, you must specify the hypothesis precisely, before you start. This may lead you to an early decision as to whether your review should look across studies to aggregate treatments (such as operations), aggregate patients, or aggregate settings (such as clinics or hospitals).

We ordinarily view the outcome of a clinical research study as being the result of interactions between the treatment, the patient, and the setting, compounded by random error. Reviews can answer many diverse questions, but we commonly seek answers to three:

1. What is the *average effect* of the treatment?
2. Are there *particular* patient *groups* or settings where the treatment works especially well?
3. *Can we implement it* in our department?

To answer the first question, we compare patients who receive the treatment with similar people who do not.

The second question asks for interactions. Do particular combinations of treatments and patients work especially well or poorly? For example, suppose a surgeon believes that a particular operation is especially valuable for elderly men, while any one of several operations is as effective in younger men. A single research design that crosses different operations with patients of various age groups can test this hypothesis. But what do you do if no study systematically considers all of the combinations of operations and patients that you wish to examine? For example, one study may have looked at large numbers of elderly men, and other studies at large groups of younger men. Taken together, these studies may give the reviewer some information about whether or not interactions exist. In other words, a collection of studies can sometimes shed light on complex interactions, when studies considered individually do not.

The third question concerns implementation. Strictly speaking, studies tell us only what happened to the patients or the participants in the investigation. We are ordinarily interested in generalizing these findings to similar patients under our care. If we know from the start that a review is to inform a local policy decision, the reviewer will look for studies that bear particularly on the local circumstances. Information can be sought that would help us to decide how an operation is likely to work in our hands, at our hospital, on our kinds of patients.

Both qualitative and quantitative conclusions from meta-analysis can be updated as new study results become available. A wide array of descriptive, etiological, intervention, clinical tool validation, or diagnostic method testing studies may be the subject of meta-analysis. The general objectives of meta-analysis are as follows.[7]

To confirm information (hypothesis, proof, initial findings)
To find errors
To search for additional findings—to develop new ideas (hypotheses) for further research and future original studies

Origin and Types of Meta-Analysis

During the past 20 years scholars, particularly in the social sciences, have developed the notion of quantitative meta-analysis in a robust way. After the first stimulating article on the subject by Light and Smith,[8] Glass put forward his first definitions of meta-analysis:[3] the "analysis of analyses," or better, "the statistical analysis of a large collection of analyses results from individual studies for the purpose of integration of the findings." The methodology for combining evidence from different studies stems from work in the 1950s.[9,10] Quantitative methods and techniques were further developed by Rosenthal,[11,12] Hedges,[13] and others. The 1983 annual review of *Evaluation Studies*, edited by R. Light,[14] brought together an important array of methodological articles and many important original studies. Basic methodological textbooks,[15–19] monographs dealing with

statistical methods,[20] and computer software[21] soon followed.

Since 1989, "meta-analysis" has been a MeSH term (i.e., a keyword in MEDLINE). After having reached a peak of nearly 400 publications in 1991, about 150 meta-analyses annually are found in medical journals today. Many surgical problems have been addressed by means of meta-analysis,[22–30] and further investigations will undoubtedly follow.

The usual purpose of quantitative or "classical" meta-analysis was to assess effectiveness of treatments, programs, and interventions and, less often, to study pathogenesis. To obtain reliable answers, meta-analysts gathered as many published and unpublished studies as possible. They did not, however, give enough consideration to the *quality* of the studies and were subsequently criticized on that score.[16] Problems of heterogeneity, experimental design, and execution—especially in fields such as education and medicine—soon demanded that a *qualitative* meta-analysis be added to the *quantitative* approach, "classical meta-analysis." The former is not only a systematic accumulation of the information in and characteristics of different studies, but also an assessment of quality, uncertainty, missing data, random error, and bias across relevant studies. In medicine, the greatest challenge of meta-analysis lies in the integration of the qualitative and quantitative assessment of given information (e.g., scoring of quality, weighing of the effect size by quality score).

When should you perform a meta-analysis? First of all, you must recognize that a meta-analysis, if performed adequately, is an enormous amount of work. The time and effort needed are comparable to that required for planning and conducting a clinical trial. Therefore, the question you want to answer with a meta-analysis should have comparable importance. If you plan to do a new study or if you want to establish a new research project, it would be an ideal starting point to conduct a meta-analysis. A thorough presentation of existing evidence avoids repetition and clearly focuses the project on those questions that still need an adequate answer. This holds true also if you are applying for a grant or if you are trying to get your research project funded. If you intend to set up diagnostic or therapy guidelines for your clinic, or if a society intends to define "rules" for a broader group of users, a meta-analysis can serve as a scientific basis. Consensus conferences can work more efficiently, and recommendations achieve a broader rate of acceptance if their findings are based on a meta-analytic examination of existing evidence (evidence-based medicine).

However, there are certain prerequisites that have to be fulfilled before a meta-analysis can be performed. First of all, there must be a sufficient amount of previous work on that specific problem, for example, clinical studies must have been conducted, because meta-analysis integrates only existing results. A new technology, for example, with hardly any data about its effectiveness cannot be assessed by means of a meta-analysis. Second, you need a team with at least two attributes. You require clinical experts who are thoroughly familiar with the problem under investigation; they guarantee the required completeness of information and are able to pose the relevant questions. And you need at least one person with competence in methodology who provides the necessary tools for combining information. A statistician with minimal understanding of the problem or a clinician without experience in methodology will, each working alone, produce poor results.

Qualitative Meta-Analysis

Qualitative meta-analysis, or best-evidence synthesis,[31,32] in medicine, has been defined as a "method of assessment of the importance and relevance of medical information coming from several independent sources through a general, systematic and uniform application of pre-established criteria of acceptability to original studies representing the body of knowledge of a given health problem or question."[33] The objectives of qualitative meta-analysis, according to Jenicek,[7] are as follows.

To determine the prevalence, homogeneity, and distribution of quality attributes
To expand the knowledge of missing and/or imperfect "outliers" (e.g., observation beyond a customary range)

Almost any clinical question or controversy can be subjected to qualitative meta-analysis, but the

objectives for each meta-analysis *must* be clearly formulated *before* analysis. As in any research endeavor, development of a working protocol will formalize the decisions made at the design stage, to achieve the objectives. For each general objective, investigators can also identify such secondary objectives as determining the age groups for which a treatment may be most effective.

A valid meta-analysis includes as many relevant studies as possible, but the authors should provide details of their search procedures. At present, sole reliance on computer searches of the literature is not sufficient because they may yield less than two-thirds of the relevant studies.[34] Efforts to minimize this bias include working from references of published studies, searching databases of unpublished material, and questioning experts in the particular field. The meta-analysis will be clear only if the studies are chosen according to predefined inclusion and exclusion criteria whose rationale is clearly stated. Each meta-analysis should list the studies analyzed, the studies excluded, and the reasons for exclusion.

Qualitative meta-analysis calls for an adequate dimensional assessment of the quality of studies. Several methods of assessment of the quality of original studies are available.

Table 38-1 lists selected authors who have proposed criteria checklists, or other methods, to evaluate different types or parts of clinical studies; a recent review by Moher[50] gives a thorough overview.

Mahon and Daniel[35] proposed a four-step method to evaluate reports of drug studies. Their process consists of applying only four criteria:

1. Were adequate controls used?
2. Were treatments randomized?
3. Were drug effects measured objectively? (This usually involves double-blind techniques.)
4. Were results analyzed statistically?

In 1970 Lionel and Herxheimer[36] presented the checklist they used to evaluate 141 clinical studies in four medical journals. Their checklist constitutes a formal assessment of whether an article is definitely acceptable, probably acceptable, or unacceptable. In 1979 Horwitz and Feinstein[37] proposed a set of 12 standards to be applied to retrospective case-control research; the standards

Table 38-1. Formal approaches of several authors for evaluating the quality of published clinical trials.

Author(s)	Year	No. of items	Applicability	Reference
1. Mahon and Daniel	1964	4	General	(35)
2. Lionel and Herxheimer	1970	42	Therapeutical studies	(36)
3. Horowitz and Feinstein	1979	12	Case-control studies	(37)
4. Levine	1980	29	Clinical studies	(38)
5. Chalmers et al.	1982	36	RCT[a]	(39)
6. Weintraub	1982	55	Drug trials	(40)
7. DerSimonian et al.	1982	11	Clinical studies	(41)
8. Bailar et al.	1984	5	General	(42)
9. Evans and Pollock	1985	33	RCT	(43)
10. Neugebauer et al.	1987	9	Experimental studies	(1,26,44)
11. Colditz et al.	1989	9	Clinical trials	(45,46)
12. Ter Riet et al.	1990	18	Clinical studies	(47)
13. Oxman et al.	1993	8	Clinical reports	(48)
14. Goodman et al.	1994	34	Clinical studies	(49)

[a]RCT, Randomized controlled trials.

were successfully used in the evaluation of 85 studies.

There may be sound reasons for a study not having adequate external, or even internal, controls and having to rely on controls outside the study (e.g., historical controls). Bailar and colleagues[42] proposed a series of five questions for assessing the value (i.e., strength of evidence) of externally controlled studies and used them to evaluate a group of 20 publications in the *New England Journal of Medicine.*

Neugebauer and coworkers[44] used a decision tree (Figure 38-1) in their meta-analysis of the current status of histamine as a causal chemical factor in the pathogenesis of septic/endotoxic shock. All published studies investigating the presence of histamine release in septic/endotoxic shock in vivo, and its absence in a state of health were evaluated by the criteria defined by the test nodes in the decision tree. All criteria and methodological standards at the test nodes were tabulated and set up in detail before the analysis was started. This meta-analysis suggested that, despite decades of histamine research, there is still no acceptable answer to the question of whether histamine plays a pathogenetic role in septic/endotoxic shock.[44]

In many cases, it may not be enough to list present or absent attributes of each study; these facts must have an appropriate dimension, where necessary. Scoring of quality is of particular interest. Evans and Pollock[43] proposed a qualitative assessment of clinical trials, based on the method of Chalmers and colleagues,[39] where—from a total score of 100—up to 50 points are given for the database, design, and "protocol," with emphasis on blinding; up to 30 points are allowed for statistical analysis; and up to 20 points are given for the way the study is presented (Table 38-2). They used this method to rate 36 randomized controlled studies and found only 16 that scored more than 70 points. The same method was successfully used, recently, in two meta-analyses about steroid therapy for trauma patients[28] and in sepsis and septic shock.[26]

The Trial Assessment Procedure Scale (TAPS) of Levine[38] is one of the most detailed trial assessment procedures with a scoring system. It involves an analysis of each report (e.g., trial protocol, completed study report, or journal article) in terms of attributes that reflect trial quality. The attributes are clustered into eight categories, each covering two to five related characteristics, to facilitate independent assessment of the quality of the various components of a trial—that is, to rate trial quality without regard to findings on treatment efficacy or safety. This form should be used only by very experienced raters.

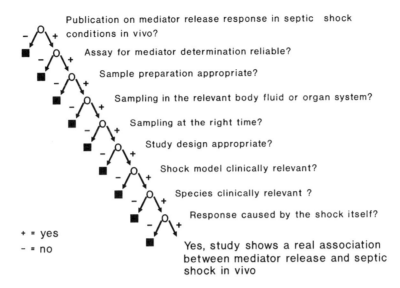

Figure 38-1. Decision tree for investigating a real, existing association between mediator release and septic/endotoxic shock under in vivo conditions.[1,44]

The sequence followed in all the approaches above is qualitative assessment of studies, then selection of acceptable or best evidence, and finally, if possible, quantitative meta-analysis of the latter. Frequently, quantitative meta-analysis is not feasible because few studies fulfill the current standards of trial methodology[44] and survive the systematic qualitative assessment, or because the studies with acceptable quality are so heterogeneous (i.e., they used widely differing research designs, treatments, and target populations). Unacceptable studies must be rejected, for stated reasons, before quantitative meta-analysis is undertaken. Acceptable studies may undergo quantitative meta-analysis according to the rules stated next.

Quantitative Meta-Analysis

In medicine, quantitative meta-analysis can be defined as a general, systematic, and uniform evaluation of dimensions across studies dealing with topics such as the following:

The magnitude of a health problem
The strength and specificity of a causal relationship in etiological research
The strength and specificity of the impact of a preventive or therapeutic intervention

The internal and external validity of clinical tools (e.g., diagnostic methods)
The costs and benefits of diagnostic methods and treatments

Quantitative meta-analysis was developed to overcome the weakness of previous methods of research integration. Like any other scientific work, each meta-analysis should begin with a plan that clearly states the question to be answered and the methods to be employed. There is no single "correct" method for performing a meta-analysis, but several attempts have been made to define the basic methodological issues. The workshop on methodological issues in overviews of randomized clinical trials, sponsored by the National Heart, Lung, and Blood Institute and the National Cancer Institute,[51] and the Potsdam International Consultation on Meta-Analysis[52] were two recent examples. Sacks and colleagues[53] have evaluated the quality of 86 meta-analyses of randomized controlled trials, using a scoring method that considered the most important elements of meta-analysis (i.e., a meta-meta-analysis). The generally accepted issues in a quantitative meta-analysis are portrayed in Figure 38-2 and explained, briefly, in subsequent paragraphs.

Table 38-2.   Method of Evans and Pollock for evaluating controlled clinical studies. Reprinted with permission from Evans M, Pollock AV[43] (1985).

Steps in evaluation	Yes	No
Design and conduct		
Is the sample defined?	2	0
Are exclusions specified?	2	0
Are known risk factors recorded?	3	0
Are therapeutic regimens defined?	5	0
Is the experimental regimen appropriate?	5	0
Is the control regimen appropriate?	5	0
Were appropriate investigations carried out?	2	0
Are endpoints defined?	5	0
Are endpoints appropriate?	5	0
Have numbers required been calculated?	2	0
Was patient consent sought?	1	0
Was the randomization blind?	3	0
Was the assessment blind?	4	0
Were additional treatments recorded?	4	0
Were side effects recorded?	2	0
Analysis		
Withdrawals:		
Are they listed?	3	0
Is their fate recorded?	4	0
Are there fewer than 10%?	4	0
Is there a compatibility table?	3	0
Are risk factors stratified?	3	0
Is the statistical analysis of proportions correct?	3	0
Is the statistical analysis of numbers correct?	3	0
Are confidence intervals reported?	2	0
Are values of both test statistics and probability given?	1	0
In negative trials, is the type II error considered?	4	0
Presentation		
Is the title accurate?	2	0
Is the abstract accurate and helpful?	3	0
Are the methods reproducible?	3	0
Are the sections clear-cut?	2	0
Can the raw data be discerned?	2	0
Are the results credible?	3	0
Do the results justify the conclusions?	3	0
Are the references correct?	2	0

Methodological Elements of a Quantitative Meta-Analysis

Aim

A meta-analysis usually addresses sharper questions than a literature review and seeks quantitative answers; thus its objectives must be clearly formulated before the study begins. A review of care for stoma patients might discuss treatment methods available, changing uses, and the pros and cons of different methods. A meta-analysis might take such a specific measure as the proportion of patients rehospitalized within 1 year of release under various conditions, combine the relevant evidence from several studies, and try to compare performance of different treatments. A distinction between two levels of questions lead-

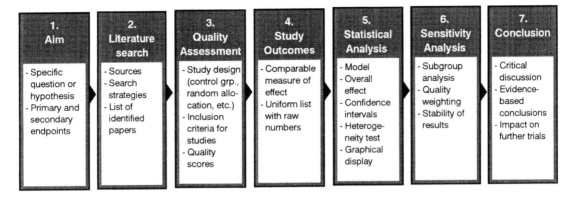

Figure 38-2. Sequence of methodological steps of qualitative and quantitative meta-analysis.

ing to two different types of hypothesis can be made: (1) a search for tentative answers and their verification, and (2) verification or hypothesis testing.

Literature Search

As many relevant studies as possible should be included in a qualitative meta-analysis; details of the computerized and manual search procedures used to find them should be described. Computerized searches are not always straightforward and consistent, and several articles have examined this problem[54,55] (see chapter 10). A professional librarian who specializes in literature searches of clinical topics should be involved.

Literature searches will not find unpublished studies, and published studies may differ, systematically, from unpublished studies. Meta-analyses based on literature searches alone may display "publication bias."

Authors are more likely to submit, and editors are more likely to publish, work with statistically significant versus nonsignificant results. As a consequence, a reviewer who focuses on published studies will likely overstate treatment effects.

A computer search should be supplemented by consulting *Current Contents,* reviews, textbooks, and people with relevant expertise, and by reviewing the references cited in the trials found.[53] Publication bias is one of the main criticisms leveled at meta-analysis, but sampling bias and data retrieval limitations are inherent in any literature review.

Selecting Studies for Inclusion

Studies for meta-analysis are chosen on the basis of inclusion and exclusion criteria. How you select studies for inclusion depends on the availability of research reports, the number and frequency of different designs, and the specific questions driving your analysis. Including everything you can find has the advantage of avoiding criticism for neglecting some work or including one study while excluding another, but it does present some problems. If you discover 1,100 studies, such an embarrassment of riches will almost certainly sink your project and you must find some appropriate way of reducing the number. For example, you could draw a random sample of all the studies available and use the sample for your review.

It is important to include a wide variety of research designs and treatment variations, but if a particular study clearly has obvious, substantial, fundamental flaws, exclude it and state why. Wrong information is much worse than no information.

You may have trouble finding some studies; for example, it may be difficult to find a translator for a paper in a particular language, and certain monographs may be out of print. You may have to decide how much digging is warranted on the basis of a title or an abstract.

Another approach is to stratify your sample by dividing the available studies into categories for review. This procedure guarantees inclusion of each important type of study but requires you to analyze in detail only the shorter list of selected studies.

Experimental design is often a strong predictor of research outcomes. In a review of almost 100 studies of portacaval shunt, Chalmers[56] found a clear negative relation between the degree of control in a research design and the level of success attributed to the surgical intervention; the higher the degree of control, the less enthusiastic the investigators were about an operation's effectiveness. Similar findings were reported by Gilbert, McPeek, and Mosteller[57,58] in a study of innovations in surgery and anesthesia. Such results support the "law" enunciated by the famous statistician Hugo Muench, that nothing improves the performance of an innovation more than the lack of controls.[59] Some papers suggest this rule is not universal,[60–62] but there is much evidence that it often applies in medicine and surgery.

Research design is not the only basis for stratification. You may wish to stratify by geography, treatment, type of operation, type of clinic or hospital, or the sociodemographic or clinical characteristics of patients.

In summary, we are not aware of standardized criteria for inclusion of studies in meta-analysis. Universal criteria are not appropriate, because meta-analysis can be applied to a broad spectrum of topics, and criteria may need to vary for different objectives; disagreement on inclusion and exclusion criteria is to be expected among the readers of the published report of a particular meta-analysis. For this reason, *criteria and their rationale should be stated, and all studies found, whether included or excluded, should be listed.*

Study Characteristics

After the studies have been collected and selected, it is helpful to record the key descriptive characteristics of each study on data abstract forms. The reader needs to be convinced that the results of separate trials have been meaningfully combined. Common methodological characteristics included in meta-analyses are type and year of publication; study design; type, dosage, route, frequency, and duration of treatment; control; sample size; and subject randomization and loss. Studies may differ in any of the foregoing characteristics. In general, the meta-analyst should note any differences be-

tween the primary studies and discuss how they affect the conclusions.

Study Outcomes

Similar data abstract forms are useful for *study outcome characteristics,* because various endpoints or outcome variables are used to assess treatment effects. The outcome of interest may be measured by a continuous variable such as blood pressure, by categorical variables such as mortality or complication rates, by an ordinal variable such as tumor stage, or by time-related variables expressed in life tables. Meta-analysis has the advantage of being able to take several different dependent variables into account.[63] If you are reviewing the literature on the effects of selective vagotomy with antrectomy in patients with peptic ulcers, such outcome measures as mortality, recurrence, pain, or quality of life can be examined. When you are extracting data, record raw numbers rather than proportions, because the process is a potential source of bias. Control this type of bias by having the extracting done by more than one observer, having each observer blinded to the various treatment groups through a coded photocopying process, and measuring the interobserver agreement.[53]

Statistical Analysis

A major feature of meta-analysis is that the unit of analysis, when the results of many studies are being assessed, is not an individual patient or clinic, but a study. To compare studies, we must measure treatment impact for each study. Meta-analysis includes transformation of multiple study findings into a common matrix. The two most common measures are *statistical significance* and *effect size.*

Most research about the effectiveness of treatments asks the question, Do the differences between the treatment and the control groups exceed those we expect due to chance alone? If each of several studies compares treatment and control groups, we can take the *p*-values as measures of statistical significance to interpret the effectiveness of treatment. This strategy has two problems. Many studies in medicine and surgery have rather few participants in each of the comparison groups.

Small investigations have weak power because their ability to detect real differences between groups is low. If a weak study reports a difference, we can assume that the difference is substantial; if no significant difference was found, we can only wonder whether the findings indicate true absence of any important difference or only failure to detect a difference that does exist, because the study is too small. Consequently, relying on a p-value may be misleading.

The sample size issue can cut the other way too. Occasionally, a study has very large sample sizes, and tests of significance, such as the p-value, are heavily influenced by sample size. In a truly large study, very small or even trivial differences can be statistically significant. "Significant" does not mean "important"!

Effect sizes provide a simple estimate of how valuable a treatment is. Suppose we wish to compare the main results between the treatment group and the control group. If the information is reported in each of the individual studies, an average effect size for the entire group of studies can easily be calculated. For each study, we need to know the mean of the treatment, the mean of the control group, and the standard deviation of the control group. With an average size across a number of studies, we have a single summary value for the effectiveness of the treatment studies. In 1976 Glass and Smith[64] computed the average effect size for psychotherapy treatment across 400 separate studies to be 0.68. They concluded that an average patient receiving psychotherapy was approximately two-thirds of a standard deviation more improved than the average control group member.[4]

A comparison of proportions will give another measure of effect size. For example, one could compare the proportion of people who live longer than 5 years following different treatments for cancer. The effect size for proportions is calculated by simply subtracting the proportion surviving in the treatment group from that surviving in the control group.

Frequently, your chosen measure of effect size will depend on what numerical information is reported in the various studies. If the standard deviation of the control group, for example, is not reported or cannot be calculated, a mean-score effect size cannot be computed.

Another method of looking at the overall impact of treatment is to try to combine the significance tests from many separate studies into one comprehensive test of a null hypothesis for the studies as a whole. Rosenthal[11] has described nine ways to accomplish this. To illustrate one technique, consider the method of adding Z-scores (standard normal deviates). If each study has two comparison groups, there is a Z-score associated with each reported p-value. The Z-scores from each individual study are simply added across studies. The sum of the Z-scores is divided by the square root of the number of studies. The probability associated with this total score gives an overall level of significance for the studies under review.

Combined significance tests are simple to compute and generally require only that we know the sample size and the probability level or the level of a test statistic, such as the value of T, Z, or F, for each individual study. The larger the overall sample size, the more likely it is that a given underlying effect size will be detected as statistically significant. For example, assume that patients with duodenal ulcer treated by vagotomy and antrectomy have slightly better results than those receiving vagotomy and pyloroplasty. If the two operations are repeatedly compared in very weak trials—small sample sizes for each group—many of the studies will not show statistically significant differences between the two operations, even if such differences exist. A traditional informal reviewer who did only a vote count would almost certainly fail to see the true effectiveness of vagotomy and antrectomy. A careful reviewer who combines the studies by adding Z-scores is much more likely to find that the overall statistical test is significant because the small numbers of patients in each weak study combine to become a much larger number of patients and produce a meta-analysis of greater power than any of the smaller studies taken individually.

Sensitivity Analysis

Because there will undoubtedly be differing opinions on the appropriate method for performing a particular meta-analysis, the investigator should always ask, "How sensitive are the meta-analysis results to changes in the way the meta-analysis was done?" This process, called sensitivity analysis, is an important element in meta-analysis methodology[65] (Figure 38-2).

You may want to study how the pooled results change when randomized *and* nonrandomized studies, instead of randomized trials only, are included in a meta-analysis. This type of study simply involves the addition of a second analysis that includes data from the nonrandomized studies. A comparison of the results of the two meta-analyses will show that the type of study has little effect on the meta-analysis results, and any disagreement about inclusion criteria is unimportant, or that the type of study is indeed an important factor in drawing conclusions from the analysis. Sensitivity analysis used as a tool within meta-analysis can help to resolve clinical controversies.

Factors influencing the sensitivity analysis can be discovered in the process of meta-analysis, such as differences between studies of young compared with old patients. By testing the effect of the more subjective elements of meta-analysis, such as the choice of inclusion and exclusion criteria, the conclusions drawn from a meta-analysis can be strengthened.

A related issue is the extent to which meta-analysis results are potentially distorted through publication bias. If one assumes that negative studies or studies showing no difference are less likely to be published than positive studies, this issue should be addressed if meta-analysis shows significant differences in outcome between treatment groups. Some published meta-analyses have estimated how many unpublished trials, showing no difference between treatments, would be required to convert a statistically significant pooled difference into an insignificant difference.[65-68] A carefully performed meta-analysis describes the different analyses used to strengthen the overall result obtained.

Study Quality Assessment

The scientific quality of the papers to be combined should be assessed and included in the sensitivity analysis. The resulting conclusion will be less reliable if the original trials were poor; see the earlier discussion of qualitative meta-analysis.

Conclusions and Recommendations

The extraction and pooling of data from published reports with the methodology of quantitative meta-analysis is time-consuming and tedious. At the end of the process, the meta-analysis must put the results in perspective and, if the data are not decisive, should recommend appropriate future studies.

Presentation of Results

There are no hard and fast rules about the format for presenting the findings of a review employing meta-analysis. The format depends, to some extent, on the purpose of the final product and the organizational framework of the individual reviewer. Cooper[69] has suggested that such reviews follow an outline similar to the one used for primary research, as follows:

1. An introduction defining the problem to be addressed and identifying the controversy in the literature
2. A methods section describing how the articles were selected, the sources tapped, and the kind of information collected about each study
3. A results section presenting the statistical procedures and findings
4. A discussion section containing a summary of the findings, a comparison with other related work, and a statement of the direction future research might take

Conclusion

Systematic reviews have an important place in the link between basic research and improved human health. The growth in the number of systematic reviews, especially meta-analyses, reflects this.[70] A network of individuals and institutions, the Cochrane Collaboration,[71] has evolved at an international level in response to Cochrane's criticism of the health professions for not having organized, systematic, and periodically updated reviews of all relevant randomized controlled trials.[72] Pilot projects began in 1993 with the creation of databases that represented existing knowledge in certain areas. It is the future intention of the Cochrane Collaboration to establish a procedure to update and present the current knowledge in many areas.[73, 74]

There is an obvious need to establish an objective and systematic way to combine existing knowledge from clinical studies or experimental findings. The qualitative and quantitative process of meta-analysis is an established procedure to achieve this integration. The crucial elements of meta-analysis are its prospective planning, complete evaluation of existing evidence, qualitative assessment and reproducible selection of relevant information, statistical combination of results with subsequent sensitivity analysis, and objective conclusions that are based on facts (rather than on opinions). Thus, meta-analysis provides an ideal tool to perform evidence-based medicine. Compared to typical narrative review articles, meta-analysis provides reproducible reasoning based on scientific methods. Results of meta-analysis can be used to set up guidelines for treatment, prepare future studies or research endeavors, or generate a scientific basis for discussions.

References

1. Neugebauer EA, Holaday JW. Handbook of mediators in septic shock. Boca Raton, FL: CRC, 1993.

2. Hedges LV, Olkin I. Vote-counting methods in research synthesis. Psychol Bull 1980;88:359–369.

3. Glass GV. Primary, secondary, and meta-analysis of research. Educ Res 1976;5:3–8.

4. Glass GV. Meta-analysis: an approach to the synthesis of research results. Res Sci Teach 1982;19:93–112.

5. University Group Diabetes Program (UGDP) Study. J Diab 1970;19(suppl. 2):740–850.

6. Moses LE, Mosteller F. Afterword for the study of death rates. In: Bunker JP, Forrest WH Jr, Mosteller F, Vandam LD, eds. The National Halothane Study: a study of the possible association between halothane anesthesia and postoperative hepatic necrosis. Washington, DC: U.S. Government Printing Office, 1969, pp. 395–408.

7. Jenicek M. Meta-analysis in medicine. Where we are and where we want to go. J Clin Epidemiol 1989;42:35–44.

8. Light RJ, Smith PV. Accumulating evidence: procedures for resolving contradictions among different research studies. Harvard Educ Rev 1971;41:429–471.

9. Cochran WG. The combination of estimates from different experiments. Biometrics 1954;10:101–129.

10. Mantel N, Haenzel W. Statistical aspect of the analysis of data from retrospective studies of disease. J Natl Cancer Inst 1959;22:719–748.

11. Rosenthal R. Combining results of independent studies. Psychol Bull 1978;85:185–193.

12. Rosenthal R. Assessing the statistical and social importance of effects of psychotherapy. J Consult Clin Psychol 1983;51:4–13.

13. Hedges LV. Statistical Methodology in Meta-Analysis. Princeton, NJ: ERIC Clearinghouse on Tests, Measurement and Evaluation, Educational Testing Service, 1982.

14. Light RJ, ed. Evaluation Studies, Review Annual. Beverly Hills, CA: Sage, 1983, p. 8.

15. Glass GV, McGraw B, Smith ML. Meta-Analysis of Social Research. Beverly Hills, CA: Sage, 1981.

16. Hunter JE, Schmidt FL, Jackson GB. Meta-Analysis: Cumulating Research Findings Across Studies. Beverly Hills, CA: Sage, 1982.

17. Borg WR, Gall MD. Critical Evaluation of Research. Educational Research: An Introduction, 4th edn. New York: Longman, 1983.

18. Light JRJ, Pillemer DB. Summing-Up. The Science of Reviewing Research. Cambridge, MA: Harvard University, 1984.

19. Rosenthal R. Meta-analytic Procedures for Social Research. Beverly Hills, CA: Sage, 1984.

20. Hedges LV, Olkin I. Statistical Methods for Meta-Analysis. New York: Academic, 1985.

21. Mullen B, Rosenthal R. Basic Meta-Analysis: Procedures and Programs. Hillsdale, NJ: Erlbaum, 1985.

22. Bollschweiler E, Feussner H, Huber F, Siewert JF. Ist die Cholezystektomie ein Risikofaktor für das kolorektale Karzinom? Eine Metaanalyse. Langenbecks Arch Chir 1993;378:304–312.

23. Cheatham ML, Chapman WE, Key SP, Sawyers JL. A meta-analysis of selective versus routine nasogastric decompression after elective laparatomy. Ann Surg 1995;221:469–478.

24. Detsky AS, Baker JP, O'Rourke K, Goel V. Perioperative parenteral nutrition: a meta-analysis. Ann Intern Med 1987;107:195–203.

25. Imperiale TF, Teran JC, McCullough AJ. A meta-analysis of somatostatin versus vasopressin in the

management of acute esophageal variceal hemorrhage. Gastroenterology 1995;109:1289–1294.

26. Lefering R, Neugebauer EAM. Steroid controversy in sepsis and septic shock: a meta-analysis. Crit Care Med 1995;23:1294–1303.

27. Meijer WS, Schmitz PIM, Jeekel J. Meta-analysis of randomized, controlled clinical trials of antibiotic prophylaxis in biliary tract surgery. Br J Surg 1990;77:283–290.

28. Neugebauer E, Dietrich A, Bouillon B, Lorenz W, Lechleuthner A, Troidl H. Steroids in trauma patients—right or wrong? A qualitative meta-analysis of clinical studies. J Theor Surg 1990;5: 44–53.

29. Nurmohamed MT, Rosendaal FR, Büller HR, Dekker E, Hommes DW, Vandenbroucke JP, Briet E. Low molecular weight heparin versus standard heparin in general and orthopaedic surgery: a meta-analysis. Lancet 1992;340:152–156.

30. Selective Decontamination of the Digestive Tract Trialists' Collaborative Group. Meta-analysis of randomized controlled trials of selective decontamination of the digestive tract. Br Med J 1993; 307;525–532.

31. Spitzer WO, Lawrence V, Dales R, Hill G, Archer MC, Clark P, Abenhaim L, Hardy J, Sampalis J, Pinfold SP. Links between passive smoking and disease: a best-evidence synthesis. Clin Invest Med 1990;13:17–42.

32. Slavin RE. Best-evidence synthesis: an alternative to meta-analytic and traditional reviews. Educ Res 1986;15:5–11.

33. Jenicek M. Meta-analyse en medecine. Evaluation et synthése de l'information clinique et epidemiologique. St-Hyacinthe and Paris: EDISEM and Maloine, 1987.

34. Dickersin K, Hewitt P, Mutch I, Chalmers I, Chalmers TC. Perusing the literature: comparison of MEDLINE searching with a perinatal trials data base. Control Clin Trials 1985;6:306–317.

35. Mahon WA, Daniel EE. A method for the assessment of reports of drug trials. Can Med Assoc J 1964;90:565–569.

36. Lionel NDW, Herxheimer A. Assessing reports of therapeutic trials. Br Med J 1970;3:637–640.

37. Horwitz RI, Feinstein AR. Methodologic standards and contradictory results in case-control research. Am J Med 1979;66:556–564.

38. Levine J. Trial Assessment Procedure Scale (TAPS). U.S. Department of Health and Human Services, Public Health Service, Alcohol, Drug Abuse, and Mental Health Administration, National Institute of Mental Health, Bethesda, MD, 1980. Available from Dr. Levine, University of Maryland, Maryland Psychiatric Research Center, P. O. Box 3235, Catonsville, MD 21228.

39. Chalmers TC, Smith H Jr, Blackburn B, Silverman B, Schroeder B, Reitman D, Ambroz A. A method for assessing the quality of a randomized control trial. Control Clin Trials 1981;2:31–49.

40. Weintraub M. How to critically assess clinical drug trials. Drug Ther 1982;12:131–148.

41. DerSimonian R, Charette LJ, McPeek B, Mosteller F. Reporting on methods in clinical trials. New Engl J Med 1982;306:1332–1337.

42. Bailar JC III, Louis TA, Lavori PW, Polansky M. Studies without internal controls. New Engl J Med 1984;311:156–162.

43. Evans M, Pollock AV. A score system for evaluating random control clinical trials of prophylaxis of abdominal surgical wound infection. Br J Surg 1985;72:256–260.

44. Neugebauer E, Lorenz W, Maroske D, et al. The role of mediators in septic/endotoxic shock. A meta-analysis evaluating the current status of histamine. Theor Surg 1987;2:1–28.

45. Colditz GA, Miller JN, Mosteller F. How study design affects outcomes in comparisons of therapy. I. Medical. Stat Med 1989;8:441–454.

46. Miller JN, Colditz GA, Mosteller F. How study design affects outcomes in comparisons of therapy. II. Surgical. Stat Med 1989;8:455–466.

47. Ter Riet G, Kleijnen J, Knipschild P. Acupuncture and chronic pain: a criteria-based meta-analysis. J Clin Epidemiol 1990;43:1191–1199.

48. Oxman AD, Guyatt GH, Cook DJ, Jaeschke R, Heddle N, Keller J. An index of scientific quality of health reports in the lay press. J Clin Epidemiol 1993;46:987–1001.

49. Goodman SN, Berlin J, Fletcher SW, Fletcher RH. Manuscript quality before and after peer review and editing at *Annals of Internal Medicine*. Ann Intern Med 1994;121:11–21.

50. Moher D, Jadad AR, Nichol G, Penman M, Tugwell P, Walsh S. Assessing the quality of randomized controlled trials: an annotated bibliography of scales and checklists. Control Clin Trials 1995;16: 62–73.

51. Proceedings of "Methodological issues in over-

views of randomized clinical trials." Stat Med 1987;6:217–409.

52. Cook DJ, Sackett DL, Spitzer WO. Methodologic guidelines for systematic reviews of randomized controlled trials in health care from the Potsdam Consultation of Meta-Analysis. J Clin Epidemiol 1995;48:167–171.

53. Sacks HS, Berrier J, Reitman D, Ancona-Berk VA, Chalmers TC. Meta-analyses of randomized controlled trials. New Engl J Med 1987;316:450–455.

54. Hewett P, Chalmers TC. Using MEDLINE to peruse the literature. Control Clin Trials 1985;6: 75–84.

55. Hewett P, Chalmers TC. Perusing the literature: methods of assessing MEDLINE and related databases. Control Clinical Trials 1985;6:168–178.

56. Chalmers TC. The randomized controlled trial as a basis for therapeutic decisions. In: Lachin J, Tygstrup N, Juhl E, eds. The Randomized Clinical Trial and Therapeutic Decisions. New York: Dekker, 1982, ch. 2.

57. Gilbert JP, McPeek B, Mosteller F. Statistics and ethics in surgery and anesthesia. Science 1977;198: 684–699.

58. Gilbert JP, McPeek B, Mosteller F. Progress in surgery and anesthesia: benefits and risks of innovative therapy. In: Bunker JP, Barnes BA, and Mosteller F, eds. Costs, Risks, and Benefits of Surgery. New York: Oxford University, 1977:124–169.

59. Bearman JB, Loewenson DB, Gullen WH. Muench's postulates, laws, and corollaries. Biometrics Note 4. Bethesda, MD: Office of Biometry and Epidemiology, National Eye Institute, National Institutes of Health, 1974.

60. Stock WA, Okun M, Haring M, Witter R. Age difference in subjective well-being: a meta-analysis. In: Light RJ, ed. Evaluation Studies Review Annual, vol. 8. Beverly Hills, CA: Sage, 1983, pp. 279–302.

61. Straw RB. Deinstitutionalization in mental health: a meta-analysis. In: Light RJ, ed. Evaluation Studies Review Annual, vol. 8. Beverly Hills, CA: Sage, 1983, pp. 253–278.

62. Yin RK, Yates D. Street level governments: assessing decentralization and urban services. Los Angeles: Rand, 1974.

63. Ottenbacher KJ, Peterson P. The efficacy of vestibular stimulating as a form of specific sensory enrichment. Clin Pediatr 1983;23:418–433.

64. Smith ML, Glass GV. Meta-analysis of psychotherapy outcome studies. Am Psychol 1976;32: 752–760.

65. L'Abbe KA, Detsky AS, O'Rourke K. Meta-analysis in clinical research. Ann Intern Med 1987;107:224–233.

66. Rosenthal R. The file drawer problem and tolerance for null results. Psychol Bull 1979;86:638–641.

67. Begg CB. A measure to aid the interpretation of published clinical trials. Stat Med 1985;4:1–9.

68. Neugebauer E, Lorenz W. Meta-analysis: from classical review to a new refined methodology. Introduction to the discussion forum about an example of meta-analysis in basic surgical research: the role of mediators in septic/endotoxic shock (Theor Surg 1987;2:1–28). Theor Surg 1989;4:79–85.

69. Cooper HM. Scientific guidelines for conducting integrative research reviews. Rev Educ Res 1982; 52:291–302.

70. Spitzer WO, ed. The Postdam international consultation on meta-analysis. J Clin Epidemiol 1995;48:1–172 (special issue).

71. Chalmers I, Haynes B. Reporting, updating, and correcting systematic reviews of the effects of health care. Br Med J 1994;309:862–865.

72. Cochrane AL. 1931–1971: A critical review, with particular reference to the medical profession. In: Teeling-Smith, ed. Medicines for the Year 2000. London: Office of Health Economics, 1979, pp. 1–11.

73. Chalmers I, Altman DG. Systematic reviews. London: BMJ, 1995.

74. Robinson A. Research, practice, and the Cochrane Collaboration. Can Med Assoc J 1995;152:883–889.

CHAPTER 39

Statistical Consultation in Clinical Research: A Two-Way Street

L.E. Moses and T.A. Louis

Introduction

The results of clinical research often rest on statistical interpretation of numerical data. Thus, effective collaboration between clinician and statistician can be crucial. Interaction in the planning phases of a project can identify tractable scientific and statistical problems that will need attention and can help avoid intractable ones. The central requirement for successful collaboration is clear, broad, specific, two-way communication on both scientific issues and research roles.

Clinical research often depends for its conclusions on the correct design and performance of studies to collect numerical data, and on the subsequent interpretation of the results. Statistical issues arise in all three of these areas, and they must be correctly addressed, or the usefulness of the whole investigation can be threatened.

Statistical issues may or may not be straightforward; the clinician may or may not be statistically experienced and sophisticated. If the com-

plexity of the statistical problem is greater than the clinician's readiness to deal with it, then recourse to biostatistical consultation is likely to advance the investigation. Some statistical problems may not be readily apparent and may therefore be discovered only through such a consultation.

The kind of transaction between the clinician and the statistical consultant that we are discussing is scientific, not primarily technical. This chapter aims to indicate—to both parties—ways to improve the prospects of successful consultation. Boen and Zahn[1] and Hand and Everitt[2] discuss aspects of statistical consultation, and Baskerville[3] proposes a plan for training consulting statisticians. All three works are bountiful sources of examples of the consultative process and of additional references.

This chapter focuses neither on the consultative interaction that takes only five minutes nor on the mature relationship between a clinical and a statistical investigator that has developed through joint work on several projects. Rather, we address situations in which the integrity of the research effort may depend on sound statistical design, analysis, and interpretation, all of which may require a joint effort extending at least over several weeks. The merit of such a cooperative undertaking rests largely on the participants' success in dealing with two classes of activities that we call scientific interaction and coordination of affairs.

Portions of this chapter have appeared elsewhere (Moses L, Louis TA. "Statistical consultation in clinical research: a two-way street" in Bailar JC and Mosteller F. *Medical Uses of Statistics,* Second Edition, 1992: 349–356. Copyright 1992 Massachusetts Medical Society) and are included with the permission of the Massachusetts Medical Society.

Scientific Interaction

The consultation may start with a question that seems limited, such as "Would you give me a reference to the Mann-Whitney test?" or "What software package can do a logistic regression on our computer?" Or the question may seem (and be) broad, as in the following examples: "We are preparing a research proposal. Would you look over the statistics part? May we name you as a consultant?" or "A journal has just rejected this paper because of the statistics. Will you help me prepare it for resubmission?" However the transaction may begin, its sound progress depends crucially on one thing: the clinician and the statistical consultant must ultimately be dealing with the same problem. At the beginning, the scientific problem is unknown to the consultant. Before he or she can be helpful, the statistician must correctly understand the investigation—its purposes, motivating questions, materials, techniques, and measurements; if he or she offers advice based on a misapprehension of these features, the advice may be wrong and useless or even damaging. Thus, a clear, mutual understanding of the problem is the single most important element in the consultation.

Step-by-step communication is necessary for success. As noted above, the statistician must first gain a correct understanding of the substantive problem. When a point seems to be understood, he or she should check it by saying, "Now, let me tell *you*—the clinician—about this point and see if I have it right." This step may have to be repeated. Similarly, the clinician needs to understand the essential statistical features of the project; the investigator can best check his or her comprehension of a concept by explaining it to a colleague or to the statistician.

Each partner should have high expectations of the other. Statistical thinking is in a large measure scientific thinking, once it is understood. Clarity from the statistician is a proper expectation. Similarly, the statistician may reasonably expect that the clinician can make clear most information that he or she understands well. The iterative style of communication helps to ensure that these high expectations will be met. Of course, jargon is an unacceptable encumbrance in the consultation.

The statistician should not use it and should not accept it from the clinician.

A broad definition of the problem can lead more quickly to a correct understanding of a highly specific concept than would a narrowly focused treatment of that concept alone. This principle applies to both clinical and statistical issues, with two main consequences. First, each collaborator should be prepared to do some reading in the other's field. Second, each partner should be wary of attempting to protect the other by not mentioning topics that may be relevant, merely to avoid what may be perceived as needless complication. Although in everyday life communication may be eased by the omission of details that seem inessential or difficult to explain, that practice can lead to trouble in scientific collaboration.

Both participants' understanding of the problem needs to be specific. The worth of a study may turn on details. For example, the difference between a sound randomized clinical trial and a collection of anecdotal material depends on the answers to questions like these: How were the patients for this investigation chosen? How was it decided which ones would receive which treatment? Did the person assessing posttreatment status know which treatment the patient had received? Did the patient know?

Specific knowledge about the measurement process can also be essential. Measurements of the same phenomenon may vary from day to day; to assess that possibility in a study, it is necessary to know which observations were made on which days, with which piece of apparatus, and by which technician or interviewer. Some measurements are actually composites of others, and the variability of the composite will depend on the variability of its components. If the statistical consultant is involved in planning the investigation, his or her understanding the details may permit a more effective and efficient experimental design.

Broad, specific, and iterative communication is, therefore, essential to the consultation. But additional measures can also help the collaboration to succeed. For instance, it can be useful at an appropriate stage for one of the partners to attend a meeting of the other's colleagues, one addressed to the subject of the investigation. The clinician may invite the statistician to staff meetings or may be invited to a seminar of statistical staff and students. From such meetings, new ideas and helpful criticism often emerge.

Frequently, the collaboration is advanced by observation. The statistician may more quickly gain a fuller understanding of the study by seeing the apparatus in use, watching the diagnostic procedure, and looking at the recording processes. Similarly, the clinician who undertakes to follow the data-editing steps and statistical calculations may gain insight from doing so.

Written communication may advance the work notably. Questions, requests, information, and tentative proposals all tend to gain specificity in written form. Memoranda are not subject to memory decay and can be discussed with knowledgeable colleagues of the recipient (and the sender). Memoranda may be used advantageously to record the current stage in the participants' thinking, the nature of an issue that urgently demands resolution, or the details of a proposal that will require consultative work. It pays to be aware of situations in which a memorandum may be the preferred method of communication.

Thorough communication may take time, but shortcuts must be avoided. This recommendation parallels good medical practice, which calls for taking a medical history before prescribing treatment. The parallel reaches further; it may be that the analysis (or treatment) will not ultimately be changed by the fuller understanding (or history). In that case, the payoff is the confidence that the right course has been taken. Boen and Zahn[1] have a similar view of the role of consultation.

Coordination of Affairs

When two or more people share a task, certain difficulties may crop up as the work goes forward. Forethought can eliminate many such problems, especially when willing participants have joined together in a mutually attractive project. Problems are likely to be fewer and smaller when partners have worked together before. In a collaboration between clinician and statistician, there may be benefit in asking certain questions in advance and agreeing on the answers. Issues that merit such consideration are the schedule, resources, decisions about acknowledgment versus coauthorship, and the use of data.

Schedule

What is the schedule for the project? Are there deadlines and can they be met? Most clinicians and many statisticians grossly underestimate the time necessary to complete the project and overestimate the time available. Data must be collected before they can be analyzed and before a report can be written, and each step takes time.

If it can be foreseen that the work will proceed in stages, the participants should decide how much time should be allowed for each stage, and who is responsible for completing it. For example, data need to be prepared for computer entry, entered, and checked for validity before analysis can begin. Generally, the clinician will have to participate in the first and third of these activities, especially by providing feedback on acceptable ranges for data and by checking on numbers that are out of range.

Resources

Are the resources (budget, computer time, and personnel) adequate, or are some changes needed? Many long-term projects require a statistical collaborator, not simply an occasional consultant. A person who is trained to use statistical computing packages should be identified early so that the analysis recommended by the statistician can be carried out. Occasionally, standard computing packages cannot perform appropriate analyses for a particular investigation, and special-purpose routines must be used or new programs must be written. However, statistical packages for microcomputers now provide all standard and many specialized analyses and graphics. Therefore, statistical input sharply focuses on what to do and what to make of results; these enterprises require a large dose of statistical input. In addition, the statistician should ensure that the requisite hardware, software, and organizational structures are available to produce valid and timely data and analyses.

If financial issues arise in relation to the work, then clarity about them is crucial. Are there to be charges for the statistical consultation? How will the services of programmers be funded? What about computing costs, data entry, secretarial support?

Acknowledgment versus Coauthorship

Sooner or later a decision about authorship of the study will need to be made. High-quality statistical input in the design and analysis phases of a project can be as important a scientific contribution as that provided by the medical team. Early discussion of authorship may lead either to an agreement to defer the decision until the participants' relative contributions can be assessed, or to a tentative decision subject to change.

If coauthorship does not seem appropriate, then acknowledgement is in order. The statistician should be acknowledged for his or her advice—if it is taken, thus establishing responsibility as well as credit. Acknowledgments that are too broad or otherwise inaccurate can be unfair; it follows that any acknowledgment should be reviewed and accepted by the statistician.

Use of the Data

It may be wise to agree in advance on arrangements concerning possible future uses of the study's data and statistical analyses. Either party may someday wish to use the material in other articles or in textbooks. What steps should be taken if such an occasion arises?

The message of this discussion of potentially troublesome issues is not that there are many ways to get into difficulty but that it is well to consider early, and to agree about, the essential steps in completing the work. The collaborators should talk about the logistics of the project, resolve any immediate problems quickly, and be aware of potential problems not yet settled. It can be helpful to record the results of these discussions in a joint memorandum that may bring to light some previously unnoticed misunderstandings. We see disadvantages to this method, too; sometimes the air is chilled by the utterance "Let's put that in writing." But the possibility of preparing a memorandum about logistics deserves explicit consideration.

The Benefits of Statistical Consultation

We began this chapter by observing that clinical investigations often present problems that demand statistical treatment—correct statistical treatment. Of course, collaboration with a biostatistician will usually help with such problems. Interaction between clinician and statistician in the planning phases of a project can identify tractable scientific and statistical problems that will need attention and can help avoid intractable ones. After the data are in, it can be too late for statistical attention. As a colleague, Helena Kraemer (personal communication), has remarked,

> If consultation is at the *Post Hoc* stage, it may be that objectives cannot be accomplished (sampling bias, poor design, etc.). It is the statistician's responsibility to state this frankly. We cannot do magic, and we can't participate in cover-ups. It is as well that researchers know our limitations in advance. This is a particular problem when the first consultation takes place after a research paper is rejected for publication because of poor methodology. Not much one can do!

A study that has been planned in the light of statistical considerations is less likely to have statistical flaws. In addition, it can occasionally be much more cost-effective, saving time, money, or both. Sometimes the scope of a study can be broadened at little or no cost by making use of familiar patterns of statistical design in experiments. Admittedly, however, a good study often costs more than a poor one. Finally, intellectual benefits often accrue to either collaborator, or both, and to their students and coworkers.

Acknowledgments. We are indebted to the Harvard study group, Helena Kraemer, Ph.D., Peter Gregory, M.D., and Byron William Brown, Jr., Ph.D., for their feedback and encouragement.

References

1. Boen JR, Zahn DA. The human side of statistical consulting. Belmont, Calif.: Lifetime Learning Publications, 1982.
2. Hand DJ, Everitt BS, eds. The statistical consultant in action. Cambridge: Cambridge University, 1987.
3. Baskerville JC. A systematic study of the consulting literature as an integral part of applied training in statistics. Am Stat 1981;35:121–123.

SECTION V

Funding

R.E. Pollock

This part of *Surgical Research: Basic Principles and Clinical Practice* provides practical information about funding surgical research. We use the United States, Canada, and Europe as our examples, listing sources as well as "how to do it" advice about compiling and submitting grant applications. Perspectives of both the applicant and the reviewer are represented. These examples provide generalizable principles that can be applied in applications to most funding sources.

Grants are important to the academic surgeon for several reasons. On a practical level, a successful grant application leads to research funds under the direct control of the investigator. These funds can be used to finance an independent basic research laboratory, and as a means to "purchase" protected time for research pursuits. They provide funds to support the research environment: utilities, housekeeping, and core facilities. These activities are supported by so-called indirect funds that are awarded to the institution on behalf of the principal investigator. Indirect funds help department chairmen negotiate from a position of strength for additional intramural resources.

The well-prepared grant is a planning document that forces the principal investigator to define how an appreciable period of time and effort will be committed over the next three to five years in pursuit of specific research goals. A grant proposal provides an additional avenue for planning because it can be used as a tool to develop and strengthen collaborations. The grant is a succinct document demonstrating that the ideas of the principal investigators are on the "cutting edge," and the investigator is well organized and deeply committed to pursuing independent research.

While independent extramural funding is difficult to achieve, surgeons have several important advantages. Surgeons are keenly aware of what constitutes the significant unresolved clinical issues. Natural strengths that surgeons bring to the grantsmanship arena include a strong work ethic inculcated during the many years of clinical training, coupled with an enthusiasm and willingness to work effectively with others. While there are scant funds available for frivolous projects, a well-conceived proposal that seeks to dissect out underlying biologic mechanisms stands a good chance of ultimate funding, provided that surgical persistence is applied to the process. This is a good struggle well worth joining. Even if not initially funded, preparing and submitting a grant provides a surgical investigator with an effective means of enhancing the understanding of a given disease process, focuses thinking about solutions, strengthens collaborations, and ultimately improves the welfare of surgical patients.

CHAPTER 40

Formulating an Initial Research Plan

R.E. Pollock, C.M. Balch, J. Roth, B. McPeek, and F. Mosteller

Much thought occurs before you are ready to formulate an initial research proposal. At the broadest level, a fertile mind must be receptive to fresh ideas, ready to nurture and support a nascent plan and, after a period of intellectual germination, able to formulate the idea into a written research proposal. The process, and this chapter, operates on two levels, one, broad, conceptual, and philosophical; the other, focused, structural, and expository.

Nurturing Scientific Creativity

Research aims at learning more about the world we live in. Ordinarily, we cannot study the world or nature without first simplifying it to make our learning assignment more manageable. We study nature by abstracting it so that it becomes possible to handle, describe, and measure in a controlled, systematic way. We try to take nature into our laboratory. We subject it to experimental manipulation using modern techniques of biology and chemistry, biostatistics, epidemiology, and so forth.

In theory, we first conceive a scientific topic or issue and then try to fashion a project we could do that would yield information on the issue. In an orderly world, one might first think about the issue, what is known about it, perhaps what's not known—and some scientists do work this way.

More commonly, we conceive of a project and then realize it could produce information bearing on nature.

A variety of strategies help bring fresh insights. Ideas or techniques from one field can be applied to another, producing information that is novel and not yet available in the second field. If you hope to do scientific work, read widely. Discuss your research ideas with a variety of people who work in different scholarly areas. The literature in your own field may have a limited view of research or approaches to your topic or issue. Make a habit of browsing and reading widely in science. Remember that social scientists as well as natural scientists and clinical scholars have much to offer that is relevant to bedside medicine and surgery. Go to national scientific meetings, particularly meetings in fields other than your own.

Teaching students offers a frequent source of new ideas or insights. Students may be less constrained by the limits we see in our present knowledge and methodology. Students often ask "Why?" They have mental flexibility and recent exposure to other fields.

You must have a skeptical attitude toward conventional wisdom. Do the explanations we offer about nature or about the problems we see in our clinic really make sense? Think about what is really known and how surely it is known. Most of us are far too confident of the state of our own knowledge.

Good Questions

What makes a good research question? A good question seems interesting; the more you think about it, the more interesting it appears. As you think about it and discuss it with your research team, you want to work on it. It sparks your curiosity and emphasizes your strengths and those of the team. Its solution seems important. You would feel rewarded for your effort.

Scientists seek questions that offer originality and answers that would aim toward the solution of a basic scientific problem or have clear clinical value. We don't always think enough about feasibility. Most of us are good at devising infeasible projects requiring the key to the national treasury, as well as collaborators, patient material, equipment, space, or knowledge that is not available. This is not just an issue of a team's strengths and weaknesses (e.g., pediatric projects are difficult to run in a veterans' hospital). It is a more general problem. Inexperienced workers constantly find themselves asking too much of a research project. We forget that there is no scientific project that our own grandiose ideas cannot inflate to the point of infeasibility.

Build on Experience

As you start to develop your research project, take advantage of past experience, talk to your friends who work in the field. Seek the help of a senior scientific mentor if you are just starting out. Try to view your project as part of a continuing research program. This will serve to focus some of your interests and help you build on previous successes. It may subtly keep you from dissipating your efforts across too wide an area.

Team Work

As you develop a project, consider working with other people. Most of us find it is fun, and it is very productive. Different people have different strengths, different experiences, different insights. As you advance an idea, a whole new formulation may occur to your partner. When you plan a joint project, try to develop a series of short-term goals. They make definite what is needed or expected of individuals at a given time. They also subtly assign guilt for not having produced work (*subtly* is an important word because nothing will end a collaboration quicker than an atmosphere of blame). On the other hand, a tiny amount of self-felt guilt may advance a project as partners take their responsibilities more seriously. Regular meetings are vital for production because they provide definite expectations and deadlines.

Let us say you have an idea that seems promising and feasible, and you think it will be fun. An initial research proposal helps structure, focus, and communicate your ideas to others.

Writing a Research Proposal

A research proposal is an internal working document—not to be confused with a grant application—used by many investigators to formulate their ideas. It facilitates original and productive research by structuring intuitive intellectual processes into a carefully defined set of plans. These plans should delineate the hypothesis to be tested, appropriate controls, and an experimental design that will promote originality and clinical relevance.

In our laboratories, we continuously develop a variety of research proposals as a means of structuring, focusing, and communicating our ideas.

General Principles

1. The proposal should address one or more hypotheses to be tested. These hypotheses should be grounded firmly in underlying biological or physiological principles. Occasionally, the necessary experiments are observational (phenomenological), and a successful outcome depends on a positive result. The more incisive studies usually address hypotheses of significant scientific interest, whether the results are positive or negative.

2. Have a clear understanding of the potential clinical relevance of your proposal. Most surgical investigations are preclinical studies in relevant animal or in vitro models that have ultimate applicability to the surgical patient, or clinical stud-

ies that use human materials in vitro or accompany clinical research protocols.

3. Use the proposal-drafting process to capture and focus your ideas. Drafts only one to three pages long provide good frameworks for organizing data and concepts as they mature over time; review and update them periodically. Circulate your drafts among laboratory workers or possible collaborators as a means of initiating later discussion.

4. Know and keep up with the literature in your field. The essence of good research is originality and significance; remaining abreast of the literature helps to ensure that your own work will maintain its originality. It also allows you to design experiments that permit comparisons with published results.

5. Establish research collaborations and mentorships wherever possible. A research proposal provides a good basis for discussion and delineation of responsibilities in a multifaceted and collaborative research effort.

Outline of a Research Proposal

The basic elements of a research proposal include title, investigators, hypothesis, objectives, research design, and budget.

Title

The title delineates the theme of the research proposal; it should be as concise and focused as possible.

List of Investigators

When multiple investigators are participating in collaborative research, it is especially important to name the principal investigators and to delineate their degrees of responsibility at the outset of a research proposal. Since the order of listing may well reflect the authorship sequence on subsequent manuscripts or abstracts, the hierarchy should be decided at the start, to avoid later conflicts about authorship.

Hypothesis

The hypothesis should be based on the specific questions to be asked. An effective hypothesis usually examines the biological or physiological mechanisms underlying an unexplained observation; it should not be global but should focus on the specific area of inquiry.

Research Objectives

No more than four or five concise, *specific* questions should be listed as objectives, and they should be compatible with the research theme reflected in the title and the hypothesis being tested.

Research Design

The section on research design summarizes the overall strategy and specific tactics to be employed in testing the hypothesis and achieving the research objective. It is an outline of the basic experimental design, including a delineation of the appropriate control sample size and statistical methods to be used, and might also include a data flow sheet in a form suitable for automation and computerized statistical analysis.

Research Budget

Make a strenuous attempt to take specific account of all the costs of conducting the research project, to ensure the availability of sufficient funds to complete the study. Funding requirements for new supplies or needed, or potentially needed, equipment to conduct the research should be identified.

Conclusion

Preparing research proposals is an integral part of the effective functioning of any research laboratory, whether the research projects are large or small. The process engenders a rigorous and analytical focusing of research ideas and minimizes the risk of wasting time and resources associated with more casual or informal approaches to laboratory research. After preliminary data have been generated, a research proposal may become the basic framework for a formal research proposal and grant application.

CHAPTER 41

Ten Tips on Preparing Research Proposals

W.O. Spitzer

New or potential investigators with good research ideas often fail to take even the first step toward exploring or implementing those ideas. This usually happens when the required resources do not appear to be available. Young investigators and even mature clinicians with strong track records in teaching and service become unduly discouraged at the thought of writing a study protocol, submitting it to peer appraisal, and overcoming all the real and imaginary hurdles associated with the preparation of grant applications.

Unfortunately, clinicians who practice outside universities and colleges, and whose ongoing contact with the "real world" makes their work particularly relevant to the needs of patients, are among those who are most easily discouraged. They assume they do not have the ability or the credentials required to generate the financial support their project needs and merits, and they make no effort to seek it.

Although some skills are necessary, and there is a "right way" to do certain things, much of what is needed to prepare a research proposal is common sense. Seasoned investigators with long careers have learned most of what they need to know about writing grant applications from the com-

ments, recommendations, and objections of the peer reviewers of their earlier proposals.

The suggestions that follow are not intended as a "checklist" that will guarantee your success in "shaking the money tree" of research foundations and other research funding agencies. They are simply some tips learned over the years from colleagues and passed on to the reader. Anybody venturing into research is certain to make mistakes at first; the suggestions that follow may help you to avoid some predictable pitfalls.

Before you consider each of the ten points, it is important that you realize that undertaking research without a protocol is irresponsible at best, and unethical at worst. Doing so is just as reprehensible as embarking on the construction of a building without approved blueprints from an architect. As a general recommendation, avoid initiating or participating in "off the cuff" or "informal" research when no effort has been made to develop a plan, rationalize it, and commit it to writing in advance. Writing a grant proposal accomplishes these goals, whether it is funded on the first submission or not.

1. State Your Objective and Study Questions Clearly

When you come upon a good idea, an intriguing hypothesis, a burning question, or an important demonstration project, write your thoughts down,

Adapted with permission from Spitzer WO. Ten tips on preparing research proposals. Can Nurse 1973; 69(3):30–33.

promptly. Then, preferably within days, carefully restate your project or study. Two important steps must now be taken; neglect of either will frequently jeopardize the quality of the rest of your work. First, write the broad objective of the study. Second, formulate the specific questions your research project seeks to answer.

Try to limit the questions to two or three; if you find yourself writing more than five or six, your objectives may be vague and your concepts woolly. Questions should be phrased to permit objective and, preferably, quantitative answers. Here are some examples:

Example I

Objective. To determine whether the introduction of a system in which a senior general surgery resident functions as a consultant in the emergency ward of a teaching hospital would expedite the handling of patients with surgical problems.

Related Study Questions

1. Is the span of time from the arrival of a patient in the triage station in the emergency ward to a disposition (i.e., discharge home or admission to hospital) reduced?
2. Are calls to other senior surgical residents and to surgical attending staff in the hospital to come to the emergency room reduced after introduction of the on-site surgical resident compared to the previous situation?
3. Does an assessment of the quality of surgical care for nonelective conditions, using a quantitative index developed specifically for surgical problems commonly seen in the emergency room, indicate any improvement following introduction of the new arrangement?

Example II

Objective. To determine whether a strategy of transporting trauma patients to hospitals that involves limiting intervention at the accident site or in transit to first aid and essential lifesaving maneuvers is preferable to deploying surgeons with sophisticated equipment to accident sites to initiate more immediate and definitive treatment.

Related Research Questions

1. What are the rates of mortality and of serious residual morbidity for cases treated with the first versus the second approach, after adjustments have been made for case mix and severity?
2. What are the direct and indirect costs of the first compared with the second approach?
3. What are the barriers to the feasibility of each approach in urban and rural areas? ("Urban" and "rural" will have been operationally defined very carefully.)

Example III

Objective. To determine whether a specific preoperative bowel preparation in conjunction with intravenous administration of antibiotic X improves the results of aortofemoral grafting in patients with selected types of aortoiliac occlusive disease and abdominal aortic aneurysms.

Related Study Questions

1. What is the immediate postoperative morbidity (i.e., within 72 hours) of patients who receive the bowel preparation plus antibiotic X compared to those who receive antibiotic X alone?
2. What is the infection rate in the aortofemoral grafts within 30 days of the operation among patients in each of the arms of the study?
3. What are the 1-year and 5-year survival rates for patients in each arm of the study?
4. Do intervening dental procedures, minor operations, or viral or bacterial infections such as pneumonia or gastroenteritis affect the survival and morbidity rates for patients in each arm of the study?

When you have rewritten your objectives and study questions several times, review them with colleagues whose opinions you respect. They are likely to give you candid comments on the clarity of your objective, the feasibility of the project, and whether your research questions are sensible and amenable to research.

2. Study the Background Literature and Summarize It in Your Proposal

It is important to determine whether the kind of study or project you propose has already been done. Those who are asked to review grant applications are usually very knowledgeable in the appropriate field and are aware of related work reported in the literature or in progress. It is unlikely that you will be granted support for a project that is equivalent to seeking to "reinvent the typewriter." Expert advice on how to review the literature is provided in chapters 7, 10, and 38.

When you have reviewed the literature, write it up briefly. If you are not breaking completely new ground, you should demonstrate how or why your project would shed new light on a problem already studied by others, how you will obtain new knowledge, or how you will test an innovative application of existing knowledge. If your emphasis is on application of existing techniques or knowledge, you should indicate the relevance of your work in such terms as *benefit to patients* or *greater efficiency attained*.

3. Decide on General Strategy

Before you consider the detailed tactics you might adopt (e.g., selection of comparison groups, delineation of criteria, selection of samples, scoring techniques), design your general strategy. Are you proposing a demonstration model? Will you be conducting a survey? Do you plan a true experiment? The nature of your objective and your research questions will usually suggest the proper strategy. When two or more approaches would be suitable, your choice should be based on which is the most feasible and practical.

A common pitfall is to seek support from a research-funding agency for a project that is clearly not research. If you are trying to establish a service or educational project, such as a counseling center for adolescents who have sustained serious skiing accidents, you should apply to granting agencies whose terms of reference include the provision of funds for service or educational programs on the basis of their merit, rather than an agency whose primary focus is on research into the pathophysiology and treatment of trauma.

4. Identify the Most Appropriate Funding Agency

You should investigate whether accepted procedures or ethical considerations justify your submitting your application to more than one funding agency for support for the same project. It is important to make a decision about possible sources of funds at this stage because the tactics you specify in your detailed research design may be influenced or even determined in part by the known policies of a funding agency. Most funding agencies publish their terms of reference, and you should obtain and study them before proceeding.

5. Seek Expert Consultations

This is the time to consult some experts. Although you may have spoken with colleagues or other advisers when you formulated your objectives and study questions, you should now consult with resource persons such as research methodologists, biostatisticians, or other experts in the field that concerns you. Too often, consultations are sought *after* a grant application has been rejected or the data have been gathered. By that time, it is usually too late for a consultation to be of much help to you. Consultation with the administration staff and with the director of the agency to which you are planning to apply is an invaluable but often neglected step. You can learn what is "fundable" under the agencies' present guidelines, and you can obtain many valuable suggestions about your application. For a major grant or contract, it is worthwhile to do this in person.

At most institutions, there are experienced investigators who have well-developed skills in the field of "grantsmanship." Do not hesitate to enlist their support in planning your grant. A critical review of the finished grant by such an adviser can be extremely valuable, even if the consultant is outside your field.

When you seek expert advice about your research design, it is wise to consider some ethical questions. Are there any risks to patients or other individuals who may become study subjects? If there are, do they outweigh the potential benefits to such individuals or to the population in general? Will the study subjects be free from invasion of their privacy or any form of personal assault? Are reasonable safeguards incorporated in the design to protect the confidentiality of personal or clinical information? Is it ethical in your particular study to withhold some treatment from a control group?

The following commitment, in these or equivalent terms, should be included in your grant application:

> The individuals and families involved in this investigation would enjoy freedom from assault: personal privacy, the ability to withdraw from the experiment at any time, and the confidentiality of all personal information obtained would be scrupulously protected. The applicants have carefully weighed the potential gains from the new knowledge that would be obtained from this investigation and have concluded that these gains vastly outweigh the risks to the individuals involved in this project. Consent to take part in this investigation will be requested only after full disclosure of the nature of the project and of any potential risks to the prospective participant associated with the delivery of health services in the proposed fashion.

Some agencies require a statement on ethics (i.e., approval of the project by a properly constituted ethics review committee) in each proposal, along with copies of the consent forms that will be used.

6. Specify the Criteria You Will Use to Evaluate the Answers to Your Study Questions and the Success of Your Project

Unless you indicate what kind of objective or quantitative answers to your research questions will constitute a particular verdict, your proposal may be regarded as a self-fulfilling prophecy.

Specifying the criteria for judging the answers to research questions, *in advance*, usually distinguishes the disciplined and rigorous investigator from the wishful thinker who is out to prove a point. If we refer back to question 3 under Example I, the criterion for success might be:

Criterion. Bowel preparation plus antibiotic X will be judged to be better than antibiotic X alone if two of the following three outcomes are demonstrated:

1. The immediate postoperative morbidity in the combined approach is not only less than that with antibiotic alone, but is less than 2% of that.
2. The rate of infection of patients treated with the combined approach is 20% less than it is in those treated with antibiotic alone, within 30 days of the operation.
3. The 1-year and 5-year survival rates for patients treated with the combined approach are at least 20% better than they are in those treated with antibiotic alone.

Although negative findings in a study tend to be viewed as evidence that it failed, it may really have been successful if it provided strong, irrefutable evidence that settled a question. *The success of a study or project is not determined by the verdict it yielded, but by the quality of the evidence it produced.* Consequently, it is wise to spell out the criteria that will determine the success of your project separately from the criteria to be used in evaluating the answers to your study question.

7. Be as Brief and Clear as Possible

Reviewers of grants are not particularly interested in reading countless typed pages. Most successful grant applications for clinical or health care research projects are not longer than 10 to 15 pages. Unnecessary verbiage reflects unfavorably on the applicant's ability to think clearly and communicate effectively. Brevity, however, should not be carried to the point of failure to communicate why your group is distinctive and able to make a significant contribution. If your proposal covers a large study involving several centers and a complex design, the detailed descriptions required may justify an application that is considerably longer.

Funding agencies take pride in identifying and supporting investigators who will be effective in solving problems. A helpful stratagem you can incorporate in the significance section of your grant application is to point out that your institution has already assembled most of the pieces of the puzzle. You can show, for example, with solid documentation, that you have access to all the patients needed for the study, most of the required laboratory equipment, and a well-developed plan with a proven record of productivity; *all you need* is support to obtain the few missing pieces of the puzzle. In other words, the granting agency can underwrite a solution to the problem very economically by supporting your research plan to provide the last few pieces of the puzzle.

Although the suggested outline for grant applications provided in Appendix 41-1 will require modification for each study and may have to be changed to conform with different requirements in various countries, it may be useful in getting your thinking started and in assembling the information you will need.

8. Keep Appendices and Supporting Documents to a Minimum

Lengthy appendices, supporting documents, and bibliographies will produce a cumbersome application. The reviewer will usually feel compelled to read them and may well be irritated when he has finished if the appendices do not contribute much. An appendix or supporting document should be included only if the proposal cannot be understood without it, and it is clearly inappropriate to include the information (e.g., the precise format of an interview form) in the main body of the application. If you are in doubt, briefly state in the text of your proposal what the document contains and indicate that it is available on request. Do not attach it.

9. Be Realistic in Your Assessment of the Available and Required Resources

Do not propose to hire categories of professionals that are not available in your setting or community. If the execution of your project depends on nonexistent human or other resources, or on equipment you cannot maintain, you should not be applying for support. On the other hand, identifying *by name* the person who will perform a task strengthens the proposal by its concreteness.

Ascertain very carefully what funds you will need for salaries, equipment, supplies, specialized services, consultants, and other items. Underestimating what you require will cause you unnecessary difficulties when you come to carry out your study. Deliberately overestimating the cost of the required resources will undermine your credibility during the first review or when you submit your annual progress report.

The peers who will judge the merits of your proposal and assess its progress when you submit renewal requests are usually aware that errors of judgment can be made in estimating the requirements for a study; most of them have experienced such embarrassments and are sympathetic. Reviewers can be expected to be reasonable about applications for amendments of budgets when such requests are sensible and caused by unforeseeable contingencies. It is much better to submit supplementary requests, if the need arises, than to "pad" a submission at the outset.

10. Prepare and Justify Your Budget Carefully

Most granting agencies provide preprinted application forms that include the required breakdown of requested funding into budgeting categories. Nevertheless many research proposals are submitted without adequate justification of the expenditures included in the various categories, or without enough detail about the budget as a whole to enable the appraiser to link listed items of expenditure with the activities described in the project.

Your justification of your budget should explain the need for each individual for whom a salary (or wages) is requested, and for every item of equipment, each category of supplies, travel, and any other special requirements.

It is wise to identify any major expenditure for which the estimates are not firm. Should budgetary difficulties concerning an uncertain estimate arise later, prior identification of the potential problem will have paved the way for approval of any necessary amendment.

Conclusion

Preparing a research proposal and applying for its support need not be dreaded as an unavoidable tournament that must precede any rewarding research activity. Designing a project, exploring feasible approaches to its implementation, identifying the resources needed, and communicating all this information in a grant application are integral components of investigative activity. If you don't win the award the first time, you have still organized your project. Seek a detailed critique from the reviewers, revise your application, and resubmit it. The whole process is intellectually challenging and can even be enjoyable.

Appendix I

Suggested Outline for a Research Protocol

A. Summary (300 words or less)
B. Main protocol
  1. The objective and research question(s)
    a. Objective
    b. Question(s)—may be restated as a hypothesis or hypotheses if desired or appropriate
    c. Significance of the problem to health care or biomedical science
  2. Review of pertinent literature
  3. General strategy of the study, including a discussion of the rationale for the choice of method(s) (e.g., historical study, survey, experiment; use or not of comparison groups)
  4. Laboratory and/or clinical facilities (if applicable)
  5. Specific procedures or tactics

    a. Kinds of information to be collected
    b. Procedures to be used in the collection of information
    c. From whom the information will be collected
    d. By whom the information will be collected
    e. Where information will be collected
    f. Schedule for collection of information
    g. Copies of letters, recording forms, interview schedules, questionnaires, and so forth should be included either in the text or appendices, as deemed appropriate
  6. Ethical considerations
  7. Methods of data preparation
  8. Method of analysis, including statistical techniques, if appropriate (for sections 6 and 7, justify any planned use of computers)
  9. Dummy tables, charts, and graphs
 10. Justification of budget
 11. Criteria for success of the project

Summary of the Ten Recommendations

1. State objective and research questions clearly.
2. Use the literature review to justify the need for the proposed project.
3. Be clear about your general strategy.
4. Identify the appropriate funding agency.
5. Seek early consultation with experts.
6. Declare criteria for evaluating answers to the research questions *and* the success of project.
7. Be brief.
8. Keep appendices and supporting documents to a minimum.
9. Assess the resources needed to implement your project realistically.
10. Justify your budget carefully.

Additional Reading

Apley AG. The Watson-Jones lecture 1984: surgeons and writers. J Bone Joint Surg (Br) 1985;67:140–144.

Dixon J. Developing the evaluation component of a grant application. J Nurs Outlook 1982;30:122–127.

Jagger J. How to write a research proposal. Grants Mag 1980;3(4):216–222.

Skodal HW. Research proposal: the practical imagi-

CHAPTER 42

Funding Research in North America: The United States

J.E. Fischer

Departmental Support

Research in departments of surgery was traditionally funded by transfer of clinical income, especially from high earners, to those doing the research. This system was never really able to fund full-time programs at the best of times. In the current economic climate, departments of surgery can provide only seed money and a modicum of support for 3 years for new faculty surgeons to develop a research program. Beyond that, each laboratory must derive its support from some of the sources described below.

Not all departments want to sponsor research, and not all chairpersons believe that research is critical to their program. However, a commitment to research must be a departmental commitment; it cannot be solely a chairperson's commitment. Most department members must believe research to be worthwhile. Even if laboratories are not supported by clinical monies, there will inevitably be some transfer from those who generate the clinical dollars to those who are spending some time in research. This money may be for core support of the department, support of those academic functions that department members agree should be funded, or for monetary rewards to the researchers if this is departmental policy. In general, researchers will never be rewarded monetarily to the extent that busy clinicians will be, but recognition of the value of what they do, similar to rewards for teaching, is essential.

If departments cannot support programs over a prolonged period, some reserve funds should be set aside for interim support of individuals who lose their grants. Unfortunately, losing support is a fact of research life that may become more common in the future. Bridging funds are essential if a departmental commitment to research is to be kept. I emphasize that this should be only "bridge" funding and cannot be a permanent part of the laboratory's support.

Collaboration with Basic Scientists

Surgeons who are excellent researchers generally can support themselves through the practice of surgery if they participate in an income-sharing practice with other productive clinicians. The laboratory, however, must be fundable from external sources. In the current scientific milieu, successful competition for funding depends on hiring first-class collaborating postdoctoral researchers to work within the department of surgery. Many departments like ours have hired such individuals, who often have their own funding. Collaborations with basic scientists are mutually beneficial. Usually a clinical problem has sparked the idea for the research project; surgeons can provide a sense of direction, defined goals, and a well-developed ability to get from point A to point B without going through point Z. In addition, surgeons in academic departments can often provide a willing and talented source of manpower: surgical residents who spend protected time in the laboratory. Basic scientists with whom we collaborate love to work with surgical residents, who approach the laboratory as if they were still on the clinical service: they come early, stay late, and are generally bright, intelligent, energetic problem solvers with a highly developed sense of morality and the value of work.

Funding Surgical Residents in the Laboratory

Fortunately, there is a fairly large number of scholarships available for surgical residents who wish to spend two years in the laboratory. The scholarships include NIH training grants in trauma and critical care, cancer, heart disease, and gastrointestinal disease, and National Research Scholarship Applications (NRSA). In addition, at least 36 surgical organizations fund scholarships for residents, giving whole or partial support for the period in the laboratory. This estimate does not include local scholarships or others such as the Shriners of North America scholarships. A list of scholarships is published in February of each year in the *Bulletin of the American College of Surgeons* as a service of the Surgical Research and Education Committee of the College. An increasing number of organizations are attempting to fund such fellowships to provide for the uninterrupted growth of surgical research.

Funding Sources

Diversity is a politically correct word. In the case of funding research, *diversity* is an essential word; diversified research funding protects continuity and productivity. Following is a diverse list of sources for research funding, including tips on successfully obtaining funding from those sources.

The National Institutes of Health (NIH)

Although becoming more difficult for everybody, including surgeons, to obtain, NIH funding remains the gold standard. It is highly respected by colleagues and prized by deans because of the substantial amount of overhead that accrues to the medical school, and the fact that it is administered under the financial control of the dean. Deans compare their various departments and make space and other resource allocation decisions based on NIH funding. While funds obtained from other organizations may have the same cash value, they do not contribute as much overhead.

NIH awards for new investigators, both the R29s (the First awards) and the K08s (Clinician Investigator awards), may have a more favorable funding percentage than the standard R01 award for more established investigators. The review process for the R29s may be somewhat less stringent for young investigators, especially on reapplication. The K08s certainly have a different review process because of the fact that these grants support a mentoring relationship. The burden of proof of merit is on the mentors and their track records rather than on the investigators. Thanks to the efforts of the Surgical Research and Education Committee of the American College of Surgeons, K08s are now available to surgeons. (See Table 44-1 in chapter 44 on writing grant applications for the NIH.)

Veterans Affairs

In previous years, the VA hospitals were an excellent resource for the funding of research of young faculty members. RRAGs, the initial research applications by VA physicians and surgeons who contributed at least 5/8 time, could provide funding for 2 years at up to $35,000 per year. Since this funding did not include the surgeon's salary, it was a valuable resource. The RRAG proposals as a source of funding have become unpredictable because VA funding is no longer secure. This formerly reliable avenue has become a source of frustration to young faculty members.

Similarly, the merit review process, which previously funded more than half of the grant applications reviewed, now funds approximately the same percentage of grants as the NIH. The review process is just as stringent. Although this avenue can be pursued, one should bear in mind that the assurance of getting funding here is considerably less than in the past. The research track of the VA may provide funding for meritorious research by basic scientists, especially those within departments of surgery.

Development Awards from National Organizations

The American College of Surgeons and the American Surgical Association both have developmental awards for young faculty members. These are highly competitive and very prestigious awards intended to support young surgical investigators. They provide comparatively long periods (up to 5 years) of funding with partial salary support. The American Association for Thoracic Surgery, The Orthopedic Foundation, the Thoracic Surgery Foundation, and other surgical foundations provide support for 1 to 2 years of research on a competitive basis.

Other nonsurgical national organizations such as the American Cancer Society, American Heart Association, Kidney Foundation, American Diabetes Association, Muscular Dystrophy Foundation, and so on all have research programs to which surgeons may apply. In the case of the American Cancer Society, while the funding is coordinated with the NIH's National Cancer Institute, the reviewers may be different. Some reviewers may view a grant differently than others, and thus one may increase the chances of being funded by submitting a nearly identical grant to both organizations, since only one of the applications can be funded.

While one may apply to the national organizations for comparatively large grants, many of these organizations, such as the Kidney Foundation, American Cancer Society, and American Heart Association, have local funding (state or chapter) that is considerably easier to obtain for smaller amounts, for example, up to $20,000. These are excellent sources for seed money for new research projects that can be used to obtain data so that one may apply to the national organizations.

Local Foundations

Every individual interested in funding should obtain a copy of the book listing local and state foundations. You will be amazed by what is available. Some fortunate schools have well-endowed local foundations specifically interested in funding new investigators. Other schools may have a built-in mechanism by which promising young investigators are funded by the institution in competitive fashion. Some schools have access to various individual philanthropic donors who may wish to provide funding for a young investigator. The research committee in the college of medicine of those schools that have taken the trouble of establishing these mechanisms can be very helpful in trying to approach such individuals.

Industry Funding

The reader may wonder why industry funding has not been mentioned earlier, because this has been an important traditional source of funding for many departments of surgery. It remains so, but industry funding has become more difficult and more goal directed. Industry is less willing than it once was to allow free-ranging research in an area rather than a specified research project that they would like to see performed. Industry money is not, as supposed by many, "easy money." It is far better to have an investigator-originated grant, such as a grant from the NIH. While it may be harder work to get it, once you have it you can do pretty much unfettered research, provided that you can produce enough results to get the grant renewed. This is not the case for industry research. There is more difficulty or "hassle factor" than with the NIH. If you develop a long-term relationship with industry, a less restricted contract or grant for a specific area of investigation may be secured, but this kind of grant is becoming increasingly more difficult to obtain.

Venture Capital

Venture capitalists are interested in research that is clinically relevant and may result in marketable products. If you have a marketable idea, take care to protect it through the intellectual properties organization of the university so that royalties from patents and so forth may accrue to you and your university. Venture capital companies may in fact be far more enlightened, compared with the remainder of industry, about seizing opportunities. If a valuable product results from a well-negotiated joint venture, there will be long-term support for the laboratory, the institution, and the department.

Department of Defense

The Department of Defense is a less well known resource that some surgical researchers have used successfully for many years. Department of Defense grants usually fund areas that are of interest to the military, including injury and metabolism, which encompass burns, trauma, and critical care. The application process is somewhat different than for the NIH, requiring a letter of intent and then, if successful, a full-fledged research grant proposal. These grants are highly competitive, but well worth considering.

Unusual Federal Areas

Getting to know the NIH and related organizations may result in the identification of additional funding sources. Certain lesser known institutes of the NIH, such as the Institute for Advanced Technology, have research funds available that in many cases go begging because people do not know about them. A thorough investigation of some of the less well known programs of the NIH may be fruitful.

North Atlantic Treaty Organization (NATO)

You may able to collaborate with colleagues in western Europe and obtain funding through NATO fellowships for research fellows working in your laboratory on a NATO fellowship. This is well worth investigating. There are other transatlantic fellowships, such as those from the Max Planck Institute; some of these programs are specifically for European fellows to work in laboratories in the United States.

The Robert Wood Johnson Foundation

I have always thought it particularly unfortunate that large organizations such as the Robert Wood Johnson Foundation have not funded traditional research avenues. However, outcomes analysis in departments of surgery is becoming a more common, valid avenue of research for young surgical investigators. Other foundations, such as the Markle Foundation, which has produced many fine individuals as Markle Scholars, have also chosen to fund other activities. However, attention to some of the programs of organizations such as the Robert Wood Johnson Foundation, Whittaker Foundation, and Pew Charitable Trust are well worthwhile.

Some Practical Suggestions on Obtaining Research Funding

1. Get to know the people who make funding decisions in your area of research. Get to know the scientific review advisor of the study section, and the program coordinators in the institute or organization to which you are applying.
2. Get to know the system and how the system works.
3. Visit the system. Allow enough time. Set up your appointments prior to arriving in Washington or wherever the organization resides. Don't expect individuals at the NIH or other organizations to devote time to you just because you are there, but set up a careful schedule with sufficient time in advance to allow them to prepare. Tell them what it is you are interested in.
4. The system is not monolithic. There are obvious variations in the individuals who are reviewing your grant. Some will be more sympathetic and helpful than others.
5. Become familiar with the study section to which your grant is likely to go, or you wish it to go. You undoubtedly will recognize the names of some of those in the study section. These are the people who are likely to review your grant. It is wise to quote their work in your grant application, no matter how re-

mote. It is not a good idea to fly in the face of their work or to challenge in a confrontational manner work that your likely reviewer has published.

6. READ THE INSTRUCTIONS. CARRY OUT THE INSTRUCTIONS.

7. If (when) you receive your study section critique, pay attention to the criticisms. Underline them and draw up a list of what you think the criticisms are. At this point it will be useful to call the scientific review advisor of the study section. Pay attention to the criticisms and address them directly, and do it quickly while the memory of your work is still fresh.

8. View the initial application as a first try. If your grant is turned down, resubmit it during the next cycle. If you send it back to the study section, it is likely to be reviewed by those individuals who reviewed it the first time. If you have addressed the criticisms squarely and fairly, it is likely that you will ultimately get funded. If you wait for 2 years, for example, the composition of the study section will be changed and there will be an entirely new set of criticisms.

9. YOU WILL NOT BE FUNDED UNLESS YOU APPLY.

10. Place yourself in the shoes of the reviewer. Make things easy for the reviewer. Do not have an impossibly long appendix that he or she has to refer to repeatedly. The closer the reviewer comes to his or her boiling point, the lower your score will be.

11. Do a precise job. No typographical errors. Make sure it looks nice and has an attractive font. Dot matrix–printed grant applications suffer the fate of dot matrix printers.

12. Do not irritate the reviewer. Do not use a series of abbreviations that even an expert in the field would not recognize. Spell everything out. Do not make your grant application look like a military exercise with an impossible number of acronyms.

13. Use a mentor. Even if your mentor is not in your field, he or she can certainly help you in preparing a proper grant application.

Conclusion

- You will not get funded unless you apply.
- Almost no one gets funded the first time.
- Getting grant support requires a sustained effort; if you continue to address the criticisms and resubmit the grant, it is likely that ultimately you will get funding.
- NIH funding remains the gold standard, but there are many other sources of funding available.

Commentary

Every investigator's dream is stable funding that will provide uninterrupted research support. The steady state is hard to attain and is reached only through a series of many small steps. The commonly held pessimistic view that research funding is not available to surgeons is invalid. One of the main reasons research funds are infrequently allocated to surgeons is that there are so few surgical grant requests. This chapter provides a multitude of sources to which the surgical investigator may look, and references for source material that will be helpful. Remember that the goal of all funding organizations is to give their money away; thoughtfully preparing an application using the techniques described in this book has the potential to yield good results, especially if you are persistent and responsive to reviewers' comments. Dr. Fischer points out the limitations of industrial research: traditionally interested in the funding of projects, industry does not provide investigators with a stable platform on which to stand.

A.S.W

CHAPTER 43

Funding Research in North America: Canada

S. Keshavjee and S. Gallinger

Research funding in Canada is similar to research funding in the United States, with some important differences. Ten years ago the breakdown of biomedical research funding sources was as follows: Medical Research Council (MRC) 39%, voluntary agencies 18%, industry 2%, local sources 2%, other 39%. By 1993 these proportions changed to the following: Medical Research Council 24%, voluntary agencies 14%, industry 22%, local sources 4%, other 36%. Although funding by the Medical Research Council has increased over the past 10 years, the major increase in research expenditure has come from private industry. For example, funding by the MRC has increased twofold from approximately $100 million per year to $200 million per year over the past 10 years (increase not corrected for inflation; all amounts are Canadian dollars, throughout this chapter). Funding from the provincial government, nonprofit organizations, and local agencies or the universities have also increased at the same rate. However, funding from private industry has increased 22-fold, bringing the amount of funding provided by industry to just under $200 million in 1993. (Proceedings of the 1994 Consensus Conference on Surgical Research in Canada).

An analysis of research funding obtained by surgical departments in Canada was presented at the Consensus Conference. The 16 departments of surgery examined had research funding totaling approximately $62 million; $51.8 million of this was from external sources and $10.3 million came from internal sources. Much of the internal support came from clinical earnings and endowments. Considerable variation exists in total funding and in the amount generated for salaries for surgeon-scientists. In many departments there is approximately a 10:1 ratio between external operating grant funds received and external salary support for staff surgeon-scientists. In some departments there is a similar relationship between internal salary support of surgeon-scientists and external operating grants received.

In summary, the departments of surgery receive considerable amounts of money for research from external and internal sources, with a ratio of about 5:1. There appears to be a relationship between the dollars obtained for salary support of faculty surgeon-scientists and dollars received for operating grants.

External salary support for surgeons to do research comes from a variety of sources, with varying duration and levels of support. Some sources are province specific, such as the Alberta Heritage Foundation for Medical Research, Fonds de la Récherche en Santé du Québec (FRSQ), and the Career Scientist Development Program of the Ontario Ministry of Health. Nationally, the Medical Research Council has recently become a significant source of salary support through its highly successful and useful Clinical Scientist Award program. The MRC has developed a Clinical-

Scientist Committee specifically designed to assist clinical-scientists and clinical departments. Members from several departments of surgery participate in this committee. The MRC Clinician-Scientist awards are especially attractive because of their long-term duration of salary support that spans the training phase and the subsequent phase as an independent investigator. Operating funds are also provided during the investigator phase. MRC scholarships have occasionally been awarded to surgeon-scientists, although these scholarships are extremely competitive and difficult to obtain because of the large number of applications received from competing basic scientists.

External funding sources utilized by Universities in Canada include the Alberta Heritage Foundation for Medical Research, Canadian Urology Scholarship, Medical Research Council of Canada, Ministry of Health Career Scientist Program–Ontario, Heart and Stroke Foundation of Canada, National Cancer Institute of Canada, University of Calgary Research Grant, Arthritis Society of Canada, Fond de la Récherche en Santé de Québec, BC Health Care Program, Miles Robinson Foundation, and others. Funding from these sources ranges from $20,000 to $80,000 per annum, with an average of $49,000 per annum.

Many surgical laboratories have nonclinician, non-M.D. scientists as faculty members who spend 75% or more of their time in research. These positions are not usually funded by the university, and developing salary support requires ingenuity. Combination funding from provincial governments, hospitals, clinical earnings, external funding agencies, and industry is commonly used. A surprisingly low amount of the total funding comes from industry.

Following is a list of some of the potential sources of funding available to surgeons. This annotated alphabetical list is not exhaustive, but it will give the reader an idea of the different types of funding sources that are available.

- *Armstrong Ontario Fellowship and Nutritional Sciences Related to Inflammatory Bowel Disease.* Provides for support of nutritional research in inflammatory bowel disease, particularly Crohn's disease. Three years of support is available at up to $40,000 per year.

- *Banting Research Foundation.* Provides support for young investigators for the establishment of new projects. Support for projects is usually for a term of 1 year and is rarely renewed. Funding is in the range of $12,000 to $20,000.

- *J. P. Bickell Foundation.* Grants are provided for biomedical research in Ontario universities, hospitals, and scientific institutions. Support is within the $10,000 to $25,000 range.

- *Canadian Association of Gastroenterology/Astra Pharma Inc. Research Initiative Award.* This award is aimed at further advancing biomedical research in Canada relevant to gastroenterology. The three following areas are funded: mucosal defense, inflammatory bowel disorders, and neuromuscular disorders of the gut. The award is $75,000 per year for 2 years and is intended to provide support for a postdoctoral fellow, plus operating expenses.

- *Canadian Association of Gastroenterology/Industry Research Fellowship Program.* Two research fellowship programs are provided in collaboration with Glaxo Canada, Jensen Pharmaceuticals, and Abbott Laboratories. The fellowships are provided to train clinical investigators in sciences, for an academic career related to gastroenterology. The applicant's supervisor must be a member of the Canadian Association of Gastroenterology.

- *Canadian Breast Cancer Foundation.* The primary purpose of the grants is to provide seed funding for new projects for the advancement of breast cancer research, treatment, education, and awareness.

- *Canadian Breast Cancer Research Initiative.* A combined effort by the MRC, National Cancer Institute of Canada, National Health Research and Development Program, and the Canadian Cancer Society. Similarly, a joint effort by various agencies has recently begun to support the International Genome Project and is referred to as the Canadian Genome Analysis and Technology (CGAT) Program. Personnel support awards are also available as joint agreements between MRC and a number of agencies in different countries including Argentina, Brazil, China, France, and Italy. These awards include a living and travel allowance for scientific visits to the host countries.

- *Canadian Cystic Fibrosis Foundation.* A large number of awards is available, including research grants, scholarships, fellowships, studentships, summer studentships, clinical incentive grants, transplant incentive grants, visiting scientists awards, special travel grants, and small conference grants.
- *Canadian Diabetes Association.* Provides research grants, scholarships, fellowships, graduate studentships, young scientists award, and Canadian Diabetes Association-Bayer Inc. fellowship in clinical diabetology.
- *Canadian Liver Foundation.* Establishment grants are available to provide start-up funds for clinical investigators and basic scientists who have recently completed their training and are taking up full-time faculty-level positions in a Canadian university. Up to 3 years of support is available, with awards of up to $60,000 per year. Canadian Liver Foundation Fellowship awards are available for salary support for qualified persons with an M.D. or Ph.D. in the fields of hepatic function or disease.
- *Canadian Orthopedic Foundation.* Research grants are available in the field of orthopedic surgery and are funded up to a level of $10,000 to $15,000.
- *Cancer Research Society Inc.* Operating grants and fellowships are available for a period of 2 years, in the range of $10,000 to $30,000.
- *Canadian Surgical Research Fund.* Established by the Canadian Association of General Surgeons to finance research in surgical diseases.
- *Crohn's and Colitis Foundation of Canada.* Grants are awarded for a maximum of 3 years, up to $50,000 per year. One clinical research fellowship is awarded yearly for training of candidates who have completed core clinical subspecialty training requirements.
- *Heart and Stroke Foundation of Canada.* Personnel support and grants are available to qualified investigators in cardiovascular and cerebralvascular research. The Heart and Stroke Foundation of Canada is responsible for personnel support, while the provincial Heart and Stroke Foundations provide grant support. A number of personnel awards are available, including junior personnel awards, research fellowships, medical scientist traineeships, senior personnel awards, visiting scientist program, and career

investigator awards. Major grants are available for up to 3 years of funding.
- *Hospital for Sick Children Foundation.* Support is available for all aspects of child health in Canada including pediatric research, health promotion, public education, and postgraduate training and community projects.
- *London Life Award in Medical Research.* An annual award of $100,000 per year for 3 years is available for a medical researcher working in Canada.
- *Medical Research Council of Canada.* This large national agency is comparable to the NIH in the United States. All forms of personnel support and research grants are available. Research personnel program awards include studentships, fellowships, centennial fellowships, and clinician-scientist awards, which have been obtained by a number of surgeons across the country. Grant funding is quite varied and includes operating grants, equipment grants, and group projects. University industry research funding is promoted with the MRC contributing $1.00 for every $2.00 provided by industry support.
- *National Cancer Institute of Canada (NCIC).* This large agency offers a number of programs for operating grants and personnel support. Granting opportunities include individual and group grants, equipment grants, molecular epidemiologic/clinical correlative studies, and feasibilities grants. The NCIC forms part of a multiagency group that supports the Canadian Breast Cancer Research Initiative. Personnel support programs include career development awards, research fellowships, clinical research fellowships, and studentships. Surgeons throughout the country have competed successfully for operating grants and fellowships offered by the NCIC. The NCIC clinical trials group supports national and international multicentered trials of cancer therapy and has collaborated extensively with the European Organization for the Research and Treatment of Cancer and other clinical trials societies.
- *National Health Research and Development Program (NHRDP).* Four primary areas are now being funded: health systems support and renewal, population health strategies for groups at risk, management of risk to the health of

Canadians (products and disease control), delivery of services to First Nations, Inuit, and the Yukon.

- *Natural Sciences and Engineering Research Council (NSERC).* This large research granting agency supports university research and the training of scientists and engineers. NSERC also provides a large budget for the Networks of Centers of Excellence Program.
- *Ontario Thoracic Society.* This agency is the medical section of the Ontario Lung Association and supports research directly relevant to human respiratory health problems.
- *Rick Hansen Man in Motion Foundation.* Fellowships and studentships are awarded to support basic spinal cord injury, rehabilitation, and prevention research.

Commentary

Approximately half of the university surgery departments in Canada have clear rules that require diversion of some of the clinical income of surgeons to research and education. Mechanisms include practice plans, a dean's tax, and so forth. These two young surgeons are technically proficient specialists in difficult areas of surgery (lung transplantation and hepatobiliary surgery). They have established enviable records of funding while maintaining a high-level clinical practice. Young surgeons can look for specific, detailed information on funding in the research office or on the web page of their university.

M.F.M.

CHAPTER 44

Applying for Funding from the NIH: A Useful Paradigm for Most Applications

R.E. Pollock, J.E. Niederhuber, and C.M. Balch

Purposes of a Grant Application

A research grant application serves a number of purposes. The most obvious is its potential as an entré to research funding, but it is also a critical planning document that can be used as a precise and detailed research "road map" for the ensuing project. By competing for a peer-reviewed research grant, the investigator receives a critique of his best efforts from other experts in the field. If the grant application is successful and funded, it becomes a very strong statement of peer approval and recognition of the quality of the applicant's research efforts.

Types of Grant

A number of organizations offer grants. Two major sources of medical research funding in North America are the National Institutes of Heath (NIH) in the United States and, in Canada, the Medical Research Council (whose grants and review process are very similar to those of the NIH). Other sources of funding include national and re-

gional grants sponsored by the American Cancer Society, Kidney Foundation, American Heart Association, and so forth. Surgical organizations such as the American College of Surgeons, Association for Academic Surgery, and Society of University Surgeons have also established training grant programs. These are discussed in greater detail in Dr. Fischer's chapter (chapter 42).

Three basic types of grant are available to investigators or aspiring investigators through the NIH (Table 44-1). Training grants, for example, the NIH Clinician-Investigator Award (K08 series) and institutional training grants, are targeted to physicians with 2 to 7 years of clinical training who are interested in academic careers but lack appropriate basic research training. Training grants usually require applicants to commit 75% or more of their time to their research training effort over the course of 3 to 5 years. The goal is to train a clinical investigator capable of functioning independently at the end of the training period. The award is made to the trainee and the training institution.

The second type of grant funds investigator-initiated research projects (e.g., the NIH R01 and R29 award series). These grants presuppose that the applicant is fully trained in research and capable of functioning independently; the surgeon-investigator has to compete with other fully trained autonomous scientists, both physicians and holders of doctorates in other disciplines. The

---

Extensively adapted from Niederhuber JE. Writing a successful grant application. J Surg Res 1985;39:277–284; and Pollock RE, Balch CM. The NIH Clinician Investigator Award: how to write a training grant application. J Surg Res 1989;46:1–3.

Table 44-1. NIH grants available to surgical investigators.

Grant mechanism	NIH series	Eligibility
Training grants, i.e. Clinician-Investigator award	K08	Physicians with 2–7 years of clinical training, lacking research training
Investigator-Initiated project	R01	Established investigators
	R29	"First Awards" for fully trained young investigators
Program project grant	P01	Established R01-funded investigators (young investigators can be coinvestigators)

award is made to the individual investigator in conjunction with his or her institution; funds are transportable to other institutions if the investigator moves to a new department.

The third type of grant is for program projects (e.g., the NIH P01 series). Applications for these grants are submitted by senior R01-funded investigators with established research track records. A younger investigator may have the opportunity to participate as a coinvestigator in a project covered by a larger program grant. The program project is developed around a unified, defined research goal encompassing a number of sound, individual complementary projects that will be strengthened by being part of the overall program. Such applications are reinforced by a convincing demonstration of the significant cost savings that will accrue from creating the facilities to support the P01-related projects. The strength and unity of the program stem from the excellence of its component projects, the focus on a common goal, and collaboration among the project investigators.

Prewriting Phase

You must accurately assess your ability to function independently versus your need for additional training prior to becoming an autonomous investigator. A project (independent or program) grant application is required if you are capable of conducting independent research; if not, an application for a training grant is appropriate. Making this decision first, in the prewriting phase, is necessary because the applications are markedly different.

To write a successful training grant application, you will need to think carefully—during the pre-

writing phase—about the four essential elements of your application: you—as the applicant, your mentor (sponsor), the research environment in which you propose to pursue your training, and your research project.

The first component is you, because your *potential* to develop independent research capacities will be evaluated. You must demonstrate a serious intention to pursue an academic research career, because the granting agency is investing its money primarily in your potential to develop into an independent investigator rather than in your project per se.

The second matter you must decide is who your mentor (sponsor) will be. It is important to select someone who is recognized as an accomplished investigator, as documented by the quality of his or her bibliography and track record in getting peer-reviewed support. The granting agency will also evaluate your mentor's ability and availability to guide and support you; that is, can he or she foster your development into an independent investigator? Evidence that your mentor has successfully trained one or more fellows who were subsequently funded as independent investigators is usually required.

The third element of your application is the quality of the research environment in which you wish to receive your training. The granting agency's reviewers are looking for proposals for training within strong, well-established, active research programs, because such programs imply the presence of a critical mass of faculty members in the clinical and basic sciences. Your proposed research training center should have a reputation for helping young investigators develop independent research careers. An important factor in evaluating the research environment is evidence that the chairperson of the department supports and protects trainees during and after their training period.

The fourth consideration is your research project. You will need to demonstrate the overall merit of a multiyear plan of research. The reviewers will examine how the project dovetails with your career plans and how likely it is that it will help you develop the skills you will need. That is, assuming you complete the project, will you be equipped to function as an independent investigator and will you have developed a research attitude that enables you to shift your focus of concentration from a project aimed at getting a single result to one that opens an area of investigation you can pursue in the future?

You must also obtain a departmental letter of support to accompany your application for a training grant. It is a binding guarantee from the chairperson of your clinical department that the required percentage of your time and effort for basic research will be protected if your proposal is funded. A vague statement from a well-meaning, but naive chairperson is insufficient; the chairperson must state exactly how you will be protected and supported while you are executing the proposed research.

nician, choose coinvestigators with strong bibliographies, their own peer-reviewed grant support, and the complementary scientific expertise needed to ensure the success of your project. Review committees are very aware of the demands on the time of clinicians, and of the buttressing value of basic science coinvestigators who need not apportion their time between clinical and investigative tasks.

Your research environment should have the space and equipment required to perform your proposed research. Your independent project application will be strengthened if you can show that other established investigators work in the same general vicinity and that cross-collaborations could develop during the project. It is essential to provide evidence that you have departmental support, especially with regard to projected time requirements.

Your project should be plausible, original, and significant; the quality of these parameters is more important than in a training grant application. The training grant project is a vehicle for the acquisition of independent investigative skills; the individual grant project must have inherent potential for significant scientific advance—its value as a training mechanism is not relevant to the review process.

PRE-WRITING PHASE

- Training grant versus independent investigator grant
- Organize your background
- Identify sponsor or mentor (only if a training grant)
- Review quality of research environment
- Plan research project
- Choose coinvestigators

The prewriting phase of an independent research grant application is different. You will be evaluated on your established strengths as an independent investigator, not on your potential to become one; you will need to recruit coinvestigators, not select a mentor. Choosing coinvestigators will require as much careful deliberation as selecting a mentor does for a training grant. It may be particularly important that you, as a cli-

Compiling the Grant Application

Although the format of an application is unique to each funding agency, the principles underlying most grant applications are sufficiently similar to warrant using the NIH as a generic example.

The detailed instructions in the booklet that usually accompanies the application form should be followed exactly; the requirements and format are frequently revised. If your institution has a grants administration office staffed by individuals who are knowledgeable about grant applications, be sure to identify them and make use of their experience. It would also be helpful to obtain a funded grant proposal from an established senior investigator and use it as a model. Respect *absolutely* all stated page limitations; applications exceeding the stipulations are frequently returned unread! Do not use photoreduction to gain space;

if the proposal is not easy to read, it may not be read at all. Use a clear, concise scientific writing style; for the NIH, the official guidelines require the type size to be 12 pitch or greater.

An important first element is the budget. You must complete 12-month and multiyear budget statements, with justifications addressing both time and money parameters. Feel free to contact the granting agency staff to gain insight into grant program restrictions. You may be tempted to inflate your budget to offset anticipated cuts during its review, but resist doing this, because an unrealistic budget reflects poorly on you and can exert a detrimental influence.

You must provide justification for each budget item (e.g., personnel, supplies, travel, equipment). Do not treat this part of your application too lightly; you must formulate your justifications thoroughly, carefully, and skillfully to ensure maximum support for your project. Ask yourself, Is the budget completely justified? Is it in keeping with grant program restrictions? Does it show, specifically and credibly, how you propose to spend both your time and the granting agency's money?

Biographical sketches for you and any coinvestigators or mentors usually come next. Present the best possible, but accurate, image of yourself and any other participants. It is important to demonstrate the adequacy of your investigative training and its relevance to the research you propose to do. Your bibliography should support your qualifications by clearly delineating a common theme in your research efforts. For R01 and First awards, your bibliography should provide evidence of independent work; and for P01 applications, evidence of existing collaborations.

Your application must document other grant support currently under your control as principal investigator, or under the control of your coinvestigator(s) or mentor, in sufficient detail to allow the reviewer to grasp your situation quickly and easily. One- or two-sentence outlines describing the objective and the distinctiveness of each listed project should make it evident that the grants are cohesive, nonoverlapping parts of an overall theme of investigation.

The granting agency's reviewers will usually be familiar with the various institutions and departments supporting your application, but you should describe in detail the laboratory resources available for your proposed project and characterize your institution's environment in terms of laboratory space, animal facilities, core equipment, and access to needed patient materials.

When you are compiling a grant proposal, you must keep institutional and granting agency deadlines in mind. At the M. D. Anderson Cancer Center, five separate M. D. Anderson forms have to be completed before a grant proposal is allowed to leave the premises. The five forms require seven signatures from seven different offices. There are also 6-page animal care approval forms and equally lengthy human surveillance clearance forms. Completing these forms requires time, and the job must be done early enough to allow sufficient time for internal peer review before submission of the application to the granting agency!

COMPILATION PHASE

- Contact grants office at home institution
- Create and justify budget
- Write focused biographical sketches of all investigators
- Identify other grant support

The most important part of your grant proposal is your research plan, in four sections with a limit of 25 pages: specific aims, significance, preliminary studies, and experimental design and methods. Your research plan has a critical bearing on the final rating your proposal will receive and will gain or lose you the most points. Despite its importance, writing the research plan is often left until last.

A successful grant application is based on a significant idea or hypothesis that is not only interesting and exciting but entirely plausible and feasible. Once your research hypothesis/objective has been carefully defined, you will need to devise a series of specific aims that will provide answers to the questions raised by your hypothesis. You are allowed to devote one page to a succinct and feasible statement of the specific aims of your proposal. The challenge is to show that the aims are achievable and are based on a sound and important biologic hypothesis. An outline (Appendix 44-1) is an excellent format for helping the reviewer understand your hypothesis and specific aims. List each aim separately, in the logical sequence you will follow when you implement the plan.

The statement of significance comes next. Your critical review of the pertinent peer-reviewed literature should be approximately 3 pages. It allows you to show that you are aware of the most critical areas of current inquiry in your chosen area of research. You must demonstrate a thorough knowledge of the subject area and the relevant and current questions surrounding your proposal, and you must relate your project's specific aims to the critical questions being asked by other scientists working in the same area. The significance section should make it clear that successful completion of your proposed experiment(s) will make a meaningful contribution to the knowledge base of your subject.

The preliminary studies section follows the one on significance and should be approximately 8–10 pages. If your application is to be successful, you must describe enough completed preliminary work to convince the reviewer that your project has an excellent chance of being carried to a successful completion. This is also your opportunity to convince the reviewer that you have the requisite skills and experience. The reviewer's expectations regarding the extent and sophistication of your preliminary studies are greater for an independent research project grant than for a training grant.

Presenting the data obtained in your preliminary studies in the form of tables, graphs, and photographs is a great help to the reviewer; these materials should be of publication quality, and it should be possible to photoreduce and insert them at appropriate places in the text to simplify the reviewer's job (Appendix 44-2). This is better than attaching the figures and tables as appendices because it relieves the reviewer of the tedium of having to go back and forth between the text and the appendices. Each table and figure should be easily understood and should have appropriate legends. The topic sentence in each paragraph should be underlined or highlighted by boldface type; for easier review, the paragraphs should be displayed in a numerical, protocol-type format.

The experimental design and methods section is possibly the most important part of your entire application; the evaluation it receives will count most heavily in determining the priority score the

review committee assigns to it. Consequently, devote at least two-thirds of your allotted writing time to this part of your application.

When you are describing your methods, provide details without being diffuse; lack of focus is one of the most frequent criticisms of grant applications. Use the first portion of the experimental design and methods section to describe the routine methods to be used, in detail, and keep it separate from the research plan. The experimental techniques you will employ should be up to date and referenced, and you must demonstrate a thorough knowledge of their use. The reviewers will judge your experimental design by asking such questions as, Does the experimental design address a significant research question? Does the design build logically on the preliminary studies? Will the design satisfy the specific aims as they have been articulated? Will the design reveal underlying biologic mechanisms, or will it hover at the superficial level of phenomenology?

RESEARCH PLAN

- Specific aims should be hypothesis-driven.
- Write background to identify unresolved issues in *current* literature.
- Preliminary studies should document your ability to do the proposed work.
- Experimental design is very critical in grant reviews.
- Identify likely problems and solutions.

You must demonstrate a thorough understanding of the difficulties you may encounter when you conduct the proposed experiments, and what alternative methods could be flexibly applied to correct or resolve such problems. The most common error is to be too descriptive; you must be able to distinguish coincidence and epiphenomena from true cause and effect.

Mechanism of Review

Some insight into the review process will help you understand why research applications are disapproved or rated poorly.[1] For example, NIH research grants are assigned to an appropriate panel of scientists—known as a study section, that is assisted by an executive secretary who assigns each application to a primary and a secondary reviewer. At the scheduled meetings of the study section, the assigned reviewers lead a discussion of the scientific merit of the proposal. The committee will be composed of investigators of national stature who are engaged in basic research and multiple professional activities that leave them very little time to devote to voluntarily reviewing of grant applications. The review committee may, or may not, include a surgical investigator.

Accordingly you must examine your application very skeptically to see whether it could be adequately digested by a primary reviewer in as little as 2 hours. Bear in mind that your primary reviewer will take 15 minutes, at most, to present your application to the entire review committee of 7 to 16 members. The success or failure of your application will depend on the primary reviewer's ability to digest its salient features quickly and present your ideas in a favorable light to the review committee. Anything you can do to make the reviewer's job easier can only help you; brevity, clarity, and logical organization are essential.

Members of the committee vote to approve or disapprove the application; if it is approved, the review committee will then vote on a priority score. A summary statement of the critique, referred to as the "pink sheet," is prepared by the executive secretary and is sent to you, the applicant.

Your application and its initial review results are then presented to the appropriate NIH advisory council responsible for program review. The council determines how well your proposed research would advance the institute's mission and what funds are available to support external applications. The council relies heavily on study section reviews and priority scores in determining which applications will be funded. The most critical determinant of success is the initial review by the primary reviewers and the panel of scientists serving as members of the study section.

If you are a new faculty member making your first application for external research funding, seek help from your more experienced and senior colleagues, especially those who are members of grant study sections. Remember that one of the major and oft-cited weaknesses of grant applications is lack of focus, especially in the presentation

of research plans. Allow enough time to complete the application and have it reviewed internally by colleagues who are thoroughly knowledgeable in your particular area. It is preferable to miss an application deadline rather than submit a proposal that has not received an internal review, because an unreviewed proposal has a much higher likelihood of being rejected.

Commonly recurring reasons for grant disapproval, identified by the NIH, are outlined in the following section.

Reasons for NIH Grant Disapproval[2]

1. Lack of new or original ideas; weak or trivial hypothesis
2. Diffuse, superficial, or unfocused research plan
3. Lack of knowledge of published relevant work
4. Lack of expertise in the essential methodology
5. Uncertainty concerning future research directions
6. Questionable reasoning in experimental design
7. Absence of an acceptable scientific rationale
8. Unrealistically large amount of work
9. Lack of sufficient experimental detail
10. Uncritical approach to current knowledge

If the application is not successful, you can usually obtain this information and the critique a few weeks after the study section meeting. If you rewrite your application, address the comments of the critique very carefully. A rewritten grant application taking adequate account of the reviewers' comments may achieve an improved priority score that will warrant funding after resubmission and review.

If your grant application is funded, you may want to apply for additional funding in subsequent years. Competitive renewal has its own set of challenges, but it is an opportunity to show that the initial funds allocated to you by the granting agency were well spent, your specific aims were met, your time and money budgets were not exceeded, you kept abreast of and integrated changes in your field of research, and, most pertinent, you contributed to progress by presenting and publishing your work in peer-reviewed forums.

In conclusion, a training grant represents an investment in the possibility that, with the proper training, you can emerge as an independent investigator. In contrast, a research project grant is an investment in the quality and potential of the project itself. An awareness of these distinctions will help you to select a mentor, coinvestigator(s), or project, astutely, and to formulate a grant application in accord with its underlying purpose. (See also chapter 41.)

References

1. Pollock RE, Balch CM. The NIH Clinician-Investigator award: how to write a training grant application. J Surg Res 1989;46:1–3.
2. Niederhuber JE. Writing a successful grant application. J Surg Res 1985;39:277–284.

Additional Reading

NIH peer review of research grant applications. Washington, DC: Department of Health and Human Services, 1988.

Appendix 44-1

Outline of a research plan that derives from underlying biological principles. Each segment is addressed by studies described in the experimental methods and design section of the research plan.

Outline of Research Plan

1.0 Specific aims
2.0 Background and significance
    2.1 Introduction
    2.2 Difficulties in diagnosis and staging
    2.3 Impact of soft tissue sarcoma biology on modes of care
        2.31 Addition of radiotherapy to surgery
        2.32 Addition of chemotherapy to radiotherapy and surgery

    2.4 Problems in soft tissue sarcoma clinical research
3.0 Preliminary results
    3.1 Preoperative chemotherapy as the initial treatment modality
    3.2 Deletion of preoperative radiotherapy in preoperative chemotherapy responders
        3.21 Relevant radiotherapy experience
        3.22 Relevant surgery experience
        3.23 Relevant chemotherapy experience
    3.3 Substitution of hyperthermic isolated limb perfusion for radiotherapy in preoperative chemotherapy nonresponders
    3.4 Development of soft tissue sarcoma molecular staging criteria
        3.41 Mutation of wild type (wt) p53 tumor suppressor gene
        3.42 Mutation of MTS1 multiple tumor suppressor gene
        3.43 Amplification of MDM2 oncogene
4.0 Experimental design
    4.1 The clinical protocol
    4.2 The integrated clinical-molecular prospective database
    4.3 The bioresource facility
    4.4 Molecular staging studies
    4.5 Correlative basic investigations
        4.51 Transfection of exogenous wt p53 into soft tissue sarcoma cells lacking wt p53
        4.52 Development of in vivo extremity sarcoma preclinical molecular therapy model
        4.53 Role of MT1 and MDM2 genes in soft tissue sarcoma progression

Appendix 44-2

In the following excerpt from a grant application, the task of the reviewer is eased because preliminary results are illustrated with publication-quality figures.

Our own studies have identified gross and subtle p53 mutations in soft tissue sarcoma. Figure 4 depicts studies of a primary synovial cell sarcoma and axillary metastasis that became clinically detectable and was resected six months after the primary tumor. The primary tumor contained wt p53, whereas the metastasis had mutated p53 where a specific point mutation could be demonstrated using single strand conformational polymorphism (SSCP) followed by sequencing (manuscript in preparation). This unusual opportunity to examine primary tumor and metachronous metastasis tissues retrieved from a single patient suggests that p53 gene mutation may play a role in soft tissue sarcoma progression, as has been suggested by Vogelstein in colon carcinoma (62). In light of these considerations, analysis of p53 gene mutations may be relevant in developing molecular staging for soft tissue sarcoma.

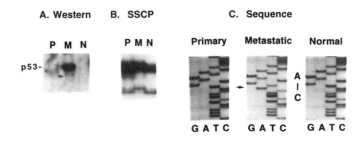

FIG. 4 A. Western blot analysis on protein lysates from synovial sarcoma primary tumor (P), metastatic tumor of the same patient (M), and normal tissue of the same patient (N). 60 µg proteins from each sample were electrophoresed on 8.5% SOS-PAGE and transferred to nitrocellulose. The primary antibody used was anti-p53 Ab-6 monoclonal antibody (Oncogene Science Inc., Manhasset, NY). The position of p53 protein is indicated. B. SSCP (single strand conformation polymorphism) analysis of exon 5 of p53 gene. A mobility shift was clearly observed in metastatic tumor (middle lane). C. Nucleotide sequence analysis of exon 5 of p53 gene. The exact site of a C to A single base mutation seen on metastatic tumor is indicated by an arrow.

Commentary

Although this chapter focuses on the NIH grant proposal format, it is broadly applicable to anyone writing a grant proposal in virtually any country. The essential elements are the same, although they may be organized differently, or the different components may have differing relative weights. The list of reasons why grants are turned down, presented in the concluding section of the chapter, is particularly helpful. Working backward is a good technique. Critically assess your own grant to see what reasons you can find for disapproval; even better, ask a critical friend or trusted colleague to do that for you.

One of the greatest pitfalls in grant preparation is doing it at the last minute; we are all guilty of such behavior, but shortcuts or a hurried approach to a single portion of the grant can make the difference between approval and disapproval. Similarly, developing investigators generally give insufficient attention to the prewriting phase of the application. This is an extremely critical time. You should be testing your grant ideas on as many people as you can. Seek criticisms in three areas: your proposed approach, the importance of the questions that you are asking, and the hypothesis that you are developing. A structurally perfect grant with precise reasoning will not be funded if the inherent area of inquiry is deemed of insufficient importance to the reviewers. You should feel comfortable about contacting the granting agency to help align your proposal with their goals. Investigators frequently forget that the whole purpose of funding agencies is to give away their money. A preliminary chat with someone from the agency will help to determine whether your area of interest is a good match for the focus of that particular agency, and useful suggestions are frequently obtained. Surgeon-scientists have a problem with writing grant applications because their clinical work interferes with consecutive thinking. Thus, the planning process must be even more careful, and there must be enough lead time to account for the unpredictable elements that arise in a surgical practice. Most surgeons who have prepared a grant proposal find that the process is difficult and lengthy, but at the end it provides them with a better understanding of their area of inquiry and an excellent road map to follow as they explore unsolved problems.

A.S.W.

CHAPTER 45

What a Grant Review Committee Looks For

I. Kron

Young surgical investigators are often told that it is impossible to get a major grant funded, particularly by the National Institutes of Health (NIH). It has been stated that most funding goes to basic scientists, and therefore it is useless to write a grant. In fact, 10–25% of individual grant proposals are presently funded by NIH. Though this sounds incredibly hard, many of these are resubmissions, and therefore, though difficult, funding still is possible. This chapter is intended to improve the chance of being funded by familiarizing readers with some of the paths and pitfalls of the review process.

Mechanisms for Grant Review

It is helpful for the investigator submitting an individual grant request to understand the mechanisms of grant review. At NIH and most other major funding agencies, there are at least two primary reviewers assigned per grant. Both individually will fully review the proposed grant and come up with a priority score. A reader is assigned at NIH to review the grant as well. The reader will review the grant in detail but does not write out a full summary. The primary and secondary reviewers present their analyses of the grant at a meeting of the study section, which usually consists of 10–20 scientists. Others with an interest in the area may also discuss the grant. If the grant is approved, as the majority are, then a priority score is given by each member by written ballot. This is the main determinant of whether the grant gets funded.

Recently the concept of triage has been added to reduce the work of the study section. Grants that are judged to be in the bottom 50th percentile by the assigned reviewers will be triaged to reduce the amount of discussion at meetings. For a grant to be triaged, there has to be agreement of the primary and secondary reviewers. A grant can also be triaged at any time during a study section meeting if all who have reviewed the grant agree that it is in the bottom 50th percentile. Even if a grant is triaged, a pink sheet, which is the critique, will be furnished to the investigator to help him or her determine what can be done to salvage the grant.

It is important for the individual applying for a grant to understand the competition. The majority of individual NIH grants beyond the initial training grants are in two categories. The R01 is a larger grant available for more senior investigators. The R29 "First award" is offered for the investigator who has not had a major NIH grant thus far. Both R01 and R29 grants compete for funds in the same pool. The major difference in judging R01 and R29 grants is that the latter requires less preliminary data and less of a track record to obtain approval.

There is a tremendous amount of work in grant

review. Most reviewers take their work very seriously and spend hours on each grant reviewed. It is critical to your success to make reading the grant as painless as possible. The majority of grants that are unsuccessful are turned down for similar reasons.

The Individual Grant from the Standpoint of the Study Section

The reviewers assigned to one's individual grant are instructed to read the grant from a supportive standpoint. Theoretically, at least one reviewer will champion your grant to the rest of the study section. Make it simple for the reviewer to read and enjoy the grant. The grant should be well written and it should not be difficult to find the material. That is, make the grant short, simple, and do not continually refer to appendices, which forces the reviewer to go from the body of the grant to the appendices. The appendices should be limited, and anything you really want to say should be in the body of the grant.

It is very important that the grant be carefully reviewed by you and your colleagues before you submit it. There should not be typing errors, misspellings, or poorly constructed sentences. Though these are often disregarded, they alienate. If you've not put in the time to edit your own grant carefully, why should you expect the reviewer to do it?

Your biographical sketch should highlight your achievements, particularly the recent publications specific to your expertise in the area in which you plan to work. You should put in your total number of publications, even if you can't list them all, so the reviewer will not have to guess or to assume the worst. In your biographical sketch, choose peer-reviewed, primarily research papers.

The hypotheses of the grant must be clear. There should be limited hypotheses and they should be specific. One of the major reasons that grants are rejected is that they are unfocused. There should be no doubt about what you are trying to accomplish and why. It helps if the subject that you are interested in has some clinical relevance, and this should be clearly stated in the abstract. Each of the aims should be keyed to a specific hypothesis and, eventually, the methodology keyed to the specific aims, at least as far as the protocols.

The background data does not necessarily have to be all-inclusive, but it should be up to date. Give a balanced overview of the area of interest. The background should state clearly why you are doing your present project.

The section on preliminary data is quite important. A major cause for grant rejection is doubt that the investigator can accomplish the project at hand. Therefore, your preliminary data should lead in a stepwise fashion to the present grant proposal. Present the work that has been done to validate the methods that will be used. I cannot emphasize enough the importance of good preliminary data, particularly some that has been published in peer-reviewed journals. One of the reviewers' major concerns is that a large amount of money will be invested in a laboratory that is not prepared or able to complete the project. This is money wasted—money that could have been used by another promising investigator. A good track record of publications helps demonstrate ability to carry a project to completion. This is true even for a relatively young investigator. There has to be evidence, and not merely testimony and hope, that the individual applying for the grant is productive.

The most important section of the grant is the methods section. The methods should be absolutely clear. State in a complete fashion the various techniques that are to be used. Mention in each of these sections that the present techniques are currently in use in your laboratory or in a collaborator's laboratory. A supportive letter is needed if a collaborator is providing an important portion of the methodology. The various protocols are then keyed to specific aims in an orderly fashion. The reviewer must be able to understand how the research is to be conducted. A timetable should be given, usually in graphic form. Research science is not perfect, so the attrition rate for the studies should be given based on the investigator's own experience. Research techniques and models are imperfect, so pitfalls must be noted and some appropriate means for their solution given. In the pitfalls section, it is very important for an investigator to state what will be done if a major hypothesis cannot be tested. The reviewer would hate to see a grant fail based on the fact that if one of the initial major hypotheses is incorrect, then the study is over.

The budget should be realistic and not excessive. Adding salary support, for example, for your entire department is unrealistic and may raise the ire of the reviewer. The number of years of funding requested is very important. Clarify why you need the time you request to do the project. More often than not, too many studies are budgeted. Unrealistic projections of 500 experiments to investigate 16 different study groups in a year's time will not be funded.

There are multiple reasons for NIH grant disapproval. The usual ones include lack of focus. Another important area is that the work is observational as opposed to hypothesis driven. Lack of clinical relevance has been a more recent issue raised. The perceived inability to perform the study is very frequently raised, particularly related to new investigators or more senior investigators trying a new area. A lack of preliminary data is often cited, and excessive numbers of studies that seem to be unrelated is a very frequent problem.

There are two other important issues that are often raised. One is adding experiments with the hope of pleasing the reviewer. For example, the investigator might have little, if any, experience in molecular biology, but feel that the grant must include a molecular biology section to get approval. The investigator is far better off using good, straightforward science, instead of adding bells and whistles in the hope that doing so will show completeness. Another common problem is doing everything possible to the experimental animal in order to be complete. If multiple studies are needed, a logical sequence must be established. Most importantly, write the grant the way you would like to read it if you were the reviewer. Tedious grants by and large do not get funded.

What Helps Reviewers to Like Your Grant Proposal

- Follow the rules.
- Minimize appendix material.
- Have the grant appear neat.
- Correct typographical errors.
- Make it easy to read.
- Recruit the reviewer.
- Demonstrate attention to prior reviews if this is a resubmission.

Resubmission of a Grant

The odds are very good that your first submission will not be funded, and a pink sheet will be sent to you summarizing the critique. You should not be put off by the concept of resubmitting your grant proposal. The better the priority score, the better your chances are on resubmission. Even a poor priority score can lead to eventual funding if the critiques are analyzed carefully. If the critique says basically to start over, then start over. However, most of the time the issues are very straightforward.

If you need more preliminary data, then it is clear that it must be obtained, usually using departmental or institutional support. Most of the time, the grant just needs to be more focused. It does not help to get angry at the reviewers. There is nothing personal in the review. Objectively analyze the critique and if you agree that the critique can improve the grant, follow the critique. Some of the critique may be inappropriate, and it is quite reasonable to state why one or two of the issues raised are not relevant to your proposal. This doesn't need to be done in a hostile fashion; rather it should be done objectively and scientifically, just as you approached the grant you have submitted. If the critique is analyzed carefully and the resubmission adheres to the critique, in theory, the priority score should improve. If the critique requires more data, the priority score will not improve unless the data is obtained.

Competitive Renewal

If you are fortunate enough to have had a major grant funded, you will eventually face the concept of competitive renewal. To continue the research you must resubmit for further funding. It is critically important to demonstrate productivity during the years of the initial grant. The various objectives should have been achieved; if they were not, explain why. It is perfectly appropriate to show that one line of investigation was not fruitful, so another line was started. If nothing has been accomplished, then it is unlikely you will get funded. By the same token, if you have fully investigated the area of interest and accomplished all goals, and no new obvious goals seem possible, then a new line of investigation must be started.

When the investigator seems to run out of ideas, funding stops, regardless of your reputation or your previous funding. If you are working in an area for eventual clinical use, then it is critically important to focus the grant on what work is necessary to complete the project. It really doesn't help to ask for funds to repeat multiple different sets of studies to corroborate what has already been found. The investigator must state what remaining questions must be answered to get the device or technique into clinical use. A submission focused on those areas should have a high likelihood of funding. Repeating old material will just irritate the reviewer.

Conclusion

Submitting a grant is a painful, "character-building" experience. However, the only way to be able to fund major research is through external grant agencies. Surgeons often fail at this mission primarily because they don't submit as many grants as basic scientists do. Grants usually get rejected on the first attempt, but that doesn't mean that funding is not possible if you are persistent. If you have a good idea and have done good work, you are likely to get funded eventually. Every successful investigator can paper his or her walls with failed grants. When Dr. Wechsler asked me to write this section, he stated, "I consider you very expert at this, since you have had the opportunity to revise your grant so many times as a consequence of the study section reviews." He was exactly right, and I have learned from the experience that persistence will allow you to maintain funding of your research.

Commentary

Dr. Kron's comments about what a review committee looks for in a grant proposal will resonate positively with the experiences of those who have served on such bodies and/or submitted grant proposals. At the outset, it is important for the new investigator to realize that preparing a grant requires a continuous 3 to 6 weeks of full-time work. It may be necessary to arrange a short leave of absence from other duties to accomplish this goal. Alternatively, a long time line for submission to incorporate this amount of preparation may be required. Part of this long time line is related to the difficulty of articulating a coherent plan for 3 to 5 years of research, as well as the logistical problems of assembling the multiple components that go into a major research proposal. In addition, time must be allowed for the work to germinate, particularly because time will be needed for internal review by other, more experienced investigators. As a final caveat, it is advisable not to rush grant preparation to meet an imminent deadline. Instead of rushing, it is a much wiser strategy to miss the first deadline, thereby allowing sufficient time for germination, internal review, and sophisticated grant preparation, all of which will enhance the likelihood of funding in the next round.

Several specific grant preparation techniques merit additional discussion. It is imperative that the budget be realistic as well as fully justified; budget justification means that the costs are broken down to the lowest common denominator units so that a reviewer can understand exactly why it is proposed to have the funding agency spent $10,000 on nude mice (nude mouse at $20 per animal $\times$ $2 per diem $\times$ 6 months of housing $\times$ X number of animals = $10,000). To facilitate budget justification completion, we maintain a laboratory computer base that includes all the current unit pricing information as well as names, addresses, and telephone and fax numbers for all suppliers. In this way the budget justification can be initially assembled by a laboratory assistant, with real time savings for the principal investigator.

The specific aims section of the proposal should be extremely succinct and limited to no more than four or five specific aims. Grant reviewers know that satisfying more than this number of specific aims is probably not achievable in a realistic time framework. Moreover, it is critical that satisfying the aims will establish a basic mechanism underlying a biological process; in addition to lack of focus, the other major reason for funding failure is that specific aims are phenomenologic rather than mechanism driven.

The significance section must include a critical

review of pertinent peer-reviewed literature. This highly focused review seeks to demonstrate an understanding of the knowledge relevant to the subject of investigation, as well as the gaps in this knowledge base. A good significance section allows direct demonstration of why such gaps will be important to fill, and therefore how the specific aims will address these holes in our understanding. The preliminary data section provides an opportunity to demonstrate mastery of relevant techniques. It is usually effective to include figures and diagrams directly in the preliminary results text; using optical scanners and current desk-top publishing software, it is possible to incorporate preliminary results directly in a visually pleasing and informative manner.

The experimental design section is arguably the most important single component in the grant. This section provides an opportunity to show how the specific aims will be satisfied. More globally, it is an opportunity to demonstrate overall control of the research project. Contingency plans should be clearly articulated in the event that a hypothesis proves to be incorrect or a specific aim cannot be satisfied. Alternative methodologies should be suggested along with a brief but cogent description of the relative value of one method compared to another, particularly if the first choice methodology is at all controversial. Any proposed method must be referenced to the appropriate current peer-reviewed literature; moreover, putative control over the methodology must be supported by results presented in the preliminary data section. A well-organized and time-line denominated experimental design section provides tangible evidence that there is good control of the experimental systems, and therefore that it is likely that reproducible information will derive from execution of this design.

It is very important to make certain that the proposal has been reviewed by animal care (IACUC) and/or the institutional review board (IRB), as appropriate to the biological systems being studied. If humans are involved, care should be taken to adequately document the minorities and gender section of the grant proposal. These intramural processes all require time. A proposal can be submitted to the granting agency pending review by the IACUC or IRB; however, the time line for completion of these reviews is usually no

more than 60–90 days, and so the investigator must remain in control of this issue.

Several other considerations may also be important to the investigator applying for an R29 (First award). While the R29 proposal is reviewed by a standing study section that also is considering R01 proposals from more senior investigators, and while the priority scores for R29 and R01 proposals are pooled, the actual payline percentile is generally higher for R29 proposals. As a result, a proposal that might not get funded as an R01 grant stands a somewhat better chance of being funded as an R29 application. This reality should be considered in decisions about applying for R29 versus R01 funding. The K08 Clinician Investigator Award grant is reviewed by an ad hoc rather than standing review committee. This is an ideal funding mechanism for an individual who is not yet capable of establishing an independent research program.

Finally, it is daunting to receive a pink sheet review, particularly if the proposal has received an unfavorable priority score. However, many proposals are ultimately funded upon resubmission if the critique is addressed in a careful, objective, point-by-point manner. Surgeons encounter difficulty in securing funding not only because we generally do not have the time to submit multiple proposals, but because we do not resubmit proposals that have been rejected for initial funding. Perseverance and a willingness to seek help from more experienced investigators will frequently enable a proposal to ultimately be funded. While the process can be anxietogenic, the opportunity to discover that is created by funding success is worth the good struggle.

R. E. Pollock

Commentary

Dr. Kron's chapter recapitulates some of the points emphasized in the previous chapter (chapter 44), but brings insight from looking at the process from the reviewer's viewpoint. Under ideal circumstances, the grant writer and the grant reviewer are precisely aligned. The writer is providing what the reviewer wants, and the result is a successful grant application. Dr. Kron makes it clear that one of the tasks of grant writers is to recruit the reviewer to their side. The reviewer then becomes the surrogate for the grant writer when presenting material to the rest of the review committee. The reviewer must be passionate about the quality of the grant if it is to be supported by the rest of the review group in the competition for funds. One or two unkind or disparaging words are enough to sink a grant proposal; the reviewer must be prepared to defend the grant against unwarranted criticism based on hasty visualization of the grant by a less-informed reviewer. In the chapter on writing the grant, there is a great deal of emphasis on substance, as it should be. In the chapter on grant review, there is significant emphasis upon form. It would be inappropriate to argue that form should take precedence over substance, but it is critical to know that both are vital components of the application. It is the form that allows easy access to the sub-stance, allows the gradual introduction of complex thoughts, and helps draw the reviewer to the same conclusions as the writer. As a reviewer, I have been impressed at how effective and convincing a grant application can be when it "tells a story." Like an illustrated manuscript, the figures and text must blend in a way that facilitates understanding and interpretation of the tale.

The grant writer says to "justify the budget"; the grant reviewer says not to be unrealistic in budgetary expectations. Alignment occurs when a realistic budget is appropriately justified. The writer says to make the specific aims hypothesis driven and convince the reviewer that the work can be done. The reviewer says to present specific aims that are not overly ambitious and that can be accomplished in the time allocated for conduct of the grant. Although there is overlap in the two chapters, this strengthens rather than weakens the presentation of this important topic.

A.S.W.

CHAPTER 46

Funding Research in Europe

W. Lorenz, A. Fingerhut, and H. Troidl

Introduction

The pursuit of funding for clinical research occupies most of the potentially fruitful time of senior scientists. It has become a professional game of its own, much abstracted from its primary goals and strongly overemphasized—a pathological state. There are several reasons why modern researchers must learn to play the game skillfully.

- Clinical departments were protected and did not depend on extramural support of clinical research when funding for the treatment of patients, provided by the health care systems, could be used for clinical research. There was no clear distinction between money for care and money for research in university clinics. For the most part, this source of funds has disappeared because of rigid cost analyses and constraints.

- About 30 years ago, extremely active researchers who needed more money than the clinical budget provided applied for funding, usually to a single organization (NIH [National Institutes of Health] in the United States, MRC [Medical Research Council] in Britain, DFG [*Deutsche Forschungsgemeinschaft*—German Research Association] in Germany, and CNRS [*Centre National de Recherche Scientifique*] in France).

Now acquiring funding from numerous sources has become a valuable skill in itself. The quality of a scientist is determined by the amount of money raised. The ultimate outcome of this money, in fact, is less important. But paperwork has to be done, and the publication machinery had to be enlarged to demonstrate to the grant-giving authorities by numbers of articles how effectively the research money was used in the clinical laboratory. In contrast, Sir James Black, who won the Nobel Prize in 1989, published only 18 papers; among them, one was on ß-blockers in *Lancet* and one on H_2-antihistamines in *Nature*.

- Money for funding clinical research is not equally valued in academic circles. There is a hierarchy: NIH money in the United States and DFG money in Germany are ranked number one, money from the Ministry of Technology number two, money from the Ministry of Health number three, and money from the pharmaceutical industry last. A scientist with a considerable portion of funding from industry is less respected.

Europeans, in general, have more critical attitudes toward the system of raising grants than Americans, but there are considerable differences among European countries. This chapter focuses on Germany, France, and the European Community.

Who Needs Funding for Clinical Research?

The Dreyfus scale of expertise[1] is used to distinguish several types of applicants for grants:

1. *The novice.* In Germany, novices enter the arena of competition after conducting work for a doctoral thesis in medicine, often after completing other studies. The novice cannot apply for a grant from DFG without a doctoral degree, but there is a chance to raise some money from private foundations (e.g., the Kempkes Foundation) or from the pharmaceutical industry. Typically, these grants do not depend on previously published work; they require only a carefully designed research plan and a request for less than $30,000 (U.S.).

2. *The advanced beginner.* The advanced beginner starts independent research about 2 years after graduation and applies for a standard DFG grant (*Normalverfahren*). This grant, if successfully secured, provides up to $100,000 for two years; it is a prestigious grant and relatively easy to administer. To get this grant, a few previously published articles in high-impact journals (Current Contents Journal Impact Index > 1.0)[2] are a prerequisite. If the grant proposal is rejected, the advanced beginner seeks funding from private foundations, which can provide similar amounts of money, or from the pharmaceutical industry. In France the novice or advanced beginner is rarely, if ever, involved in grant application.

3. *The competent clinical researcher.* Seven to ten years after graduation, the level of "habilitation" has been achieved. This procedure assesses one's capabilities to become an independent researcher and teacher at the university level (*Privatdozent,* similar to assistant professor). Several standard grants from the DFG, or research money from private foundations and industry, have been obtained. There is not only an idea for research but demonstrated competence in a research field. The investigator is able to participate in DFG research programs in a university or as a member of a clinical research group (*Klinische Forschergruppe*) or of a special research program (*Sonderforschungsbereich*). This level of researcher

can also participate in countrywide programs of the DFG (*Schwerpunktprogramm Klinische Pharmakologie*), the Ministry of Technology (BMFT), Ministry of Health (BMG), or large private foundations (e.g., *Volkswagenstiftung, Thyssenstiftung*). In the case of large, randomized, controlled clinical trials (e.g., multicenter trials), significant funding can also be raised from the pharmaceutical industry. All these grants, if successfully secured, provide a wide range of money, from $100,000 to $1 million per year for 3 to 9 years. However, these grants demand considerable adaptation and consensus; they are of moderate importance in defining academic credentials and are more difficult to administer.

4. *The expert in clinical research.* The expert is the leader in the department and the chairperson of complex research programs in which only competent researchers participate. These programs are sponsored by the DFG and the other organizations listed. In addition, joint ventures of the Federal Republic and the federated states of Germany might support larger programs requiring more expensive equipment (so-called HBFG programs). International programs, such as the German-Israeli Foundation or the Minerva Centres, the programs in the European Community, such as Biomedicine and Health Research (Biomed II) of European Commission, grants from international societies, such as OMGE (*Organisation Mondiale de GastroEntérologie*), and from NATO and EURATOM, belong to this category of grants. These grants provide considerable amounts of money, usually around $1 million per year for at least 3 years. They convey great academic credibility, power, and high prestige, and are very time-consuming to administer. In addition, they are usually complex in their structure and organization.

A special collection of grants is available for all types of applicants: funding for traveling, for congresses and visits, or for research stays in other countries supported by the Humbolt Foundation or the DAAD of the Ministry of Foreign Affairs in Bonn. Through this mechanism, the pharmaceutical industry provides funding with a minimum of bureaucracy. In Germany—in contrast to the NIH in the United States—these activities are not supported by the government. High registration fees and accommodation and travel costs prohibit participation of clinical researchers in European meetings that are, in contrast to intercontinental meetings, ineligible for support from the DFG or other grant-giving authorities. Industry pays the costs for clinical investigators, and the system would not work without it.

How Do You Get Funding for Clinical Research?

Guidelines are the new tools for problem solving in clinical medicine and are probably suitable for advice on how to obtain funding for a particular clinical research project as well. They are presented in the format of a table (Table 46-1), rather than that of a clinical algorithm because they do not contain many decision modes.

The German Position

These guidelines are based on personal experience and recommendations of grant-giving authorities and the Association of Medical Societies in Germany (AWMF). According to this association, which has 300,000 members, the most important faults in grant applications leading to rejection include the following:

- Lack of originality
- Lack of quality research (i.e., methodology)
- No stringency in presenting the state of the art
- Diffuse hypotheses as the basis for the research plan
- Superficial design of the research project
- Uncritical selection and application of methodology

The French Position

Funding of surgical research in France is ill-defined and problematic; however, progress is being made. The French government, through the *Ministère de la Santé et de la Recherche Médicale*, has made a firm engagement toward further development of research, especially in the fields of care management and cost-effectiveness but also in fundamental research, quality control, and evaluation.

The sources available, as elsewhere, are of course limited, and the paperwork enormous and complicated. Major sources of funding for medical research in France include specialized organizations such as the INSERM (*Institut National de la Santé et de la Recherche Médicale*), the CNRS (*Centre National de Recherche Scientifique*), and the *Direction des Hôpitaux* (Central Office of Hospitals, depending on the *Ministère du Travail et des Affaires Sociales*), occasionally in conjunction with INSERM, to name just a few. Research in France is conducted within the hospital (or hospitals if a collaborative study is undertaken) or in laboratories and is usually based on university budgets.

Regarding grants from INSERM, the principal investigator must first perfectly structure the research project in writing. The request for funding should not be longer than 30 pages. The project is then submitted to an INSERM committee (30 members), which decides whether the project is worthwhile. If the committee favors the proposal, funds are allocated for a maximum of 4 years. Before the grant expires, the principal investigator will usually ask for the creation of an official INSERM unit of research. To continue the investigation, the researcher must rewrite the project, usually supported by satisfactory preliminary results. It is important to include some of the permanent INSERM personnel in the suggested team to increase one's chances of obtaining the grant. The project is presented to one of ten subcommittees called the CSS (*Commission Scientifique Spécialisée*), composed of 20 to 25 members involved in the specific field of research. Members of this subcommittee tour the hospital or laboratory and listen to the investigator's presentation; well-documented accomplishments and optimistic results are prerequisites for success. This committee then reports to the Scientific Council of INSERM, composed of some 25 members, which invites the principal coordinator to present the project with appropriate data. If the unit is authorized, it is for a 4-year term, with the possibility of renewal every 4 years for a total of 12 years.

There are no more than four to five creations of this kind per year in each of the ten fields of

Table 46-1.

Flow direction and time course in algorithm	Specification
1. Development of research idea and concept; feasibility	Something new, truly original? Clinically relevant? For many? Feasibility of one researcher or only for a team? Local or multicentric? Experts form one or several research fields?
2. Selection of appropriate type of grant	Suitable for research idea? Basic research in clinic or clinical problem-solving research? Amount of money needed? Deadline for a funding program tolerable? Prestige associated with grant? Procedure of grant approval reasonably transparent? Possibilities to react? Trust in the honesty of refereeing?
3. Call in for grant protocols	Most important: make a connection with the personal contact of the grant-giving authority—telephone or even visit Develop preliminary scheme (1–2 pages) of your proposal and discuss it with the authorities.
4. Preparation of research proposal:	
4.1 General operations	Important: keep the deadline Important: be stringent, align your arguments in a *goal-oriented* way—leave no loopholes Follow the grant protocols exactly; do not exceed 30 pages Be clear enough for non-specialists: find the compromise between the general and specific in the protocol
4.2 Summary	Important: although placed at the beginning of the proposal, write it last
4.3 State of the art in the field of research.	Do not be comprehensive; carefully select the premises for your research idea (10 references) Do not mention your own work; consider possible referees
4.4 Presentation of your previous work	Emphasize your previous contributions (20 references); modesty will not help you
4.5 Research program	Develop a detailed research program—not only designs and operations, but also methods Be comprehensible—use headings and subheadings Be realistic with regard to time and money Do not make the referees suspicious about any connections of your present proposal with other research programs, especially those in industry Carefully solve problems in human ethics, animal ethics, and gene technology

(continued)

research. In 1996, for instance, there were a total of 24, out of 39 requests, in all of France. Funding can range from 400,000 to 500,000 French francs ($80,000 to $100,000) per year for small research units, to as much as 50 to 80 million French francs ($10 to $16 million) per year for the megaunits. Separate budgets are available for equipment and personnel needs. The procedures are somewhat similar for CNRS and the hospital directorate. For the latter, however, the coordinator must ask for special grant formulas from the Ministry and obtain specific authorization from the hospital director and the university center on which the hospital or hospitals depend to conduct the study. The project then has to be approved by the DRRC (*Délégations Régionales à la Recherche Cli-*

Table 46-1. Continued

Flow direction and time course in algorithm	Specification
4.6 List of funding requested: the heart of the story.	Be modest in your calculation costs, but always remain open to reduction Start with costs for staff Study Federal laws for research people (BAT) before you write Replace permanent staff (technicians) with young academic workers: they are underpaid, but have a chance for promotion Do not forget costs such as those for assurances (clinical trials) and information technology (copies, printing, reprints) Avoid flat anti-tank mines for your referees! Little or no basic equipment, no travelling, and no industry. Also, computers and software are not well appreciated. Do not mention too much about your basic equipment—your referees may become envious
5. Submission of grant proposal and waiting time	Submit well ahead of the deadline. Consider the possibility of postal delays or other catastrophes. Expect to wait 3–6 months Contact the funding authorities after two months—not before! Convey the impression of febrile activity first, the need for money last
6. Working with the grant—if funded. . . .	Report the grant approval to the University administration *and* the public Start work *immediately*. 2–3 years is shorter than you think Cooperate with the administration Be careful with all accounts
6. Working with the grant, continued.	Consider that effectiveness must be shown *before* the end of your funding time—about six months before. Grant renewal takes time Papers are superior to anything else, but abstracts, oral presentations and any kind of *documented* effectiveness must be kept preciously. Consider bridging salary costs for your co-workers—they must live as well.
7. Measures after the bad news: Not funded. . . .	Carefully analyse the referee's reports Do not waste time protesting or awaiting a change Do not give up: apply in the lower category of prestige. Transform your application format appropriately Try to get industrial money for bridging—it is more flexible

nique) and the CNRC (*Comité National de la Recherche Clinique*). The DRRC controls the methodology and coordination of the various partners involved (especially for multicenter studies). Its role is to ensure that proper evaluation has been performed before and during investigations. The DRRC is informed continually of the progress of the study once it commences. The CNRC reports on the submitted projects and presents them for final approval to the appropriate office in the Ministry. The duration of the grant depends on

the project, and funds are usually distributed, monthly or biannually, for the predetermined period, according to needs.

All projects involving research on humans must be approved by CCR in accordance with Senator Huriet's law. This law requires that written, informed consent be obtained from the patient. Another important aspect of research in France is the requirement of insurance for each project.

Other possible sources for funding medical research in France are the *Ligue Contre le Cancer*, pharmaceutical companies, medical organizations or societies, world organizations such as WHO (World Health Organization) or the International Red Cross, and the nonmedical industry. Most clinical research in France is dependent on pharmaceutical companies. Although these companies can sponsor clinical, randomized trials, like many of the medical societies, they give out specific prizes as well. The list is long, but the main awards offered in France include those from Smith Kline French, Beaufour, Fournier, Jouvinal, Ferring, Schering-Plough, Latema, Rhone Poulenc, Astra, Abbott, Allard, Glaxo, Biotherax, Lilly, Merck Sharp and Dome, Beecham, and Roche.

Among those available from the societies are the Robert Tournut Award (*Société National Française de Gastro-Entérologie*), the bourse de Recherche from the *Region Ile de France*, the Claude Bernard Award from the city of Paris, the Bourdin Award in oncology, the Andreg Prize offered by the International Rotary Club, and the Merci Prize offered by the Lion's Club. Industrial support is present in France as well; Peugeot and Renault, for example, are very active in this respect, and Hewlett-Packard and Mercedes-Benz offer funding for clinical research. All of these opportunities are announced yearly in university hospitals, and the rules for application are available upon direct request to the firm responsible. The paperwork is usually less than that required for the INSERM or CNRS research projects, but the sums allocated are also proportionally less. These grants are usually lump sums, to be used at the discretion of the investigation teams, and are inclusive of all expenses—conceptualization, accomplishment of the project, and presentation of results.

The European Position

Special conditions have to be met for multicenter grants in the European Community (EC). At least five centers are usually required, and some of them must come from the southern part of the continent. This requirement explains why EC grants are so political; the refereeing process is practically unfathomable, needs considerable adaptation and consensus, and is also quite difficult

to administer for the study leader (chairperson of the project management team). However, the amount of money is sizeable ($1 to $10 million per year for 3 to 6 years) and is generally distributed unequally among the study centers.

An example was the COMAC-BME initiative for a bipartite action on computer-aided diagnosis. Two projects are listed in this chapter: the acute abdominal pain project of the late Tim De Dombal[3] and the jaundice project of S.M. Lavelle.[4] The complicated structure of the De Dombal project is shown in Figure 46-1, including all participating centers. The entire organizational structure of the medical research program of the European Community is depicted in Figure 46-2, as taken from the jaundice project of Lavelle. The two presentations are complementary.

New programs, at present, are the Biotechnology (Biotech II) and the Biomedical and Health Research (Biomed II) programs, which comprise funding of about 500 million ECU (European Currency Units), which corresponds to about $750 million—a large sum of money. Germany felt systematically excluded from this source of research money and has implemented a special coordinating center for grant application in the European Community: the KoWi Centre of the Scientific Organisations in Germany including AvH, HGF, DAAD, DFG, FhG, HRK, MPG, and the Stifterverband. Address: D-53175 Bonn, Godeberger Allee 127 *or* Bruxelles B 1050, Rue du Trône 98.

Conclusion

Acquiring funding for clinical research has become not only a necessity for clinical researchers in all academic positions but also a social game with many negative aspects—a distortion of the original concept of supporting the realization of researchers' ideas chief among them. The research manager has overcome the innovative researcher, and funding has become an achievement in itself. Clinical researchers have to be aware of this dangerous development and handle the difficult situation professionally and ethically.

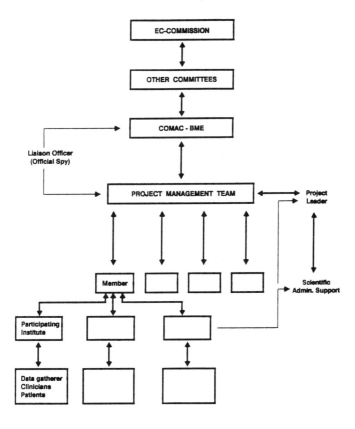

Figure 46-1. Structure of the EC/COMAC project on acute abdominal pain. Reproduced from T. De Dombal.[3]

Participating centres

Cattedra di Gastroenterologia 1, Rome
Ospedale San Filippo Neri, Rome
Università di Ancona, Faculty of Medicine, Ancona

Belgium
Stedilijk Ziekenhuis, Mechelen
O.L.V. Kliniek, Aalst
Academische Ziekenhuis Gasthuisberg, Leuven
Roeselare Hospital
Clinique St.-Elisabeth − ASBL, Bruxelles

Denmark
Rigshospitalet, Copenhagen
University of Aalborg

France
Hopital Intercommunal de Poissy, Poissy
Hopital Louis Maurier, Colombes
Hopital D'Orsay
Hopital Henri Mondor, Creteil

Germany
Chirurgische Universitätsklinik Düsseldorf
Chirurgische Klinik, Bürgerhospital, Frankfurt/Main
Chirurgische Universitätsklinik Homburg/Saar
Chirurgische Universitätsklinik Köln-Merheim
Chirurgische Universitätsklinik Marburg/Lahn

Greece
Crete University Medical School, Crete
Aretaieion Hospital, Athens

Ireland
University College, Galway
Our Lady's Hospital, Navan

Italy
Ospedale V. Cerveno, Palermo, Sicily
Ospedale E. Albanese, Palermo, Sicily
Istituto di Chirurgia d'Uregenza, Milan

Nether-lands
Stichting Deventer Ziekenhjuizen, Deventer
Zeeweg Ziekenhuis, AL Ijmuiden
Ziekenhuis ST. Annadal, Maastricht
St. Elizabeth Ziekenhuis, Tilburg

Portugal
Hospital Militar Principal, Lisbon
Hospital de St. Jose, Lisbon
Hospital Civis de Lisboa, Lisbon

Spain
Universidad de Barcelona
Hospital Clinic, Barcelona

Sweden
Hospital of Varberg

United Kingdom
District General Hospital, Ormskirk
Trafford District Hospital, Manchester
Royal Hospital, Oldham
Hope Hospital, Salford
The General Infirmary, Leeds
St. James University Hospital, Leeds
District Hospital, Dewsbury
Children's Hospital, Sheffield
Airedale District General Hospital, Keighley
Whipps Cross Hospital, London
General Hospital, Birmingham
Southend Hospital, Westcliffe-on-Sea
Steppling Hill Hospital, Stockport
Birch Hill Hospital, Rochdale

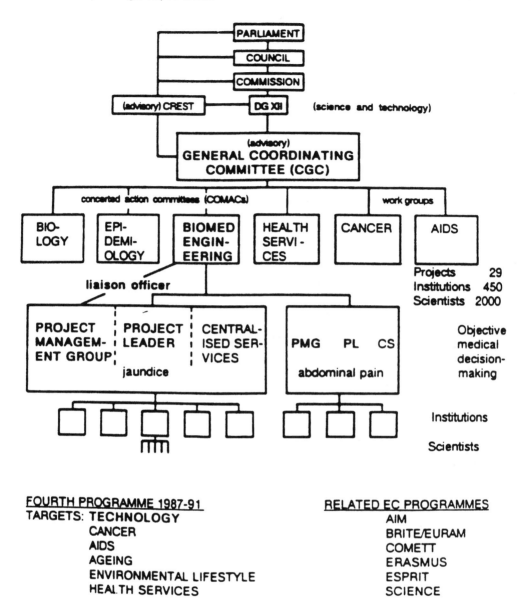

FOURTH PROGRAMME 1987-91
TARGETS: TECHNOLOGY
　　　　　CANCER
　　　　　AIDS
　　　　　AGEING
　　　　　ENVIRONMENTAL LIFESTYLE
　　　　　HEALTH SERVICES

RELATED EC PROGRAMMES
　　　　AIM
　　　　BRITE/EURAM
　　　　COMETT
　　　　ERASMUS
　　　　ESPRIT
　　　　SCIENCE

Figure 46-2. Organizational structure of medical research programs in the European Community. The elements in boldface are those more directly concerned with the objective medical decision-making projects. Of the related EC programs, that on advanced informatics in medicine (AIM) is the most cognate. COMET and ERASMUS are educationally oriented, and the remainder are industry oriented. Particulars are available from the Community national offices. BRITE, Basic Research in Industrial Technologies for Europe; EURAM, European Research on Advanced Materials; ESPRIT, European Strategic Programme for Research and Development in Information Technologies; SCIENCE, Scientific cooperation. Reproduced from Lavelle et al.[4]

References

1. Hilden J. Intuition and other soft modes of thought in surgery. Theor Surg 1991;6:89–94.
2. Garfield E. Citation Indexing: Its Theory and Application in Science, Technology, and Humans. New York: John Wiley & Sons, 1979.
3. De Dombal FT. The European Community concerted action on objective medical decision-making in patients with acute abdominal pain. Theor Surg 1990;5:112–117.
4. Lavelle SM, Dawids SG, van Beneken JEW. The initiative on medical decision-making of the Concerted Action Committee on Biomedical Engineering (COMAC-BME) of the European Community. Theor Surg 1990;5:107–111.

Commentary

This chapter brings out a pitfall of contemporary science. Investigators are becoming more preoccupied by the business of application and management of grants. They can be distracted from their primary scientific goal by this preoccupation.

H.T.

Commentary

As an American investigator I enjoyed reading this vivid account of research funding in Europe. The European population is large and diverse; attempts to coordinate investigative protocols across international boundaries must be daunting, EEC or not. It is easy to understand why this process has become highly politicized.

Several observations are as true in North America as they are in Europe. The writers point out that the quest for research dollars has become an endpoint that may be divorced from the scientific work that it is designed to support. As sums of money for investigative programs increase, the power of those holding those important grants also increases. Their political stature among colleagues rises. In the United States large grants carry prestige, offer employment for many individuals, enhance the visibility of an institution when the work is well done and published, and frequently bring secondary gains to the institution. Examples of secondary gains would include reimbursement of the indirect costs of maintaining research facilities and new money for renovation, construction, and equipping new research facilities. In a difficult fiscal environment universities are hesitant to part with investigators who demonstrate an ability to bring large sums of money to the institution, just as professional sports teams do not like to lose players who attract large crowds and thus enhance profitability. Total grant support becomes a bargaining chip used by successful investigators to increase their worth during job negotiations. Frequently it is a tool by which powerful scientists and chairpersons retain their positions at universities even in the absence of filling the multiple mandates that accompany such positions.

Substantial support for clinical research or laboratory investigation also provides the appropriate backing for dedicated scientists of high quality to pursue their work in a relatively unfettered fashion. Large clinical research trials have led to reduction in the mortality of myocardial infarction, have supported the use of one or another treatment modality, have increased cure rates among cancer patients, and frequently provide the scientific infrastructure for advances in epidemiological approaches to public and world health. At the level of populations, small differences may translate into large gains and savings of vast sums of money.

Human investigation is costly. Money and the power that it brings have a tendency to corrupt, and only the inherent qualities of the individuals in the system can maintain appropriate scientific integrity and scholarship based on the healing and teaching of others.

A.S.W.

SECTION VI

Implementation

CHAPTER 47

From Concept to Clinical Reality: Implementing Pancreatic Transplantation

L. Rosenberg

This chapter is about the development of a research-based clinical program. How does an institution decide to develop a new program? Should it be done? Can it be done? How can we ensure success? I will describe the gradual evolution of the program in pancreatic islet transplantation in the department of surgery at McGill University as an example.

We could simply describe the conventional scientific proposal and business plan approach to program development. I suspect that this would be unsatisfying to many in our intended audience of young surgeon-scientists. Such a presentation would not provide narrative continuity and nuance. It would leave many important questions unanswered. For example, why was islet transplantation chosen as the subject of a discussion on program planning? Why did this occur at McGill? And how did the author come to be involved? These questions expose issues that are fundamental to career planning and faculty development. The business and research plan in the process of program development will not be neglected; I will return to these important elements later in the chapter.

The evolutionary path of my research into the cell biology of the pancreas began more than 15 years ago. This chapter is a personal account of my own adventures in surgical research; my colleagues and I gained many valuable insights that contributed to our successes and helped us to overcome our failures. This work represents a practical application of many of the ideas expressed in other parts of the book. It illustrates the scope of surgical research and how surgeons approach a research program.

At the time of this writing, we are poised to initiate the program of human islet transplantation at McGill University. All the required elements are falling into place. It could only have happened at this point in time. In several different disciplines, novel lines of investigation into the biology of the islet cell have begun to converge. As a result we now find ourselves on the threshold of a new treatment for type I diabetes mellitus.

But this is the end of the story. Back to the beginning.

In the Beginning: Identifying a Clinical Problem

Our work began in 1980 with the study of pancreatic carcinogenesis. I was in the third year of general surgery residency and was about to enter the laboratory for our program's traditional research year. I had cultivated an interest in pancreatic cancer because of the abrupt death of a close relative. I approached our department's pancreatic surgeon, Dr. Rea Brown, to ask for his support and supervision during my year of research. He quickly agreed but then introduced me to Pathologist-in-Chief Dr. Bill Duguid, who would cosupervise the project. I originally felt I was being farmed out, but this decision on the part of Dr. Brown was critical to my future development as a surgical investigator. The relationship with Dr. Duguid proved to be a fertile one that continues after all these years.

Characterization of the Problem

The first issue was to decide what aspect of the problem we would study. At this time, pancreatic cancer was recognized as the second most common gastrointestinal (GI) malignancy, with an incidence that equaled the annual mortality rate.[1] Not much was known about the predisposing factors, and only a few animal models existed with which to investigate pathogenesis. Although these models seemed to have little direct clinical relevance, the hamster model was the most promising.[2]

In a previous series of studies, Drs. Biron, Brown, and Duguid had developed a canine model of chronic partial pancreatic duct obstruction in which Dr. Duguid noticed that duct epithelial hyperplasia was a prominent feature.[3] Since pancreatic cancer usually occurred against the backdrop of chronic pancreatitis, and since chronic duct obstruction was a common accompanying feature, the question arose whether duct epithelial hyperplasia was a precursor lesion for pancreatic duct carcinoma.

Determining the Research Question

Two questions were then formulated: (1) Could the canine model for pancreatic duct epithelial hyperplasia be adapted to the hamster? and (2) Could it then be used to create a new model of pancreatic carcinogenesis?

The technique for partial obstruction of the canine pancreatic duct, by placing cellophane tape over a needle placed alongside the exposed duct, was not directly applicable to the hamster pancreas because the duct was too small. While trying to circumvent this problem, I wrapped the tape

around the entire head of the pancreas, serendipitously developing the technique now known as cellophane wrapping of the pancreas.[4,5] This modified technique recreated the chronic partial obstruction produced in the dog but without the associated chronic inflammation and atrophy that had characterized the canine model.

This was an opportune time to begin these studies, because the National Institutes of Health (NIH) in the United States had just initiated a request for applications for the study of pancreatic cancer. We submitted a proposal to develop a model of partial duct obstruction in order to study the subsequent cellular changes as possible precursors to the development of cancer. To our surprise, the initial attempt to secure external funding was successful. With this support, we were able to develop the first experimental model for carcinoma of the head of the pancreas.[6] This model was important for understanding the problem because it demonstrated for the first time that partial obstruction, and the resulting duct epithelial hyperplasia in particular, were important predisposing factors for the development of pancreatic cancer.[6] After this first year of investigation, I was encouraged by the departmental chair, Dr. Mulder, to consider remaining in the laboratory to pursue a graduate degree in research. I stayed on, and the second chapter of the story took a surprising turn.

"Chance Favors the Prepared Mind" (Louis Pasteur)

The pancreas of the hamster was known to be histologically very similar to the human gland. It was not fully appreciated at the time that the cells of the hamster pancreas were particularly sensitive to trophic stimuli, making it an ideal organ in which to study factors that regulate cell proliferation and differentiation. Serendipity intervened once again.

Although the cellophane wrap model of partial obstruction produced duct epithelial cell hyperplasia, we were astonished to observe that this partial obstruction was followed by the induction of islet cell differentiation and new islet formation. We had stumbled onto a new way to induce islet neogenesis in an adult animal in the absence of tissue destruction, atrophy, or chemical agents.[5]

These were exhilarating and highly productive years. Additional peer-reviewed funding was received from the Cancer Research Society, and I was awarded a Medical Research Council (MRC) Fellowship for personal salary support. Most important, however, was the continued active support of the leadership of the departments of pathology and surgery. Additional resources were made available as circumstances required, and I was given the freedom to pursue an area of research that was entirely new to both departments.

Midcourse Correction: From Cancer to Diabetes, From Residency to Junior Faculty Member

The observation that partial duct obstruction led to new islet formation prompted redirection of our focus from pancreatic carcinogenesis to islet neogenesis. Would the induction of islet cell proliferation and differentiation be sufficient to reverse a diabetic state?

Hamsters rendered diabetic by the administration of the beta-cell toxin streptozotocin underwent the cellophane wrap procedure. Six weeks later, we had our answer. Partial obstruction of the pancreatic duct could induce islet neogenesis in a hyperglycemic environment, and the new islet tissue functioned to reverse the diabetic state.[7,8] This was the last experiment I was to conduct as a surgical resident. After three years in the laboratory, it was time to complete my clinical training in general surgery.

At the end of this period, three things occurred that were to establish my career path in academic surgery as a clinician-scientist. First, I successfully defended a thesis entitled "Cell Proliferation in the Pancreas of the Syrian Golden Hamster," for which I was awarded a Ph.D. degree. Second, I was invited to join the faculty of the department of surgery at McGill, on condition that additional postgraduate clinical and research work be completed. My clinical interest in general surgery now centered primarily on pancreatic disease. This shift was not mere coincidence; I felt that such a

clinical focus would complement and facilitate my future research on pancreatic cell differentiation. This alignment has yielded dividends ever since, and the field is still ripe for further investigation. Third, the research collaboration with Dr. Duguid that facilitated many of the studies and led to my completion of the Ph.D. provided more than expert supervision and advice; he became a mentor, a role model, and eventually a good friend. Both the mentoring and the friendship continue to this day. This ongoing cross-disciplinary collaboration remains the basis for our research successes, both past and present.

Midcourse Correction (II): From General Surgery to Transplantation. What Is the Mechanism of Induction of Islet Neogenesis?

Upon completion of my residency, I was awarded a McLaughlin Travelling Fellowship to pursue postgraduate studies. The important decision was where to spend the next 2 years. This time would be pivotal, for both my research and my credibility as a clinical surgeon on my return to McGill. After careful deliberation, I chose to pursue a combined clinical and research transplant fellowship in the department of surgery at the University of Michigan (U of M), under the supervision of the chair, Jeremiah Turcotte. He was a transplant surgeon, with interests in chronic pancreatitis and portal hypertension, and an appealing role model.

There were two primary reasons for this decision. The U of M Medical Center was a large faculty with diverse interests and abundant resources. The section of general surgery in particular was renowned for its work in pancreatic surgery, an academic environment in which I would thrive. Despite the long tradition of pancreatic surgery, pancreas transplantation, which was under the expert guidance of Don Dafoe, was still in its infancy. The experience of going through the learning curve along with some of the pioneers in the field was an unparalleled opportunity. Not only did I acquire new surgical skills that applied to the pancreas, but I also learned how to manage the development of a new clinical program.

The second reason for choosing Michigan was the excellent research facilities and the presence of several well-known investigators whose interests lay in the pancreas. Two clinician-scientists who were the most influential during my stay in Ann Arbor were in fact not surgeons but internists. Tachi Yamada, then head of gastroenterology, was a superb sounding board and an excellent source of advice and innovative ideas. Arthur Vinik, an endocrinologist, had expertise in islet cell tumors, growth factors, and diabetes. Arthur gradually assumed a mentoring role and eventually became an important collaborator in the research on islet neogenesis. My association with him was largely responsible for setting the future direction of both our research programs, a productive collaboration that continues to this day.

While in Ann Arbor, I began a series of investigations that focused on two fundamental questions. First, did the newly formed islets in the cellophane wrap model function in a regulated manner and produce a normal molecular form of insulin? In vitro perfusion of islets isolated after neogenesis confirmed that their insulin secretory response to glucose stimulation was normal.[9] Using reverse-phase high-performance liquid chromatography (HPLC), we demonstrated that these islets synthesized and secreted two molecular forms of insulin, as opposed to the one normally produced by adult hamster islets.[9] At the time, it seemed reasonable to speculate about whether the additional molecular species of insulin represented a fetal form of the molecule, but the issue was never pursued.

The second question, why did partial duct obstruction lead to the induction of islet neogenesis, was obviously multifactorial and very complex. To begin to address it, we generalized the question to ask whether the control mechanisms for initiation of proliferation, differentiation, and growth maintenance of islets were centrally mediated or could be achieved by local influences. To answer this question, I turned to the concept of parabiosis (common cross-circulation between animals).

An experiment was designed to determine whether humoral factors were involved in islet neogenesis and, in particular, to ascertain whether the trophic effect of obstruction was the result of the local release of growth factor(s). The surgical technique of parabiosis in small animals had been described some 50 years earlier and was easily adapted to the hamster. The results of these studies suggested that the induction of islet neogenesis by partial obstruction was mediated locally by an autocrine or paracrine mechanism.[10,11]

If it were true that islet neogenesis was regulated locally, then it was conceivable that partial obstruction produced trophic factors that, by some unexplained sequence of events, induced islet neogenesis. Assuming this to be true, I set out to identify the active factors. A tissue extract, subsequently named ilotropin, was prepared from the partially obstructed hamster pancreas and was demonstrated by in vivo bioassay to have trophic effects on normal pancreatic tissue.[12] This was the first hint that we might have stumbled onto something of considerable clinical significance. Unfortunately, just as these observations were being made, it was time to leave Ann Arbor and return to the Montreal General Hospital and McGill University.

The move back to Montreal presented many new challenges. In a short space of time and without prior specific instruction or training for the tasks, I was expected to set up a clinical practice, assume the leadership of the nascent renal transplant program, and develop a pancreas transplant program. With respect to research, I had to reestablish my laboratory and again seek external peer-reviewed support. The transition was eased by the division chief, the departmental chair, Bill Duguid in pathology, and the hospital's executive director. Three key elements were quickly put in place: adequate laboratory space, start-up research funds, and protected time.

With these problems receding, I could once again concentrate on a question that would preoccupy me, Arthur Vinik, and Bill Duguid for the next 8 years: What is the key to islet neogenesis? Enough preliminary work had been published in the preceding 4 years that, within a year of my return, I was able to secure external funding for the research, initially from the American Surgical Association Foundation and then from the Medical Research Council and the Canadian Diabetes Foundation.

In our next two studies, ilotropin itself, in the absence of duct obstruction, was shown to lead to the induction of islet neogenesis[13] and the reversal of a diabetic state.[14,15] This study was an enormous financial undertaking due to the cost related to the preparation of ilotropin. Ultimately, additional financial support from the Montreal General Hospital Foundation and the departments of surgery and pathology was required to sustain the effort. Their support and encouragement were unwavering at this critical juncture, and the gamble to place all our resources into this one project seemed to have succeeded.

In 1990 we published the concept of the duct-islet axis,[16] in which we emphasized that the ontogenetic relationship between ducts and islets carried over to the adult pancreas. We speculated that it was perhaps not premature to envisage new approaches to the treatment of diabetes mellitus. We suggested that identification of the factor or factors that regulate islet cell proliferation and differentiation in our model might permit proto-undifferentiated cells and islets to be grown in culture. This concept could be extended to induce endocrine cell differentiation in vivo as well. Furthermore, islet cell growth factors could be used to provide "trophic support" to islet transplants as a means of maintaining graft viability. There may also be greater scope for gene therapy when the growth factor or factors have been isolated, purified, sequenced, and cloned. This period marked the first time that I began to think seriously about islet transplantation as a therapeutic option for type I diabetes.

Limitations and the Need to Expand the Collaboration

With the demonstration that our research may have clinical applicability, it became clear that an expansion of activity was required. It was also apparent that our existing capabilities at Montreal General were limited and that any expansion would have to establish new interdisciplinary collaborations. Luckily, the opportunity for such a collaboration arose when Arthur Vinik moved in 1991 from Ann Arbor to the Diabetes Research Institute at Eastern Virginia Medical School in Norfolk.

An expanded investigative team was formed that now incorporated protein chemists and molecular biologists. In this new, larger group, Montreal became responsible for studies that related to cell biology and islet physiology, while Norfolk assumed the responsibility of identifying and purifying growth factors in the partial obstruction model.

Different Pathways of Investigation Converge

Over the ensuing 3 years the collaborative effort generated a number of new observations. The growth factors induced by partial obstruction began to be characterized,[17–20] new culture techniques were developed to study individual pancreatic cell populations,[22–24] and we used these to demonstrate a previously unappreciated trophic interaction between pancreatic ducts and islets.[23] This latter observation gave further credence to our concept of the duct-islet axis.[16]

As a result of these studies, I began to wonder if we had not perhaps found one reason for the apparent lack of success of human islet transplantation-purification. If a trophic interaction existed between islets and ducts (and perhaps acinar cells), then might the effort at islet purification be detrimental to the long-term survival of the islet graft? This question would remain just a thought for another year.

Our understanding of islet neogenesis in the adult pancreas has continued to increase.[25,26] Novel growth factors that appear after duct obstructions have been identified, and the cells in which these are synthesized, as well as the target cells on which they act, are being characterized.[27,28] Another significant progression has been the shift to human pancreatic tissue for in vitro studies. This move was prompted by the need to confirm our previous observations in human tissues and to acquire experience in the digestion of the human pancreas for islet isolation in preparation for islet transplantation.

Shortly after work with human tissue was begun, it became apparent that human adult islets possessed a potential for further differentiation.[29] Under appropriate conditions, their genetic program could be switched and the cells transformed to primitive ductlike cells. As we began to explore the mechanisms involved, we were compelled once again to change direction in order to concentrate on the issue of islet cell survival.

Restoration of an islet cell mass that continues to synthesize and secrete insulin and that reestablishes the normal intra-islet cellular interactions is the ultimate objective in the treatment of insulin-dependent diabetes mellitus. The Holy Grail of the diabetologist is how best to accomplish this goal.

The experience to date with islet transplantation is disappointing. An unexpectedly large islet mass is required to achieve demonstrable serum levels of C-peptide, let alone successful restoration of normal glucose homeostasis. As a consequence, more than one pancreas is required to produce a graft of sufficient cell mass. Furthermore, it is becoming apparent that the inability to sustain graft viability may represent a major unforeseen problem.

Although these shortcomings highlight the need to pursue alternative therapeutic options, it becomes important to understand why whole pancreas transplantation is so successful in reversing hyperglycemia but transplants of purified islets ultimately fail in the long term. Certainly, some or all of the following factors must be pertinent: (1) inadequate cell mass at the time of islet transplantation; (2) inadequate islet cell mass at the site of implantation; and (3) inability to diagnose rejection sufficiently early, leading to a loss of functional islet tissue. Relevant as these issues may be, they do not address the fundamental difference between grafts of whole pancreas and purified islets: the contribution of the nonendocrine cell compartment. A fourth cause of islet graft failure, the loss of trophic support, needs to be considered. This last point offers an important insight into the very nature of the pancreas itself, an issue that has dominated my work for the last 6 months.

I am more confident than ever that the puzzle of successful islet transplantation may be ready for solution. Various lines of investigation are beginning to converge: the existence of trophic interactions between ducts and islets; the identification of INGAP, a new trophic factor that appears during islet neogenesis;[27,28] the recognition of the transdifferentiation potential of human adult islet cells;[29] and new information about apoptosis and islet cell survival. Finally, a clearer understanding of islet biology is emerging.

Midcourse Correction (III): From Bench to Bedside— Islet Transplantation

As the focus of my research has been drawn back to clinical transplantation, new issues have surfaced. There is a need to further expand our existing collaboration. New areas of investigation must be explored, and once again I am forced to recognize my limitations and those of the institution. This minicrisis, for that is the way I perceive it, comes at an opportune time. The MRC and the JDFI (Juvenile Diabetes Foundation International) are funding new networks of centers of excellence in diabetes research in Canada. I have been fortunate to be able to collaborate with experts in metabolism, growth factors and extracellular matrix, nutrition, and immunology on one such proposal. Regardless of whether the application is accepted, new friendships have been established and new research collaborations have already been put in place. This is a mutually beneficial arrangement for all members of the proposed network, who will be able to pool their different expertise and resources with the aim of developing winning strategies for successful islet transplantation.

RESEARCH-BASED CLINICAL PROGRAM DEVELOPMENT

- Choose an area of clinical expertise that parallels your research interests.
- Develop colleagues in related disciplines.
- Design precise needs to accomplish career goals.
- Recognize the limitations of your own environment.
- Supplement institutional capabilities with geographically distant collaborators when necessary.

Back to the Future

While the science seems to be taking care of itself, I must now concentrate on planning for a human islet transplantation program at McGill. As you will now appreciate, this could only be happening at this time. Several new questions, not related to research per se, have assumed importance: What programs does the hospital need to develop? Is islet transplantation on the list?

The planning process began with exploratory discussions with the chairperson of the department of surgery, the director of the division of general surgery, the director of the division of endocrinology, the director of professional services of the hospital, and the scientific director of the Research Institute. Tentative approval for proceeding with an islet program was received and a preliminary budget submitted to the director of professional services. Funding for this project is also being sought as part of the MRC-JDFI Network of Centers of Excellence Program. In the interim, space for a dedicated human islet isolation laboratory has already been provided by the MGH Research Institute. This will permit us to continue to perfect the technique of islet isolation in advance of our first transplant.

An impact analysis will be carried out in the coming months to determine whether we can actually put a program in place and what we need to assure its success. This is a comprehensive and time-consuming process. On completion, however, we will have a road map of where we are going and how we are going to get there. The issues addressed by the impact analysis are summarized in Table 47-1. Finally, in parallel with these efforts, an islet transplant trial protocol was drafted. This document has been reviewed by internal and external referees and had received tentative approval from the institutional ethics review board. The key players are all engaged and the pieces are slowly falling into place.

Conclusion: Some Personal Observations

It has often been said that it is difficult to know what lies at the end of a long road; this is especially true of research. I began 15 years ago to investigate pancreatic carcinogenesis and now find myself ready to apply what I have learned to human islet transplantation, not only in terms of conventional transplantation but also by inducing

Table 47-1. Islet transplantation at McGill: summary of impact analysis questions.

1. **Patient impacts**
   What are the impacts on
   - quality of care?
   - anticipated outcomes?
   - coordination of care across the continuum of services?
   - the patient's group (i.e., family)?
   - clinical ethical issues?

2. **Staff and employee impacts**
   What are the impacts on
   - physician resource planning?
   - other personnel redistribution/numbers?
   - mix of personnel and their roles?
   - teamwork?
   - work standards/techniques/range of activities?
   - management and organizational structure?

3. **Systems impacts**
   What are the impacts on the regional health care system by
   - community support services, such as home care programs?
   - other academic centers outside the McGill network?

   What are the impacts on McGill's hospital system by
   - closely related programs?
   - hospital stay and bed requirements?
   - operating room utilization and equipment?
   - day care or day surgery?

islet neogenesis. This is what Joseph Murray referred to, in his Churchill Lecture to the Excelsior Society, as the fourth phase in the evolution of surgery, that is, inductive surgery.[30]

Several years after having written my doctoral thesis, I encountered a series of intriguing studies reported by de Takats, a New York surgeon.[31–34] In these studies, which date from the late 1920s, he relates surgical attempts to "increase sugar tolerance" in children with juvenile onset (type I) diabetes. What is remarkable is that the surgical procedure he describes is exactly the same as the cellophane wrap technique, and it appears to have been partly successful.

Why should surgeons carry out clinical research, rather than leave this task to others? The surgeon-investigator has a major advantage over the scientist confined to the laboratory. By virtue of our training and experience, we understand the questions that need to be asked about surgical conditions. In clinical practice, we observe biological events that can stimulate us to seek better ways to help our patients. Research and clinical practice do not compete, they reinforce each other.

References

1. Wynder EI, Mabuchi K, Maruchi N, Fortner JG. Epidemiology of cancer of the pancreas. J Natl Cancer Inst 1973;50:645–667.
2. Pour P, Kruger FW, Althoff J, Cardesa A, Mohr U. Cancer of the pancreas induced in the Syrian golden hamster. Am J Pathol 1974;76:349–358.
3. Biron S, Brown RA. Les effets d'une obstruction chronique et progressive du canal pancreatique principal sur l'epithelium des canaux et sur le tissu pancreatique exocrine. Can J Surg 1978;21:548–552.
4. Rosenberg L, Brown RA, Duguid WP. Induction of experimental nesidioblastosis: a study of islet differentiation and function. Surg Forum 1982;33: 227–230.
5. Rosenberg L, Brown RA, Duguid WP. A new model for the development of duct epithelial hyperplasia and the initiation of nesidioblastosis. J Surg Res 1983;35:63–72.
6. Rosenberg L, Brown RA, Duguid WP. Development of experimental cancer in the head of the pancreas by surgical induction of tissue injury. Am J Surg 1984;147:146–151.
7. Rosenberg L, Duguid WP, Brown RA. Effect of experimental nesidioblastosis on streptozotocin-induced diabetes. Surg Forum 1983;34:48–51.
8. Rosenberg L, Duguid WP, Brown RA, Vinik AI. Induction of islet cell proliferation will reverse diabetes in the Syrian golden hamster. Diabetes 1988;37:334–341.
9. Rosenberg L, Vinik AI. Induction of endocrine cell differentiation—a new approach to the management of diabetes. J Clin Lab Med 1989;114:75–83.
10. Rosenberg L, Duguid WP, Vinik AI. Regulation of pancreatic islet growth and differentiation—evidence for paracrine and/or autocrine growth factor(s). Clin Res 1990;38:271A.
11. Rosenberg L, Kahlenberg M, Vinik AI, Duguid WP. Paracrine/autocrine regulation of pancreatic islet cell proliferation and differentiation in the hamster—studies using parabiosis. Clin Invest Med 1996;19:3–12.
12. Rosenberg L, Thomas D, Dafoe DC, et al. Stimulation of pancreatic growth by a cytosol extract derived from the cellophane wrapped pancreas. Surg Forum 1986;37:168–169.
13. Clas D, Rosenberg L, Duguid WP, Malashenko I. Islet cell differentiation and proliferation induced by a pancreatic cytosol extract. Surg Forum 1988; 39:620–624.
14. Rosenberg L, Duguid WP, Healy M, Clas D, Vinik AI. Reversal of diabetes by the induction of islet cell neogenesis. Transplant Proc 1992;24: 1027–1028.
15. Rosenberg L, Vinik AI, Pittenger GL, Rafaeloff R, Duguid WP. Islet cell regeneration in the diabetic hamster pancreas with restoration of normoglycemia can be induced by a local growth factor(s). Diabetologia 1996;39:256–262.
16. Rosenberg L, Clas D, Dagged WP. Trophic stimulation of the ductular-islet cell axis: a new approach to the treatment of diabetes. Surgery 1990;108: 191–197.
17. Pittenger G, Rosenberg L, Vinik AI. Partial purification and characterization of ilotropin, a pancreatic islet–specific growth factor. J Cell Biol 1991;115:270A.
18. Rafaeloff R, Qin XF, Barlow SW, Rosenberg L, Vinik AI. Identification and differentially expressed genes induced in pancreatic islet neogenesis. FEBS Lett 1996;378:219–223.
19. Rosenberg L. Ilotropin—a novel pancreatic growth factor. Partial characterization and trophic effects. J Jpn Surg Soc 1993;93:151.
20. Rafaeloff R, Barlow SW, Rosenberg L, Vinik AI. IGF-II but not IGF-I is involved in islet neogenesis in adult pancreas. Diabaetes 1993;42(suppl 1): 137A.
21. Rafaeloff R, Barlow SW, Rosenberg L, Vinik AI. Expression of *Reg* gene in a hamster pancreatic islet regeneration model. Diabetologia 1996;38:906–913.
22. Rosenberg L, Vinik AI. In vitro stimulation of hamster pancreatic duct growth by an extract derived from the "wrapped" pancreas. Pancreas 1993; 8:255–260.
23. Metrakos P, Yuan S, Agapitos D, Rosenberg L. Intercellular communication and maintenance of islet cell mass—potential implications for islet transplantation. Surgery 1993;114:423–428.

24. Yuan S, Metrakos P, Duguid WP, Rosenberg L. Isolation and culture of intralobular ducts from the hamster. In Vitro Cell Dev Biol Anim 1995;31: 77–80.

25. Rosenberg L. In vivo cell transformation: neogenesis of beta cells from pancreatic ductal cells. Cell Transplant 1995;4:371–384.

26. Rosenberg L, Rafaeloff R, Clas D, Kakugawa Y, Pittenger G, Vinik AI, Duguid WP. Induction of islet cell differentiation and new islet formation in the hamster—further support for a ductular origin. Pancreas 1996 (in press).

27. Pittenger GL, Rafaeloff R, Yan B, Rosenberg L, Vinik AI. INGAP and reg proteins stimulate proliferation of pancreatic duct epithelial cells but not insulin-secreting HIT cells. Diabetes 1995;44 (suppl 1):210A.

28. Rafaeloff R, Barlow SW, Qin XF, Rosenberg L, Vinik AI. Cloning and sequencing of a hamster novel gene involved in pancreatic islet neogenesis (INGAP). Diabetes 1995;44(suppl 1):75A.

29. Yuan S, Paraskevis S, Duguid WP, Rosenberg L. Phenotypic transformation of isolated human islets in collagen matrix culture. Transplant Proc 1996 (in press).

30. Murray J. The origins and consequences of organ transplantation. Am Coll Surg Bull 1995;80: 12–25.

31. de Takats G, Cuthbert FP. Surgical attempts at increasing sugar tolerance. Arch Surg 1933;750–764.

32. de Takats G, Wilder RM. Isolation of tail of pancreas in a diabetic child. JAMA 1929;93:606–610.

33. de Takats G. Ligation of the tail of the pancreas in a diabetic child. Endocrinology 1930;14:255–264.

34. de Takats G. The effect of ligating the tail of the pancreas in juvenile diabetes. Surg Gynecol Obstet 1931;53:45–53.

Commentary

Dr. Rosenberg's odyssey along the first steps of his career path is fun to read. Readers should be certain to read between the lines; there were difficult and seminal decisions to be made. His recognition of the need for further training was critical to his success. He experienced doubt over his initial mentor's judgment, although in retrospect it proved to be excellent. We can imagine nights of discussion, worrying whether this would be a productive environment in which to acquire knowledge. (As Yogi Berra has been credited with saying, "Prediction is difficult, especially about the future.") The choice of a research target can only be made with one's limited ability to see the importance of an area of interest for the foreseeable future. If enough wisdom is expressed in the selection, other opportunities will appear along the way and may ultimately become the dominant force for future investigation.

Dr. Rosenberg gives credit to serendipity and preparation to take advantage of opportunities as they appeared. Opportunities come to those who seek them aggressively. It is clear that he was persistent and accurate in defining career and investigative goals. The importance of functioning in an appropriately interactive environment is well presented. Junior faculty should not be afraid to move to alternate situations when necessary. It is interesting that a career that began in a basic laboratory is now at the stage of dealing with contemporary forces that shape medical decision making. Integrating the clinical investigative plan must be rationalized to gain funding in the market environment. The same skills and thoughtful analysis that went into planning the basic laboratory research experiments and won institutional and grant support to fund them will later sustain the surgeon as administrator and leader of a research-based clinical unit.

A.S.W.

CHAPTER 48

Animal Experimentation

W.H. Isselhard and J. Kusche

Animal experimentation and research with animals is integrated into surgical research at two levels: perplexing problems encountered in clinical practice are taken to the animal laboratory for simplification and solution, and animals generally serve as the first subjects for testing and development of new methods and approaches to the cure and alleviation of disease and disability. Animal experimentation is to be understood as research that will benefit both humans and animals.

Scientific and biomedical research employing animals has a long, productive, and exciting history. To pass over this history in a single paragraph does an injustice to many researchers and their innumerable accomplishments. The long list of names may be represented by John Hunter (1728–1793), the surgeon, anatomist, and naturalist, and by Claude Bernard (1813–1878), the physiologist. Hunter introduced arterial ligation for treating aneurysms, after the study of collateral circulation in the deer. He also conducted transplantation experiments in fowl, in the hope of establishing a technique for transplanting the human tooth. At the end of the Age of Enlightenment, he anticipated the value of research in animals for medical activities in humans. Bernard elucidated functions of liver and pancreas and advocated the still-modern concept of the *milieu intérieur*. At the threshold of modern natural sciences and medicine, he contributed to the development of medical sciences by insisting on the use of strict experimental methods in the study of biological problems. This history provides convincing proof that progress in clinical medicine is, in large part, linked to advances in other "basic" sciences and that animal experimentation often was, and still is, the absolutely necessary key. A large body of facts and a remarkable knowledge of interactions in physiology, pathophysiology, biochemistry, microbiology, and normal and pathological morphology, stem from research in animals, the value of which cannot be overestimated. They provide the fundamental scientific basis for contemporary medicine and surgery.

The scientist working with animals as a scientific tool must be aware of, and prepared for, the fact that research with animals and animal experimentation give rise to scientific, ethical, legal, and technical problems and controversies. These problems and the controversy they generate have existed for a long time. They change with time. To a large extent, they present themselves differently in different cultures and social communities. In countries where animal research has grown to major dimensions, questions concerning animals and animal experimentation have attracted considerable public interest. Unfortunately, the discussion of totally opposite views on, and interests in, animals has become emotionalized. This attitude is regrettable, because it makes mutual consent nearly impossible and hinders pragmatic solutions.

Every scientist working with animals should be familiar with the problems of animal experimentation and local legal and ethical requirements for animal care. Animal experimentation demands the highest level of scientific and humane responsibility.

While it is not possible to provide the reader with a complete list of books, protocols, and statements on animal experimentation, references 1–18 provide coverage of relevant publications.

- Investigators using animals assume responsibility for ethical, humane care.
- Institutional and local laws govern standards of care.
- Each animal species is subject to specific pathologies that may impact research observations.
- Extraordinary care is required in planning experiments on living creatures capable of experiencing pain.

The Role of Animal Experimentation in Clinical Research

Animal experimentation has made it possible for surgery and most other disciplines of human and veterinary medicine to reach their present high standards. An enumeration of the achievements made in surgery alone with the help and sacrifice of animals is beyond the scope of this chapter; a catalog of surgical developments accomplished without animal experimentation would be much shorter. Our relatively vast knowledge of facts and interactions in physiology, pathophysiology, biochemistry, and morphology is largely the result of research in animals and provides the roots of today's surgery. Careful and judicious research in animals of various species preceded the introduction and accompanies the continuous amendment of surgical procedures and other therapeutic measures.

Examples of the contributions such research has made include development of gastrointestinal surgery, including gastrectomy for the treatment of ulcers and malignancies; development of mod-

ern thoracic and pulmonary surgery; elaboration of essential components of our knowledge of peri- and postoperative pathophysiology and its consequences for prophylaxis and therapy; establishment of open heart and coronary artery surgery, including development of the heart-lung machine, hypothermia, induced cardiac arrest, and myocardial protection; advances in microsurgery; treatment of terminal renal insufficiency by dialysis or transplantation; transplantation of tissues and such life-supporting organs as the kidney, liver, heart, and pancreas; preservation of live tissues and organs; development of neurosurgery; analysis and therapy of the various forms of shock; pilot preparation of the open reduction and internal fixation (ORIF) techniques and other techniques of osteosynthesis; testing of artificial joints; and biological and synthetic replacement of bone defects.

Research involving animals will continue to be necessary in the future if we wish to enjoy the advantages of innovation, widening knowledge of biological processes, and the possibility of curing as-yet incurable diseases and disorders. The development of animals with targeted gene alterations (e.g., "knockout" mice with specific enzymes or cytokine deficiencies) extends the possibilities of solving pressing biomedical problems with the help of animal experimentation.

At present, crucial biomedical research activities are centered on molecular biology, immunology, and genetics. Medicine will undoubtedly benefit considerably from the rapidly accumulating knowledge in these fields. Molecular processes and interactions are the ultimate underlying material principle of all life. This current accentuation, however, does not render classical animal experimentation less important or obsolete. For example, further optimization of organ transplantation is needed to accomplish an unrestrained, lasting function of the donor organ with fewer inconveniences to the recipient. The future use of xenotransplants as an interim or long-term treatment to overcome shortages of human donor organs would alleviate some of the psychological strains and molestations related to living donor allografts. In addition to necessary new ethical reflections, xenotransplants will require elucidation of the molecular and cellular mechanisms of graft versus host disease and selective inhibition of the reactions generating the expression of these mechanisms. In vivo animal models are needed to generate graft versus host disease and xenotransplant rejection and to validate therapeutic approaches before their application in clinical medicine.

Research in animals is usually the first step in attempts to make established operative interventions less cumbersome and stressful for patients. The development of endoscopy, from a technique for direct inspection and diagnosis to a method for curative surgical intervention, is an example. Many affected regions of the body can now be reached via natural apertures or small incisions, in comparison with earlier approaches that involved substantial disturbances to, or even destruction of, normal tissues. Similarly, animal experimentation has played an essential role in the development of lithotripters and their routine application in patients with nephrolithiasis.

Work with and in animals is also an important constituent of teaching and learning before practice involving humans. The acquisition of medical and surgical skills, the avoidance of mistakes and wrong reactions that may have unfortunate consequences, and the development of sensitivity based on personal experience with extremely complex biological systems can be achieved only by means of intensive study of living organisms. Books, films, models, and modern audiovisual teaching methods are undoubtedly helpful in the teaching and learning processes, but they cannot completely replace work with living matter. The mandate and ethics of medicine require that the restoration and improvement of health be sought with the least possible risk to human patients. Lofty as this goal is, it does not absolve the investigator from a deep and continuing moral obligation to handle other-than-human life with care, responsibility, consideration, and respect.

The Differentiation of Living Matter

To appraise the importance, usefulness, and yield of experimentation in intact animals versus the use of alternative methods, it is worth devoting some discussion to the differentiation of living matter.

All living matter is subject to very similar, if not identical, biological laws; that is, all living matter functions according to very similar principles and mechanisms, even though the degree of differentiation is extremely wide.

The cell is the smallest entity of self-supporting life. It may exist as a separate unicellular organism comprising all the attributes required to maintain its own existence and the continuation and evolution of its species. Alternately, the cell may be bound to the coexistence and cofunctioning of many different cells whose number may be uncountable and whose potentialities for differentiation and performing different specific functions may be neither known nor understood definitively. The latter statement can be easily illustrated by a little reflection.

What information and conclusions could a physician derive from a white blood cell count and a differential blood smear 30 years ago compared to the early hints the specialist now gets for discriminating an early episode of rejection from a viral or bacterial infection after organ transplantation? Only one generation ago, the endothelium was assigned hardly any roles other than separating the blood from tissues and participating physiologically in the blood clotting processes and pathophysiologically in some vascular diseases and disorders. Today, biomedical science has started to realize that the endothelium has many differentiated physiological attributes like an organ and may initiate or contribute to numerous pathologic processes.

A multicellular living system originates from unicellular living matter. In its unicellular state, it comprises all the species-specific characteristics of all the cells in the eventual multicellular organism. Multicellular living systems are able to exist independently and to continue the propagation and evolution of their species only after they have reached a sufficiently differentiated multicellular state of ontogenesis, as determined by phylogenesis.

An increase in the differentiation of cells usually means an enhancement of abilities and specialized functions that accompanies the evolution of the special cells, tissues, organs, and organ systems that, with their multiple interdependencies, constitute the body of the organism. For most of the specialized cells and organs, differentiation implies the loss of certain properties; for example, many differentiated cells totally lack potential for regeneration. As a rule, more differentiated living systems are considered to be higher forms of animal life than less differentiated forms. This view does not negate the fact that lower animal life has given rise to remarkable differentiations and capabilities. Human life can be rightfully regarded as the most differentiated living system.

Surgery is the art of palliative, curative, or restorative intervention in highly differentiated organisms. It cannot be learned or taught, nor can it progress, without access to adequately differentiated living systems.

Alternatives to Animal Experimentation?

So-called alternative methods, as originally defined, are alternatives to animal experimentation. A definition that classifies such methods and approaches as substitutes that will reduce animal experimentation is more realistic.[10,13,16,17] An animal experiment is defined as an intervention in, or treatment of, a living animal under strict scientific conditions. In the past few decades, the so-called alternative methods have been persistently propagated, often in an irrelevant way on the basis of an overvaluation of their efficiency. The apparent aim is to represent animal experimentation as being useless and needless. The excessive zeal of antivivisectionists sometimes causes occupational and personal defamation and discrimination against the experimental investigator.[18]

For more than a century, biomedical research has taken advantage of experiments with living matter other than animals. It continuously improves these methods and designs new approaches. The scientific community distinguishes between in vivo studies in living animals and in vitro experiments with tissues or organs from sacrificed animals. The culturing of cells and the controlled growth of fetal organs, in whole or in part, are now established laboratory procedures, and studies in these preparations must be classified as in vitro experiments.

The important distinction between *schmerzfähiger und nicht schmerzfähiger Materie* (matter capable of suffering and not capable of suffering) is fully accepted by expert investigators[10] although it

did not originate in the scientific community.[15] An in vivo experiment with animals is an experiment with living matter capable of suffering, whereas an in vitro experiment makes use of living matter that is no longer capable of suffering.

Current biomedical and surgical research employs the following approaches, when they are appropriate:

1. Experiments with surviving cells, tissues, organs, parts of organs, and organ systems.
2. Experiments with cultured cells, tissues, and organs.
3. Experiments with lower organisms.
4. Work with nonbiological materials.
5. Calculations in immaterial models.
6. Experiments involving a large variety of chemical, biochemical, molecular biological, microbiological, physical, and immunological methods of in vitro analysis.

It must be recognized, nevertheless, that cells, tissues, and organs for in vitro studies have their origin in living animals. It should also be realized that numerous animal experiments are still needed for development, testing, quality control, and comparative studies.

The prohibition of all animal experimentation and the exclusive use of alternative methods are not feasible, given the present state of scientific knowledge. This is particularly true for surgical research and experimental surgery. Problems such as the care of the polytraumatized organism; elaboration of more effective therapeutic approaches to different kinds of shock; management of multiorgan failure; effect of rejection of organs, in whole or in part; tissue or organ substitution by biological or nonbiological matter; improvement of existing and development of new devices, including the heart-lung machine or the artificial heart; and trial of new concepts of surgical interventions can only be studied in whole animals.

Results obtained in an in vitro study cannot always be transferred directly to the in vivo situation; for example, an early cardioplegic agent[19] proved to be rather toxic in in vitro studies with isolated cells,[20] but under in vivo conditions it was found to be only slightly inferior to more modern therapeutic agents.[21,22] The scientific value of in vitro research must not, however, be underestimated. In vitro studies can reveal biological facts that may remain unrecognized in whole-animal experiments due to their complexity. Even in surgical research, in vitro experiments may be of help in the solution of special problems—for example, for the screening of cardioplegic and organ-protecting solutions and principles and the determination of tolerances to various forms of deprivation (e.g., ischemia, anoxia, hypoxia, and hypoperfusion). Work with isolated or cultured cells, such as the preservation and transplantation of islets of Langerhans or the preoperative "endothelialization" of vascular prostheses is part of surgical research. The researcher has to be aware of the advantages, the disadvantages, and the limits of this scientific tool.

In 1959 Russell and Burch[20] enunciated the three Rs for research in animals: replacement, reduction, and refinement. Replacement, as originally defined, refers

> to a wide range of techniques in which animals were not required at all in the actual experiment or in which they were exposed to no distress. For example, a terminal experiment in which the animal is always under anesthesia until it is humanely killed would fall into the category of replacement. The use of tissue cultures and computer modeling represent the former category. The concept of reduction focused on reducing the number of animals required by better experimental planning, statistical design, and statistical analysis.... The trial and error approach is less desirable than the hypothetico-deductive approach in which the researcher formulates a testable hypothesis.... Refinement dealt exclusively with experimentation in which the animal was subjected to some degree of stress during the investigation. The 3 R's principle thus centers mainly on the question of stress research.

Within the concept of the three Rs "it is permissible to use an animal in research provided that the animal suffers no pain whatsoever."[16] Rowan[16] finds this concept to have changed its meaning "with the advent of the term 'alternatives' to laboratory animals." Now,

> the main thrust is aimed at the total numbers of animals used, rather than at the question of stressful research. As a result, replacement and reduction refer solely to the number of animals

used while refinement refers to the overall question of reducing the stress suffered by the laboratory animal.... An "alternative" includes any system or method that covers one or more of the following:

1. Replacing the use of laboratory animals altogether.
2. Reducing the number of animals required.
3. Refining an existing procedure or technique so as to minimize the level of stress or pain endured by the animal.

But, there is also the statement that "any 'alternative' must provide information or results which allow the investigator to draw the same conclusions with at least the same degree of confidence."[16] Smyth[13] has argued similarly.

It is important to know that not only the in vitro methods but also the commitment to humane in vivo experimentation with animals originated in the scientific community. Renowned scientific societies and science-promotion societies have supported animal-protection laws in various countries.

Animal Models

For clinical and surgical research, Wessler's definition of an animal model of human disease may be useful. An animal model is "a living organism with an inherited, naturally acquired or induced pathological process that in one or more respects closely resembles the same phenomenon in man."[24]

A more general definition covering all aspects of biomedical research was adapted from this definition by the Institute of Laboratory Animal Resources (ILAR).[25] An animal model might vary from a one-cell protozoan, the study of which can lead to a better understanding of cellular function, to the chimpanzee, one of the species phylogenetically closest to humans, which may be the only species other than humans susceptible to a particular infectious agent.[26] Animal models, according to Gill,[27] are used mainly for three reasons:

1. To elucidate host defense mechanisms.
2. To point the way for subsequent studies in humans.

3. To screen substances for effectiveness or toxicity.

There is no doubt that animal models have great merit in relation to the first and second points. An early example is the work of Edward Jenner (1749–1823), who observed that milkmaids affected by cowpox did not contract the malignant smallpox, then epidemic in England. Another important example is the finding of Robert Koch that guinea pigs are highly susceptible to tuberculosis. He used it to establish the causal relationship between the tubercle bacillus and tuberculosis. Koch's postulates concerning infectious diseases cannot be fulfilled without a susceptible animal model. For further important historical animal models, see the paper by Jones.[28]

The third point in the preceding list is the subject of much debate, because it is doubtful whether animal experiments can accurately predict the toxicity of substances in humans, whether the current extent of animal experiments is necessary, and whether alternatives can replace animal experiments.

If animal models are used, they should be appropriate for the situation that is to be studied. For instance, a model of prostatic cancer that depends on a tumor growth that is insensitive to hormonal influence is not relevant to the clinical situation, nor is an animal model of duodenal ulcer production that occurs without elevated acid output in the stomach.

There is probably no ideal model for any disease. The disease itself may be variable and may have many facets so that more than one animal model may be required. Although the ideal model may not exist, we should seek "its more modest cousin"[26] (i.e., the most appropriate model available).

During a workshop on needs for new animal models, Leader and Padgett[29] listed nine criteria for a good animal model:

1. It should accurately reproduce the disease or lesions under study.
2. It should be available to multiple investigations. Sharing of animals and data among institutions has been an important factor in many research successes. It allows monitoring of the scientific validity of observations and stimulates further investigation.
3. It should be exportable.
4. If the disease under study is genetic, the species should be polytocous—producing multiple young at each birth.
5. The animal should be large enough for multiple biopsy samples.
6. It should fit into the available animal facilities of most laboratories. The accelerating costs of any changes in animal housing and care standards make this criterion particularly relevant.
7. The animal should be easily handled by most investigators. However, convenience should not be the determining factor in the selection of the model.
8. It should be available in multiple species.
9. The animals used in the model should survive long enough to be usable.

To ensure maximum comparability of results, another point should be added to the list of criteria. The animals for induced or spontaneous models of human disease should be genetically defined.

Although several populations of animals can be distinguished and their use has special advantages and disadvantages,[27] it is difficult to say which is the most appropriate for mimicking a particular disease or effect of therapy in a human population.

1. *Randomly mating animal populations.* There are two types, those that are colony bred and those found in the wild. The major use of the first type is testing the effects of drugs; the second type may be useful for developing studies relevant to human disease, because it generates mutants and mimics a disease process.[27]
2. *Outbred populations.* These animals are systematically bred to maintain maximal genetic heterogeneity and are useful for drug screening.
3. *Inbred strains.* An inbred strain is defined as being the product of 20 generations of brother-sister matings. Inbreeding implies a genetic drift. When an inbred strain has been separated from its primary source for eight or more generations, it should be identified as a subline by giving it a laboratory designation that follows the strain name. For the mouse, a standardized nomenclature exists,[30] but it does not for other species, such as the rat. The same rules for listing inbred strains should be used for species other than the mouse.[31] The major

use of inbred strains is the study of specific questions, such as drug effects on a tumor, in a genetically defined population.

4. *F₁ hybrids.* Two progenitor inbred strains are mated to form F_1 hybrids, which are more resistant to environmental influences than the parent inbred strains. The F_1 hybrid provides a well-defined population with limited genetic diversity.

5. *Coisogenic and congenic strains.* Two isogenic (i.e., genetically identical) strains that differ only at a single locus, the differential locus, are known as coisogenic strains. Such strains arise as a result of mutation within an inbred strain. Strains that approximate the coisogenic status can be developed by backcrossing a gene from a donor strain into an inbred strain (the background strain of the inbred partner). The resulting partially coisogenic strains that differ at the differential locus and an associated segment of chromosome are known as congenic strains.[30] The major use of these animals is to study the effects of one specific gene.

This chapter is not the place to describe the characteristics of the various animal models described in the literature. Bustad and coworkers[32] embarked on this task when they wrote a chapter in *The Future of Animals, Cells, Models, and Systems in Research, Development, Education, and Testing.* When they exceeded 6,000 references for animal models, they decided to publish their list as an appendix. We have limited ourselves to preparing Table 48-1 to give you some help in finding the animal model you need in a special situation. If you intend to study duodenal ulcer disease, for example, you can look for spontaneous animal models[33] or for an experimentally induced model that was presented as a chemically induced duodenal ulcer by Szabo.[34,35] Even if your search does not produce the ideal animal model of this human disease, there are some models that come close to the human situation (e.g., the "Executive Monkey"[36]) or resemble human duodenal ulcer disease in many ways (e.g., the cysteamine ulcer;[37] see Table 48-2).

Remember that when a human disease is to be studied, you should reflect on the criteria for the appropriateness of an animal model, study the information available, and not leave animal models as a "neglected medical resource."[38]

Quality Control

Quality of Experiments

In several studies, the quality of publications has been evaluated by reporting the frequency and accuracy of the statistical data and criteria published in them.[3,40] In a similar exercise that focused on experimentation in animals, Juhr[41] investigated some volumes of *Laboratory Animal Science.* The result of his study (Table 48-3) provides a useful checklist of criteria that should be adhered to in a well-designed animal experiment. Control groups were described in only 14% of papers. Aspects of breeding, sex, and age of the animals are frequently reported, but the conditions of animal care are rarely given. The environment and the handling of animals can have an important input on study parameters of interest. If these factors are not recognized and controlled, the validity of the research results may be questioned. For example, transportation of test animals affects such factors as total leukocyte counts and ACTH levels.[42]

The principles of experimental design are discussed in Part IV of this textbook, but Table 48-3 shows that the calculation of sample sizes, or the choice of statistical tests, is not very different from those for clinical trials. Many people mistakenly assume that random allocation of animals is not necessary, because the animals represent a random sample taken from a well-defined population. Immich[43] has demonstrated that this technique is as necessary in animal experiments as it is in clinical trials.

Besides skillful design and presentation of the results, the optimum utilization of animal experiments includes attention to the possibility of reducing the number of animals necessary for each experiment. In every laboratory where several groups are performing animal experiments, information about planned studies should be exchanged to enable more than one research group to participate in a project. Sacrificing one rat today to obtain a colon sample and another tomorrow

Table 48-1.   A selection of animal models in the literature.

Animal Models of Human Disease	Handbook published by the Registry of Comparative Pathology, U.S. Armed Forces Institute of Pathology, continuing series of fascioles.
Experimental Cardiovascular Diseases	Salye H. New York: Springer-Verlag, 1970.
Naturally Occurring Animal Models of Human Disease	Appendix to the paper: "Animal Models" by Bustad UK, Hegreberg GA, Padgett GA. The Future of Animals, Cells, Models and Symptoms in Research, Development, Education and Testing. Washington, DC: National Academy, 1975.
Animal Models for Biomedical Research VI-Metabolic Disease	Fed Proc 1976;35:1992–1236.
Animal Models of Thrombosis and Haemorrhagic Diseases	National Institute of Health, Bethesda, MD, 1976.
Experimental Models of Chronic Inflammatory Diseases	Glynn LE, Schlumberger HD, eds. Heidelberg, New York: Springer-Verlag, 1977.
Spontaneous Models of Human Diseases	Andrews EJ, Ward EJ, Altman NH, eds. New York: Academic, 1979.
Animal Quality and Models in Biomedical Research	Spiegel A, Ericks S, Vollevald HA, eds. New York: 8 Fischer Verlag, 1980.
Animal Models for Diabetes Mellitus: A Bibliography	ILAR News, 1981;24:5–22.
Animal Models for Research on Aging	Washington, DC: National Academy, 1981.
Animal Models and Hypoxia	Stefanovich V, ed. New York: Pergamon, 1981.
Bibliography of Naturally Occurring Animal Models of Human Diseases	Hegreberg GA, Leathers C, eds. Pullman, WA: Human Student Books, 1982.
Bibliography of Induced Animal Models of Human Disease	Hegreberg GA, Leathers C, eds. Pullman, WA: Human Student Books, 1982.
Animal Models for Tumor Progression	Leibovici J, Wolman M. Anticancer Res 1984;4:165–168.
Recent Advances in Molecular Pathology. Animal Models in Athereosclerosis Research	Jokinen MP, Clarkson TB, Prichard RW. Exp Mol Path 1985;42:1–28.
Animal Models of Gastrointestinal Diseases	Pfeiffer JC. Boca Raton: CRC Press, 1985.
Animal Models of Human Diseases	Cohen D. Boca Raton: CRC Press, 1985.
Experimental Models of Exocrine Pancreatic Tumors	Longnecker DS. In: Go VWL et al., eds. Pancreas: Biology, Pathobiology, and Diseases. New York: Raven Press, 1986.
Animal Models: Assessing the Scope of Their Use in Biomedical Research	Kawamata J, Melby EC, eds. New York: Alan R. Liss, 1987.
Use of Animal Models for Research in Human Nutrition	Bayan AC, West CE, eds. Basel: S. Karger AG, 1988.
Animal Models in Chronic Renal Failure	Gretz N, Strauch M, eds. Basel: S. Karger AG, 1988.
Animal Models for Human Nutrition Physiology	Kirchgessner M, ed. Berlin-Hamburg: Verlag Paul Parey, 1990.

to get a piece of muscle is wasting animals. Every effort should be made to reduce the number of animals needed by such measures as using a two-step experimental design or a sequential trial, or the replacement of a time- and animal-consuming dose-response curve by the up and down method of Dixon,[44] when the determination of an LD_{50} is required.

Last, but certainly not least, the quality of animal experiments depends on the correct handling and care of animals and the proper use of anesthetics, analgesics, and tranquilizers. If a proce-

Table 48-2.   Comparison of chemically induced duodenal ulcer with human duodenal ulcer.

Condition	Experimental duodenal ulcer	Human duodenal ulcer
Localization of the ulcer	Anterior and posterior wall	Anterior and posterior wall
Tendency to perforate	Yes	Yes
Penetration into the liver and/or pancreas	Yes	Yes
Occurrence of "giant ulcer forms" and massive bleedings	Yes	Yes
Presence of chronic healed and/or active ulcers	Yes	Yes
Occurrence of pyloric ulcers with deformities of the pylorus	Yes	Yes
Accompanying adrenocortical necrosis	Frequent	Rare(?)
Presence of functional and/or organic brain disorders	±	+
Increased gastric acid output	±	±
Elevated basal serum gastrin levels	+	±
Supersensitivity of serum gastrin to food intake	Yes	Yes
Response to		
Antacids	+	±
Antisecretory agents	+	+
H$_2$-receptor antagonists	+	+
Vagotomy	+	+
Availability to study preulcerogenic and very early ulcerogenic functional and morphologic changes	Yes	No

Reprinted with permission from Szabo S[40] (1980).

dure must be conducted without the use of an anesthetic, analgesic, or tranquilizer, because such an agent would defeat the purpose of the experiment, the responsible investigator must personally supervise the procedure to ensure that it is carried out in accordance with institutional policies and local, state, or federal regulations. Muscle relaxants or paralytic drugs (e.g., succinylcholine or other curariform drugs) are not anesthetics, and they should not be used alone for surgical restraint.

Appropriate facilities and equipment should be available for surgical procedures. A facility intended for aseptic surgery should be maintained and used for that purpose only, and its cleanliness should be assured. Surgery on animals should only be performed by persons who are properly qualified by training and experience and should be conducted in the same formal and respectful manner that characterizes the operating theater during surgery on humans.

Postsurgical care should include observation of the animal until it has recovered from anesthesia, administration of supportive fluids and drugs, care of surgical incisions, and regular monitoring to ensure the animal's physical comfort and optimal

Table 48-3.   Frequency of items reported in papers involving animal experiments.

		%
General declarations		
Strain		91
Genetics		70
Origin		67
Sex		61
Age		80
Class of age		80
Experimental design		
Total number		94
Number of		61
Body weight		31
Bacteriological state		43
Selection		22
Randomization		14
Environment and care		
Adaptation to environment		27
to humans		14
to the experiment		27
Light/dark change		14
Temperature		20
Animal laboratory		20
Humidity		16
Air change		8
Noise		0
Feed		49
Drinking		22
Animals per cage		16
Cage material		29
Size of cages		18
Litter		10
Change of litter		18
Course of the experiment		
Duration		71
Mortality		12
Diagnosis		12
Analysis of the experiment		
Number of groups		71
Animals/groups		59
Controls		14
Animals/control groups		18
Statistical tests		34
Statistical significance		39

Scale: 20   40   60   80   %

Modified with permission from Juhr[44] (1980).

recovery. Appropriate medical records should be maintained.

Euthanasia should be performed by trained persons in accordance with institutional policies and applicable laws. The choice of method depends on the species of animal and the project in which the animal was used (i.e., it should not interfere with postmortem examinations). Procedures for euthanasia should follow approved guidelines, such as those already established by the American Veterinary Medical Association Panel on Euthanasia. Animals of most species can be killed quickly and humanely by the intravenous or intraperitoneal injection of a concentrated solution of barbiturate. Mice, rats, and hamsters can be killed by cervical dislocation or by exposure to gaseous nitrogen or carbon dioxide in an uncrowded chamber. Ether and chloroform are effective, but their use is hazardous to personnel; ether is flammable and explosive, and chloroform is toxic and possibly carcinogenic. If animals are killed by ether, special facilities and procedures are required for storage and disposal of carcasses. Serious explosions can result from storage in refrigeration equipment that is not explosion proof and disposal by incineration.

The environment and dietary regimen should be suitable for each species. The components of the diet should be known and standardized and should be adapted to the age of the animals when necessary. Young animals usually need a diet richer in protein than that given to adults. Information about normal values for the species used in an experiment can be very helpful in arriving at a first estimation of the reliability of your own measurements.

Quality of Animals

A quality assurance program to define and characterize research animals adequately is important. Various commonly occurring microorganisms cause subclinical infections in animals that may flare to produce high morbidity or mortality when the animals are stressed by an experiment. Such incidents frequently complicate the research results, invalidate the scientific data collected or their interpretation, and cause loss of money, time, and other research resources.[41] Rodents, for example, should be free from sendai virus, mouse hepatitis virus, Reo 3 virus, lactic dehydrogenase elevating virus, lymphatic choriomeningitis virus, ectromelia, *Salmonella, Hexamita, Pneumocystis, Haemobartonella, Eperythrozoon, Syphacia, Aspiculuris,* ectoparasites, and the microorganisms listed in Table 48-4. When these pathogens infect and proliferate in animals, they cause subtle, long- or short-term changes in organ and cell function, metabolism, and physiology, even though the animals appear to be clinically healthy. A sampling plan for the microbiological or pathological monitoring of animals to detect the presence of diseased animals, within adequate confidence limits, has been published by Hsu,[45] along with a list of the pathogens and parasites that may be encountered.

All laboratory animals should be observed daily for clinical signs of illness, injury, or abnormal behavior by a person trained to recognize such signs. All deviations from normal, and all deaths from unknown causes, should be reported promptly to the person responsible for animal disease control.

The most important link in a quality assurance program is probably the producer of the animals. Producers must ensure proper breeding systems for both the inbred strains and outbred stocks to maintain their genetic integrity and characteristics. They should periodically perform health characterization and genetic monitoring of their animal colonies and make their findings available at regular intervals or on request by those who purchase their animals. The methods used in genetic monitoring are listed in Table 48-5. Research animals should always be obtained from a reliable vendor who consistently supplies high-quality, genetically defined animals. Vendors should be periodically evaluated according to the management, economic, and other criteria listed in Table 48-6.

The aim of all these measures is to lower costs, reduce the number of animals necessary for an experiment, and improve the reliability of the re-

Table 48-4.   Bacteria for which routine monitoring is recommended.

Mice	Rats	Guinea pigs	Hamsters
Salmonella	*Salmonella*	*Salmonella*	*Salmonella*
Pseudomonas	*Pasteurella*	*Streptococcus*	*Pasteurella*
Corynebacterium	*Diplococcus*	*Zooepidemicus*	*Bordetella*
Pasteurella	*Klebsiella*	*Bordetella*	
Klebsiella	*Pseudomonas*	*Klebsiella*	
Bordetella bronchiseptica	*Corynebacterium*	*Diplococcus*	
Diplococcus pneumoniae	*Bordetella*		
Mycoplasma	*Mycoplasm*		

Modified with permission from Hsu CK, New AE, Mayo JG[48] (1980).

Table 48-5. Methods for genetic monitoring.

A. Breeding methods
B. In vivo histocompatability testing
   1. Skin grafting
   2. Lymphoid tissue transplantation
   3. Tumor transplantation
C. In vitro histocompatability testing
   1. Mixed lymphocyte reaction (MLR)
   2. Cell-mediated lympholysis (CML)
   3. Serology
D. Biochemical marker analysis
E. Embryo cryopreservation
F. Chromosomal banding
G. Mandible analysis

Modified with permission from Hsu CK, New AE, Mayo JG[48] (1980).

Table 48-6. Vendor evaluation.

1. Type of practice (producer or dealer)
2. Type of facility (barrier or conventional)
3. Management and operation (accredited or not)
4. Professional and technical staff
5. Availability of animal quality data
6. Genetic uniformity and compatibility
7. Methods of transporation
8. Number, strain, and species that can be supplied
9. Reliability in meeting ordering specification
10. Cost
11. Quality of animals

Modified with permission from Hsu CK, New AE, Mayo JG[48] (1980).

sults. Experimenters will feel better about a well-designed experiment when they have taken care to avoid any unnecessary injury to, and sacrifice of, whatever creatures have been involved.

The "Guide for the Care and Use of Laboratory Animals"[51] will help "in caring for and using laboratory animals in ways judged to be professionally and humanely appropriate." It is not an exhaustive review but is widely accepted. The recommendations cannot be fulfilled completely in all respects and everywhere; different cultures and communities vary in their valuation of the animals' status and thus have developed different ways of handling animals. Striving for realization of the goals of the guide has many benefits, not least of which would be the scientific value of universally comparable animal experimentation of high standards and responsibility.

Conclusion: Some Personal Comments

Learning to use animals in clinical and surgical research, recognizing the possibilities and limits of animal experimentation, and accepting the attendant responsibilities should be seen as privileges. Competence in animal experimentation has to be learned like any other skill. The fact that living matter is involved, whatever its place in the classification of living organisms, imposes a particular obligation on you, as the investigator. The

recent broadening of biomedical research methods to include the development of targeted alteration of animal genes increases this responsibility.

The researcher and all coworkers—those involved directly in the experiment and those taking care of the animals in the animal quarters—ought to be aware that animals have their joys and feel discomfort, are sensitive, are capable of suffering and enduring pain, can be afraid, and have memory. Members of the team who lack and cannot be taught respect, responsibility, and correct treatment of the animal as a fellow living being should not be allowed to use or handle animals.

You should go beyond the legal regulations in meticulously scrutinizing the scientific necessity, value, and mode of implementing each experiment.[11] You bear ultimate moral responsibility for your actions and choices related to animal experimentation.[46] There must always be a reasonable expectation that your study will contribute significantly to clinical knowledge and progress.

Experiments in animals should always be carefully thought out. A study of the literature relevant to the topic should precede the planning, and especially the implementation, of any series of experiments. Helpful information can almost always be gained about the selection of relevant parameters, adequate methods of analysis, and appropriate animal model species. An animal species should not be used just because it is the one most readily available and most familiar to you. You should not find it repugnant to ask for advice and help. The animal is to be the surrogate of humans.

The conception, planning, preparation, and performance of animal experiments is a major scientific responsibility. It requires time. It can rarely be discharged properly by adding it onto the end of a long day's work.

In vivo experiments and the sacrificing of animals without pain or fright at the end of experiments, or to obtain tissues or organs for in vitro experiments, must be performed by, or under the immediate and continuous supervision of, an appropriately qualified scientist. Experiments in animals should be performed with the assistance of a sufficient number of properly trained personnel; individual research has given way to the team approach. Work on a do-it-yourself basis using self-taught techniques in a distant corner of a laboratory is contrary to the principles of experimentation in animals. Surgical research in animals should be confined to specialized and adequately equipped institutes, departments, or units.

The three Rs—replacement, reduction, refinement[17]—are important guides for research in animals. Animals should be used only after careful consideration has convinced you that no method other than an animal experiment can solve a problem or provide the information needed. The scientific question should be formulated in such a way that a clear and valid answer can be reached with a minimum number of experiments. As much data as possible should be collected in each experiment, provided overinstrumentation does not invalidate the model.

> The care and use of animals for experimental purposes should be based on the principle that pain and discomfort must be avoided. To this end, anesthetics and analgesic agents should be employed in an appropriate manner, unless specifically withheld as a requirement of the experiment. Pain-relieving drugs should be continued as long as necessary. Experiments in which pain and discomfort are an unavoidable consequence should be undertaken only when, on the basis of expert opinion, there are reasonable expectations that such studies will contribute to the ultimate enhancement of our knowledge of life. The degree of pain should never exceed that determined by the humanitarian importance of the problem to be solved by the experimental study.[47]

Surgical research and postoperative care, particularly in higher animals, should be conducted according to the same standards as surgery in humans.

The decision on the fate of an animal depends on the purpose of an experiment. Either the animal must be sacrificed when the experiment is completed or its subsequent life must be free from pain, grief, and discomfort.

References

1. American Association of Pathologists. A workshop on needs for new animal models of human disease. Am J Pathol 1980;101(suppl. 3):S1–266.
2. Tierexperimentelle Forschung und Tierschutz/Dt. Forschungsgemeinschaft, Mitteilung III. Boppard: Boldt Verlag, 1981.
3. Gärtner K, Hackbarth H, Stolte H, eds. Research Animals and Concepts of Applicability to Clinical Medicine, vol. 7. Basel: S. Karger, 1982.
4. Hoel DG. Animal experimentation and its relevance to man. Environ Health Perspect 1980;32:25–30.
5. Hoff, C. Immoral and moral uses of animals. New Engl J Med 1980;302:115–118.
6. IABS 16th Congress for Biological Standardization. The standardization of animals to improve biomedical research. Basel: Production and Control S. Karger, 1980.
7. ILAR Symposium. The Future of Animals, Cells, Models, and Systems in Research, Development, Education, and Testing. Washington, D.C.: National Academy of Sciences, 1977.
8. Kübler K, ed. Der Tierversuch in der Arzneimittelforschung (interdisziplinäres Fachgespräch im Bundesgesundheitsamt) bga-Berichte, vol. 1. Berlin: Dietrich Reimer Verlag, 1980, pp. 1–111.
9. McDaniel CG. Animal rights or human health? Med J Aust 1984;141:855–857.
10. Merkenschlager M, Wilk W. Gutachten über tierschutzgerechte Haltung von Versuchstieren. Gutachten über Tierversuche, Möglichkeiten ihrer Einschraenkung und Ersetzbarkeit. Recommendations for the Keeping of Laboratory Animals in Accordance with Animal Protection Principles. Berlin-Hamburg: Verlag Paul, Parey, 1979.
11. Riecker G. Aerztliche Ethik und Tierversuche. Arzt Krankenhaus 1984;11:306–312.
12. Sechzer JA, ed. The role of animals in biomedical research. Ann N Y Acad Sci 1983;406.

13. Smyth HD. Alternatives to Animal Experimentation. London: Scolar Press, 1978.
14. Sontag KH. Der Tierversuch nach dem Stand der wissenschaftlichen Kenntnis. Pharm Ind 1982; 44:4.
15. Weihe WH. Das Problem der Alternativen zum wissenschaftlichen Tierversuch. Fortschr Med 1982;100:2162–2166.
16. Ullrich KJ, Creutzfeldt OD, eds. Gesundheit und Tierschutz. Wissenschaftler melden sich zu Wort. Düsseldorf-Wien: ECON Verlag, 1985.
17. Sedlacek H. Tierschutz: Güterabwägung oder Gleichheitsprinzip Klinikarzt 1986;15:508–510.
18. The Ethics of Animal Experimentation: Proceedings of the Second CFN Symposium. Acta Physiol Scand 1986;128(Suppl. 554):4–250.
19. Rowan AN. The concept of the three R's, an introduction. 16th IABS Congress: the standardization of animals to improve biomedical research, production, and control, San Antonio, 1979. Dev Biol Stand 1980;45:175–180.
20. Russell WMS, Burch RL. The Principle of Humane Experimental Technique. London: Methuen, 1959.
21. Stiller H, Stiller M. Tierversuch und Tierexperimentator. München: F. Hirthammer Verlag, 1977.
22. Kirsch U. Untersuchungen zum Eintritt der Totenstarre an ischamischen Meerschweinchenherzen in Normothermie. Arzneimittelforschung 1970;20:1071–1074.
23. Carrentier S, Murawsky M, Carpentier A. Cytotoxicity of cardioplegic solutions: evaluation by tissue culture. Circulation 1981;64(Suppl. II):II90–II95.
24. Isselhard W, Schorn B, Hügel W, Uekermann U. Comparison of three methods of myocardial protection. Thorac Cardiovasc Surg 1980;28:329–336.
25. Hügel W, Lübbing H, Isselhard W, Hohlfeld T, Jötten HU, Daleihau H, Guldner N. Hemodynamics and metabolic status of the human heart after application of different forms of cardioplegic solutions. In: Isselhard W, ed. Myocardial Protection for Cardiovascular Surgery. München: Pharmazeutische Verlagsgesellschaft, 1981.
26. Rowan AN. Laboratory animals and alternatives in the 80s. Int J Study Anim Probl 1980;1:162–169.
27. Wessler S. Introduction: what is a model? In: Animal Models of Thrombosis and Hemorrhagic Diseases. Bethesda, Md.: National Institutes of Health, 1976, pp. xi–xvi.
28. ILAR National Research Council Committee on Animal Models for Research on Aging. Mammalian Models for Research on Aging. Washington, D.C.: National Academy Press, 1981.
29. Held JR. Appropriate animal models. Ann N Y Acad Sci 1983;406:13–19.
30. Gill THJ. The use of randomly bred and genetically defined animals in biomedical research. Am J Pathol 1981;100:21–32.
31. Jones TC. The value of animal models. Am J Pathol 1981;101:3–9.
32. Leader RW, Padgett GA: The genesis and validation of animal models. Am J Pathol 1981;101:11–17.
33. Festing FW. Inbred Strains in Biochemical Research. London and Basingstoke: Macmillan, 1979.
34. Jay GE. Genetic strains and stocks. In: Durdette WJ, ed. Methodology in Mammalian Genetics. San Francisco: Holden-Day, 1963, pp. 83–126.
35. Bustad LK, Hegreberg GA, Padgett GA. Animal models. In: The Future of Animals, Cells, Models, and Systems in Research, Development, Education, and Testing. Washington, D.C.: National Academy of Science, 1977.
36. Andrews EJ, Ward BC, Altman NH, eds. Spontaneous Models of Human Diseases. Academic Press, 1979.
37. Szabo S. Animal model of human disease: duodenal ulcer disease. Animal model: cysteamine—induced acute and chronic duodenal ulcer in the rat. Am J Pathol 1978;93:273–276.
38. Szabo S, Haith LR Jr, Reynolds ES. Pathogenesis of duodenal ulceration produced by cysteamine or proprionitrile: influence of vagotomy, sympathectomy, histamine depletion, H_2-receptor antagonists, and hormones. Am J Dig Dis 1979;24:471–474.
39. Brady JV. Ulcers in "Executive" Monkeys. Sci Am 1958;199:99–100.
40. Szabo S. Discussion. Am J Pathol 1980;100:78–82.
41. Cornelius CE. Animal models: a neglected medical resource. New Engl J Med 1969;281:933–944.
42. McPeek B. Darstellung von Elementen des Designs und derer Analyse in klinischen Studien. In: Rohde H, Troidl H, eds. Das Margenkarzinom. Stuttgart: Thieme Verlag, 1984, pp. 35–39.
43. Pollock AV. Design and interpretation of clinical trials. Br Med J 1985;290:243.
44. Juhr NC. Die Optimierung des Tierversuchs—

Aufgabe einer Tierversuchskunde. In: Kübler K, ed. Der Tierversuch in der Arzneimittelforschung bga-Berichte, vol. 1. Berlin: Dietrich Reimer-Verlag, 1980, pp. 57–62.

45. Held JR. Mühlbock memorial lecture: consideration in the provision and characterization of animal models. In: Spiegel A, Erichsen S, Solleveld HA, eds. Animal Quality and Models in Biomedical Research. Stuttgart and New York: G. Fischer Verlag, 1980, pp. 9–16.

46. Immich H. Medizinische Statistik. Stuttgart and New York: Schattauer Verlag, 1974.

47. Dixon WJ. The up-and-down method for small samples. Am Statis Assoc 1965;60:967–978.

48. Hsu CK, New AE, Mayo JG. Quality Assurance of Rodent Models. 7th ICLAS Symposium. Stuttgart and New York: G. Fischer Verlag, 1980, pp. 17–28.

49. Bonnod J. Principles of ethics in animal experimentation. 16th IABS Congress: the standardization of animals to improve biomedical research, production and control. Dev Biol Stand 1980;45: 185–187.

50. Rowsell HC. The ethics of biomedical experimentation. In: The Future of Animals, Cells, Models, and Systems in Research, Development, Education, and Testing. Washington, D.C.: National Academy of Science, 1977.

51. U.S. Department of Health and Human Services. Guide for the Care and Use of Laboratory Animals. Public Health Service, National Institutes of Health NIH Publication No. 86-23 revised, 1985.

Commentary

Although there will always be pressure from groups opposed to animal experimentation, most scientists agree that animal experimentation is required for the advancement of human health. Drs. Isselhard and Kuche outline the special obligations incumbent upon investigators who use animals for research. An animal experiment should be performed only when it is clear that no other method will provide the information required and when the conditions discussed in this chapter are met.

One methodologic issue in animal investigation was not discussed. Although not usually done, blinded experiments lend further credibility to the scientific conclusions drawn from animal studies. Investigators should build as many elements of blinding into the study design as possible, just as one would do in a prospectively randomized human clinical trial.

A.S.W.

CHAPTER 49

The Isolated Organ in Research

T. Yeh Jr. and A.S. Wechsler

Introduction

Technological advances in artificial perfusion allow effective isolated perfusion of a wide variety of organs and tissues, including, but not limited to, brain, heart, lung, heart-lung, liver, kidney, spleen, pancreas, thymus, gastrointestinal tract, urinary tract, reproductive tract, skeletal muscle, nerves, and blood vessels. The option of extended pharmacological or surgical treatment of animals before organ isolation makes this technique extremely powerful. To the uninitiated, isolated organ perfusion may conjure up images of Frankensteinian surgery, machinery, and complexity; however, surgeons are particularly well equipped to implement these models, which actually are much simpler today than they were historically.

Tissue similarities make evaluation of certain phenomena, that is, metabolic or biochemical processes and their related enzyme systems, oxygen consumption, organ weight, water content, electrolyte content, tissue compartment size, and measurement and analysis of organ blood or lymph flow, possible in virtually any organ system. Perfusion with disaggregating solutions subsequently dissociates cells for molecular biological analysis, cell culture, cellular separation, and subcellular fractionation.[1] Direct perfusion of tissue with fixatives or histochemical stains, such as vital dyes, provides excellent material for light or electron microscopy. Modification of perfusate composition or administration conditions permits the study of drugs, toxins, hypoxia, ischemia, hypotension, or hypertension on organ function.

Organ-specific investigations depend on the presence of specialized organ function such as exocrine secretion by the liver or pancreas or endocrine secretion (hormone production) in the pancreas, thymus, or adrenal. Kidney or liver preparations permit evaluation of organ clearance capacity for drugs, metabolites, or toxins. Beating hearts, peristalsing gastrointestinal tracts, or isolated tissues (muscles, nerves, or vessels) permit the study of mechanical or electrical function, including depolarization, automaticity, or rhythmicity. The possibilities are endless.

Advantages and Disadvantages of Isolated Perfusion

Isolating an organ for study confers several experimental advantages over in vivo studies. First, surgical access to the organ is simplified. Arteries are easily cannulated for perfusion and precise drug administration. Lymphatic effluent, venous blood, and/or exocrine secretions are easily obtained for analysis simply by cannulating the appropriate system. The entire organ can be continuously weighed, biopsied, or monitored for mechanical or electrical function.

Precise control of experimental variables with intrinsically high variability is a second advantage. In vivo, the nature of systemic homeostasis demands that each organ adapt to changing conditions (e.g., parasympathetic versus sympathetic stimulation and resultant changes in blood flow) as required for organism survival. Unpredictable physiologic responses of individual animals confounds the study of phenomena in which exacting reproducibility is critical. The parameters of isolated organ perfusion (e.g., perfusate composition, oxygenation, pressure, flow, and temperature) are rigorously controllable (at physiologic or pathophysiologic levels) and not subject to homeostatic fluctuations. Drug or toxin levels can be strictly maintained, eliminating systemic metabolism that may unpredictably change levels of or produce unwanted metabolites. Loading conditions of cardiac, skeletal, or smooth muscle can be standardized. Cellular depolarization can be electronically stimulated for in vitro analysis of electrical activity or mechanical contraction. Because isolated preparations are free of hemodynamic instability, as well as homeostatic neural and hormonal influences, organ response is unaffected by systemic responses of the intact organism.

A third advantage is economy. The preparation of isolated organs is generally faster and less expensive than preparing intact animals. A single preparation of the apparatus often permits multiple studies, conserving investigator resources and time. An isolated preparation is ideal for screening new hypotheses before initiating more extensive experiments. Finally, because organs are rapidly excised and the donor animal immediately sacrificed, isolated preparations may be a more humane form of animal experimentation.

Isolating an intact organ also confers advantages not achievable in tissue culture or cellular homogenates. The anatomic and physiologic division of the organ into compartments (vascular, interstitial, extracellular, intracellular, secretory-excretory, and luminal) are maintained. Such separation is physiologically critical in proper organ functioning. Normal cell-cell relationships allow the potential for undisturbed study of autocrine and paracrine effects. Leakage of intracellular enzymes into the experimental preparation medium (perfusate in this case) is minimal.[2]

The major disadvantage of isolated perfusion is the unstable nature and, hence, limited viability of the preparations. The etiology and prevention of organ death are fundamental questions that unfortunately will not be answered in this chapter. Humans do not completely understand the physiologic requisites for survival in artificially perfused systems. Even in state-of-the-art clinical applications, patient deterioration is unavoidable in prolonged extracorporeal membrane oxygenation, and organ grafts for transplant have limited viability after removal and perfusion for storage.

The causes of this instability are debated. Perfusates are either nonblood or modified blood preparations and are administered with artificial pumps, conduits, and oxygenators without benefit of normal systemic homeostasis. Blood cellular elements and proteins are damaged. Platelets are destroyed and clump, forming microaggregates; red blood cells are hemolyzed; white blood cells are lysed and enzymes released. Serum proteins are denatured and adhere to tubings, resulting in hypoproteinemia and edema, which, if severe, can lead to compromised plasma membrane integrity. Microemboli of these elements, as well as of crystalloid-based perfusion solutions and small bubbles in perfusate solutions, may contribute to deterioration. Nonspecific activation of pathophysiologic inflammatory mediators and the immune system in blood-based models may result in organ injury. Activation of cellular lysozomes and abnormal gas concentrations may also contribute. It is interesting that clinically these effects from artificial surfaces are minimized in vivo in devices that have the opportunity to form pseudoendothelium (e.g., prosthetic grafts and left ventricular assist devices with special surfaces that permit this phenomenon).

Also, in a less well-understood phenomenon, isolating an organ from the body may result in critical deficits in undelineated but important metabolites, substrates, hormones, or neural control that could result in cellular dysregulation. Hypothetically, these deficits may disturb normal cellular homeostasis, possibly by disrupting enzymatic, transcriptional, or translational processes that eventually culminate in cell death. Apoptotic death is distinct from necrosis both at the morphological and molecular levels and has been likened, in colloquial terms, to cellular "suicide" rather than "murder." Necrosis typically results when cells are exposed to severe and sudden injury (e.g., ischemia, trauma), with changes in mitochondrial morphology and rapid loss of ability to maintain homeostasis. It results in a significant inflammatory response. Apoptosis, also known as programmed cell death, occurs in response to more subtle signals from the environment, that is, "planned" morphogenetic death during embryonic development, elimination of self-reactive T cells, or withdrawal of a hormone or growth factor, thermal stimuli (heat or cold), poison, glucocorticoids, or low-dose ionizing radiation. Spillage of intracellular contents does not occur because cells that break into a series of membrane-bound apoptotic bodies are phagocytosed and thus inflammation is minimal. The process requires new gene expression (c-myc, p53, Fas, to name a few) and can be protected by expression of other intracellular suppressors (bcl-2, bcl-x). Apoptosis has obvious implications far beyond the scope of this chapter, but for our purposes should affect the interpretation of studies done using organs withdrawn from their native environments.[3,4]

These unavoidable limitations inevitably cause deterioration in organ function, making extended or chronic isolated perfusion impractical. Finally, because experimental results are obtained from isolated systems, results may not be entirely applicable to in vivo organ response.[5] Historically, it was suggested that isolated perfusion was really the study of a dying organ,[6] but today results are widely accepted as reliable and relevant, provided the organ is studied within a reasonable time window and the scientist is able to demonstrate stability of the system.

The Isolated Organ	
Advantages	Disadvantages
Simple surgical access	Instability (limited viability)
Control of experimental variables	Abnormal perfusion
Freedom from systemic reflexes	Loss of trophic hormones
Economy	Blood damage

System Design, Implementation, and Maintenance

As typified by clinical surgery, the implementation of isolated organ research is best learned by doing. Isolated organs are widely employed in university environments, and an academic colleague who employs a similar model will often teach or collaborate with a novice. Even if the precise model differs, many of the techniques can be generalized.

Choice of Animal Species

Conservation of resources requires careful planning in the early stages of any experiment. The need for well-attended, healthy animals in obtaining meaningful data is self-evident.[5] Although smaller animals may be more cost-effective in evaluating biochemical or cellular phenomena, the chosen species must allow adequate assessment of the parameter of interest. Tissue, metabolites, exocrine secretions, or endocrine products must be available or produced in sufficient quantities for subsequent analysis. Organ size must permit cannulation of small vessels, ducts, lymphatics, or organ chambers of interest. Biochemical and physiologic responses may vary among species, and the investigator must determine whether a given species is appropriate for investigating a particular hypothesis.

Anesthesia

To avoid hypoxia or respiratory arrest, consider the use of ventilatory support. Choose anesthetic agents rationally, avoiding those with detrimental effects on the organ of interest, such as irreversible myocardial depression when halogenated hydrocarbons are used in studies of cardiac physiology.[7] Short acting agents are preferable since organ removal is generally rapid and residual anesthetic effects should be minimized. Precision in dosage is required. Underdosage is not only inhumane, but concomitant pain-associated catecholamine release may have profound and undesirable effects on organ vasculature.[8] If muscle relaxants are used, their interference with assessment of anesthetic adequacy may have the same ultimate outcome as underdosage.[5] After induction, overdosage may prematurely kill the donor or unnecessarily depress the organ of interest.

Route of administration is generally a matter of convenience. Intraperitoneal administration is often simplest in smaller animals. Intravenous administration is usually possible in larger animals, although intramuscular injection may enhance investigator safety with ferocious carnivores. Inhalational methods require calibrated vaporizers and close monitoring but are also an option.[5]

In protracted organ harvests, even closer monitoring of ventilatory, hemodynamic, hydration, thermal, and metabolic status is indicated. The same holds true for parabiotic systems in which a support animal supplies oxygenated blood perfusate to an isolated organ for the duration of the experiment.

Surgery

Although surgical preparation of isolated organs varies among specific organs, animal species, and experimental protocols, minimizing organ hypoxia with rapid, consistent harvest and expeditious reperfusion is absolutely essential for reproducible results.[5] Fortunately, protocols to expedite harvest and minimize ischemia exist for most organs (e.g., liver harvests can be performed without any period of total ischemia). Mechanical organ trauma should also be minimized by avoiding unnecessary tissue handling.

Perfusion System Design

Choice of Perfusate

Design a perfusion system that meets experimental requirements but simplifies daily use and maintenance. In choosing one of the many available formulations, basic requirements include oxygenation of tissue, provision of nutrients, removal of metabolic wastes, appropriate buffering, physiologic concentration of principal ions, and adequate colloid osmotic pressure to limit edema.

Perfusates are generally classified as (1) nonblood perfusates or (2) blood-based perfusates. In studies of cardiac physiology, Langendorff in 1895 first demonstrated that sufficient quantities

of oxygen could be dissolved in crystalloid solution to support isolated rat hearts.[9] Such nonblood perfusates are generally more economical and convenient than blood-based perfusates but are, not surprisingly, less physiologic. First, the oxygen-carrying capacity of pure crystalloid is limited.[10] Second, aqueous solutions are less viscous and yield higher flow rates than blood-based perfusates.[1] Finally, crystalloid is without the normal complement of cells and proteins found in blood. Nevertheless many important, well-accepted studies have been executed with nonblood perfusates. The composition of a commonly employed formulation, modified Krebs-Henseleit buffer, is given in Table 49-1, but many solutions have been formulated for specific uses.[1]

Meticulous preparation of nonblood perfusates is imperative. All components must be accurately measured and, once in solution, adequately filtered. In Figure 49-1, a filter used for nonblood perfusate demonstrates that even analytical grade chemicals have impurities that can form microemboli in organ capillaries and compromise performance.[1,11] Filters of silk, wool, or membrane[1,12,13] are recommended; paper filters are unacceptable because they release cellulose fibers. Finally, advance preparation of sufficient quantities of perfusate is strongly advised. Nothing is more disheartening than a smoothly running preparation that suddenly runs out of perfusate for a period of unwanted ischemia whose duration is limited solely by the investigator's land speed.

The second class of perfusates, blood-based perfusates, are generally more costly and troublesome but are also more physiologic. Use of any blood-based perfusate necessitates anticoagulation. Heparin is most commonly employed, but others are available if heparin is contraindicated.[14] Be cognizant of alterations in blood components

Table 49-1. Modified Kreb's–Henseleit solution.

NaCL	118.0 mmol/L
KCl	4.70 mmol/L
CaCl$_2$	2.52 mmol/L
MgSO$_4$	1.64 mmol/L
NaHCO$_3$	24.88 mmol/L
KH$_2$PO$_4$	1.18 mmol/L
Glucose	5.55 mmol/L

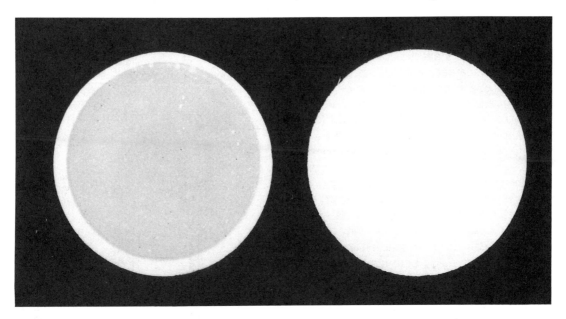

Figure 49-1.   Used filter. Five-micron membrane filter (left) used to filter crystalloid perfusates prepared with analytical grade chemicals vs. unused filter (right). Even though prepared perfusate was clear to visual inspection, the necessity for filtration is apparent.

that occur in any extracorporeal system and degrade tissue perfusion.[15] These alterations include protein denaturation,[16] fat embolism,[17] erythrocyte and platelet aggregation,[18] viscosity changes,[19] and cellular disruption of erythrocytes, leukocytes, and platelets.[5]

Regardless of perfusate class, the concentration of perfusate components, such as sodium, potassium, chloride, calcium, magnesium, and glucose, as well as experimental additives, should be analyzed periodically. Blood-based perfusates are prone to hemolysis, which lowers hematocrit and raises potassium and plasma-free hemoglobin, all of which should be assessed when using blood-primed systems.[5,20–23] Remember that free hemoglobin is damaging and is cleared by liver preparations. Blood-based perfusates are also more prone to hyperkalemia (from hemolysis) and fluctuations in calcium levels with changes in pH.

If blood from a second animal is used, blood-tissue incompatibility may result. To avoid this phenomenon, autologous blood is preferable, some claim essential, for success.[5] The use of autologous blood presents the logistical difficulty of increasing organ ischemia since organ and per-fusate must be simultaneously obtained from the same subject.[5]

Constant-Pressure or Constant-Flow Perfusion

An important advantage of isolated perfusion is that either pressure or flow can be strictly controlled. The superiority of either is debated. As illustrated in Figure 49-2, a constant-pressure system is implemented by the action of gravity on a column of perfusate that is maintained at a constant height above the perfused organ with a mechanical pump. In this method, perfusion pressure remains constant, but flow varies with the vascular resistance of the organ. Proponents of constant-pressure perfusion argue that mean perfusion pressure is constant in intact circulations and is therefore physiologically more relevant in isolated systems.[1]

As illustrated in Figure 49-3, a constant-flow system is implemented by pumping perfusate directly to an isolated organ. Flow remains constant, but perfusion pressure varies with the vascular resistance of the organ. Perfusion pressures are gen-

Figure 49-2. Simple constant-pressure preparation (crystalloid perfusate, nonrecirculating). Constant pressure is effected by maintaining a column of perfusate at constant height above the organ. Perfusate is continuously pumped from the runoff reservoir to the constant-pressure reservoir. After the desired level is achieved (e.g., 100 cm above the heart), perfusate overflows to the runoff reservoir through the overflow conduit. In this system, perfusate is discarded after one pass through the organ and is replenished by adding warmed, oxygenated perfusate to the runoff reservoir. Perfusate temperature is monitored and controlled by water jacketing of perfusate conduits. System oxygenation and pH are maintained by bubbling both reservoirs with a mixture of 95% O_2 and 5% CO_2. The organ chamber maintains constant temperature (with water jacketing) and hydration (by bathing the organ in its effluent). Continuous in-line filtration (e.g., 5 μ) removes residual particulate matter from the perfusate before it reaches the constant-pressure reservoir. Auxiliary inputs of the organ cannula allow other columns to be added in parallel for rapid or repetitive switching of perfusates, drugs, and so forth. An intraventricular balloon attached to a pressure transducer is used to monitor ventricular function.

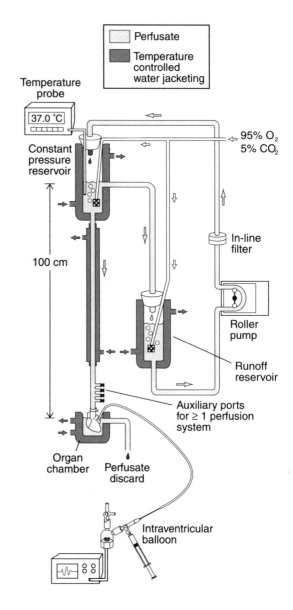

erally lower than in vivo arterial pressure, probably a result of autonomic denervation, the absence of circulating catecholamines,[5] and decreased perfusate viscosity (in crystalloid or diluted blood-based perfusates). Proponents of constant-flow perfusion argue that loss of normal neural and endocrine mediation of vascular tone,[5] as well as altered vascular reactivity, leads to abnormal vascular resistances and that only constant-flow perfusion assures flow rates in the physiologic range.[1]

Overperfusion should be carefully avoided, or irreversible damage, in the form of edema, increased vascular resistance, petechial hemorrhage, or frank hematoma, may result. Exocrine secretions may become tinged with blood. Underperfusion is generally less serious and many organs will tolerate brief periods of moderately reduced flow.[5]

Whether constant flow or constant pressure is utilized, pumps must be of adequate capacity. Perfusate flow and pressure should be monitored during experimentation. Pulsatile flow, an option in constant-flow preparations, mimics the function

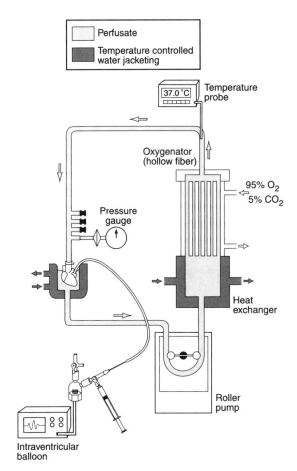

Perfusate

Temperature controlled water jacketing

37.0 °C

Temperature probe

Oxygenator (hollow fiber)

95% O$_2$
5% CO$_2$

Pressure gauge

Heat exchanger

Roller pump

Intraventricular balloon

Figure 49-3. Simple constant-flow preparation (blood-based perfusate, recirculating). Many features of this preparation (temperature control, oxygenation, and pH control) are similar to the constant-pressure preparation. Remarkable differences are that a commercially available hollow-fiber oxygenator oxygenates blood. An occlusive roller pump supplies constant flow (rather than constant pressure) to perfuse the organ, and perfusate pressure is monitored with a pressure gauge (or pressure transducer). Because of expense and limited availability, blood is usually recirculated rather than discarded. Note that these illustrations are only two of many examples, depending on one's experimental needs.

of the intact cardiovascular system with pumps that simulate arterial pressure waveforms. Several studies have shown its benefit in isolated organs[24–27] as well as in cardiopulmonary bypass surgery.[28–30] The use of pulsatile flow may be more important in vascular system studies.[5] Pulse pressure must be monitored closely, because the poor compliance of artificial tubing may transmit undampened system pressures and damage the organ. A side arm in the circuit filled with a column of air or incorporation of excess aorta into the perfusion circuit functions as an effective compliance chamber. The advantages of pulsatile perfusion must be weighed against its cost, complexity, and the additional blood trauma introduced.[5]

Recirculation versus Nonrecirculation of Perfusate

If perfusate is recirculated, waste products accumulate and nutrients or substrates are depleted,

not only with time but also in proportion to the size and metabolic rate of the organ being studied. Although nonrecirculating systems eliminate these problems, recirculation may be required to study minute changes in perfusate composition or if expensive admixtures or blood-based perfusates are used.[1,11,31,32] The sheer volume of perfusate required by organs from larger animals may prohibit a one-pass system. Regardless of the method chosen, the supply of perfusate in a nonrecirculating system, or losses from recirculating preparations, must be monitored and repleted as necessary.

Choice of Oxygenator

For reproducible results, accurate standardization of perfusate gas tensions between studies is essential and requires that an oxygenator be of sufficient size to handle maximum anticipated flow while maintaining adequate gas exchange. Oxygenators have evolved into two commonly employed designs: bubble oxygenators and membrane oxygenators. Bubble oxygenators are less expensive and ideally suited for pure crystalloid perfusates; however, they are more destructive to the blood cells and proteins present in blood-based perfusates.[5] For pure crystalloid perfusates, a bubble oxygenator is easily implemented with commercially available aquarium aerators (generically known as "airstones") that deliver fine gas bubbles into any chamber.[33] Membrane oxygenators are more costly but minimize blood element damage[34] and require smaller priming volumes.

A particularly ingenious and inexpensive "membrane" oxygenator was brought to our attention by Dr. Carl Apstein and colleagues (Figure 49-4). In this system, fresh bovine blood is heparinized (15,000 units/L) and washed three times by centrifugation with Krebs-Henseleit solution. Gentamicin is added to the packed cells (final concentration 2 mg/L) and the mixture refrigerated (1 to 3 days). When ready for use the erythrocytes are resuspended (260 mL packed erythrocytes/240 mL Krebs-Henseleit) and brought to a volume of 600 mL with stock solutions (final concentrations: 4% albumin, 0.4 mM/L palmitate, and 1 unit/mL heparin).

The erythrocyte suspension is oxygenated by pumping through two serially connected long coils of silicone elastomer tubing (inner diameter 0.058 inches, outer diameter 0.077 inches),* each coiled inside a water-jacketed open-topped glass cylinder and pumped from bottom to top of the cylinder for optimum gas exchange. Oxygen (95% O_2, 5% CO_2) is passed in the base of each glass cylinder and diffuses through the silicon tubing. Oxygenation (pO_2 typically 200–300 mm Hg) is increased by increasing gas flow rate and pCO_2 (typically 35–45 mm Hg) increased by partial coverage of glass cylinders as required by system blood gases. Oxygenated blood is passed through 20-μ, water-jacketed transfusion filter† and is maintained at constant pressure as described previously. This system provides relatively atraumatic oxygenation for small organ research.[35]

A parabiotic system, first described in 1904[36] and depicted in Figure 49-5, directly perfuses an isolated organ with arterial blood from a support animal. Several variations on this method exist,[37–39] but, in general, venous blood is captured and returned via the jugular vein to the support animal, which not only functions as a living oxygenator but also maintains perfusate homeostasis. One disadvantage is the risk of an incompatibility reaction between blood and isolated organ tissue.[1]

The gas typically employed for oxygenation and buffering of nonblood perfusates is a 95% oxygen–5% carbon dioxide mixture,[5] although carbon dioxide is generally not required in blood-based systems. Verify gas supplies before experimentation for the same reason adequate quantities of perfusate are prepared in advance. Continued gas flow is imperative for oxygenation and is assessed visually in bubble oxygenators or tactually at the exhaust port of membrane oxygenators. Periodically monitor perfusate gas tensions and pH during experimentation, adjusting gas flows as necessary. Extracorporeal gassing allows precise control of oxygenation. Hypoxia is induced by bubbling perfusate with nitrogen.

Conduits, Cannulae, and Reservoirs

Choose tubing of sufficient caliber to handle anticipated flow rates without undue turbulence but within that limit minimize caliber and length to reduce priming volume. Silicon rubber and polyvinyl chloride (PVC) tubing are commonly employed. Silicone rubber has the advantage of being inert and is more compliant than PVC tubing; however, it is expensive and, because of its permeability to gases, is more prone to bubble formation if flow ceases for moderate periods of time. PVC tubing is cheaper and impermeable but is relatively rigid and can harbor detrimental contaminants from the manufacturing process.[40,41] Its use may be more deleterious with whole blood than with crystalloid solutions.[41,42]

Choose tubing connectors that minimize turbulence and are air- and watertight, particularly on the arterial side of the circuit, to prevent leakage of perfusate or aspiration of air into the system (Venturi effect). Banding of connections may alleviate these problems.[5]

Cannula tips should have a lip or groove so that cannulated structures can be secured with ties. If a metal cannula is used, a groove can be ground

---

*Bentec Medical Inc., Boston, Massachusetts
† Statcorp. Jacksonville, Florida.

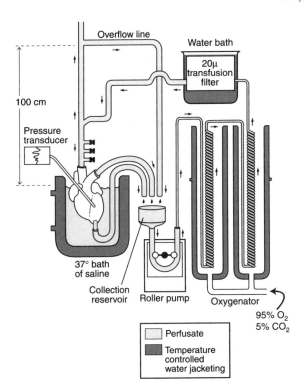

Figure 49-4. Blood-perfused isolated heart. An easily constructed and inexpensive oxygenator allows use of blood-based perfusate to partially counteract the unphysiologic aspects of crystalloid-based perfusion. The implementation beyond the oxygenator is quite similar to previously described models.

on a lathe. If a plastic or glass cannula is used, flaming the tip and touching it to a cool surface will form a satisfactory lip. Cannulae should be carefully positioned so as not to obstruct smaller supply arteries (e.g., the coronary ostia when cannulating the ascending aorta of the heart).[1] Consider, also, that a metal cannula may serve as a grounding electrode for electrical stimulation or for monitoring electrical depolarization.

If the venous circulation is cannulated, particularly in recirculating systems, larger tubing is generally required than for arterial cannulation to achieve adequate venous drainage.[5] The venous reservoir should accommodate necessary volumes and flow without increasing venous hydrostatic pressure, be of adjustable height, allow exclusion of air, and minimize stagnation of blood.[5] Some investigators believe that preservation of normal venous pressure is important in successful long-term perfusion, and monitoring venous pressure (e.g., portal venous pressure in liver perfusions) therefore becomes important.[43]

Avoidance of Emboli

Microscopic or macroscopic emboli can be troublesome in artificial perfusion. Microemboli can

be avoided with appropriate filtration of perfusate. For crystalloid systems, filtration can be performed in line with a 5-μ filter. Blood-based systems generally require a 15-μ filter. During extended perfusions, filter clogging occurs and manifests itself, at best, as decreased forward flow or, less ideally, as sudden tubing decompression that showers everyone within range. In-line filters occasionally rupture and seed an organ with microemboli; the only manifestation may be a precipitous deterioration in organ function. Regular replacement and careful seating of the filter in its holder may prevent such incidents.

Macroscopic emboli are usually air bubbles that can be avoided by carefully priming the system, using air traps where appropriate, securing tubing connections, and inspecting conduits after periods of perfusate stasis. Foaming and protein denaturation[16] can be problematic in colloid- or blood-primed systems and may require the use of anti-foaming agents.[5]*

---

*Silicone MS Anti-foam A, Hopkins and Williams Ltd., Chadwell Heath, Essex

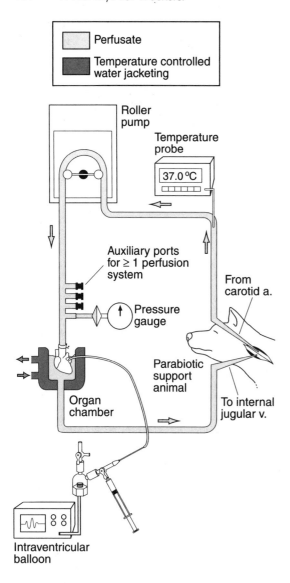

Figure 49-5. Parabiotic isolated heart (constant-flow, blood-based perfusate, recirculating). This ingenious variation employs a parabiotic support animal to supply arterial blood (with a pump) to an isolated organ. After perfusion, venous blood is recaptured and returned to the support animal in which it is oxygenated and homeostatically regulated. Constant pressure or constant flow can be implemented. If desired, the support animal's arterial pressure can directly supply the isolated organ.

Temperature Control

An organ chamber is required to control organ temperature and prevent tissue desiccation.[1] Two varieties of chambers are commonly used: (1) a temperature-controlled, humidified gas chamber and (2) a physiologic fluid bath into which the organ is immersed for temperature and humidity control. The fluid bath may confer hydrostatic advantages and limit the edema formation inherent in isolated preparations by increasing tissue pressure (see later section).[1] Organ chamber and perfusate temperature are generally controlled with supplemental water baths and some combination of water jackets, heat exchangers, or warming blankets (in parabiotic systems).

On System Stability

In an isolated system, physiologic homeostasis and organ stimulation become the responsibility of the investigator. During experimentation all system parameters (arterial pressure and flow, venous pressure [if applicable], perfusate levels, gas flows, temperature, oxygenation, acid-base status, perfusate chemistry, and electrical stimulators and recorders), as well as functional stability of the organ, must be continuously monitored.

A period of stabilization is mandatory as an isolated organ adjusts to its new environment. Depending on the organ, 15 to 60 minutes are required, but experimental parameters of interest (e.g., ventricular mechanical function, hepatic bile production) should be assessed to confirm that stabilization has occurred. Documentation of stability with extended trial perfusions is essential before bona fide experimentation begins, so that results are not merely a reflection of system instability. Many investigators perfuse control organs at regular intervals to ensure quality control. At any point during actual experimentation, deteriorating organ function may indicate a problem in the system. Once this relatively late alarm has sounded, the further experimental validity of that preparation is suspect. Remember that organ function inevitably deteriorates and that experimentation should be performed within an organ's window of stability.

Some organs have idiosyncratic reactions to isolated perfusion: Livers develop hepatic venous spasm. Kidneys tend toward arterial spasm. Lung's are prone to edema formation. These problems can generally be circumvented, if their existence is known.[5]

System Maintenance

The importance of appropriately maintaining and cleaning the system cannot be overstated. In blood-primed or protein-containing systems, disassemble the apparatus, discard disposable items, scrub the reusable apparatus to remove blood residues, and soak overnight in hydrogen peroxide. The next day copiously rinse the apparatus with hot running tap water and recirculate with distilled water, followed by saline, and finally by physiologic crystalloid.[5]

When using crystalloid primes, the regimen can be simplified. Before and after use, copiously rinse the apparatus with hot tap water, then with filtered, deionized water. Some advocate boiling water for removal of residual glucose used in most perfusates. Change all filters before priming with crystalloid perfusate. On a periodic basis, depending on usage or for unexplained system instability,

soak all glassware and nondisposable items in chromic sulfuric acid for 24 hours, then in reagent grade water for 24 to 48 hours.[44] After copious rinsing, reassemble the system, preferably with new tubing.

Although sterility is unnecessary for most short-term studies, bacterial contamination of the apparatus may occur, especially in nutrient-rich, blood-primed systems. Consider sterilization for persistent unexplained instability.

Physiology of Isolated Organs

Isolated organs have a time-dependent tendency to acquire weight. With protein-free crystalloid solutions, water gradually escapes from the vascular bed and interstitial edema develops. This phenomenon can be limited in two ways: (1) Increase the colloidal osmotic pressure of the perfusate with albumin,[5] other colloids, or osmotic agents;[45,46] or (2) increase tissue pressure, as is commonly done in isolated hearts, by immersion (1 to 2 cm) into a bath filled with perfusate. Immersion is believed to increase hydrostatic pressure, thereby reducing transcapillary fluid escape and minimizing tissue edema. Without immersion, the dry weight (weight of dried tissue/weight of wet tissue) of guinea pig hearts after perfusion with saline solution decreases from 20–21% (in situ) to 16.0% after 30 minutes.[1] Rat hearts perfused with Krebs-Henseleit solution increase their extracellular volume by 2% after 15 minutes, 5% after 30 minutes, and 17% after 60 minutes.[47] After 4 hours of perfusion combined with immersion, the dry weight of the left ventricular myocardial tissue is limited to 17.2 ± 0.2% and viability is extended.[1]

Eventually, the function of all isolated organs deteriorates, presumably because normal homeostasis is absent and the perfusates and apparatus of isolated perfusion are unphysiologic. In blood-primed systems, the gradual destruction of cellular elements and proteins contributes to this deterioration. Distinguishing unphysiologic deterioration from physiologic response to experimental manipulation is critical.

Examples

Two examples are presented. For comprehensive details of implementation refer to the bibliography; these details are much more easily read than rediscovered.

Heart

Oscar Langendorff was the first to devise a method for investigating the isolated mammalian heart. He demonstrated that retrograde perfusion of the ascending aorta in the presence of a competent aortic valve closed the valve and perfused the coronary arteries. Except for coronary venous drainage, the cardiac cavities remained empty. An excellent technical reference to Langendorff's original technique and modern modifications is H. J. Doring and H. Dehnert's *The Isolated Perfused Warm-Blooded Heart according to Langendorff.*

A wide variety of parameters are assessed in isolated hearts. Coronary flow and autoregulation in response to endogenous or exogenous vasoactive substances may be assessed with or without the modulation of endothelium.[48] Myocardial rate, rhythm and rhythm disturbances, electrical potentials and depolarization, and refractory period can be studied in response to cardioactive drugs, hypoxia, ischemia, or electrical stimuli. Biochemical, metabolic, and histologic investigations discussed in the introduction are all possible. Pharmaceutical pretreatment, experimentally induced myocardial infarction, chronic cardiac overload, and transplantation are all fertile areas for investigation.

Historically, cardiac contractility was difficult to evaluate because fluctuations in heart rate, perfusion pressure, afterload, and preload often confounded the evaluation of true changes in contractility. The isolated heart allows precise standardization of such variables so that ventricular function can be accurately assessed, typically with one of two basic models: (1) the nonworking heart or (2) the working heart.

In both models, crushing or excising the sinus node and external pacing produces a constant heart rate. Right atrial pacing, either with two atrial microelectrodes or a metal aortic cannula and a single atrial microelectrode, is preferable for normal ventricular conduction and contraction.

Stimulus amplitude should not exceed 4 volts, because norepinephrine release from cardiac sympathetic nerve fibers may exert a positive inotropic effect.[1]

The nonworking heart standardizes preload and afterload with a left ventricular balloon that is also used to assess ventricular function.[1,49] As illustrated in Figure 49-6, construct the balloon by tying an appropriately sized piece of latex (latex condom) onto a semirigid (polyethylene) catheter attached to a stopcock. Prime the balloon with fluid to eliminate air bubbles, withdraw the fluid, and connect the apparatus to a mechanoelectrical pressure transducer. Confirm air- and watertightness of the balloon by adding volume (thus applying a test pressure) and observe for a pressure drift indicative of a leak. Potential leakage sites are a hole in the balloon (condom rubber ages and eventually leaks), the ligature holding the balloon on the catheter, the catheter, the stopcock, the transducer dome, the transducer itself, or connections between any parts of the apparatus. Insert the balloon via a left atriotomy through the mitral valve into the left ventricle for accurate assessment of ventricular pressure and performance assessments. Make certain that, after placement, the catheter tip does not press on the apex of the heart and impede pressure recording.[1]

Incremental increases in balloon volume effectively increase left ventricular preload and allow independent assessment of diastolic and systolic ventricular function. Analyze diastolic function by (1) plotting compliance curves of end diastolic pressure versus balloon volumes or (2) comparing end diastolic pressure at the baseline volume that generates a predetermined end diastolic pressure (e.g., 5 or 10 mm Hg) and remeasuring end diastolic pressure at that same volume after an intervention. Similarly, assess systolic performance by comparing (1) peak systolic pressures or developed pressures (maximal systolic pressure minus end diastolic pressure) at the same volumes described previously or (2) maximal developed pressure over a range of balloon volumes.[50] Electronically differentiating the pressure signal yields the rate of ventricular contraction (a measure of systolic function) and relaxation (a measure of diastolic function). Normal functional parameters are known for many species.[1] Of particular interest is that the isovolumic left ventricular balloon does

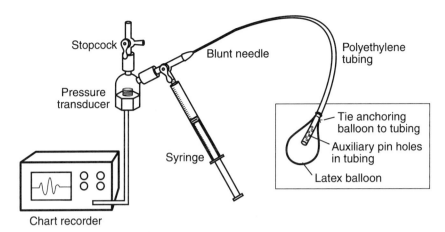

Figure 49-6. Construction and use of intraventricular balloons. A blunt needle is used to attach poly-ethylene (PE) tubing to stopcock. Additional pinholes are made in the end of the tubing that is to be within the balloon so that fluid flow (from the syringe) and transmission of pressure waves to transducer is unimpeded by the latex itself. Latex balloons may be purchased commercially or constructed from condom rubber. They should be slightly larger than the ventricle of interest so that no pressure is generated by the balloon itself at maximal volume. A silk tie firmly secures balloon to polyethylene tubing. Intraventricular pressure is transmitted from the balloon to a standard electromagnetic pressure transducer. An appropriately sized syringe is used to precisely vary balloon volume and is subsequently isolated from the system (with the stopcock) when measurements are made.

not cause recognizable myocardial lesions and that at even relatively high preloads (up to 60 mm Hg) coronary flow is unimpeded.[1]

The second basic model for assessing ventricular function is the working heart. As illustrated in Figure 49-7, the working heart is implemented by inserting a second cannula into the left atrium and allowing perfusate to flow under constant pressure (i.e., constant preload) through the mitral valve into the left ventricle. During systole, perfusate is ejected against constant afterload (i.e., a column of perfusate in the aortic cannula), and work is performed. System design allows easy switching between nonworking and working modes. Working hearts require a compliance chamber to prevent injury from pumping against noncompliant tubing.[5] They may be more physiologic because the heart actually pumps perfusate and is forced, by system design, to supply its own perfusion pressure. However, consider also that constant-pressure atrial filling does not standardize ventricular volumes in the presence of changing ventricular compliance. Ventricular function is assessed by simply measuring cardiac output or

with more sophisticated dimensional analyses of cardiac function (i.e., sonomicrometric crystals and pressure transducers or impedance catheters).[51]

Liver

The isolated liver permits the study of standard biochemical processes, blood flow, lymph flow, oxygen consumption, tissue composition, or histology; however, other unique opportunities also exist to study hepatic bile flow and composition (bilirubin, bile salts, alkaline phosphatase, pH, and electrolytes), liver regulation of perfusate composition, hepatocyte function (glycogen metabolism), and metabolism and clearance of drugs or toxins, as well as subsequent excretion of metabolites into the bile. Animal pretreatment with drugs or surgery to alter liver parenchyma or the biliary tree add tremendous potential to the technique.[95]

The isolated perfused liver went through its own technical evolution largely because of its pre-

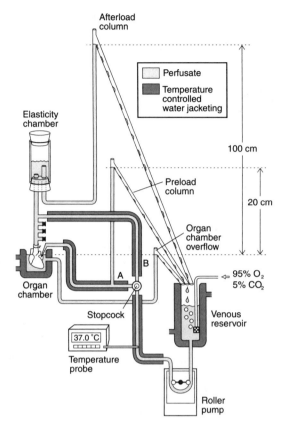

Figure 49-7. Working heart preparation (constant pressure, recirculating). The intraventricular balloon has been criticized for the unphysiologic (isovolumic) load it places on the heart. The working heart preparation forces the heart to supply its own perfusion pressure and pump blood, thereby performing work that can be measured. With the stopcock open to the left atrium (A), oxygenated perfusate enters the left atrium under a constant pressure controlled by the height of the preload column, traverses the mitral valve, and is pumped by the left ventricle into the aortic cannula. Ejection occurs against an afterload determined by the height of the afterload column. This same column also supplies a constant-pressure head that retrogradely perfuses the heart with oxygenated perfusate.

Closing the stopcock to the left atrium (A) and opening the stopcock to the aortic cannula (B) converts the system to a nonworking preparation. Perfusate is delivered to the coronaries in the usual retrograde fashion.

Note that the design of this apparatus requires that perfusate be pumped faster than the coronary flow (in the nonworking mode) or faster than cardiac output (in the working mode) so that perfusate continuously overflows the constant-pressure columns. This design minimizes perfusate oxygen desaturation or temperature loss by avoiding stagnation. Also note that construction of the preload column prevents aspiration of air into the left atrium in the nonworking mode, even after the preload column pressure has dropped to zero. Clamping the preload column instantaneously eliminates preload from the heart. Finally, note that overflow columns (afterload, preload) have air inlets that promote free runoff and prevent lowered column pressures from siphoning effects.

disposition to develop a phenomenon known as hepatic venous outflow block. The problem was first reported in 1915, in response to histamine or peptone in constant-pressure, crystalloid-perfused canine livers.[52] In 1928 blood-based, constant-pressure perfusion improved organ survival,[53] but constant-pressure perfusion was eventually criticized because progressively increasing organ resistance diminished portal venous flow. As a result, constant-flow perfusion was attempted.[54] In 1951 a description of constant-flow, sanguineous perfusion was published[55] and subsequently modified in 1953, with autologous blood, adjustable pumps, and avoidance of any total ischemia, in a preparation that became firmly established as a model for physiologic studies.[56] H. D. Ritchie and J. D. Hardcastle's *Isolated Organ Perfusion* provides an excellent review of the specifics of isolated liver perfusion.

Hepatic venous outflow block is variably evident after initiation of perfusion by edema, cyanosis, and mottling of the organ. Serous fluid streams from the liver surface as portal pressure rises and bile flow diminishes in a virtually irreversible process. In early preparations, venous outflow block occurred within 30 minutes of initiating perfusion.[53] Current techniques afford several hours of stability before the onset of serious deterioration. Many factors, including histamine, endotoxin, pharmacological agents,[57] and a rise in hepatic venous pressure, are thought to precipitate this phenomenon. Its physiologic basis may be spasm of smooth muscle in the walls of small hepatic venous radicles.[58]

Minimize hepatic venous outflow block by observing several salient points. Surgically, avoid unnecessary organ manipulation and any period of total ischemia with staggered cannulation of portal vein and hepatic artery.[5] Some consider the use of autologous blood essential. The addition of homologous blood that is not cross-matched to a porcine liver preparation causes a marked fall in total hepatic blood flow.[59] Even with cross-matching, early outflow block occurs when homologous blood is used.[8] Fully oxygenated, diluted blood is also preferred since a lower hematocrit facilitates perfusion and lessens hemolysis. A mixture of autologous blood and modified Kreb's solution is usually employed to obtain a hematocrit of 35% for isolated greyhound livers.[5] Maintaining pH over 7.30 may also aid in maintaining stable vascular resistance. Constant-flow perfusion has proven more successful than constant pressure. Steady portal venous pressure is useful in confirming stability. With initiation of artificial perfusion, portal venous pressure is high but gradually settles to less than 10 cm H_2O. Pressures that steadily rise or are greater than 15 cm H_2O indicate a deteriorating preparation and impending outflow block.[5] Meticulous maintenance of the perfusion apparatus is essential to prevent contamination by substances or foreign proteins that precipitate hepatic venous outflow block. The excessive blood trauma and protein denaturation of bubble oxygenators may contribute to hepatic venous outflow block.[16] Silastic tubing is preferred over PVC tubing because vasoconstrictor substances can be leached out of the latter by the perfusate.[42]

Livers generally require 1 hour of stabilization. Stability is achieved after portal venous pressure falls and plateaus, bile flow rises and plateaus, and bile composition stabilizes. Plasma potassium and glucose concentrations usually rise from parenchymal cell loss and then stabilize. Studies should not be undertaken before stability is achieved.[5]

Conclusion

The isolated organ is a model rich in possibilities. Its limitations are few and, for the most part, reflect deficient knowledge of the physiologic requisites necessary for extended survival in isolated systems. Consequently, markedly extended perfusion is currently not practical. Furthermore, caution is required in generalizing results obtained in isolated systems to in situ organ response. Nevertheless, for the meticulous investigator, isolated perfusion is an extremely powerful tool, economically conferring a host of experimental advantages in a model whose potential is limited primarily by the imagination.

References

1. Doring HJ, Dehnert H. The isolated perfused warm-blooded heart according to Langendorff. In: Methods in Experimental Physiology and Phar-

macrology, vol 5. Biological Measurement Techniques. West Germany: Biomesstechnik-Verlag, 1985, pp. 89–90.

2. Ross BD. Perfusion Techniques in Biochemistry. A Laboratory Manual in the Use of Isolated Perfused Organs in Biochemical Experimentation. Oxford: Clarendon, 1972, p. 6.

3. Cohen JJ. Apoptosis. Immunol Today 1993; 14:126–130.

4. Ueda N, Shah SV. Apoptosis. J Lab Clin Med 1994;124:169–177.

5. Ritchie HD, Hardcastle JD. Isolated Organ Perfusion. Baltimore: University Park, 1973, p. 9.

6. Baggiolini M, Dewald B. Stoffwechsel von Pharmaka in der isoliert perfundierten Rattenleber. In: Staib W, Scholz R, eds. Untersuchungen über dad Methylhydrazinderivat Ibenzmethyzin. Stoffwechsel der isoliert perfundierten Leber. Berlin: Springer-Verlag, 1968, p. 200.

7. Doring HJ. Reversible and irreversible forms of contractile failure caused by disturbances of general anesthetics in myocardial ATP utilization. In: Fleckenstein A, Dhalla NS, eds. Recent Advances in Studies on Cardiac Structure and Metabolism. Basic Functions of Cations in Myocardial Activity. Baltimore: University Park, 1975, pp. 395–403.

8. Andrews WHH, Hecker R, Maegraith BG, Ritchie HD. The action of adrenaline, 1-noradrenaline, acetyl choline, and other substances on the blood vessels of the perfused canine liver. J Physiol (Lond) 1955;128:413–434.

9. Langendorff O. Untersuchungen am überlebenden säugetierherzen. Arch f d ges Physiol 1895;61: 291–332.

10. Kammermeier H, Rudroff W. Funktion und energiestoffwechsel des isolierten herzens bei variation von pH, pCO_2 und HCO_3. Pflugers Arch 1972; 334:439–449.

11. Bleehen NM, Fisher RB. The action of insulin in the isolated rat heart. J Physiol (Lond) 1954;123: 260–276.

12. Fallen EL, Elliott WC, Gorlin R. Apparatus for study of ventricular function and metabolism in the isolated perfused rat heart. J Appl Physiol 1967; 22:836–839.

13. Taylor IM, Huffines WD, Young DT. Tissue water and electrolytes in an isolated perfused rat's heart preparation. J Appl Physiol 1961;16:95–102.

14. Cole CW, Bormanis J. Ancrod: a practical alternative to heparin. J Vasc Surg 1988;8:59–63.

15. Miller JH, McDonald RK. The effect of hemoglobin on renal function in the human. J Clin Invest 1951;30:1033–1040.

16. Lee WH Jr, Krumhaar D, Fonkalsrud EW, Schjeide OA, Maloney JV Jr. Denaturation of plasma proteins as a cause of morbidity and death after intracardiac operations. Surgery 1961;50: 29–39.

17. Miller JA, Fonkalsrud EW, Latta HL, Maloney JV Jr. Fat embolism associated with extracorporeal circulation and blood transfusion. Surgery 1962;51: 448–451.

18. Long DM Jr, Folkman MJ, McClenathan JE. The use of low molecular weight dextran in extracorporeal circulation, hypothermia, and hypercapnia. J Cardiovasc Surg 1963;4:617–641.

19. Rand PW, Lacombe E, Barker N, Derman U. Effects of open-heart surgery on blood viscosity. J Thorac Cardiovasc Surg 1966;51:616–625.

20. Cahill JJ, Kolff WJ. Hemolysis caused by pumps in extracorporeal circulation (in vitro evaluation of pumps). J Appl Physiol 1959;14:1039–1044.

21. Ferbers EW, Kirklin JW. Studies of hemolysis with a plastic-sheet bubble oxygenator. J Thorac Surg 1958;36:23–32.

22. Indeglia RA, Shea MA, Varco RL, Bernstein EF. Mechanical and biologic considerations in erythrocyte damage. Surgery 1967;62:47–55.

23. Paton BC, Grover FL, Herson MW, Bess H, Moore AR. The use of a nonionic detergent added to organ perfusates. In: Norman JC, Folkman J, Hardison WG, Rudolf LE, Veith FJ, eds. Organ Perfusion and Preservation. New York: Appleton-Century-Crofts, 1968, pp. 105–120.

24. Brodie TG. The perfusion of surviving organs. J Physiol (Lond) 1903;29:266–275.

25. Hooker DR. A study of the isolated kidney: the influence of pulse pressure upon renal function. Am J Physiol 1910;27:24–45.

26. McMaster PD, Parsons RJ. The effect of the pulse on the spread of substances through tissues. J Exp Med 1938;68:377–399.

27. Giron F, Birtwell WC, Soroff HS, Deterling RA. Hemodynamic effects of pulsatile and non-pulsatile flow. Arch Surg 1966;93:802–810.

28. Trinkle JK, Helton NE, Bryant LR, Word RC. Metabolic comparison of pulsatile and mean flow for cardiopulmonary bypass. Circulation 1968; 38(suppl. 6):vi–196.

29. Trinkle JK, Helton NE, Bryant LR, Griffen WO.

Pulsatile cardiopulmonary bypass: clinical evaluation. Surgery 1971;68:1074–1078.

30. Shepard RB, Kirklin JW. Relation of pulsatile flow to oxygen consumption and other variables during cardiopulmonary bypass. J Thorac Cardiovasc Surg 1969;58:694–702.

31. Bacaner MB, Lioy F, Visscher MB. Induced change in heart metabolism as a primary determinant of heart performance. Am J Physiol 1965; 209:519–531.

32. Brink AJ, Lochner A. Work performance of the isolated perfused beating heart in the hereditary myocardiopathy of the Syrian hamster. Circ Res 1967;21:391–401.

33. Rebeyka IM, personal communication, 1988.

34. Lee WH Jr, Krumhaar D, Derry G, Sachs D, Lawrence SH, Clowes GHA Jr, Maloney JV Jr. Comparison of the effects of membrane and non-membrane oxygenators on the biochemical and biophysical characteristics of blood. Surg Forum 1961;12:200–202.

35. Lorell BH, Isoyama S, Grice WN, Weinberg EO, Apstein CS. Effects of ouabain and isoproterenol on left ventricular diastolic function during low-flow ischemia in isolated, blood-perfused rabbit hearts. Circ Res 1988;63:457–467.

36. Heymans JR, Kochmann M. Une nouvelle méthode de circulation artificielle à travers le coeur isolé de mammifère. Arch Int Pharmacodyn Ther 1904; 13:27–36.

37. Osher WJ. Pressure-flow relationship of the coronary system. Am J Physiol 1953;172:403–416.

38. Mendler N, Hagl S, Sebening F, Theobald KP. Metabolite des energiestoffwechsels im parabiotisch perfundierten rattenherzen während und nach kardioplegie durch ischämie, kaliumchlorid und kalium-magnesium-aspartat. Arzneimittelforschung 1972;22:909–912.

39. Weiss M, Zehl U, Förster W. Koronare autoregulation des isolierten kaninchenherzens. Acta Biol Med Germ 1978;37:291–299.

40. Little K, Parkhouse J. Tissue reactions to polymers. Lancet 1962;2:857–861.

41. Guess WL, Stetson JB. Tissue reactions to organotin-stabilized polyvinyl chloride catheters. JAMA 1968;204:580–584.

42. Duke HN, Vane JR. An adverse effect of polyvinylchloride tubing used in extracorporeal circulation. Lancet 1968;2:21–23.

43. Fisk RL, Brownlee RT, Brown DR, McFarlane DF, Budney D, Dritsas KG, Kowalewski K, Couves CM. Perfusion of isolated organs for prolonged functional preservation. In: Norman JC, Folkman J, Hardison WG, Rudolf LE, Veith FJ, eds. Organ Perfusion and Preservation. New York: Appleton-Century-Crofts, 1968, pp. 217–227.

44. David Hearse, personal communication, 1986.

45. Ferrans VJ, Buja LM, Levitsky S, Roberts WC. Effects of hyperosmotic perfusate on ultrastructure and function of the isolated canine heart. Lab Invest 1971;24:265–272.

46. Weisfeldt ML, Shock NW. Effect of perfusion pressure on coronary flow and oxygen usage of nonworking heart. Am J Physiol 1970;218:95–101.

47. Fisher RB, Williamson JR. The oxygen uptake of the perfused rat heart. J Physiol (Lond) 1961; 158:86–101.

48. Furchgott RF, Zawadzki JV. The obligatory role of endothelial cells in the relaxation of arterial smooth muscle by acetylcholine. Nature 1980; 288:373–376.

49. Gottlieb R, Magnus R. Digitalis und herzarbeit. Nach versuchen am überlebenden warmblüterherzen. Arch Exper Pathol Pharmakol 1904;51: 30–63.

50. Coulson RL, Rusy BF. A system for assessing mechanical performance, heat production, and oxygen utilization of isolated perfused whole hearts. Cardiovasc Res 1973;7:859–869.

51. Sagawa K, Maughan L, Suga H, Sunagawa K. Cardiac Contraction and the Pressure-Volume Relationship. New York: Oxford University, 1988, pp. 428–444.

52. Mautner H, Pick EP. Ueber die durch schockgifte erzeugten zirkulations-störungen. Münchener Medizinische Wochenschrift 1915;62:1141–1143.

53. Bauer W, Dale HH, Poulsson LT, Richards DW. The control of circulation through the liver. J Physiol (Lond) 1932;74:343–375.

54. Trowell OA. Urea formation in the isolated perfused liver of the rat. J Physiol (Lond) 1942;100: 432–458.

55. Brauer RW, Pessotti RL, Pizzolato P. Isolated rat liver preparation. Bile production and other basic properties. Proc Soc Exp Biol Med 1951;78: 174–181.

56. Andrews WHH. A technique for perfusion of the canine liver. Ann Trop Med 1953;47:146–155.

57. Greenway CV, Stark RD. The hepatic vascular bed. Physiol Rev 1971;51:23–65.

58. Arey LB. Throttling veins in the livers of certain mammals. Anat Rec 1941;81:21–33.
59. Eiseman B, Knipe P, Koh Y, Normell L, Spencer FC. Factors affecting hepatic vascular resistance in the perfused liver. Ann Surg 1963;157:532–547.

Additional Reading

Doring HJ, Dehnert H. The isolated perfused warm-blooded heart according to Langendorff. Methods in experimental physiology and pharmacology. Biological measurement techniques. West Germany: Biomesstechnik-Verlag, 1985. This is an excellent technical reference with a wealth of practical information and advice on the isolated heart preparation. An excellent summary of crystalloid perfusate solutions is given, as well as variations on the Langendorff preparation and many modalities of assessing the isolated heart.

Ritchie HD, Hardcastle JD. Isolated Organ Perfusion. Baltimore: University Park Press, 1973. This is a helpful reference of general principles in the implementation of isolated organs and a valuable technical reference for specific concerns in isolated livers.

Norman JC, Folkman J, Hardison WG, Rudolf LE, Veith FJ. Organ Perfusion and Preservation. New York: Appleton-Century-Crofts, 1968.

Bartosek I, Guaitani A, Miller LL. Isolated Liver Perfusion and Its Applications. New York: Raven, 1978.

Ross BD. Perfusion Techniques in Biochemistry. A Laboratory Manual in the Use of Isolated Perfused Organs in Biochemical Experimentation. Oxford: Clarendon, 1972.

Commentary

A textbook defining the successful conditions for perfusion of each specific organ is impractical, but the fundamental information for anyone wishing to use an isolated organ as a research model is readily available and well referenced. Perhaps the most difficult aspect is making the initial decision to use an isolated organ in an in vitro setting rather than in vivo. Any experimental conclusions will always have to be qualified by the realization that the organ has been studied in isolation. Isolated organs are highly idiosyncratic in their requirements and responses; establishing successful organ perfusion that does not introduce an undesired element precipitating its own pathology is difficult. Consistency of the preparation must always be maintained; this can be facilitated by consultation with laboratories that have had success with the particular technique. We had great difficulty in setting up an isolated blood-perfused heart model until we visited Dr. Apstein's laboratory. His generosity in sharing with us the minute details and nuances of successful heart perfusion stands as a model of scientific cooperation; its importance cannot be overemphasized. If you are considering setting up a complex system in your own laboratory, visit someone who has been able to make it work rather than relying on reading the methods put forward in even the most carefully detailed scientific manuscript. Making an isolated organ system work is a lot like cooking; reading the recipe simply is not the same as seeing how it is done.

A.S.W.

CHAPTER 50

Computer Models

K.S. Kunzelman and R.P. Cochran

Introduction

Why Use Computer Modeling for Surgical Research?

Most early surgical advances were made by astute clinical researchers in the operating room or at the bedside. In this early era of surgical research, Halsted described the hospital as the "surgeon's laboratory."[1] Practical and ethical limitations on the use of the bedside "laboratory" and the human as the subject of the experiment led in the early portion of the twentieth century to the use of animal models for developing surgical techniques, defining physiologic responses, and testing new interventions.

Just as the limitations in bedside research drove surgical researchers to seek animal model alternatives, limitations in using animal models have driven surgeons to seek another avenue to advance their art and science. Some notable disadvantages of using animal models include differences in anatomy and physiology,[2,3] rising costs for purchase and care, and increasing interference from animal rights activists.[4,5]

Computer models offer the new generation of surgical researchers advantages similar to those that bedside researchers found in animal models and much more. Computer modeling offers the surgical researcher opportunities only dreamed of in animal models. Computer models allow the study of the function of precisely isolated systems, with all unwanted systems removed. In addition, computer models allow an isolated system to be integrated into a new environment and then be evaluated as to how the system will function under new conditions. The same isolated or integrated system can be tested time and again without fatigue or variability, or, if desired, the effects of fatigue and variance may be included and further examined. The rapid evolution of the computer and software industries makes computer modeling an exciting scientific tool, with nearly unlimited potential for surgical investigators.

Origins of Computer Models

Computer modeling has been applied to a variety of problems in industry, including aerospace,[6–9] sail design,[10] and parachute design,[11] as well as piping and fluid transport.[12,13] The common factor in these diverse industries is the need to evaluate the interaction of complex dynamic systems. Computer modeling has been applied to these systems to evaluate and solve problems, as well as to design new products. The most striking use for computer modeling for newly designed products was demonstrated by the aerospace industry. The Boeing 777, recently produced and flown commercially, was designed and tested solely using computers.[14,15] No actual prototypes were tested in a wind tunnel, and all preconstruction testing, including test flights, was simulated before manufacturing was begun.

Although not initially embraced by the medical field, computer analysis and modeling have expanded from aerospace and other industries into some areas of medicine. Medical imaging is one field in which computer use has been the major factor in advancing the state of the art. Computerized tomography (CT) scan systems, magnetic resonance imaging (MRI), and echocardiography all rely heavily on computer manipulation of data.

Applications of Computer Models in Surgery

Computer modeling can be applied to advance the state of the art of surgical education using demonstration, hands-on simulation, or teaching through questions and answers. In basic research, models may be used to verify hypotheses or to determine whether additional tests will further elucidate the mechanisms of the system under study. In clinical applications, models may be utilized for making diagnoses, to aid in the testing of newly proposed surgical or medical interventions, or to evaluate prostheses or pharmaceutical regimens.

Types of Models

There are several different types of computer models, including anatomic models, mathematic representations, and finite element models. The choice of which model to use depends on time, money, expertise, and software, as well as the outcome and accuracy desired.

Anatomic Models

Anatomic computer models, the most basic and appealing of the computer models, are well suited to educational applications.[16] They are essentially graphical representations of three-dimensional objects. The three-dimensional data points that represent the surface or volume of the object are stored in the computer, and a two-dimensional

view is displayed on the screen. Computer graphics allow shading and other methods that make the object appear to be three-dimensional, and the objects may be rotated, sectioned, and so forth, just as if they were physically real. Models of the brain,[17-20] thoracic viscera,[21,22] hand,[23] knee,[24] and human fetus[25] have been generated. Several groups are committed to the development of combined models that represent all anatomic regions in the human body.[26,27] These types of anatomic models are used extensively in the field of virtual reality[28,29] and are presently used more for surgical education than for surgical research.

Mathematic Representations

Mathematical computer models are the most familiar of the three computer model types for most surgical researchers. Mathematical modeling is suited to both basic research and clinical applications. A mathematical model of a physiologic system provides a description of the system in terms of sets of equations. The equations are usually differential and constructed to describe the mechanics and dynamics of the system. The complexity of these differential equation sets usually dictates the use of computers and numerical analysis software. In addition to modeling the behavior of physiologic systems, mathematic representations have been used for population studies, such as evaluating outcome variables,[30-32] for predicting risk of surgery,[33,34] and recently for evaluating cost-effectiveness.[35]

Finite Element Models

The most complex but versatile type of computer modeling is finite element modeling. This type of model represents an advanced level, combining both anatomic and mathematic modeling, and involves very large sets of complex differential equations. This method was originally developed in the aerospace industry and recently has been applied to surgical problems. Finite element modeling can be used for education, research, or clinical applications and serves as an excellent example for describing the ways in which computer modeling can be applied in surgical research.

Finite Element Method

Rationale

To solve very complex physical or physiologic problems, the finite element method takes a complicated problem and subdivides it into many simpler ones. Each simple problem can then be defined by a solvable mathematical relationship. The solutions to each small problem are then combined to obtain an answer that approximates how the whole complicated structure will behave. In finite element terms, this means that a structure is divided into small areas or volumes (elements) fitted to the natural geometry. These elements are connected at common points (nodes). The result is the recreation of the whole structure from smaller mathematically defined parts. Since all biological structures are subject to a changing environment, the laws that control this environment must be identified in the model. The physical laws that determine force and movement due to applied loads or physical movement are specified. Based on applied loading, the resulting deformation and stresses at each node can then be calculated and displayed, in either table or graphical form. This process allows analysis of large or complex structures that are subjected to complex loading or environmental fluctuations. Many different variables can be evaluated separately or in combination, depending on the local and global effect each variable has on the structure.

Finite element analysis was first developed to solve engineering problems. The surgical problems that most readily lend themselves to this type of analysis are those involving elements of engineering, such as solid mechanics, fluid dynamics, heat transfer, electromagnetics, steric alteration, and surface interaction. Since surgical research has a long and integral history with applied engineering, there has been a natural cross-fertilization between the two fields, and finite element modeling has been applied to many surgical problems that involve engineering. In the solid mechanics area, diverse surgical issues have been evaluated, such as prosthetic hip replacement,[36,37] lithotripsy,[38] and prosthetic heart valve replacement.[39-42] In fluid mechanics, the finite element processes that were originally applied for pipe analysis have been utilized to examine blood flow in arteries[43-45] and blood flow around heart valves.[46-49] In heat transfer, problems relating to burn injury,[50-52] radiofrequency ablation,[53,54] and laser[55] have been analyzed. Electromagnetic analyses have recently been used to examine and optimize defibrillation protocols[56-58] and microwave injury and treatment.[59,60] Steric alteration and surface interaction have been used to analyze protein function.[61]

The creation of a finite element model in each of these areas follows a stepwise course. First, the system components are defined, the model geometry is established, the material properties are assigned, and the simplifying assumptions are identified. The appropriate element types are then applied to the geometry. Next, the boundary and initial conditions are established, loading and displacements are prescribed, and the solution method is chosen. After solution, the output variables of interest are identified, and the results are evaluated. Finally, the model is verified and the limitations acknowledged.

This process can be illustrated using an example of its application to cardiac surgery. For the past 10 to 15 years, cardiac surgeons throughout the world have embraced mitral valve repair as a superior alternative treatment to mitral valve replacement.[62-64] Chordal manipulation is an essential element of mitral valve repair. Many reparative techniques that alter the native tissue, including chordal shortening, transfer, excision, and fenestration, have been described.[65] However, one of the limitations of mitral valve repair arises when there is inadequate chordal tissue available for repair. In these cases, the replacement of ruptured or elongated chordae with polytetra fluoroethylene (ePTFE) suture is being advocated by many surgeons. This technique has been described in experimental animals,[66-68] as well as used clinically.[69,70] This represents a complex clinical problem that is especially difficult to evaluate experimentally. It does not lend itself readily to an animal model. However, the determination of whether chordal replacement with ePTFE suture is an appropriate and durable surgical maneuver is an excellent example for demonstrating the application of finite element analysis to a surgical problem.

Process

Define System Components

To begin a finite element model, it is first necessary to select the physical components essential to the model. For example, the physical components for parachute analysis are relatively straightforward and consist of the canopy and the shrouds. Conversely, in studying the mitral valve, the physical components are more complex. The primary components are the annulus, leaflets, chordae tendineae, and papillary muscles (Figure 50-1). In addition, one could consider including the physical environment of the mitral valve, which would include atrial and ventricular muscle, as well as the blood within the chambers. Including all of these components makes for an extremely complex analysis. One of the first decisions to make is what level of complexity is necessary and appropriate to answer the questions posed. As model complexity increases, so does the necessary degree of computer sophistication and computational time. For the mitral valve problem, a somewhat simplified system was chosen that would reduce computational time but still ade-

quately answer the questions posed. This simplified system included the primary physical components (annulus, leaflets, chordae tendineae, and papillary muscles), for which the geometry was then defined.

Model Geometry

The geometry for finite element models can be defined in many ways. A fluid transport model may require only the diameter and length of the conduit used. In a hip prosthetic replacement model, more complex information is required, including length, diameter, angles, thickness, and taper. How these data are obtained for each model varies with the complexity of the geometry. Geometry for the more complex biologic models is more difficult to obtain but can be determined from physical specimens in several different ways.

Classically, physical specimens have been fixed by freezing, cast with plastic resins, or immobilized by other methods, and then thinly sectioned. Next, the dimensional coordinates for the anatomical cross sections are meticulously determined by overlaying grids, digitizing the outlines, or using computerized image analysis. Since there is no clinically applicable technique that presently yields sufficiently detailed data to recreate the geometry of the mitral valve for a finite element model, this classic technique was used. The coordinates obtained were used to reconstruct the valve structure (leaflets and chordae) as a static three-dimensional computer representation (Figure 50-2). ANSYS structural analysis software was used (Swanson, Inc., Houston, Penn., Version 4.4a) using a DEC station 5000/200 (Digital Equipment Corporation, Bellevue, Wash.).

To assess the efficacy of ePTFE suture replacement for ruptured posterior chordae tendineae, three mitral models with differing geometry were required. The three models are termed normal,[71] chordal rupture,[72] and ePTFE replacement. The normal model was defined with all anatomic structures intact. Chordal rupture was simulated by removing four marginal and four basal chordae from the central portion of the posterior leaflet. ePTFE replacement was simulated by replacing the ruptured chordae with two 2-0 ePTFE sutures.

This classical approach of sectioning physical specimens is tedious, time-consuming, and the

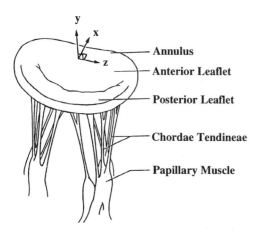

Figure 50-1. Mitral valve structure. The primary components of the valve are the annulus, anterior and posterior leaflets, chordae, and papillary muscles. The coordinate system for the FEM model is shown in relation to the valve. The x-z plane is in the plane of the annulus, with the positive x-axis directed toward the anterior annulus. The positive y-axis is directed toward the atrium.

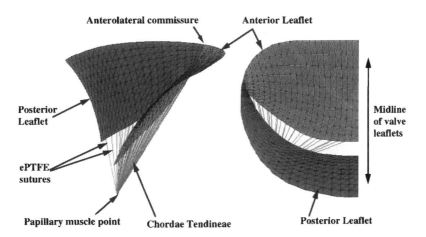

Figure 50-2.   Finite element discretization of the mitral valve system, including placement of ePTFE suture replacements. Only the anterolateral half of the valve was modeled due to symmetry. Panel a shows an oblique view with the commissural area at the top of the panel, and the valve leaflet midlines shown as the slightly curved edges at the bottom half of the panel. Panel b shows a view from the atrium toward the ventricle, with the commissural area on the left and the valve leaflet midlines on the right. Each triangle represents an individual element within the leaflet, and the chordal elements are shown as lines extending from the leaflets to the papillary muscle point.

tissue is destroyed. In the near future, clinical imaging methods may replace this classical approach. Presently, technology is evolving that will allow CT, MR, or transesophageal (TEE) images to be used for automatically creating the three-dimensional geometry coordinates. CT, MR, TEE, and other imaging techniques offer several advantages. These techniques are routinely applied clinically, are nondestructive, and therefore may be applied to living systems. These image formats may be directly applicable for finite element modeling in the near future.

Material Properties

Once the geometry of a structure is established, the physical properties of the structural materials can be assigned. The physical properties of any material, such as steel, rubber, or canvas, can be expressed as numbers (constants), which will numerically describe how the material responds under loads or deformations. For mechanical modeling, the material properties necessary for finite element analysis are Young's modulus, Poisson's ratio, and density. Young's modulus is a measure of the force necessary to produce a certain elon-

gation of a specimen (Figure 50-3). Specifically, one can plot the stress (force/cross-sectional area) versus the strain (change in length/original length) to identify the representative stress-strain curve for the material (Figure 50-4). The slope of this curve is the Young's modulus. Poisson's ratio is a measure of how much the material will contract in one direction, if there is a tensile force in a perpendicular direction. Density is a measure of the mass per volume of the material and becomes important in applications that involve dynamic forces and movement. In other applications, such as fluids analysis, parameters such as fluid density and viscosity are the material properties of interest. In electromagnetic applications, conductivity and resistivity are important. Parameters such as Young's modulus, Poisson's ratio, and viscosity are highly measurable by many techniques and are essential to the construction of a finite element model.

For the mitral valve model, it was necessary to obtain the material properties for the leaflets and chordae tendineae tissue. These tissues are complex structures composed of several components (collagen, elastin, and glycosaminoglycans). For the purposes of this model, the material properties

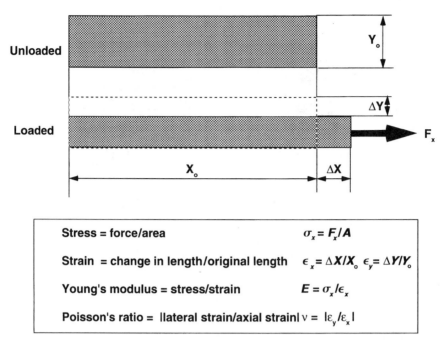

$$\sigma_x = F_x / A$$

Stress = force/area

Strain = change in length/original length $\epsilon_x = \Delta X / X_o \quad \epsilon_y = \Delta Y / Y_o$

Young's modulus = stress/strain $E = \sigma_x / \epsilon_x$

Poisson's ratio = |lateral strain/axial strain| $\nu = |\epsilon_y / \epsilon_x|$

Figure 50-3.   Graphic representation of a beam under a tension force F. A represents the cross-sectional area of the beam. The mathematical definitions of stress, strain, Young's modulus, and Poisson's ratio are given.

of the leaflet or chordal tissue as a whole were determined. The Young's moduli for the leaflets and chordae were determined by calculating the slope of the stress-strain curves for leaflet and chordal tissue.[73,74] Mitral valve tissue, like most biologic tissues, is nearly incompressible due to the high water content. This characteristic would be represented by a Poisson's ratio of 0.5, indicating that the volume remains constant regardless of the loading. However, most finite element programs will not accept a value of 0.5 for this parameter because of computational requirements, and thus it must be approximated as 0.45. Finally, the density of the tissue is nearly that of water, 1.04 g/cm³, which could be directly assigned to the model. Blood density must also be considered; since the density of the blood was not explicitly included in the model, it can be implicitly included by making a simplifying assumption that incorporates it in the density of the tissue.

Simplifying Assumptions

To solve problems involving complex geometry, nonlinear material properties, or time-dependent loading in a reasonable period of time, computer modeling requires that simplifying assumptions be made. First, complex geometry may be simplified by identifying planes of symmetry within the structure, with the assumption that the same outcome is mirrored on the other side of the plane. Second, if the material properties are nonlinear, it is important to determine the range of function on the stress-strain curve for the model. Third, if there is time-dependent loading, loading rate and material density must be considered. These assumptions, if correctly made, may significantly reduce computational time.

For the finite element model of the mitral valve, assumptions regarding symmetry, tissue material properties, and time-dependent loading were defined. First, the mitral valve is relatively symmetric about a plane through the anterior and posterior leaflet midlines;[75] this plane of symmetry divides each leaflet into equivalent halves. Accordingly, only half of both leaflets and one papillary muscle were analyzed. Second, the stress-strain curves and resultant material properties are nonlinear for the leaflet and chordal tissue. Based

CHORDAL STRESS/STRAIN SUMMARY
(10 mm/min)

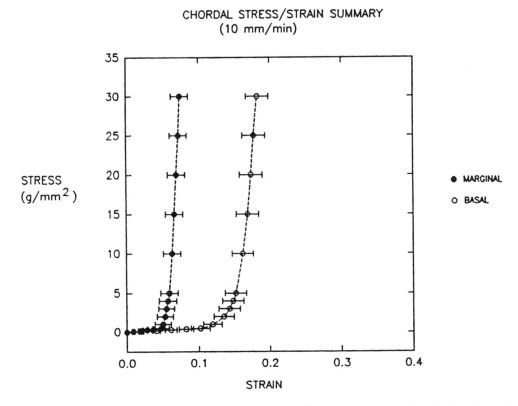

Figure 50-4. Representative stress-strain curve for biological tissue. In general, under low loads there is little resistance to extension. At higher loads, the collagenous fibers in the tissue have become straightened and offer significant resistance to extension. This resistance results in a typical two-phase curve (pretransition and posttransition phases).

on physiologic data, it was assumed that the tissue functions on the second half (or posttransition part) of the curve during systole. Therefore the Young's moduli assigned for the model were the slopes of the posttransition part of the curve. Third, the pressure loading in the mitral valve system is time dependent, and, as such, loading rate and material density were considered. The loading rate was assumed to be decreased by three orders of magnitude because if the actual rate were used, the number of substeps necessary to solve the mathematical equations would be enormous. Next, since motion of the leaflets results from the pressure forces applied to the leaflet mass, the tissue density was considered. The density of the blood was implicitly included by incorporating it in the density of the tissue. Therefore, an effective leaflet and chordal mass density of 10.4 g/cm³ was assigned, which is ten times that of the actual tis-

sue. By increasing the density, the leaflets themselves would have the necessary increased inertia to resist dynamic motion. This technique has been used in aortic valve models.[76]

Elemental Representations

Once the model geometry and appropriate assumptions are defined, the types of elements that will be used to represent the structure may be chosen. The geometry of the system is subdivided into a mesh of finite elements. For linear objects, the elements are generally rod or cable elements. For surfaces or relatively thin membranous structures, the elements might consist of triangular or quadrilateral shell elements. For solid objects, pyramidal or cubic solid elements could be used. The choice of element type and shape depends on what is most appropriate for the part of the model to be represented.

Mitral valve components were represented by several different types of elements. The anterior and posterior leaflets were represented by a mesh of triangular thin-shell elements. The marginal and basal chordae and ePTFE sutures were represented by two-noded, tension-only cable elements. The papillary muscle was represented by a single node (with no associated physical or material properties). Finally, the physical barrier at the coapting surface of the anterior and posterior leaflets was represented by two-noded, three-dimensional interface elements.

Boundary and Initial Conditions

Once the components are defined, the geometry established, and the material properties assigned, the environmental surroundings of the model can be considered. Boundary and initial conditions both concern environmental factors such as pressure, physical location, and temperature. The difference is that boundary conditions remain constant throughout time, whereas initial conditions are specified at a single time point before any loading of the model.

For the mitral valve, many boundary conditions are necessary to simulate normal physical restraints. For example, at the annular attachments of the leaflets, a hinge condition was established, allowing the leaflets to rotate. As another example, basal and marginal chordae tendineae were freely hinged at the sites of attachment to the leaflets and papillary muscles. There were many other boundary conditions necessary to fully simulate the environmental conditions. There was only one initial condition necessary for this model, which was a low static pressure (0.001 mN/mm²). This was necessary to smooth out the initial finite element mesh before physiologic loading was applied.

Loading and Displacement

Once the constants of boundary and initial conditions are established, the changing environmental conditions such as load and displacement are identified. Loads may be represented by pressures, forces, temperature gradients, fluid flows, magnetic fields, or other variables. The magnitude of the loads and the time over which the loads are applied must be explicitly defined. Displacements must be defined by prescribing certain nodes to move from point to point or rotation about a certain axis.

In the mitral valve model, pressure loads were applied to simulate the isovolumic contraction and rapid ventricular ejection phases of the cardiac cycle (Figure 50-5). Isovolumic contraction was simulated by a linear pressure relationship, rising from 0 to 80 mm Hg over a 70-ms period. However, rapid ventricular ejection was simulated by a sinusoidal relationship from $t = 71$ to 250 ms.[77] As described previously, the rate of loading was assumed to slow by three orders of magnitude.

Displacement conditions were then defined to simulate annular and papillary muscle contraction. The posterior annular nodes were defined to move within the annular plane in a direction normal to the local curvature such that the total decrease in posterior annular length was 8%.[78] The papillary muscle was defined to shorten 16.4% from an initial length of 10 mm during the systolic interval.[79–81]

Solution Method

At this point, all of the known factors, including geometry, material properties, boundary and initial conditions, and loads and displacements, have

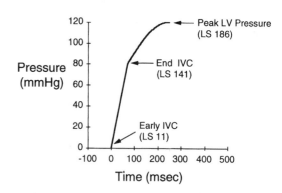

Figure 50-5.   Pressure-time relationship used in the loading of the finite element mechanical model of the mitral valve.

been established. Now the equations that describe the physiologic system may be solved for the unknowns, which are the resultant displacements, stresses, and strains. Appropriate solution methods will vary depending on the types of elements in the model and particularly on the time dependency of the loading. Quite often, the loading must be broken down into many substeps, with multiple iterations necessary to obtain convergence to a stable, accurate solution.

For the mitral valve model, several factors dictate what type of solution method is necessary. First, several element types in the model have nonlinear behavior. For example, the chordal elements will not resist compression but will resist extension under tension. Second, the pressure loading is time dependent, and the solution method must take into account the transient nature of the pressure and solve at multiple load steps as if the model were in equilibrium at each step. Therefore, a nonlinear transient equilibrium analysis was necessary.

Outcome Variables

Due to the complexity of the systems modeled, the multiple variables considered, and the mathematical sophistication required, the amount of data generated by a finite element solution may be overwhelming. When planning and using finite element models, it is important to choose the output variables that are of greatest relevance to the problem at hand. These variables could include motion of the system components, stress or strain in particular parts of the system, fluid flow patterns, or developed pressures. In addition, the crucial time points for analysis must be chosen carefully to avoid excessive data collection or memory overload.

Displacement, stress, and strain were recorded for the leaflets, chordae, and suture replacements in each mitral valve model. Of the 186 time points that could have been chosen for analysis, three time points were identified as the most crucial. These were early in isovolumic contraction, end of isovolumic contraction, and peak loading. In addition, the time to leaflet closure was observed, as well as the degree of leaflet coaptation.

Evaluate Results

The results may be evaluated as raw numerical data, X-ray graphs, or three-dimensional representations. Since many models are complex geometric entities, it is often most informative to view the results as a three-dimensional representation in which the deformed geometry can be rotated to be viewed from any direction. The use of color coding for stress or strain values in the model greatly simplifies the interpretation of vast amounts of numerical data. Once the method for examining the results is chosen, it is absolutely critical to assess whether the results are reasonable in terms of physical reality or known data from other sources.

For the mitral valve, both three-dimensional representation and x-y plotting were necessary for appropriate evaluation. The three-dimensional representations, particularly with color contours, aided with interpretation of stress distribution differences in the normal, chordal rupture, and ePTFE models. In the normal mitral valve model (Figure 50-6a), it was found that the anterior leaflet was subject to tensile stress in all directions, with the highest levels at the commissure. This is consistent with the presence of the fibrous trigone, which is capable of carrying high loads because of its collagenous makeup. Interestingly, the posterior leaflet was subject to much lower levels of tensile stress. In the circumferential direction the posterior leaflet was actually subject to compressive stresses, resulting in buckling or folding of the tissue. This is consistent with the buckled appearance of the posterior leaflet under normal conditions. In the normal valve model at peak loading, the leaflets were fully coapted and the edges of the anterior and posterior leaflet were even.

In the chordal rupture model, the stress distribution in the leaflets was surprisingly similar to the normal model. However, there was a notable change in the region where the marginal and basal chordae were removed. In that region, the posterior leaflet edge was unrestricted and prolapsed toward the atrium (Figure 50-6b). As a result, there were stress concentrations at the attachment points of the adjacent remaining chordae.

In the ePTFE chordal replacement model, the prolapse of the rupture model was corrected (Figure 50-6c) and the leaflet stress patterns were re-

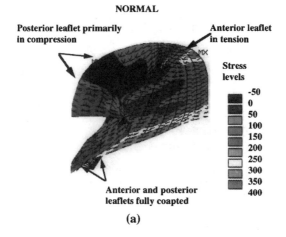

NORMAL

Posterior leaflet primarily in compression

Anterior leaflet in tension

Stress levels

-50
0
50
100
150
200
250
300
350
400

Anterior and posterior leaflets fully coapted

(a)

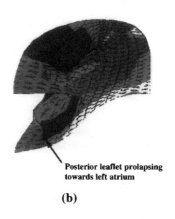

CHORDAL RUPTURE

Posterior leaflet prolapsing towards left atrium

(b)

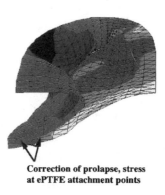

ePTFE REPLACEMENT

Correction of prolapse, stress at ePTFE attachment points

(c)

Figure 50-6.   Contours of maximum principal stress for the mitral valve models at peak loading (oblique view of the valve, indicating the change in leaflet position with respect to the annulus). The color key indicates the stress level, where negative numbers indicate compressive stress and positive numbers indicate tensile stress. (a) Normal model, (b) chordal rupture model demonstrating posterior prolapse, (c) ePTFE replacement model demonstrating correction of prolapse.

turned to a state similar to that of the normal model. However, at the area of suture attachment to the leaflet, stress concentrations were evident, particularly at the suture closest to the midline, which does not have natural chordae adjacent to it.

To analyze chordal stress, x-y plotting proved most beneficial. In the normal model, it was observed that the stress in the anterior chordae was greater than in the posterior chordae (Figures 50-7a and 50-8a), consistent with the higher anterior leaflet stress. In addition, the peak stress was at the location where the "strut" chordae are located. The strut chordae are specialized chordae noted to be thicker than the other chordae and would be suited to carry the higher stress.

In the posterior chordal rupture model, the stress distribution in the anterior chordae (Figure 50-7b) was not significantly altered. However, for the posterior chordae, where the first four marginal and basal chordae were removed, the stress was elevated in the chordae immediately adjacent to the rupture site (Figure 50-8b).

Finally, in the posterior ePTFE suture replace-ment model, the stress distribution in the anterior chordae (Figure 50-7c) was similar to the normal and chordal rupture model. Not surprisingly, the stress elevation seen in the posterior chordae in the rupture model was significantly reduced with ePTFE replacement and a large amount of the stress was carried by the suture (Figure 50–8c).

Model Verification

Finite element models, like all experimental models, must be validated.[82] Unfortunately, it is often almost impossible to measure the outcome variables in the biological system directly, and it is difficult to validate them directly. It is for this very reason that some models have been created. Nevertheless, it is essential to attempt to verify the results. For finite element models, verification can be accomplished by either analysis of data from the biological system or comparison to *closed-form* solutions. Closed-form solutions are mathematical equations that can be directly solved for simpler known geometry and loading, without the

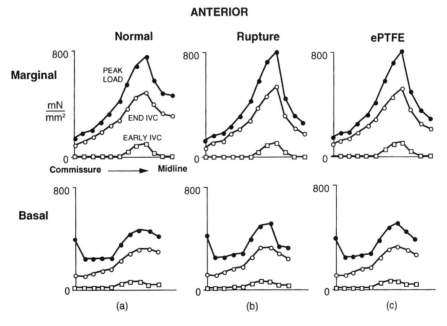

Figure 50-7. Stress levels in the anterior mitral valve chordae at three intervals: early in the loading cycle, end isovolumic contraction, and peak loading. Individual chordae are represented along the x-axis, from commissure to midline: (a) normal model, (b) chordal rupture model, (c) ePTFE replacement model.

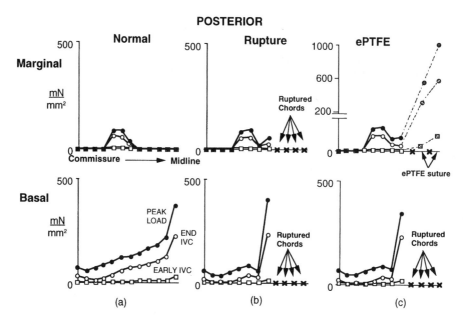

Figure 50-8. Stress levels in the posterior mitral valve chordae at three intervals (early in the loading cycle, and isovolumic contraction, and peak loading): (a) normal model, (b) chordal rupture model, (c) ePTFE replacement model.

iterative numerical approximations utilized by the finite element method.

As an illustration of the dilemma of model verification, the overall stress distribution on the mitral valve components in vivo is not available for comparison to the predicted results. Even though our finite element mesh was based on the actual three-dimensional geometry and the anisotropic material properties, it is not guaranteed that the resulting stress distribution represents the actual in vivo magnitudes. It is unlikely that we will ever be able to measure the entire stress pattern for all components in the in vivo valve, because the presence of instrumentation required to do so would severely distort the natural patterns. Some less direct comparisons can be made between the finite element models and the in vivo valve. For instance, the predicted leaflet deformations at 120 mm Hg were consistent with that seen in porcine specimens that were resin fixed at the same pressure. The stress patterns calculated for the leaflets were consistent with the collagen fiber orientation observed in natural specimens. The predicted stress and strain values did not exceed any of the tissue-failure stress levels for either leaflet or

chordal tissue. Finally, the predicted chordal stress was consistent with that measured for in vivo specimens. For purely mathematical verification, individual components (leaflet and chordal tissue) were modeled separately with simple geometry and loading, and the predicted results were exactly as calculated from closed-form solutions.

Limitations

Since all finite element models of biological systems require simplifying assumptions, some limitations result. It is essential to acknowledge these limitations and to justify the assumptions made in developing the model.

Although several assumptions in the mitral valve model result in limitations, the assumptions can be justified based on the questions the model was designed to answer. For example, the valve was assumed to be symmetric about the midplane and only half of the valve was analyzed. The limitation is that asymmetric pathologic conditions cannot be analyzed with this particular model. However, this model was designed to analyze techniques of repair in which asymmetry is not an issue. As another example, only the posttransition material properties were considered for this model. This choice limits the analysis to the systolic period of loading. However, the posttransition period is when the greatest stress values will be encountered, which is critical to repair techniques.

Resources Required

Computer modeling is a tremendously valuable tool now available to surgical research. Appropriate application requires careful selection of the model's type and construction. Many choices and assumptions must be made to attain the maximal benefit in a reasonable time frame. The resources necessary for computer modeling are available in various forms to almost all surgical researchers.

The choice of which type of model to use depends on the application, as well as on the available time, money, expertise, software, and accuracy desired. There are unavoidable tradeoffs between these issues, particularly of time, money, and expertise. Most surgical researchers have expertise in medicine, not engineering or computer programming: It may be unrealistic for one individual to attempt to master all the principles and practices of medicine, engineering, and mathematics that are needed to generate complex computer models. Outside consulting firms specialize in such modeling. This service is generally quite expensive; thus, collaboration is essential. At most academic medical centers, it is often possible to form a working alliance among surgeons, engineers, and computer specialists to tackle the surgical problems that can be addressed with computer models. In addition, it is often valuable to obtain input from disciplines such as physiology and anatomy, biochemistry and biophysics, instrumentation and measurement, and applied mathematics.

Once the appropriate collaboration is formed, the necessary software and desired accuracy of the model can be considered. For example, most commercially available finite element software packages were originally designed for industrial applications; some can be adapted relatively easily for physiologic analysis, others cannot. Certain software packages are directly suited for mechanical analysis, while others are designed for fluid flow. Some handle nonlinear problems better than others. Compatibility among software packages for combined analyses is limited and specific. These issues must be kept in mind when choosing software. In some cases, it may be necessary to have specific code written for a particular problem that cannot be handled by the commercially available software. Due to the intense computational requirements, most of the commercially available packages run best on workstations. PCs may be used, but the interactive and solution run times may be extremely high (days), as opposed to on workstations (hours) or supercomputers (hours or minutes).

Future Applications

The ability of finite element modeling to electronically reproduce complex systems and integrate vast amounts of data make it an exciting and powerful tool for future research. The potential exists for significantly increased sophistication, and there are many new areas of possible application.

As an example of increased sophistication, models of heart valves and surgical repair may lead to on-line tools for planning of clinical interventions. The resolution of clinically available noninvasive testing continues to increase, and soon we will be able to accurately define geometry for an individual patient's valve. As finite element software continues to improve and computational times are reduced, the time required for solution of complex analyses may be reduced to a matter of minutes. Envision the cardiologist with the ability to obtain three-dimensional echo images and translate those exact images as coordinates for the finite element model. Next, the surgeon will simulate the proposed surgical repair, akin to a high-tech video game. The model will take into account all of the variables, including the specific disease process in the tissue, surgical alterations, and any prosthetic material planned for implantation. The model will determine whether the repair corrects the physiologic problem and whether the new stress distribution for the repaired valve is optimal. In the highest evolution, the computer model could advise the surgeon in particular cases whether replacement may be more advantageous than repair or whether surgical intervention should be delayed if risks such as reoperation or anticoagulation are considered to outweigh the benefits of the intervention.

Another futuristic application of finite element modeling will be in the area of surgical simulation for education and training. Presently, anatomic models exist for training for particular surgical interventions, such as video-assisted thoracoscopic surgery. As virtual reality technology improves and is combined with the finite element method, the ability to critically evaluate surgical procedures will be significantly enhanced. The ability to teach the surgical decision-making processes that historically have been conducted primarily by trial and error will be a major use for these tools.

As cellular biologists push back the frontier of intercellular and intracellular interactions, there will be increased demand for means of analyzing the rapidly occurring events in an infinitesimally small and delicate environment. Computer modeling, particularly finite element modeling, offers an optimal tool for analysis of this type of system. As the cell and its myriad roles are unraveled, researchers will want to consider biochemical interactions, temperature regulation, steric alterations, flow dynamics, and much more. The complexity of these issues could be staggering without carefully chosen and well-orchestrated computer models.

The use of computer models as on-line tools for planning surgical intervention, or for shedding light on the behavior of currently unseeable microsystems, may appear to border on the realm of science fiction. However, the reality of the technology explosion combined with the phenomenal growth in computer science implies that what is science fiction today could be clinical practice tomorrow. Computer-aided DNA analysis continues to reveal, characterize, and record the sequences rapidly; it is estimated that the entire human genome may be logged by the turn of the century. With this knowledge, more and more disease processes are being defined as genetic mutations, either inherited or of a spontaneous nature. The ability to manipulate or reverse these defects will certainly require computer models,

rather than human or animal models, for temporal, fiscal, and ethical reasons.

The evidence is compelling that computer modeling is the future of surgical research. It is imperative that all surgical researchers, present and future, become familiar with the techniques, the technology, and the applications. Few surgical research projects today could not benefit from the addition of some form of computer modeling. A literature search of MEDLINE articles since 1990 using the key words *finite element* produced 675 references. As we enter the next millennium, a surgical scientist will rarely be without ease in the art and science of computer modeling. With increasing patient awareness and sensitivity regarding clinical research, with animal costs escalating and animal rights activism high, and with the complexity of surgical questions continually growing, the natural progression will be the union of surgical research and computer modeling. Were Halstead to practice at the turn of the twenty-first century, he would perhaps change his famous quote to "your hard drive is your laboratory."

References

1. MacCallum WG. William Stewart Halsted, Surgeon. Baltimore: The Johns Hopkins Press, 1930.
2. Renegar KB. Influenza virus infections and immunity: a review of human and animal models. Lab Anim Sci 1992;42:222–232.
3. Report of a WHO informal consultation on animal models for evaluation of drugs and vaccines for HIV infection and AIDS. Biologicals 1990;18: 225–233.
4. Johnston C. Researchers, animal rights activists fight public relations war at Western. Can Med Assoc J 1993;148:1349–1353.
5. Erickson D. Blood feud—researchers begin fighting back against animal-rights activists. Sci Am 1990;262:17–18.
6. Crytser T, Nandi G, Hinman-Sweeney EM, Dwivedi SN, Tobbe PA, Lyons DW. Finite element design of manipulator-coupled spacecraft for a research testbed. J Intellig Robotic Sys 1995; 13:75–91.
7. Ross DC, Volakis JL, Anastassiu HT. Hybrid finite element-modal analysis of jet engine inlet scattering. IEEE Trans Ant Prop 1995;43:277–285.

8. Chuban VD, Kudryashov AB. 'Integral' finite elements for designing the strong frames of highly maneuverable airplanes. Comput Struct 1994;53: 473–483.

9. Prudhomme SM, Haj-Hariri H. Investigation of supersonic underexpanded jets using adaptive unstructured finite elements. Finite Elements Anal Design 1994;17:21–40.

10. Hansen J. The demystification of flow and membrane: North's computer design system. North News, Winter 1986–1987, pp. 5–8. North Sails Group, Milford, Conn., 1986.

11. Mullins WM, Reynolds DT. Stress analysis of parachutes using finite elements. J Spacecraft 1971; 8:1068–1073.

12. Roidt RM, Kim JH. Analytical and experimental studies of a stratified flow in a pipe. In: Courtland M, Delhaye JM, eds. Sixth International Topical Meeting on Nuclear Reactor Thermal Hydraulics, vol. 1. Grenoble, France: Commissariat a l'Energie Atomique, 1993, pp. 541–547.

13. Frid A. Fluid vibration in piping systems: a structural mechanics approach. I. Theory. J Sound Vibration 1989;133:23–38.

14. Lapin M. Boeing brings the skies inside. Test Meas World 1995;15:53–58.

15. Riter R. Modeling and testing a critical fault-tolerant multi-process system. Boeing Commercial Airplanes, Seattle, Wash. Digest of Papers: Twenty-Fifth International Symposium on Fault-Tolerant Computing. Los Alamitos, Calif.: IEEE Computing Society, 1995, pp. 516–521.

16. Rosse C. The potential of computerized representations of anatomy in the training of health care providers. Acad Med 1995;70:499–505.

17. Narayan S, Sensharma D, Sontori EM, Lee AA, Sabherwal A, Toga AW. Animated visualization of a high resolution color three-dimensional digital computer model of the whole human head. Int J Biomed Comput 1993;32:7–17.

18. Zachman HH. Interpretation of cranial MR images using a digital atlas of the human head. In: Lemke HU, ed. Proceedings of the International Symposium on Computer Assisted Radiology. Berlin: Springer-Verlag, 1991, pp. 191–198.

19. Grietz T, Bohm C, Holte S, Eriksson L. A computerized brain atlas: construction, anatomical content, and some applications. J Comput Assist Tomogr 1991;15:26–38.

20. Lemoine D, Barillot C, Gibaud G, Posqualini E. An anatomical based 3-D registration system of multimodality and atlas data in neurosurgery. In: Colchester ACF, Hawkes DJ, eds. Proceedings of the 12th International Conference on Information Processing in Medical Imaging. Berlin: Springer-Verlag, 1991, pp. 154–164.

21. Conley DM, Kastella KG, Sundsten JW, et al. Computer generated three-dimensional reconstruction of the mediastinum correlated with sectional and radiological anatomy. Clin Anat 1992;5: 185–202.

22. Conley D, Rosse C. Animation of thoracic viscera (Digital Anatomist Series videodisc). Seattle: University of Washington Health Sciences Center for Educational Resources, 1994.

23. Meals RA, Kabo JM. Computerized anatomy instruction. Clin Plastic Sur 1986;13:379–397.

24. Ratiu P, Rosse C. 3-D animation of knee anatomy (Digital Anatomist Series CD-ROM). Seattle: University of Washington Health Sciences Center for Educational Resources, 1994.

25. Richter E, Kramer H, Lierse W, Maas R, Hohne KH. Visualization of neonatal anatomy and pathology with a new computerized three-dimensional model as a basis for teaching, diagnosis, and therapy. Acta Anat 1994;150:75–79.

26. Ackerman MF. The visible human project of the National Library of Medicine. In: Degoulet P, Remme TE, Rienhoff O, eds. MEDINFOR 92: Proceedings of the Seventh World Congress on Medical Informatics. Amsterdam, The Netherlands: North Holland Elsevier Science Publications, 1992, pp 366–378.

27. Rosse C. Anatomical knowledge sources for enhancing applications of the UMLS. National Library of Medicine Contract NO1-LM-4-3546, 1994.

28. Satava RM. Emerging medical applications of virtual reality: a surgeon's perspective. Artif Intell Med 1994; 6:281–288.

29. Merril J, Allman S, Merril G, Roy R. Virtual heart surgery: trade show and medical education. Virtual Reality World 1994;2:55–57.

30. Miles BJ, Kattan MW. Computer modeling of prostrate cancer treatment: a paradigm for oncologic management? Surg Oncol Clin N Am 1995; 4:361–373.

31. Chang RWS, Bihari DJ. Outcome prediction for the individual patient in the ICU. Unfallchirurg 1994;97:199–204.

32. Weiss MH, Harrison LB, Isaacs RS. Use of decision analysis in planning a management strategy for the stage NO neck. Arch Otolaryngol Head Neck Surg 1994;120:699–702.

33. Albertsen PC. Computer modeling and decision making: clinical applications in bladder cancer. Sem Urol 1993;3:171–176.

34. Fisher WS. Selection of patients for surgery. Neurosurg Clin N Am 1993;4:35–44.

35. Watcha MF, Smith I. Cost-effectiveness analysis of antemetic therapy for ambulatory surgery. J Clin Anesth 1994;6:370–377.

36. Kang YK, Park HC, Youm Y, Lee IK, Ahn MH, Ihn JC. Three dimensional shape reconstruction and finite element analysis of femur before and after the cementless type of total hip replacement. J Biomed Eng 1993;15:497–504.

37. Verdonschot NJ, Huiskes R, Freeman MA. Preclinical testing of hip prosthetic designs: a comparison of finite element calculations and laboratory tests. Proc Inst Mech Eng [H] 1993;207:149–154.

38. Chuong CJ, Zhong P, Preminger GM. A comparison of stone damage caused by different modes of shock wave generation. J Urol 1992;148:200–205.

39. Krucinski S, Vesely I, Dokainish MA, Campbell G. Numerical simulation of leaflet flexure in bioprosthetic valves mounted on rigid and expansile stents. J Biomech 1993;26:929–943.

40. Black MM, Howard IC, Huang X, Patterson EA. A three-dimensional analysis of a bioprosthetic heart valve. J Biomech 1991;24:793–801.

41. Huang X, Black MM, Howard IC, Patterson EA. A two-dimensional finite element analysis of a bioprosthetic heart valve. J Biomech 1990;23:753–762.

42. Chandran KB, Kim SH, Han G. Stress distribution on the cusps of a polyurethane trileaflet heart valve prosthesis in the closed position. J Biomech 1991;24:385–395.

43. Satcher RL, Bussolari SR, Gimbrone MA, Dewey CF Jr. The distribution of fluid forces on model arterial endothelium using computational fluid dynamics. J Biomech Eng 1992;114:309–316.

44. Lou Z, Yang WJ. A computer simulation of the blood flow at the aortic bifurcation. Biomed Mater Eng 1991;1:173–193.

45. Xu XY, Collins MW. A review of the numerical analysis of blood flow in arterial bifurcations. Proc Inst Mech Eng [H]1990;204:205–216.

46. Dubini G, Pietrabissa R, Fumero R. Computational fluid dynamics of artificial heart valves. Int J Artif Organs 1991;14:338–342.

47. Reif TH. A numerical analysis of the backflow between the leaflets of a St Jude Medical cardiac valve prosthesis. J Biomech 1991;24:733–741.

48. Peskin CS, McQueen DM. Cardiac fluid dynamics. Crit Rev Biomed Eng 1992;20:451–459.

49. McQueen DM, Peskin CS. A three-dimensional computational method for blood flow in the heart. II. Immersed elastic fibers in a viscous incompressible fluid. J Comput Phys 1989;82:289–297.

50. Torvi DA, Dale JD. A finite element model of skin subjected to a flash fire. J Biomech Eng 1994;116:250–255.

51. Tropea BI, Lee RC. Thermal injury kinetics in electrical trauma. J Biomech Eng 1992;114:241–250.

52. Russo G, Kicska G, Lee RC. Effectiveness of surface cooling in reducing heat injury. 3-D finite-element model of the arm. Ann N Y Acad Sci 1994;720:79–91.

53. Shahidi AV, Savard P. A finite element model for radiofrequency ablation of the myocardium. IEEE Trans Biomed Eng 1994;41:963–968.

54. Anderson G, Ye X, Henle K, Yang Z, Li G. A numerical study of rapid heating for high temperature radio frequency hyperthermia. Int J Biomed Comput 1994;35:297–307.

55. Moreira H, Campos M, Sawusch MR, McDonnell JM, Sand B, McDonnell PJ. Holmium laser thermokeratoplasty. Ophthalmology 1993;100:752–761.

56. Panescu D, Webster JG, Stratbucker RA. Modeling current density distributions during transcutaneous cardiac pacing. IEEE Trans Biomed Eng 1994;41:549–555.

57. Jorgenson DB, Haynor DR, Bardy GH, Kim Y. Computational studies of transthoracic and transvenous defibrillation in a detailed 3-D human thorax model. IEEE Trans Biomed Eng 1995;42:172–184.

58. Karlon WJ, Eisenberg SR, Lehr JL. Effects of paddle placement and size on defibrillation current distribution: a three-dimensional finite element model. IEEE Trans Biomed Eng 1993;40:246–255.

59. Oleson J, Samulski T, Clegg S, Das S, Grant W. Heating rate modeling and measurements in phantom and in vivo of the human upper extremity in

a defective 2450 MHz microwave oven. J Microw Power Electromagn Energy 1994;29:101–108.

60. Martin GT, Haddad MG, Cravalho EG, Bowman HF. Thermal model for the local microwave hyperthermia treatment of benign prostatic hyperplasia. IEEE Trans Biomed Eng 1992;39:836–844.

61. Berger RL, Davids N, Perrella M. Simulation of hemoglobin kinetics using finite element numerical methods. Methods Enzymol 1994;232:517–558.

62. Tischler MD, Cooper KA, Rowen M, Le Winter MM. Mitral valve replacement versus mitral valve repair. A Doppler and quantitative stress echocardiographic study. Circulation 1994;89:132–137.

63. Enriquez-Sarano M, Schaff HV, Orszulak TA, Tajik AJ, Bailey KR, Frye RL. Valve repair improves the outcome of surgery for mitral regurgitation. A multivariate analysis. Circulation 1995; 91:1022–1028.

64. Yun KL, Miller DC. Mitral valve repair versus replacement. Cardiol Clin 1991;9:315–327.

65. Carpentier A. Cardiac valve surgery—the "French correction." J Thorac Cardiovasc Surg 1983;86: 323–337.

66. Zussa C, Polesel E, Rocco F, Galloni M, Frater RW, Volfre C. Surgical technique for artificial mitral chordae implantation. J Cardiac Surg 1991; 6:432–438.

67. Vetter HO, Burack JH, Factor SM, Macaluso F, Frater RWM. Replacement of chordae tendineae of the mitral valve using the new expanded PTFE suture in sheep. In: Bodnar E, Yacoub M, eds. Biologic and Bioprosthetic Valves. New York: Yorke Medical Books, 1986, pp. 772–784.

68. Revuelta JM, Garcia-Rinaldi R, Gaite L, Val F, Garijo F. Generation of chordae tendineae with polytetrafluoroethylene stents. J Thorac Cardiovasc Surg 1989;97:98–103.

69. David TE, Bos J, Rakowski H. Mitral valve repair by replacement of chordae tendineae with polytetrafluoroethylene sutures. J Thorac Cardiovasc Surg 1991;101:495–501.

70. Zussa C, Frater RWM, Polesel E, Galloni M, Valfre C. Artificial mitral valve chordae: experimental and clinical experience. Ann Thorac Surg 1990; 50:367–373.

71. Kunzelman KS, Cochran RP, Chuong CJ, Ring WS, Verrier ED, Eberhart RC. Finite element analysis of the mitral valve. J Heart Valve Dis 1993;2:326–340.

72. Kunzelman KS, Cochran RP, Chuong CJ, Ring WS, Verrier ED, Eberhart RC. Finite element analysis of mitral valve pathology. J Long Term Effects Med Implants 1993;3:161–179.

73. Kunzelman KS, Cochran RP. Stress/strain characteristics of porcine mitral valve tissue: parallel versus perpendicular collagen orientation. J Card Surg 1992;7:71–82.

74. Cochran RP, Kunzelman KS. Comparison of the viscoelastic properties of suture versus porcine mitral valve chordae tendineae. J Card Surg 1991;6:508–513.

75. Kunzelman KS, Cochran RP, Verrier ED, Eberhart RC. An anatomic basis for mitral valve modeling. J Heart Valve Dis 1994;3:491–496.

76. Hamid MS, Sabbah HN, Stein PD. Vibrational analysis of bioprosthetic heart valve leaflets using numerical models: effects of leaflet stiffening, calcification, and perforation. Circ Res 1987;61:687–694.

77. Miller GE, Marcotte H. Computer simulation of human mitral valve mechanics and motion: a tool for clarifying mitral valve prolapse. Texas J Sci 1983;35:4–36.

78. Tsakiris AG, von Bernouth G, Rastelli GC, Bourgeois MJ, Titus JL, Wood EH. Size and motion of the mitral valve annulus in anesthetized intact dogs. J Appl Physiol 1971;30:611–618.

79. Burch GE, DePasquale NP. Time course of tension in papillary muscles of the heart: theoretical considerations. JAMA 1965;192:701–704.

80. Grimm AF, Lendrum BL, Lin H. Papillary muscle shortening in the intact dog. Circ Res 1975;36: 49–59.

81. Hirakawa S, Sasayama S, Tomoike H, Crozatier B, Franklin D, McKown D, Ross J Jr. In situ measurement of papillary muscle dynamics in the dog left ventricle. Am J Physiol 1977;233:H384–H391.

82. Sargent RG. Verification and validation of simulation models. In: Celier FE, ed. Progress in Modeling and Simulation. New York: Academic Press, 1982, ch. 9.

Commentary

Drs. Kunzelmann and Cochran have chosen the technique of finite element analysis applied to function of a cardiac valve as a paradigm for computer analysis of an experimental problem. This process can be translated with equal efficacy to the function of cells, balances between synthesis and degradation of specific gene products, or the process of rejection of a transplanted organ. The specific requirements for finite element analysis allow substitution of terms. In some instances the model will become more complex and in others simpler. For example, to model the geometry of a cell may be relatively simple and described as "cuboidal," or it might be extraordinarily complex if one were trying to define the capacity for cell membranes with multiple convolutions to modulate activity as a consequence of surface area exposed at any instant. Boundaries that are described by the author have to do with anatomic structure, whereas boundaries in initial conditions of other systems could be rates, for example, of enzymatic reactions or oxygen consumption. Their approach is not limited to the study of physical properties of a system but should be understood as a broadly applicable approach to biologic and mechanical phenomena.

A.S.W.

CHAPTER 51

The Operating Room as a Laboratory

V. Rao, G.T. Christakis, and R.D. Weisel

The collection and documentation of data from patients undergoing concurrent surgical treatment has been one of the most useful but least used methods of surgical clinical research. The advantages of intraoperative clinical research are obvious, whether it involves a descriptive cohort study or a randomized controlled clinical trial. Clinical application of new surgical techniques increases rapidly following perioperative documentation of their benefits. For example, the use of blood cardioplegia in cardiac surgery at our institution increased from approximately 10% in 1980 to almost 100% in 1995. This increased utilization of blood cardioplegia followed the intraoperative documentation of its metabolic and functional benefits, along with an improvement in morbidity and mortality rates associated with its use.[1]

Although most surgical techniques are first evaluated in the laboratory, only the availability of clinical information allows for their widespread adoption. For example, extended tracheal resections were performed for years in the dog laboratory, but Grillo[2] and Pearson[3] needed to validate these observations in patients to popularize the current surgical techniques for tracheal resection.

The relative paucity of interventional surgical clinical research, especially intraoperative experimentation, is likely a result of the extraordinary organizational skills required for intraoperative experimentation.

Organization of a clinical research program necessitates a logical stepwise progression beginning with identification of clinical problems to be studied, formulation of mechanisms and hypotheses to explain clinical observations, construction of an experimental protocol to address the hypotheses, evaluation of the experimental protocol on both scientific and ethical grounds, and finally an appropriate statistical analysis of the experimental data to accept or reject the initial hypotheses.

Identification of Clinical Problems

All experiments must begin with clear identification of a clinical outcome or problem that is clinically or scientifically significant enough to warrant the interest of other surgeons and scientists and that may improve the understanding of a disease process or patient problem. The clinical outcome of interest must be related in some way to a surgical intervention. An example of a clinical problem that may be addressed is the incidence of ventricular dysfunction or cardiac low-output syndrome following coronary bypass surgery. The prevalence of postoperative low-output syndrome may be related to perioperative myocardial protection.[4] To investigate alternative surgical techniques aimed at reducing morbidity such as the incidence of low-output syndrome, the clinical outcome must be carefully and systematically defined. For example, if one classified any patient with a systolic blood pressure below 90 mm Hg as having low-output syndrome, one would erroneously include patients with high cardiac outputs and low systemic vascular resistance. A stricter definition of low-output syndrome, such as the one used by the Warm Heart Investigators,[5] would specify patients with poor ventricular function, such as those who require inotropic or intraaortic balloon pump support to maintain a cardiac index above 2.1 L/min/m². Alternative techniques of myocardial protection may improve results in this latter group but would not be expected to improve results in the former group.

In addition to well-specified endpoints, the researcher must ensure that the endpoints chosen are accurately and reliably measured with available resources. Finally, before embarking on a clinical study, one must perform sample-size or power calculations to determine whether one is able to detect significant differences if they exist.

Evaluation of Mechanisms: Hypothesis Formulation

Once a clinical problem has been selected for investigation, hypotheses must be formulated to explain how intraoperative events are related to postoperative outcome. For example, inadequate cardioplegia distribution during the cross-clamp period may account for the impaired postoperative ventricular function leading to low-output syndrome.

Hypotheses can be based on previous laboratory or clinical literature, known physiological or biological principles, or empirically observed correlations between the hypothesized mechanism and clinical outcomes.

Descriptive studies can be constructed to document possible cause-and-effect relationships. For example, retrograde delivery of cardioplegia via the coronary sinus may lead to a higher incidence of low-output syndrome compared to antegrade delivery via the aortic root. When a hypothesis has been previously tested or documented in the literature, descriptive studies can be employed to elucidate the mechanism of injury by identifying in-

traoperative clinical, biochemical, or pathological processes. For example, documentation of cardioplegic distribution, flows, volumes, and temperatures may allow one to formulate a potential mechanism for the poorer results associated with retrograde cardioplegia delivery.

Unfortunately, attempts to prove cause-and-effect relationships in descriptive studies are prone to error. Clinical outcomes are often based on multifactorial variables that are rarely controlled in a descriptive study. For example, patients receiving retrograde cardioplegia may be more likely to be undergoing reoperative surgery, may have poorer preoperative left ventricular function, and may be an older patient population than those receiving antegrade cardioplegia. These factors will obviously result in poorer outcomes for patients receiving retrograde cardioplegia, but the actual direction of cardioplegic delivery may have had only minimal impact on postoperative outcomes.

A more powerful protocol to investigate cause-and-effect relationships would involve a prospective randomized trial. Randomizing patients by the use of a sealed envelope, computer-generated randomization schedule, or other methods removes the confounding effect of different baseline characteristics and reduces the bias inherent in a retrospective trial. Comparing antegrade and retrograde cardioplegic delivery in a prospective fashion provides much stronger evidence for a cause-and-effect relationship between the route of cardioplegic delivery and the development of low-output syndrome.

Constructing a Protocol

A protocol is a mandatory summary completed before any clinical experiment and is designed to communicate the thought processes involved in the design and conduct of an experiment. The protocol should be designed to clearly define the hypotheses to be tested, the rationale behind the hypotheses, the experimental technique, and the primary and secondary study endpoints, including methods of measuring the endpoints. In addition, a sample-size calculation should be performed and presented to convince the reader that the investigator has a sufficient sample size to detect the differences specified in the hypotheses.

Introduction

The precise definition of a clinical problem and its significance to the patient must be stated. The hypotheses to be tested should be defined clearly at the beginning of the protocol in order to orient the reader. For example, the development of low-output syndrome following coronary bypass surgery is associated with a high mortality. Interventions aimed at reducing the incidence of low-output syndrome or at elucidating the mechanisms underlying its development would obviously be of importance in helping to reduce the morbidity and mortality associated with coronary bypass surgery. A potential hypothesis is that the use of tepid (29°C) cardioplegia would reduce the incidence of low-output syndrome compared to cold (10°C) cardioplegia. A prospective, randomized trial comparing cold and tepid cardioplegia would then be instituted to look for differences in the incidence of low-output syndrome following these two interventions. Secondary endpoints in this study may include perioperative myocardial infarction, postoperative strokes, and operative mortality.

Rationale

In the rationale section of a protocol, the scientific merit of a particular intervention should be discussed. A prior complete review of the literature is mandatory to support the investigator's hypothesis and compare it with others. For example, there is an abundance of literature comparing different cardioplegia strategies. It would be important to compare the incidence of low-output syndrome in these published reports to the expected incidence in the proposed study. Similarly, the magnitude of beneficial effects with different strategies should be taken into consideration when hypothesizing the effect of a new intervention or when calculating sample sizes.

The basic science literature should be reviewed to explore potential mechanisms that may account for the beneficial effect of a particular intervention. For example, one might support the use of tepid cardioplegia by noting that recovery of myocardial metabolism and function is delayed following cold cardioplegia. Tepid cardioplegia may therefore lead to improved postoperative myocar-

dial metabolism and ventricular function with a preservation of high-energy phosphates. A review of the literature may also provide alternative endpoints to those originally proposed. For example, using the hypothesis that tepid cardioplegia will reduce the incidence of postoperative low-output syndrome, one may explain this benefit by a preservation of high-energy phosphates such as adenosine triphosphate (ATP). A secondary endpoint may include a direct measurement of myocardial ATP stores.

Methods

Detailed information must be given regarding patient selection, inclusion, and exclusion criteria; the method of randomization (if appropriate); and informed consent. A detailed description of the conduct of surgery highlighting any deviations from the normal practice, such as additional data acquisition or measurements, modified or new techniques of surgery, insertion of catheters, withdrawal of blood specimens, and procurement of patient tissue, must be given.

Validation of the techniques of data acquisition may also be indicated and should be provided in this section of the protocol. The risks and benefits of the proposed study should be clearly defined.

Between 1979 and 1995, we performed intraoperative studies on more than 1,000 patients. The primary focus of our clinical research involves improving myocardial protection during cardiac surgery. We use metabolic, functional, and clinical endpoints in our studies. These measurements usually involve the placement of catheters into the coronary sinus, the aortic root, and the left ventricle. Figure 51-1 is a schematic diagram illustrating our intraoperative measurement protocol.

Pediatric feeding tubes are placed into the coronary sinus to sample coronary venous blood. A blood-sampling line is also connected to the aortic root. Using this system, we are able to measure lactate, glucose, oxygen, and pH in both coronary arterial and venous samples. Measurements of coronary sinus blood flow using a thermoresistor flow probe allow for the calculation of myocardial oxygen consumption, glucose and lactate consumption, and acid production. We have found that these sensitive measurements of myocardial

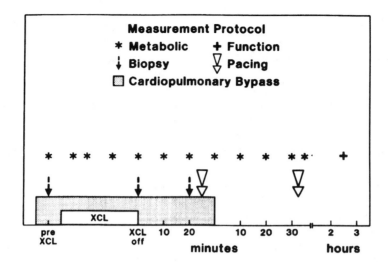

Figure 51-1. Schematic diagram illustrating the intraoperative measurement protocol.

metabolism correlate to clinical outcomes such as the development of postoperative low-output syndrome.

In addition to assessment of cell metabolism, we have performed transmural left ventricular biopsies for measurement of the myocardial high-energy phosphate ATP, creatine phosphate, myocardial lactate, and glycogen levels. Biopsies were performed at baseline on institution of cardiopulmonary bypass, immediately after cross-clamp release, and following 30 minutes of myocardial reperfusion. Myocardial biopsies have also been performed to assess myocardial deposition of [111]indium-labeled white blood cells and technetium-labeled platelets. Figure 51-1 illustrates the clinical protocol we have used for measurements of intraoperative myocardial metabolism and function.

Recently, we have employed myocardial contrast echocardiography to assess the distribution of cardioplegia.[9] Using sonicated albumin, we are able to compare the right and left ventricular distribution of cardioplegia when given in a retrograde fashion versus the standard antegrade approach.

All proposed blood sampling must be estimated and quantitated in the protocol. All measurements to be made on these samples should be described with precision.

We have employed intraventricular Millar micromanometer catheters to measure both left and right ventricular pressures.[6] In conjunction with measurements of intraventricular volumes, we have been able to construct pressure-volume relations to make sensitive measurements of cardiac function. In patients, measurements of intraventricular volume are difficult. Some investigators have reported the use of epicardial and endocardial tantalum markers to estimate ventricular volumes at all phases of the cardiac cycle.[7] Using multiplane fluoroscopy, they are able to measure end-systolic and end-diastolic volumes for both right and left ventricles. At our institution, we have used gated nuclear ventriculography to estimate intraventricular volumes.[8]

Statistics and Sample Size

Investigators should decide prospectively on the appropriate statistical analysis to be employed once the data have been acquired. Sample-size calculations should be performed routinely for all endpoints to be measured. An estimation of the results to be obtained should be made based on the prior literature review or previous experience. Investigators may also wish to perform a power calculation in the event of a negative result. A power calculation determines the magnitude of the type-2 β-error when accepting the null hypothesis (i.e., the probability of falsely accepting the null hypothesis). The completion of a sample size and power calculation before the institution of a trial will support the feasibility of the study and may prevent the commencement of a trial of insufficient size to detect the differences proposed in the hypotheses. For example, to detect a 20% decrease in the incidence of low-output syndrome from 10% to 8%, one would require 1,571 patients to achieve an α-level of 5% (the probability of falsely rejecting the null hypothesis). If an investigator is unwilling or unable to enroll a sufficient sample size, then it is unscientific and unethical to even begin the study.

Administration

A prerequisite to any experiment involving patients is approval of a surgeon's protocol by the hospital- or university-based human experimentation committee. Most committees demand a structured proposal similar to the one described earlier. External funding agencies often require an analysis of costs in addition to the scientific proposal.

Establishing intraoperative experimentation in a university-affiliated hospital creates administrative problems that must be addressed before a research schedule can be initiated. The use of patients in clinical studies may influence the referral practice and confidence of the referring physicians. Personal biases may influence the enrollment of patients in a randomized trial (i.e., if a surgeon is unwilling to subject his or her patients to a particular arm of a randomization schedule).

To encourage collaboration and cooperation of operating room nurses, anesthetists, and residents, research techniques should be tailored to be implemented with ease and slowly modified over time. Obviously, immediate introduction of surgical techniques and measurements that prolong operative time significantly and are complex will not promote collaboration. However, if intraoperative research is introduced slowly, with very simple measurements and efficient organization of blood and tissue sampling, these techniques eventually become accepted as routine by the operating room personnel. Perfusionists and nurses must be made aware of the protocol so that additional equipment such as catheters, tubing, and special sutures are made available for use on a routine basis. Alteration or modification of cardio-

plegic techniques is futile unless perfusionists understand the technical modifications and the aim of these changes. The intraoperative study of blood cardioplegia at our institution between 1982 and 1985 required that a new system of cardioplegia delivery be introduced by the perfusionists. The introduction of blood cardioplegia also necessitated the pharmacy to formulate a new crystalloid cardioplegic solution for mixing with blood. Had these modifications been involved simultaneously with the initiation of intraoperative research, collaboration would not have been forthcoming.

The key to intraoperative research is to begin with simple, uncomplicated measurements followed by slow buildup of the protocol with more measurements and interventions. Once a routine has been set and accepted by operating room personnel, additions and modifications to the protocol can be made with ease. An average of 30 to 60 minutes may be added to each surgical procedure with intraoperative studies; therefore, surgical scheduling may be necessary to guarantee that the operating day schedule ends between 3 and 4 P.M. on the day of research studies. Simple, less time-consuming operations can be scheduled on the days of research studies. The ability to designate specific days for intraoperative research will permit an efficient scheduling of operating room time and will also prepare the operating room personnel for a study case on a regular basis.

Opportunistic Cost of Intraoperative Research

Intraoperative experimentation creates increased surgical costs that include equipment (e.g., catheters, solutions, tubing, and needles) increased nursing hours, operating room time utilization, and use of biochemistry and pathology resources. Unfortunately, the current fiscal situation has caused many institutions to review their operating costs, and nonessential services are continually being eliminated. At the University of Toronto, we are fortunate to have a clear directive toward both basic and clinical research. Research programs are not eliminated on the basis of cost savings alone.

Intraoperative research is not possible without the cooperation and support of the hospital and university administration. To gain support for the increased costs related to operating room utilization, services, and equipment, administrators must be convinced that a clinical problem exists and that intraoperative research may contribute to improved patient care, surgical outcome, and frequently cost savings. For example, the mean length of stay for patients who develop low-output syndrome is 15.2 days compared to 9.9 days for those patients who do not develop the syndrome. Therapies aimed at reducing the incidence of low-output syndrome would obviously lead to improved surgical outcomes and an economic benefit by reducing hospital stays.

Clinical practice efficiency is clearly affected by the additional operating time required for intraoperative studies. In centers in which specific operating rooms are designated for research, this is less of a problem. However, most centers do not have the luxury of such designated operating rooms, and investigators are at the mercy of the operating room administrators. Once again, the strength of the research protocol with the potential positive impact on patient care and surgical outcome can be used to justify the increased resource utilization. Some administrators may request external funding to pay for the additional costs involved. Clearly, these decisions are partly dependent on the complexity of the proposed study and the potential additional fiscal liability.

The use of blood cardioplegia in our institution has resulted in a decreased morbidity and mortality associated with coronary bypass surgery (Figure 51-2). This reduction in morbidity and mortality has had a definite financial impact on the delivery of cardiac surgery in our institution. Our ongoing clinical studies involving alternative myoprotective strategies are justified on the basis that further reductions in morbidity and mortality will result in additional financial savings.

Ethics and Intraoperative Experimentation

Risk versus Benefit

Intraoperative experimentation must be designed on the philosophy that no complication to patients can be tolerated. Complications can be prevented by strategic experimental design and strict control and adherence to the protocol. Additional risks imposed on patients as a result of a clinical study must be carefully weighed against the potential benefits offered to the patient. We have attempted to ensure complication-free experiments by appropriate patient selection. For invasive studies of myocardial metabolism and function we have used only low-risk patients who presented electively for surgery. In studies requiring the use of a high-risk population, we have refrained from invasive investigation and have instead relied on clinical outcome measures. The use of low-risk patients for invasive studies ensures that any possible complication related to the research protocol is better tolerated by the patient. The interventions we have employed must be at least comparable to standard treatment and must have been previously employed in laboratory investigations. Blood loss due to sampling for research purposes must be kept to a minimum, with strategic sampling times incorporated into the experimental design. Patients who become unstable at induction of anesthesia or who develop technical problems during surgery are immediately withdrawn from further involvement in the research project. Such patients would be less likely to tolerate the insult of a research-related complication no matter how unlikely the event may be.

All patients involved in surgical research are closely observed for complications, both by the surgeon in charge and by the research physicians, intraoperatively and postoperatively. The presence of a physician may allow for the earlier detection of abnormalities and permit prompt treatment. Patient care must supersede experimental protocols at all times. Patient sedation and comfort, optimization of fluid balance, control of bleeding, and stabilization of hemodynamic parameters all supersede research-related activities. This practice occasionally results in protocol violations, but it is a mandatory component of any clinical research project.

Informed Consent

All patients enrolled in intraoperative research must give an informed consent to participate. Such consent requires that the patient be in-

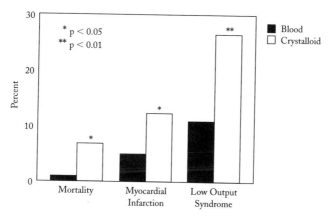

Figure 51-2. Blood vs. crystalloid cardioplegia in urgent coronary bypass surgery. Blood cardioplegia decreased the incidence of operative mortality, perioperative myocardial infarction, and postoperative low-output syndrome.

structed on how the proposed study differs from standard practice and what additional diagnostic or therapeutic maneuvers will be required. All of the potential risks and benefits must be carefully explained to the prospective study patient.

In most of our intraoperative metabolic and functional studies, we require the insertion of intracardiac catheters that frequently remain in place for several hours after the patient has arrived in the intensive care unit. Preoperatively, the patient is made aware of the risk of bleeding when the catheters are removed (less than 1:1,000 in our experience). There is a potential for extrasystoles caused by intraventricular catheters. The patient is informed that these extrasystoles may be effectively treated with medication and the catheters will be removed promptly should the extrasystoles persist despite medical treatment. Despite their use in more than 1,000 patients, we have not had to prematurely remove these catheters in a single patient.

Patients undergoing ventricular biopsies are informed of the slight risk of bleeding due to this procedure. The use of a Trucut biopsy needle has reduced the risk of bleeding associated with myocardial biopsies by limiting the size of the perforation to the heart. The use of rosette configuration–pledgetted sutures at biopsy sites and coronary sinus line insertion sites has also been instrumental in preventing postoperative

bleeding. Techniques for procuring biopsies and inserting lines into the heart were perfected in laboratory animals before being applied to humans.

Studies requiring nuclear ventriculography demand that the patient be informed of the additional radiation exposure incurred as a result of the study, despite the fact that the additional exposure is slight (equivalent to approximately 1 year of background radiation).

Lastly, an attempt is made to educate the patient as to the merits of the particular study and how the findings of each study may help to improve patient care in the future. In addition, patients are reassured that their refusal to participate in a study will in no way prejudice the quality of their care and that they are free to withdraw from a study at any time. Using these logistic approaches, we have received consent for participation in our clinical studies by more than 95% of all patients approached.

Collaboration and Consultation

By its nature, surgical research cannot be accomplished by the concerted efforts of a single individual. Close collaboration and consultation with other colleagues and health-related professionals is mandatory. In a period of 15 years we have performed more than 60,000 assays in blood for arterial and coronary sinus lactates, oxygen, and glucose levels. Thousands of myocardial biopsies have been assayed, employing high-performance liquid chromotography for high-energy phosphates, creatine phosphate, glycogen, and lactate levels. These measurements would have been impossible without the close cooperation of colleagues in clinical biochemistry. Our use of nuclear ventriculography to measure intraventricular volumes would have been impossible without the help of colleagues in the division of nuclear cardiology. Similarly, our use of intraoperative echocardiography is highly dependent on the expertise of our fellow collaborators.

Constant communication with collaborators is necessary to ascertain the feasibility of performing assays, logistics of scheduling and delivery, preparation and storage of specimens, and interpretation of the results of studies with appropriate quality control.

With time, innovations in the method of assays or in the development of new, more sensitive assays have occurred. In addition to our standard measurements of myocardial oxygen and lactate consumption, as well as myocardial high-energy phosphate levels, we have been able to estimate oxygen free radical injury with assays of blood and tissue for lipid peroxidation products and conjugated dienes.[10] The measurement of high-energy phosphates has been superseded by assays for total adenine nucleotides and degradation products. Close collaboration with experts in biochemistry ensures that new developments in this field are quickly applied to clinical research programs.

Cooperation with anesthetists, perfusionists, residents, and operating room and ICU staff is critical to conducting research successfully. All of these individuals must receive copies of experimental protocols and be included in discussions of patient care and research strategies. Anesthetists and nurses must be made aware of the reason for and timing and goals of blood sampling before research personnel can be interposed between them and the patient. Cooperation from coworkers in the operating room is essential since experimental study patients invariably require longer periods of surgery due to the instrumentation and measurements performed.

Training Surgeons for Intraoperative Experimentation

Training surgeons to perform intraoperative experimentation requires an appropriate mentor and a background in clinical epidemiology. Surgical residents should perform clinical trials under the close supervision of an experienced surgical investigator. This training would provide the best role model and expose the young surgeon to a well-established collaborative clinical research program.

Future Trends in Intraoperative Research

Techniques in intraoperative research will continue to evolve as newer technologies become available to both the basic and clinical scientist. Undoubtedly, the molecular era will have an impact on the practice of surgery. Many laboratories, including our own, are conducting experiments at the basic science level to explore the possibility of cellular cardiomyoplasty. Intraoperative gene transfer or viral transfection may be another avenue for future therapeutic strategies. Clinical transplantation is another area in which intraoperative experimentation may have a significant impact. Unfortunately, due to the logistic difficulties in scheduling studies on transplant patients, a single study may require many years for completion unless a study coordinator who can maintain close communication to all participants in the study is employed.

Prerequisites for Training

Previous training in trial design, statistics, and other aspects of clinical epidemiology would be a tremendous asset when contemplating the initiation of a clinical research program. The design of the trial requires careful consideration and an appreciation of sample-size and power calculations. The surgeon in training must have the full support of the departmental chairperson, the divisional head, and the staff surgeons. Most importantly, the surgeon in training must have the full support, cooperation, and guidance of a mentor who has a breadth of experience in clinical trials.

Intraoperative research has been and will continue to be a cornerstone in bridging the gap between surgical research performed in the laboratory and its implementation in a clinical setting. The added costs, both actual and opportunistic, of intraoperative research performed successfully by an experienced team are easily offset by the improvements in patient care.

The ability to adequately assess new surgical techniques will require fundamental training in the principles of intraoperative research. Successful clinical investigators will have a background in basic science that will enable them to adeptly transform their respective operating rooms into clinical laboratories.

Acknowledgments. Supported by the Heart and Stroke Foundation of Ontario (Grant B2267) and the Medical Research Council of Canada (Grant MT 9829).

V.R. is a Pharmaceutical Roundtable Research Fellow of the Heart and Stroke Foundation of Ontario. G.T.C. is a Research Scholar of the Heart and Stroke Foundation of Ontario. R.D.W. is a Career Investigator of the Heart and Stroke Foundation of Canada.

References

1. Fremes SE, Christakis GT, Weisel RD, Mickle DA, Madonik MM, Ivanov J, Harding R, Seawright SJ, Houle S, McLaughlin PR, et al. A clinical trial of blood and crystalloid cardioplegia. J Thorac Cardiovasc Surg 1984;88:726–741. Dr. Fremes performed this prospective clinical trial as a surgical resident in Dr. Weisel's laboratory. Dr. Fremes wrote the protocol, performed the study, and published the paper. As a result of this study, all surgeons at the University of Toronto now employ blood cardioplegia in their technique of myocardial protection.

2. Grillo HC. Primary reconstruction of airway after resection of subglottic laryngeal and upper tracheal stenosis. Ann Thorac Surg 1982;33:3–18.

3. Pearson FG, Cooper JD, Nelems JM, Van Nostrand AWP. Primary tracheal anastomosis after resection of the cricoid cartilage with preservation of recurrent laryngeal nerves. J Thorac Cardiovasc Surg 1975;70:806–816.

4. Rao V, Ivanov J, Weisel RD, Ikonomidis JS, Christakis GT, David TE. Predictors of low output syndrome following coronary bypass surgery. J Thorac Cardiovasc Surg 1996;12:38–51. Dr. Rao performed this retrospective, descriptive study as a surgical resident in Dr. Weisel's laboratory. Dr. Rao was able to show that the development of low-output syndrome correlates with operative mortality, thereby justifying its use as an alternative clinical outcome measure.

5. The Warm Heart Investigators. A randomized trial of normothermic vs. hypothermic blood cardioplegia for coronary bypass surgery. Lancet 1994;343: 559–563.

6. Christakis GT, Weisel RD, Mickle DAG, Ivanov J, Tumiati LC, Zuech PE, Madonik MM, Liu P. Right ventricular function and metabolism. Circulation 1990;82(suppl. IV):IV332–IV340. Dr. Christakis performed this prospective clinical trial as a research fellow in Dr. Weisel's laboratory. Dr. Christakis wrote the protocol, performed the study, and published the paper. This study describes in detail the methods employed to measure ventricular function that have been used in all subsequent trials.

7. Hansen DE, Daughters GT, Alderman EL, Ingels NB, Miller DC. Torsional deformation of the left ventricular midwall in human hearts with intramyocardial markers: regional heterogeneity and sensitivity to the inotropic effects of abrupt rate changes. Circ Res 1988;62:941–952.

8. Burns RJ, Nitkin RS, Weisel RD, Houle S, Prieur TG, McLaughlin PR, Druck MN. Optimized count-based scintigraphic left ventricular volume measurement. Can J Cardiol 1985;1:42–46.

9. Rao V, Ikonomidis JS, Weisel RD, Hayashida N, Shirai T, Ivanov J, Carson S, Kitching A, Rakowski H. Inhomogeneous retrograde cardioplegia. Can J Cardiol 1994;10(suppl. C):85C. Abstract.

10. Weisel RD, Mickle DAG, Finkle CD, Tumiati LC, Madonik MM, Ivanov J, Burton GW, Ingold KU. Myocardial free-radical injury after cardioplegia. Circulation 1989;80(suppl. III):III14–III18.

Commentary

As the authors point out, special skills are required to perform research in the operating room because of the time pressure and the complexity of the simultaneous interventions of anesthesia, the stresses of surgery, and the responses they elicit in the patient. (See chapter 65, "Surgical Research Around the World," by Lorenz and coworkers for more on the analysis of complexity.)

Safety monitoring is critical. An independent monitoring committee must be used to oversee safety and maintain objectivity. When comparing two operative techniques, it is easy for one intraoperative misadventure or poor outcome to lead the team to conclude prematurely that one approach is inferior. The oversight committee should be prepared to terminate the study when the accumulated evidence would convince the larger medical community that a valid difference has been demonstrated.

The authors raise another extraordinary important issue. When operating room investigations add to the time of the operation, they increase cost. The operating room is one of the most costly environments in a hospital, and this factor should be recognized in the design of research projects. Hospitals are under enormous pressure to minimize cost. Some hospitals may be willing to underwrite the cost of investigation, believing that there is an inherent gain further down the road or that it constitutes a critical part of their mission. In a highly competitive environment, appropriate funding to compensate the hospital for experimental time should be part of the research proposal.

W.A.S.
M.F.M.

CHAPTER 52

Research in the Intensive Care Unit

J.C. Marshall, D.J. Cook, and P.C. Hébert

Biomedical research seeks to apply insights gleaned from the study of biologic processes to the clinical care of the ill—a model alliteratively embodied in the concept of bench to bedside investigation. Nowhere is the distance from the laboratory bench to the bedside shorter than in the contemporary intensive care unit (ICU). The management of the critically ill patient can legitimately be seen as a continuous experiment in applied physiology. The monitoring of physiological processes in the ICU enables the intensivist to generate hypotheses regarding cause, to test them through therapeutic intervention, and to support or reject them through continuing evaluation of clinical response.

The intensive care unit is a particularly attractive venue for clinical research. The problems encountered in the critically ill patient are acute and life threatening; therefore, insights gained through research may be significant and immediately relevant to clinical practice. The ICU generates substantial costs—8% of total inpatient hospital costs and 0.2% of the gross national product (GNP) in Canada and 20% of all inpatient hospital costs and 0.8% of the GNP in the United States.[1] Finally, large amounts of data are gathered during the management of the critically ill patient, providing the investigator with a comprehensive and complete information base covering a defined time period during a disease process. This chapter reviews the unique opportunities and challenges encountered in ICU-based clinical research.

The Hypothesis and the Research Question

Good research proceeds in an apparently effortless fashion from a clearly formulated *hypothesis*, to one or more specific *questions* that the hypothesis generates, to a specific *research design* that is optimal to answer the study question (Table 52-1). Care in formulating each of these three components is critical to the success of a research venture.

A hypothesis is a scientifically testable assertion that provides a reasonable explanation for a body of observations about a biologic state or disease process. A hypothesis must be consistent with known data. However, it is more than a simple reiteration of what is known since it integrates available information into a premise whose study will generate new knowledge. For example, recognition that the critically ill surgical patient manifests a spectrum of immunologic alterations,[2] and that the presence of these alterations is associated with an increased risk of infectious morbidity and mortality,[3] led MacLean, Meakins, and Christou to hypothesize that the surgical patient is an immunocompromised host who might benefit from strategies to bolster immune function.[4] Studies arising from that hypothesis have done

Table 52-1.   ICU-based research: from hypothesis to study design.

Hypothesis	Question	Research design
ICU-acquired infections can arise as a result of gut bacterial overgrowth	1. Are the organisms producing ICU-acquired infection simultaneously present in the upper GI tract?	Descriptive study of quantitative proximal gut bacteriology in a group of ICU patients at risk for nosocomial infection[48]
	2. Can viable microorganisms translocate across an intact gut mucosa?	Case report of *Candidemia* and *Candiduria* following oral ingestion of *Candida*[49]
	3. Does maintenance of normal gastric acidity reduce rates of nosocomial pneumonia?	Randomized clinical trial comparing effects of an H_2-blocker and a gastric cytoprotective agent on rates of nosocomial pneumonia[50]
	4. Does eradication of gut luminal pathogens reduce ICU mortality or rates of nosocomial infection?	Randomized clinical trial of effects of topical, nonabsorbed antibiotics on rates of mortality and nosocomial infection[51]
Occult tissue hypoxia contributes to morbidity and mortality in critical illness	1. Is there evidence of regional hypoxia in patients in whom measures of systemic oxygenation are normal?	Descriptive study of measures of adequacy of total body and splanchnic perfusion in critically ill patients[52]
	2. Are biochemical markers of anaerobic metabolism evident in patients in whom oxygen delivery is measurably adequate?	Descriptive study of serum lactate levels in population of critically ill patients[53]
	3. Do therapies that increase oxygen delivery to supranormal levels result in improved ICU outcome?	Randomized trial evaluating effects of pulmonary artery catheter–directed augmentation of oxygen delivery[54] or dobutamine[55] on ICU survival

much to clarify the nature of host-pathogen interactions in the critically ill surgical patient, but the original hypothesis has been profoundly transformed in the process, and this group now considers the unsolved challenge to be that of immunologic overactivation rather than suppression.[5] A hypothesis can never be definitively proven or disproven and is commonly transformed as the studies it suggests proceed.

The hypothesis serves as an intellectual framework for the specific question that the research is designed to answer. The question, in turn, defines the study design, suggesting the population to be studied, the intervention to be employed, and the outcomes to be measured (Table 52-2), as well as ultimately determining whether the information that results will be of interest or relevance to clinical practice. The best research starts with a question that is clearly formulated, clinically important, and of interest, whether the answer is positive or negative.

The importance of a carefully articulated question cannot be overemphasized. Work that starts from an unfocused question such as "What is our experience with disease X or therapy Y," an unfortunately common approach for the inexperienced investigator, is doomed to produce results that are of limited interest and of uncertain relevance to patient care.

The Study Population

The study question usually suggests the appropriate population of subjects to be studied. In general terms, the investigator wishes to study a group

Table 52-2. Elements of the research question.

Component	Examples
Population	All patients admitted to a surgical ICU
	All patients meeting clinical criteria for sepsis syndrome
	All patients with an APACHE II score >15
Intervention	None
	Placement of gastric tonometer
	Administration of a monoclonal antibody or placebo
	Measurement of IL-8 in BAL fluid
	Transfusion before ICU admission
Outcome	ICU survival
	Cardiac output
	Development of pneumonia
	Requirement for dialysis

of patients that is diverse enough to be representative of the entire population of interest (to maximize the generalizability of the results) but that is restricted to those patients who might be affected by a risk factor, a test, or an experimental intervention. Moreover, he or she will want to limit the investigation to a population that is at low risk of adverse side effects from the experimental maneuver. Thus the investigator must define the group of patients to be studied (the study population) and the specific circumstances that might preclude the inclusion of subsets of these (exclusion criteria).

If, for example, we wish to determine rates of and risk factors for clinically important stress bleeding in a contemporary ICU, we will want to study all patients admitted to the ICU and to maximize the generalizability of our conclusions by studying patients admitted to a cross section of units. However, we will likely want to exclude patients admitted with upper gastrointestinal (GI) bleeding (because the endpoint has been reached before ICU admission) or patients in previously defined high-risk groups (head injury, burns).[6] On the other hand, if we wish to determine the efficacy of a novel form of stress ulcer prophylaxis,

we will restrict our study to patients at increased risk of bleeding, whereas if we wish to evaluate a diagnostic test for stress ulceration, we will evaluate only those patients who have bled.

Selection of the appropriate population for study can be challenging, and decisions made at this juncture can have a significant impact on the conclusions reached. A number of factors render the definition of an appropriate study group potentially difficult.

Patient Heterogeneity

Patients are admitted to an intensive care unit with a highly heterogeneous group of diagnoses and disease processes that result in a relatively limited spectrum of physiologic consequences. ICU care is directed to these physiologic consequences more than to the diseases that triggered them, and ICU-based research tends to mirror this focus. In contradistinction to studies of coronary artery disease or cancer, for example, where patients have a readily definable anatomic and pathologic disease process, patients are commonly enrolled in ICU studies on the basis of sharing symptom complexes such as acute respiratory distress syndrome (ARDS) or a hyperdynamic circulatory state. These symptom complexes typically arise from highly variable anatomic and pathologic causes, with the result that study populations are intrinsically heterogeneous.

Patient heterogeneity results in greater variability in baseline status and in response to therapeutic intervention, with the result that sample sizes must be larger. Heterogeneity in a patient population may mask a potentially beneficial effect for two separate reasons. The study population may include both patients who might benefit from the experimental intervention and those for whom it has no effect; however, a highly heterogeneous population may also include patients who may actually be harmed by the intervention. Both factors appear to have contributed to the disappointing and often contradictory results obtained from clinical trials of experimental mediator-directed therapy.

A well-designed randomized controlled trial of an anti-endotoxin monoclonal antibody showed survival benefit in patients with Gram-negative infection,[7] but a follow-up study of the same agent using identical entry criteria failed to confirm this benefit.[8] Similarly, a phase II study of antagonism of the proinflammatory cytokine, interleukin 1, demonstrated a striking effect on survival.[9] In a much larger phase III study, a statistically significant effect on mortality was confined to a subgroup of the most severely ill patients;[10] an unpublished follow-up study failed to support even this limited degree of efficacy. Entry criteria for these trials comprised a constellation of clinical parameters termed *sepsis syndrome,* characterized by hyper- or hypothermia, tachycardia, tachypnea, and evidence of altered function in at least one organ system, occurring in association with clinical suspicion of infection.[11] However, these physiologic criteria are not specific for a single disease process but can occur in disease states ranging from overwhelming infection to trauma and congestive heart failure. Analyses of more homogeneous subgroups of patients enrolled in these studies have suggested both differential efficacy in different patient groups and even the possibility of harm in certain subgroups.[12]

Measurement of Illness Severity

An important advance in ICU research has been the development of simple, validated methods of providing an objective measure of illness severity across a heterogeneous group of disease processes. Three similar models are widely used— APACHE (Acute Physiology, Age, Chronic Health Evaluation),[13,14] SAPS (Simplified Acute Physiology Score),[15,16] and MPM (Mortality Prediction Model).[17] Each combines the influence of a number of readily measured physiologic and biochemical variables available early during the course of the ICU admission to produce a score that reflects illness severity and predicts the probability of hospital survival.

Severity-of-illness scoring has facilitated ICU-based research by providing an objective measure of initial illness severity that permits comparisons between patient populations and stratification within clinical trials. It provides an estimate of illness acuity within a population and so has become an integral component of the demographic characterization of an ICU population. By identifying a cohort of patients at increased risk of

mortality, scoring has been used widely as an entry criterion for clinical trials or as a stratification variable within trials. Application of severity-of-illness measures to heterogeneous patient populations such as those with sepsis has been advocated as a strategy for defining a population more likely to benefit from experimental interventions.[16,18] Finally, severity-of-illness measures have found use as a method to explain variability in post hoc subgroup analyses.[10] Disease-specific severity indices such as Ranson's criteria for acute pancreatitis[19] have proven useful for prognostication and stratification in clinical practice. Generic severity-of-illness measures are probably preferable in the context of research because of their methodologic sophistication and the greater generalizability that they offer.

The Intervention

Specification of the intervention of interest is the crux of the research question. The intervention may be a particular pharmacologic agent or an invasive procedure, but it may also consist of an exposure or a diagnostic test. Most ICU-based clinical research is undertaken to characterize the natural history and risk factors of a particular process or to evaluate therapy or a diagnostic maneuver. The purpose of the investigation determines the intervention of interest; the intervention may be neither active nor deliberate.

For a study of risk factors for an ICU complication such as stress GI bleeding, pneumonia, or pulmonary embolism, the intervention is exposure to the particular risk factors of interest. Similarly, in a study to develop or validate a prognostic scoring system or outcome measure, the intervention is the presence of the intervals of abnormality of the particular variables that comprise the score. Designation of the intervention or interventions of interest is what differentiates a study from an audit. An audit merely enumerates rates of events in a population (the number of patients developing stress bleeding or deep venous thrombosis); by systematic evaluation of the impact of an intervention, a study is able to suggest an explanation for the outcome.

For a trial to evaluate the effects of therapy (for example, early tracheostomy or enhanced enteral nutrition), the intervention is the study variable of interest. However the intervention may also consist of a specific test or tests if we are evaluating a diagnostic procedure (for example, protected specimen brush bronchoscopy, bronchoalveolar lavage, and sputum culture in the diagnosis of ventilator-associated pneumonia).

Outcome Measures and Study Definitions

Like the determination of an appropriate study population, the selection of optimal outcome measures has been a particular problem for ICU-based studies, because the disorders of interest tend to be syndromes and symptom complexes rather than disease processes that are readily diagnosed by objective anatomic or laboratory criteria. Indeed the complexities of the clinical syndromes that arise through the interaction of life-threatening physiologic derangements with the invasive measures needed to support and monitor them create a series of challenges for the investigator who must establish objective definitions for study-entry criteria, interventions, and endpoints.

Definition of Clinical Events and Interventions

Careful articulation of the definitions of all significant clinical events, interventions, and outcomes is particularly important in ICU-based studies. Diagnoses such as sepsis, shock, and ARDS are notoriously subjective, and satisfactory pathologic or consensus definitions are still not generally available.[20–22] In the interests of maximizing the reproducibility of the results of a study, it is essential that the investigator specify definitions for all study variables, using objective criteria as much as possible. A study of ARDS defined as a PO_2/FIO_2 ratio of less than 200, in association with bilateral pulmonary infiltrates on chest X ray and a pulmonary capillary wedge pressure of less than 18, will provide more useful information than one in which ARDS is defined on unspecified clinical grounds. Nonetheless, even objective and reproducible definitions may fail to provide a reproducible reflection of a single underlying pathologic process.

Studies of the prevention and therapy of pneumonia provide an informative example of the problems associated with establishing a pathologic diagnosis on the basis of clinical criteria in the intubated, critically ill patient.[23] Airway colonization is common, while noninfectious processes such as pulmonary edema, increased capillary permeability, and atelectasis can produce chest X-ray evidence of a new or changing infiltrate. Systematic manifestations such as fever and leukocytosis are nonspecific, and the results of history and physical examination are unreliable. Quantitative bacteriologic techniques applied to distal airway specimens obtained through the use of the protected specimen brush or by bronchoalveolar lavage have emerged as the most reliable means of establishing the diagnosis of pneumonia,[24] but their use involves an invasive intervention that may not always be feasible. It is recognized that the technique used to diagnose pneumonia has an impact on the conclusions reached by a study; one of the few studies demonstrating improved outcome with appropriate antimicrobial therapy of ventilator-associated pneumonia relied on the results of bronchoscopically obtained quantitative cultures.[25] Similarly, a meta-analysis of studies of the efficacy of selective decontamination of the digestive tract showed that studies with the least rigorous definitions of pneumonia yielded the largest estimate of therapeutic efficacy.[26]

Even apparently simple physiologic states can prove frustratingly difficult to quantify objectively in an unstable critically ill patient. It is a common finding of descriptive[27] and interventional studies of sepsis[10] that the coexistence of clinical sepsis with physiologic evidence of cardiovascular instability (sepsis with shock) defines a population at increased risk of mortality. However, establishing criteria to define such states as entry criteria for clinical trials is difficult. Should one use blood pressure to measure hemodynamic instability, and, if so, should the systolic or mean pressure be used? Is the appropriate criterion a single value (for example, a systolic pressure of less than 80 mm Hg) or a change from the patient's own baseline? Should the value selected represent the worst value, the best value, a representative value, or a mean value? Since transient hypotension can result from the use of sedation, should the definition be modified by specifying a minimum time interval during which hypotension must be present? Moreover, since the therapeutic response is to correct the physiologic abnormality (often with some measure of success), should the definition incorporate a therapeutic response such as the use of fluids or vasopressors, and, if so, how much? Similar considerations make the establishment of definitions for dysfunction of other organ systems difficult and result in considerable variability in published criteria.[28]

Outcome Measures

In general terms, study endpoints may be *patient* or *disease* specific, although the distinction is not absolute (Table 52-3). Patient-specific outcomes (for example, 28-day mortality following administration of anti-endotoxin monoclonal antibody or the development of clinically important GI bleeding) reflect events of direct clinical relevance, making their interpretation straightforward. Disease-specific outcomes (serum levels of an inflammatory mediator or endoscopic evidence of gastric erosions, for example) describe physiologic or pathologic changes and therefore cast light on the biologic basis of a process; however, their relevance to patient care must be inferred. As a rule, patient-specific outcome measures are less sensitive, so larger sample sizes are required to establish or rule out an effect. Often an investigator will evaluate both patient- and disease-specific outcomes, using a clearly important endpoint such as mortality as the primary endpoint for determination of sample size and the disease-specific endpoints as supportive observations or hypothesis-generating data.

Patient-Specific Outcomes

The disorders leading to ICU admission are by definition life threatening. Mortality rates in a typical ICU generally exceed 10%, depending on the case mix, and may exceed 50% for certain syndromes (septic shock or ARDS with acute renal failure, for example). It is intuitively reasonable that mortality should be the most important patient-specific outcome for an ICU-based study,

Table 52-3.   Outcome measures for ICU-based studies.

Patient related	
Mortality	All causes (e.g., 7, 14, 28, 60 days)
	ICU/hospital
	Attributable or cause specific
Morbidity	Major clinical events (e.g., pneumonia, renal failure)
	Duration of therapy (ICU stay, ventilation)
	Aggregate measures of organ dysfunction or failure
Quality of life	Objective
	Subjective (e.g., pain scores)
Disease related	
Physiologic	e.g., cardiac output, mucosal pH, pulmonary compliance, CO_2
Biochemical	e.g., cytokine levels, lactate
Radiographic	e.g., chest X-ray findings
Economic	
Cost-effectiveness	
Cost per survivor	

although the use of mortality as an outcome measure is not without its problems.

The optimal time interval for the determination of mortality or survival is controversial. Critically ill patients spend variable amounts of time in the ICU and in the hospital. Moreover, they usually have comorbid conditions, complications of which have led to ICU admission, that may ultimately be fatal, even in the absence of the acute complication that led to ICU admission. Consider, for example, the dilemmas encountered in designing a study of the effects of an anti-endotoxin monoclonal antibody on mortality from Gram-negative infection. A typical study subject might be a 70-year-old man with ischemic heart disease and chronic lung disease, admitted with peritonitis secondary to a perforated sigmoid diverticulum, who receives aggressive surgical and supportive care, as well as appropriate antibiotic therapy for 7 days, and the experimental agent for 3 days. If he dies within the first week of therapy, we can probably agree that he should be considered a treatment failure. But death from sepsis syndrome is not sudden, and it is not uncommon for patients to survive for prolonged periods before ultimately succumbing. Should the patient be considered a survivor if he or she is alive at 14 or 28 days with florid multiple organ dysfunction syndrome and active therapy is withdrawn on day 35? Should the patient be considered a treatment failure if he or she is discharged from the ICU but dies on day 12 of a pulmonary embolism? What if a patient survives his or her ICU stay but ultimately dies after 63 days in the hospital of a myocardial infarct or because he or she remains lethargic and confused and supportive care is withdrawn?

Regulatory agencies have indicated a preference for the use of 28- or 30-day all-cause mortality as the primary endpoint for clinical trials of mediator-directed therapy. From the patient's perspective, survival to hospital discharge is the only truly relevant endpoint. But it is clearly unreasonable to expect that a single intervention undertaken at the time of hospital admission will prevent delayed complications such as a myocardial infarction or the sequelae of ventilator-induced lung injury and pneumonia. In methodologic terms, mortality is a responsive measure but not necessarily a reproducible measure, given the heterogeneity of patient populations and the enormous impact of other confounding variables on ICU outcome. Even the generalizability of a study finding may be affected when mortality at a fixed time serves as the primary outcome measure, since the majority of deaths in an ICU occur as a result of a conscious decision to withhold or withdraw life support, and the timing of such decisions is heavily affected by religious and cultural factors that vary widely from one area to the next.[29]

The lack of reproducibility of mortality as a study endpoint has had a significant impact on the outcome of a number of well-designed interventional studies in sepsis. Treatment with monoclonal antibody against endotoxin, for example, showed significant efficacy measured as ICU mortality at 28 days in a subgroup of patients with Gram-negative bacteremia.[7] However, when the same study was repeated in a group of patients meeting the same entry criteria, the previously documented 28-day efficacy was no longer found.[8] Studies of interventions to treat cancer commonly use survival curves to demonstrate prolongation of survival with an intervention. This approach is inappropriate for ICU-based studies; dying in an ICU after an extra week on the ventilator can hardly be considered a therapeutic success.

Mortality as an endpoint has other shortcomings.[30] The heterogeneity of ICU populations, and the unavoidable confounding influence of intercurrent disease and interventions, makes it improbable that any single intervention will result in a large decrement in ICU mortality. Equally, patients are admitted to an ICU at varying points in the course of their illnesses; for some, the disease process may be sufficiently advanced that the intervention being evaluated may no longer be capable of exerting a biologic effect. An ICU study using mortality as its primary endpoint must enroll large numbers of patients, making the study costly and logistically complex. Such studies must of necessity be undertaken in many different centers, increasing the heterogeneity of the study population and commonly introducing significant variability from one center to the next; as a result, it is more difficult to demonstrate benefit. Studies of thrombolytic intervention in myocardial infarction, undertaken in a relatively homogeneous patient population in whom there is a direct pathologic relationship between coronary thrombosis and mortality, have required tens of thousands of patients to demonstrate efficacy, showing a net reduction in mortality of approximately 1%.[31] Such large sample sizes are not feasible in ICU-based studies.

Assessing mortality attributable to the disease process of interest is difficult because of the inherent problems in assigning or rejecting causality in a complex disease process. A myocardial infarction occurring 10 days after administration of a mediator-directed agent could conceivably be an adverse effect of the medication; to eliminate these data from analysis would be to run the risk of missing unrecognized adverse effects of the experimental agent. An approach used in retrospective studies has been to evaluate attributable mortality by matching a patient group of interest with unexposed control subjects who share other potentially confounding comorbid conditions (see later section). However, adequate randomization procedures should accomplish the same objective in a prospective study.

Measures of morbidity can serve as useful outcomes for ICU-based studies. Such measures include rates of objectively defined complications, duration of therapy or ICU stay, or aggregate measures of organ failure or organ dysfunction. Length of ICU stay is a simple measure of morbidity that correlates with ICU costs. As a study endpoint it suffers from two major deficiencies: it is commonly affected by variables other than severity of illness (for example, the availability of ICU beds or the demands of the admitting physician or the patient's family), and it is often shorter for patients who are sicker and die in the ICU. There is increasing interest in the use of objective measures of organ dysfunction as an endpoint for ICU studies,[32–34] but experience with these is limited. Measures of morbidity carry a significant risk of bias and are most reliable when the individual determining the outcome is blinded to the intervention.

Disease-Specific Outcomes

Disease-related outcomes are appropriate for physiologic studies or for hypothesis-generating studies to establish preliminary data for larger studies of clinical efficacy. These endpoints generally entail objective biochemical, physiologic, or radiographic measurements, rather than measures of clinical effect. Such measures can be both more sensitive to change and more objective in their definition. However, it must be remembered that the mere detection of a biologic effect does not imply clinical benefit or harm.

Study Designs

Two factors—random error and systematic error or bias—introduce uncertainty into the results of a scientific investigation; the rationale for a rigorous study methodology is to minimize their influence. Random error reduces the accuracy of an observation, whereas bias limits its applicability.

Random error arises as a result of intrinsic biological differences between individuals and the inherent inaccuracies of measurement techniques. The effects of intrinsic biological variability are minimized by the selection of a homogeneous study population and by maximizing the sample size. Precise definition of study endpoints can reduce measurement error, as can the use of sensitive and accurate measurement techniques. For

example, if our objective is to determine whether inhaled surfactant can prevent the development of ARDS, random error will be minimized if we study as large a population as feasible, using criteria that will eliminate unwanted patient heterogeneity and yield a patient group that is uniformly at high risk for the endpoint of interest. Measurement error will be reduced if our study endpoint is a sensitive functional measure of gas exchange or compliance rather than, for example, the blinded grading of chest X ray changes.

Systematic error or bias arises through the unrecognized influence of a variable other than the one being explicitly evaluated. Bias is minimized through adherence to principles of optimal trial design, including random assignment of the experimental intervention and blinding of therapeutic intervention and outcome.

A number of different study designs are appropriate for ICU-based clinical research (Table 52-4). For convenience, these designs can be differentiated on the basis of whether there is a control group and whether there is prospective evaluation of outcome (i.e., the outcome of interest is not known at the time the patient is enrolled in the study).

The Randomized Controlled Trial

The randomized controlled clinical trial is the best study design to minimize bias. Random assignment of patients to one of two or more study groups serves to minimize bias resulting from the presence of a systematic confounding variable in one of the groups, while blinding prevents bias in outcome evaluation.

Techniques of randomization must ensure that the assignment of patients to study groups is truly random; if there are two study groups, each consecutive patient must have a 50/50 chance of being allocated to either of these groups. The use of a variable that is known before treatment assignment (e.g., initial of last name, year of birth, or date of admission) introduces the potential for bias, since the investigator can decide in advance whether a particular patient will be included in a trial. In addition, systematic bias may be introduced. For example, a study comparing crystalloids with colloids in the resuscitation of critically ill patients allocated treatment based on which of

Table 52-4.   Study designs.

| | Control Group | |
	Yes	No
Prospective outcome	Randomized controlled trial	Natural history (cohort) study Evaluation
Outcome known at study entry	Case-control study	Case report

two teams was admitting patients.[35] Since patients in one group were managed according to a clearly defined protocol, whereas patients in the second group were not, beneficial effects seen in the study group may well reflect the superiority of protocol-based resuscitation rather than a beneficial effect of the particular intervention. It has been shown that estimates of treatment effect are larger in studies in which randomization has been inadequately concealed;[36] knowledge of treatment allocation may lead to alterations in patterns of care that may independently affect outcome either positively or negatively.

Blinding of therapy is desirable whenever possible. Even if it is not possible to blind the therapeutic intervention, outcome evaluation should be performed in a blinded fashion. This is particularly important when there is an element of subjective judgment involved in determining whether the endpoint of interest has been reached (as, for example, in the diagnosis of pneumonia). However, even in clinical trials in which an apparently hard endpoint such as mortality is used, striking differences have been observed between the results of blinded and unblinded studies,[9,10] and it has been estimated that unblinded studies exaggerate treatment effect by 17% compared with blinded studies.[36]

Studies of Natural History or Prognosis

A study of natural history or prognosis (also called a cohort study) evaluates a single group of patients followed over time. Because there is no control group, it is not possible to evaluate an intervention using a cohort design, nor to establish a cause-effect relationship. On the other hand, a cohort study can provide a longitudinal description of a disease process in a discrete group of patients and is ideally suited to epidemiologic studies addressing the natural history of a disease process or evaluating the prevalence of a disorder in a group of patients. A well-designed natural history study should start with an inception cohort (a group of patients at risk for the outcome of interest, but in whom the outcome has not yet occurred at the time of study entry) and should account for all patients at the study conclusion.

The ready availability of large amounts of clinical and laboratory data has made cohort designs popular for ICU-based research. Cohort studies can provide important information on the prevalence of, and risk factors for, a disease process. Cook and colleagues, for example, undertook a multiinstitutional study to define the prevalence of clinically important upper GI bleeding and to define clinical factors identifying a subpopulation of patients at increased risk for bleeding.[6] Their observation that the rate of clinically important bleeding has dropped below 4% in the contemporary ICU suggests that routine stress ulcer prophylaxis is unwarranted, while the definition of a high-risk subgroup (patients requiring mechanical ventilation for more than 48 hours or patients with coagulopathy) defines a population that may benefit from prophylaxis.

The choice of a study population has a significant impact on the conclusions reached by a cohort study. A recent study of the prevalence of significant upper GI stress bleeding in intubated, hypotensive surgical patients documented a rate of 7.9%,[37] while in a population of postoperative cardiac surgery patients the rate was only 0.35%.[38] Generalizability is maximized by evaluating a large and heterogeneous group of patients; on the other hand, this heterogeneity may mask associations of potential interest to the investigator.

Equally important to the choice of a study population in a cohort study is the careful articulation of definitions for study variables and endpoints. When stress bleeding is defined as the presence of coffee ground emesis in the nasogastric tube, reported rates of bleeding are higher than when a more conservative and clinically relevant definition of upper GI bleeding such as hemodynamic compromise or need for transfusion is used.[39]

Ensuring data accuracy is essential to any clinical study but is a particularly important issue in cohort studies. Data collected by the patient's nurse, the ward clerk, or the clinical caregivers, or data extracted from a retrospective review of a clinical file, are inevitably less reliable and complete than data collected by a dedicated study coordinator using a systematic approach and well-defined diagnostic criteria. Errors, omissions, and incomplete data increase variability and weaken associations that might otherwise be evident. Systematic errors (such as might occur when APACHE II scores are consistently miscalculated) introduce bias. A well-trained study coordinator, working with detailed data sheets, and preferably with a mechanism to review the data collection process and measure interobserver variability, provides the surest guarantee of reliable data.

Case-Control Studies

Case-control studies are commonly used to infer causality. *Cases* (patients with the outcome of interest) are matched on the basis of potentially confounding variables with a group of *controls* who do not have the outcome of interest; demonstration of differing rates of a putative risk factor in the two groups suggests the possibility of a cause-effect relationship. For example, Durbin and Kopel studied a group of patients who required readmission to a surgical intensive care unit.[40] Each readmitted patient was matched by age, gender, unit, and diagnosis (to ensure that these explanatory variables were equally distributed between the two groups) to a patient who was not readmitted. Cases were significantly more likely to have an increased respiratory rate and positive fluid balance, leading the authors to conclude that pulmonary failure is an important cause of readmission and that the use of an intermediate care unit focusing on respiratory therapy might reduce rates of ICU readmission. Confirmation of this hypothesis would require a clinical trial, but the inference drawn from a much simpler and cheaper study design may be all that is needed to result in a change in practice.

In a classical case-control study, cases share a common outcome of interest and are compared with controls to define risk factors that may account for that outcome. A variation on the case-control design permits estimation of the extent to which a given outcome can be accounted for by exposure to a risk factor: Patients with a risk factor of interest are matched to a control group that lacks that risk factor, then the outcomes of the two groups are compared. Martin and associates, for example, matched a group of patients with nosocomial bacteremia with coagulase-negative *Staphylococci* to a group of patients of comparable age, gender, primary diagnosis, operative procedure, and date of admission[41] and showed an augmented risk of mortality (risk ratio 1.8; 95% confidence interval, 1.2–2.7) and an excess hospital stay of 8.5 days. They concluded that coagulase-negative bacteremia results in a significant increase in attributable morbidity and mortality, independent of the risk factors that might have predisposed the patient to infection.

Case-control studies are subject to bias resulting from the unmeasured influence of some confounding variable. The results of the study of Martin and coworkers,[37] for example, may be explained by a greater severity of illness in the cases, since cases were not matched by a severity-of-illness measure. Case-control designs frequently overestimate an effect and are primarily hypothesis-generating studies.

Case Reports

Case reports lack both a control group and a systematic intervention, and the information they provide is limited. A report of a significant and unusual or unexpected complication may be important for other practitioners. However, case reports do not pose questions and therefore can provide only a description of patient outcomes.

Ethical Issues in ICU-Based Research

Any ICU investigation that involves the imposition of a systematic approach to patient care, or the performance of tests or measurements outside those routinely indicated for clinical care, must be reviewed by the institutional review board or human ethics committee of the hospital or university. Indeed most contemporary journals will not even review a manuscript if it does not include an explicit description of the process of obtaining consent (or of the decision of the institutional review board to waive the need for consent), and virtually all granting agencies require the applicant to submit proof of ethical review before releasing funds.

Clinical research in an intensive care unit generally involves patients who are sufficiently ill that they cannot give informed consent to participate in a trial, and the investigator must approach a surrogate (commonly a spouse or other relative) for third-party consent. Acceptance of the principle of third-party consent for clinical research varies among institutions, granting agencies, and regulatory bodies. Many accept the principle that third-party consent is both ethical and appropriate if incompetent patients are not to be denied the potential benefits (both individually and as a group of patients) of well-done research. Others, however, require that consent for research be provided by the potential subject, arguing that this provides the surest safeguard to the patient's well-being. Local approaches must be investigated before undertaking ICU-based research.

Constraints on the performance of research with third-party consent may significantly alter the results and interpretations of such research. A study of corticosteroids in shock[42] performed in American Veterans Administration (VA) hospitals required first-party consent for study enrollment. Baseline mortality was therefore much lower than commonly seen in other sepsis trials, and patients with encephalopathy, a population known to be at particularly high risk of an adverse outcome,[43] were systematically excluded.

Industry-funded studies in the ICU present the investigator with an additional potential conflict of interest. Since funding is based on the number of patients recruited into a trial (and since ongoing research activities in the ICU are commonly dependent on externally generated revenues), the potential exists for entry criteria to be stretched and for patients to be inappropriately entered into trials.[44] Similarly, the desire of an investigator to recruit patients to a trial, usually as a result of a conviction that patients enrolled in a trial receive the best therapy currently available, may result in inappropriate patient recruitment. The scientific and political consequences of this transgression, appropriately considered to be a serious form of scientific misconduct, are considerable.[45] The investigator must be vigilant to the potential for such misconduct and should actively involve other coinvestigators or study personnel in decisions regarding enrollment of patients in whom questions of study eligibility may arise.

Implementation of ICU-Based Research: A Multidisciplinary Challenge

ICU-based research presents a number of logistical as well as methodologic challenges. The resolution of these can be difficult but rewarding and commonly leads to the creation of a better climate for overall patient care.

Research is only ethical if the benefits of the intervention are truly unknown, either because the intervention is experimental and untested or because there is genuine disagreement among practitioners as to which approach is best (a state termed *clinical equipoise*). In designing a trial testing two different transfusion strategies, Hebert and colleagues first ascertained that a state of clinical equipoise exists among Canadian intensivists.[46] If there was consensus preferring one approach or the other, regardless of how well grounded that consensus was, a clinical trial would not be clinically acceptable.

Tensions between study personnel and the ICU caregivers are not uncommon. Attending surgeons and physicians may be reluctant to consider their patients for experimental therapy and may be reluctant to allow crucial clinical decisions to be made on the basis of random allocation. Education and communication is the key to resolving these problems. Rounds and written communications to clinicians whose patients might be enrolled in a trial are a powerful tool to allay concerns and to garner one's colleagues as allies rather than as adversaries. Moreover, ongoing communication throughout the trial is critical to creating a truly collaborative intellectual climate.

Nursing staff, too, may feel threatened because a trial imposes a change in practice or an increased workload, and educational efforts must address their concerns and priorities. It has been our experience that most ICU nurses become strong supporters of clinical research and can galvanize the ICU staff to promote multidisciplinary collaborative research, if they are convinced that the work will benefit patient care. Employing an ICU nurse as study coordinator facilitates ongoing interactions with the clinical nurses in the ICU.

ICU residents must be encouraged early in their rotations to become active participants in the research process, and education is again the key to success. Residents occupy a critical role in the research process, because they are often the first to make management decisions and as a result can identify suitable patients for a trial. Conversely, residents may institute measures that render a potential study patient ineligible for study if they are not recruited as active participants in the research process.

Pocket cards outlining entry and exclusion criteria for clinical trials, posters publicizing ongoing research projects, and teaching rounds are all important tools in raising the profile of ICU-based research and of winning the maximal support of the ICU team. Ideally, research should become an intrinsic part of the ICU routine, to be reviewed during clinical rounds and integrated into an overall objective of providing the best possible clinical care.

Multicenter ICU Research: A Canadian Model

Multicenter clinical trials are the best vehicle to maximize the generalizability of an investigation and to permit its completion in a timely fashion. Clinical research in oncology and cardiovascular sciences has been immeasurably aided by the establishment of cooperative multicenter groups that define important questions for study and mobilize resources for large-scale investigation. Although industry-funded studies have led to the development of multicenter collaborative interactions, the focus of these has been the investigation of a single commercially exploitable agent or device. In contrast, ongoing peer-driven multicenter ICU research collaborations have been few.

An exception, and a model for collegial academic interaction, has been the Canadian Critical Care Trials Group (CCCTG). Founded in 1989 by a group of academic intensivists under the auspices of the Canadian Critical Care Society, the CCCTG has emerged as a powerful vehicle for developing and conducting high-quality ICU-based clinical research. The organization has attracted intensivists from most of the major academic centers in Canada, as well as a number of individuals with independent expertise in epidemiology, clinical trials design, and biostatistics. Through semiannual general meetings, the membership reviews proposals for studies, critiques study design, and facilitates interinstitutional academic collaboration. Sponsorship by the CCCTG has been viewed favorably by funding agencies, which has permitted the group to publish trials addressing the rates of, and risk factors for, clinically important GI bleeding in the ICU,[6] the optimal threshold for the transfusion of packed red blood cells in ICU patients,[47] and attitudes of Canadian practitioners to the withdrawal of life support.[29] Four more large multicenter studies are in progress, with additional projects in varying stages of development.

Collaborative multicenter research presents a number of challenges—geographic, logistical, and political. But the rewards are great. Research questions can be designed by the intensivist based on scientific and clinical interest rather than commercial potential. The intellectual stimulation derived from the interactions of a group of committed investigators is invigorating, and the availability of a large number of patients for study makes investigations both feasible and valid.

Conclusion

ICU-based research presents unique challenges and opportunities to the investigator. Challenges stem from the complexity of the clinical disorders present, the heterogeneity of the patient population, and the ongoing demands of the clinical care of critically ill patients. But intensive care units treat problems on the frontiers of medical possibility and, in the process, generate enormous costs. ICU-based research must continue to expand in scope and improve in caliber if the clinical resource is to be used optimally.

References

1. Jacobs P, Noseworthy TW. National estimates of intensive care utilization and costs: Canada and the United States. Crit Care Med 1990;18:1282–1286.

2. Maclean LD, Meakins JL, Taguchi K, Duignan JP, Dhillon KS, Gordon J. Host resistance in sepsis and trauma. Ann Surg 1975;182:207–217.

3. Meakins JL, Pietsch JB, Bubenick O, Kelly R, Rode H, Gordon J, Maclean LD. Delayed hypersensitivity: indicator of acquired failure of host defenses in sepsis and trauma. Ann Surg 1977;186:241–250.

4. Christou NV, Meakins JL. Neutrophil function in surgical patients: in vitro correction of abnormal neutrophil chemotaxis by levamisole. Surgery 1979;85:543–548.

5. Tellado JM, Christou NV. Critically ill anergic patients demonstrate polymorphonuclear neutrophil activation in the intravascular compartment with decreased cell delivery to inflammatory foci. J Leukoc Biol 1991;50:547–553.

6. Cook DJ, Fuller H, Guyatt GH, Marshall JC, Leasa D, Hall R, Winton T, Rutledge F, Royy P, Willan A. Risk factors for gastrointestinal bleeding in critically ill patients. New Engl J Med 1994;330:377–381.

7. Ziegler EJ, Fisher CJ, Sprung CL, Straube RC, Sadoff JC, Foulke GE, Wortel CH, Fink MP, Dellinger RP, Teng NNH, Allen IE, Berger HJ, Knatterud GL, LoBuglio AF, Smith CR, the HA-1A Sepsis Study Group. Treatment of gram-negative bacteremia and septic shock with HA-1A human monoclonal antibody against endotoxin. New Engl J Med 1991;324:429–436.

8. McCloskey RV, Straube RC, Sanders C, Smith SM, Smith CR, the CHESS Trial Study Group. Treatment of septic shock with human monoclonal antibody HA-1A. A randomized double-blind, placebo-controlled trial. Ann Intern Med 1994;121:1–5.

9. Fisher CJ, Slotman GJ, Opal SM, Pribble JP, Bone RC, Emmanuel G, Ng D, Bloedow DC, Catalano MA, the IL-1ra Sepsis Syndrome Study Group. Initial evaluation of human recombinant interleukin-1 receptor antagonist in the treatment of sepsis syndrome: a randomized, open-label, placebo-controlled multicenter trial. Crit Care Med 1994; 22:12–21.

10. Fisher CJ, Dhainaut J-FA, Opal SM, Pribble JP, Balk RA, Slotman GJ, Iberti TJ, Rackow EC, Shapiro MJ, Greenman RL, Reines HD, Shelly MP, Thompson BW, LaBreque JF, Catalano MA, Knaus WA, Sadoff JC, the Phase III rhIL-1ra Sepsis Syndrome Study Group. Recombinant human interleukin 1 receptor antagonist in the treatment of patients with sepsis syndrome. Results from a randomized, double-blind, placebo-controlled trial. JAMA 1994;271:1836–1843.

11. Bone RC, Fisher CJ, Clemmer TP, Slotman GJ, Metz CA, Balk RA, the Methylprednisolone Severe Sepsis Study Group. Sepsis syndrome: a valid clinical entity. Crit Care Med 1989;17:389–393.

12. Marshall JC. Infection and the host septic response contribute independently to adverse outcome in critical illness: implications for clinical trials of mediator antagonism. In: Vincent JL, ed. 1995 Yearbook of Intensive Care and Emergency Medicine. Berlin: Springer-Verlag, 1995, pp. 1–13.

13. Knaus WA, Draper EA, Wagner DP, Zimmerman JE. APACHE II: a severity of disease classification system. Crit Care Med 1985;13:818–829.

14. Knaus WA, Wagner DP, Draper EA, Zimmerman JE, Bergner M, Bastos PG, Sirio CA, Murphy DJ, Lotring T, Damiano A, Harrell FE. The APACHE III prognostic system. Risk prediction of hospital mortality and critically ill hospitalized adults. Chest 1991;100:1619–1636.

15. Le Gall JR, Loirat P, Alperovitch A, Glaser P, Granthil C, Mathieu D, Mercier P, Thomas R, Villers D. A simplified acute physiology score for ICU patients. Crit Care Med 1984;12:975–977.

16. Le Gall J-R, Lemeshow S, Leleu G, Klar J, Huillard J, Rue M, Teres D, Artigas A, the Intensive Care Unit Scoring Group. Customized probability models for early severe sepsis in adult intensive care patients. JAMA 1995;273:644–650.

17. Lemeshow S, Klar J, Teres D, Avrunin JS, Gehlbach SH, Rapoport J, Rue M. Mortality probability models for patients in the intensive care unit for 48 or 72 hours: a prospective, multicenter study. Crit Care Med 1994;22:1351–1358.

18. Knaus WA, Harrell FE, Fisher CJ Jr, Wagner DP, Opal SM, Sadoff JC, Draper EA, Walawander CA, Conboy K, Grasela TH. The clinical evaluation of new drugs for sepsis: a prospective study design based on survival analysis. JAMA 1993; 270:1233–1241.

19. Ranson JHC, Rifkind KM, Roger DF, Fink SD,

Eng F, Spencer FC. Prognostic signs and the role of operative management in acute pancreatitis. Surg Gynecol Obstet 1974;139:69–81 .

20. Sprung CL. Definitions of sepsis: have we reached a consensus? Crit Care Med 1991;19:849–851.

21. Members of ACCP/SCCM Consensus Conference Committee. Definitions for sepsis and organ failure and guidelines for the use of innovative therapies in sepsis. Crit Care Med 1992;20:864–874.

22. Murray JF, Matthay MA, Luce JM, Flick MR. An expanded definition of the adult respiratory distress syndrome. Am Rev Respir Dis 1988;138:720–723.

23. Bonten MJM, Gaillard CA, Wouters EFM, Van Tiel FH, Stobberingh EE, Van der Geest S. Problems in diagnosing nosocomial pneumonia in mechanically ventilated patients: a review. Crit Care Med 1994;22:1683–1691.

24. Cook DJ, Brun-Buisson C, Guyatt GH, Sibbald WJ. Evaluation of new diagnostic technologies: bronchoalveolar lavage and the diagnosis of ventilator-associated pneumonia. Crit Care Med 1994;22: 1314–1322.

25. Fagon JY, Chastre J, Domart Y, Trouillet JL, Pierre J, Darne C, Gibert C. Nosocomial pneumonia in patients receiving continuous mechanical ventilation. Prospective analysis of 52 episodes with use of a protected specimen brush and quantitative culture techniques. Am Rev Respir Dis 1989;139: 877–884.

26. Heyland DK, Cook DJ, Jaeschke R, Griffith L, Lee HN, Guyatt GH. Selective decontamination of the digestive tract. An overview. Chest 1994; 105:1221–1229.

27. Knaus WA, Sun X, Olof Nystrom P, Wagner DP. Evaluation of definitions for sepsis. Chest 1992; 101:1656–1662.

28. Marshall JC. Multiple organ dysfunction syndrome (MODS). In: Sibbald WJ, Vincent JL, eds. Clinical Trials for the Treatment of Sepsis. Berlin: Springer-Verlag, 1995, pp. 122–138.

29. Cook DJ, Guyatt GH, Jaeschke R, Reeve J, Spanier A, King D, Molloy DW, Willan A, Streiner DL, the Canadian Critical Care Trials Group. Determinants in Canadian health care workers of the decision to withdraw life support from the critically ill. JAMA 1995;273:703–708.

30. Petros AJ, Marshall JC, van Saene HKF. Should morbidity replace mortality as an endpoint for clinical trials in intensive care? Lancet 1995;345: 369–371.

31. Van de Werf F, Topol EJ, Lee KL, Woodlief LH, Granger CB, Armstrong PW, Barbash GI, Hampton JR, Guerci A, Simes RJ, et al. Variations in patient management and outcomes for acute myocardial infarction in the United States and other countries. Results from the GUSTO trial. Global usage of streptokinase and tissue plasminogen activator for occluded coronary arteries. JAMA 1995;273:1586–1591.

32. Hebert PC, Drummond AJ, Singer J, Bernard GR, Russell JA. A simple multiple system organ failure scoring system predicts mortality of patients who have sepsis syndrome. Chest 1993;104:230–235.

33. Fink MP. Another negative clinical trial of a new agent for the treatment of sepsis: rethinking the process of developing adjuvant treatments for serious infections. Crit Care Med 1995;23:989–991.

34. Marshall JC, Cook DJ, Christou NV, Bernard GR, Sprung CL, Sibbald WJ. Multiple organ dysfunction score: a reliable descriptor of a complex clinical outcome. Crit Care Med 1995;23:1638–1652.

35. Shoemaker WC, Schluchter M, Hopkins JA, Appel PL, Schwartz S, Chang PC. Comparison of the relative effectiveness of colloids and crystalloids in emergency resuscitation. Am J Surg 1981;142: 73–84.

36. Schulz KF, Chalmers I, Hayes RJ, Altman DG. Empirical evidence of bias. Dimensions of methodological quality associated with estimates of treatment effects in controlled trials. JAMA 1995;273:408–412.

37. Martin LF, Booth FVMcL, Reines HD, Deysach LG, Kochman RL, Erhardt LJ, Geis GS. Stress ulcers and organ failure in intubated patients in surgical intensive care units. Ann Surg 1992;215: 332–337.

38. Rosen HR, Vlahakes GJ, Rattner DW. Fulminant peptic ulcer disease in cardiac surgical patients: pathogenesis, prevention, and management. Crit Care Med 1992;20:354–359.

39. Lacroix J, Infante-Rivard C, Jenicek M, Gauthier M. Prophylaxis of upper gastrointestinal bleeding in intensive care units: a meta-analysis. Crit Care Med 1989;17:862–869.

40. Durbin CG, Kopel RF. A case control study of patients readmitted to the intensive care unit. Crit Care Med 1993;21:1547–1553.

41. Martin MA, Pfaller MA, Wenzel RP. Coagulase-negative staphylococcal bacteremia. Mortality and hospital stay. Ann Intern Med 1989;110:9–15.

42. The Veterans Administration Systemic Sepsis Co-operative Study Group. Effect of high dose glu-cocorticoid therapy on mortality in patients with clinical signs of systemic sepsis. New Engl J Med 1987;317:659–665.

43. Sprung CL, Peduzzi PN, Shatney CH, Schein RMH, Wilson MF, Steagren JN, Hinshaw LB, the Veterans Administration Systemic Sepsis Coopera-tive Study Group. Impact of encephalopathy on mortality in the sepsis syndrome. Crit Care Med 1990;18:801–806.

44. Eidelman LA, Sprung CL. Why have new effec-tive therapies for sepsis not been developed? Crit Care Med 1994;22:1330–1334.

45. Angell M, Kassirer JP. Setting the record straight in the breast cancer trials. New Engl J Med 1994;330:1448–1450.

46. Hebert PC, Wells G, Marstin C, Tweeddale M, Marshall J, Blajchman M, Sandham D, Schweitzer I, Boisvert D, Calder L. A Canadian survey of transfusion practices in critically ill patients. Crit Care Med 1997 (in press).

47. Hebert PC, Wells G, Marshall J, Martin C, Tweeddale M, Pagliarello G, Blajchman M, the Canadian Critical Care Trials Group. Transfusion requirements in critical care. A pilot study. JAMA 1995;273:1439–1444.

48. Marshall JC, Christou NV, Meakins JL. The gas-trointestinal tract. The "undrained abscess" of mul-tiple organ failure. Ann Surg 1993;218:111–119.

49. Krause W, Matheis H, Wulf K. Fungaemia and funguria after oral administration of Candida al-bicans. Lancet 1969;1:598–599.

50. Driks MR, Craven DE, Celli BR, Manning M, Burke RA, Garvin GM, Kunches LM, Farber HW, Wedel SA, McCabe WR. Nosocomial pneu-monia in intubated patients given sucralfate as compared with antacids or histamine type 2 block-ers. The role of gastric colonization. New Engl J Med 1987;317:1376–1382.

51. Blair P, Rowlands BJ, Lowry K, Webb H, Arm-strong P, Smilie J. Selective decontamination of the digestive tract: a stratified, randomized, prospective study in a mixed intensive care unit. Surgery 1991;110:303–310.

52. Gutierrez G, Bismar H, Danzker DR, Silva N. Comparison of gastric intramucosal pH with mea-sures of oxygen transport and consumption in criti-cally ill patients. Crit Care Med 1992;20:451–457.

53. Roumen RMH, Redl H, Schlag G, Sandtner W, Koller W, Goris RJA. Scoring systems and blood lactate concentrations in relation to the develop-ment of adult respiratory distress syndrome and multiple organ failure in severely traumatized pa-tients. J Trauma 1993;35:349–355.

54. Gattinoni L, Brazzi L, Pelosi P, Latini R, Tognoni G, Pesenti A, Fumagalli R. A trial of goal-oriented hemodynamic therapy in critically ill patients. New Engl J Med 1995;333:1025–1032.

55. Hayes MA, Timmins AC, Yau EHS, Palazzo M, Hinds CJ, Watson D. Elevation of systemic oxygen delivery in the treatment of critically ill patients. New Engl J Med 1994;330:1717–1722.

Commentary

There are many ways to categorize clinical re-search; one method is to identify the locus of the studies. The fundamental principles and methods of clinical research are well defined in this text-book. On the other hand, experiments in each environment have their own set of challenges. Dr. Marshall and colleagues explain with great clarity the unique aspects of research conducted in an intensive care unit. Informed consent in critically ill patients, definition of endpoints when so many of the disease processes are multifactorial, and separating the effects of an intervention in such complex illnesses are special problems in ICU re-search. From an economic viewpoint interven-tions performed in ICU settings, though poten-tially lifesaving, are frequently costly. Thus, conclusions drawn from studies performed in the ICU have potential major economic and social impact. Acquiring sufficient numbers of compa-rable patients in order to make meaningful com-parisons is a problem requiring cooperative studies between different intensive care units. After read-ing this chapter carefully I came to appreciate an aspect of ICU research that I had not previously considered. Given the critical nature of patients in such environments, a remarkable level of trust between families and physicians must exist; one of the important ingredients for successful ICU investigation is an investigator-physician who cares not only for patients but for their families.

A.S.W.

CHAPTER 53

Research in Surgical Education

H.M. MacRae, R. Cohen, R. Reznick, C. Jamieson, and M.F. McKneally

Patient care, teaching, and research are the traditional functions of an academic unit. Of these, education has long been the orphan child of academic surgery, receiving less prestige and support from the department than other areas. Recently, however, departments of surgery have begun to recognize the role of educational research and leadership in the development and maintenance of a dynamic, well-rounded department. Progressive departments have directed energy and resources toward the enhancement of educational practice, leading to the emergence of a formal role for the surgeon-educator and the practicing surgeon with a scientific approach to the teaching and learning process.

Research in the basic science and clinical arena has the goal of advancing frontiers of knowledge and ultimately enhancing patient care. However, "the work . . . becomes consequential only as it is understood by others."[1] Antman and colleagues[2] have demonstrated that more than 10 years may pass between proof that a clinical intervention is beneficial and its appearance in standard textbooks as accepted therapy, implying that an important step in the dissemination of knowledge is missing. At a time when surgical knowledge is rapidly expanding, surgical education research may enable us to bridge the gap and enhance the translation of research findings into the clinical care of surgical patients.

Changes in health care delivery are affecting surgical education dramatically. For example, surgical departments need to restructure their teaching programs to accommodate education in the outpatient setting. Departments of surgery with a strong focus in education can anticipate, evaluate, and respond to the effectiveness of change. Research on how programs can best respond and adapt to changing learning needs is also required.

A surgeon with expertise in education is able to identify the important issues in surgical training at each stage of the learning continuum, to pose meaningful research questions, and to take a proactive role in anticipating the direction of change in the future. The goal of research in surgical education, like that of all surgical research, is ultimately to enhance surgical practice.

Surgical education research may involve any stage of learning in surgery, from undergraduate training to continuing education. Surgical education as a discipline is still relatively new, and in most areas research opportunities abound. Following are some of the focal points of current research in surgical education.

Curriculum

Traditional surgical curricula have been left largely to chance. The patient population on the hospital ward determined the learning opportunities for students at all levels. The apprenticeship model assumes that a broad spectrum of surgical problems will be encountered in the hospital, ultimately leading to a comprehensive surgical learning experience. This haphazard approach to curriculum planning is not in the best interests of students. The curriculum should provide a road map, outlining realistic expectations of what students should be able to do on completion of a course of education.

In designing a curriculum, one of the first steps is to carry out a needs assessment. A learning need is the gap between the current and optimal competence or performance. Needs assessments have been an important component of curriculum research at the undergraduate and postgraduate levels. For example, a study of the learning needs of surgical residents asked surgeons who had recently graduated from general surgery programs in Canada to identify areas in which they felt their programs had not adequately prepared them. Communication skills were a widely cited area of deficiency.[3]

In continuing medical education, an important function of program design is to identify true learning needs, enabling programs to target deficits most effectively. Surveys, practice audits, pre- and posttests, and local epidemiologic data are all tools that can be used in research on learning needs. This type of research can lead directly to modification of programs to meet the needs of participants.

Research in curriculum development and planning at all levels of surgical training is needed to enable us to identify learning needs and develop programs that are able to meet those needs.

Assessment of Competence

Accountability of the profession to the public, with pressures to ensure that licensure and certification decisions are valid, has generated interest in the assessment of competence. Although the ability to ensure a candidate is capable of handling all aspects of job-related problems is an important aspect of certification and licensure decisions, these decisions have traditionally relied only on the assessment of cognitive skills. When evalu-

ating an examination, one must assess whether the tasks required on the examination are related to competent performance on the job, with validity checks ensuring there is a relationship between what is assessed in the evaluation and what constitutes the profession's theory of competence or what will be expected of the practitioner in day-to-day functioning.

Evaluation techniques include ward ratings, written tests such as multiple-choice examinations, oral examinations, and, more recently, performance-based assessments such as the Objective Structured Clinical Examination (OSCE) and its variants. Research in assessment has focused primarily on the psychometric properties (the reliability and validity) of these evaluation tools. The reliability of a measurement tool can be described as the consistency, stability, or repeatability of the measurement. Validity asks whether the test actually measures what it says it is measuring. Reliability is necessary but not sufficient for validity.

Despite the great amount of literature that has been developed in the area of assessment, validation of methods, especially in relation to how well test results predict performance in practice, has not been well established. Those interested in assessment research require familiarity with the concepts of reliability and validity, because they are the primary means by which a testing technique is judged.

A starting point in the development of research on assessment is to examine the goals and objectives of a program and to determine which ones are not evaluated in the current system of assessment. Areas such as ethics, communication skills, and technical skills are most poorly evaluated at present. The next step is to decide which of the various examination formats would be most suitable to evaluate the objectives in question. An examination can then be developed and tested to determine its reliability, validity, and feasibility.

Clinical Teaching

Evaluations of effective clinical teaching in the health professions have asked students to identify teacher characteristics and behaviors they find effective. For example, Irby[4] found six dimensions of effective clinical teachers via factor analysis of a survey: organization/clarity, enthusiasm/stimulation, knowledge, clinical supervision, clinical competence, and group instructional skills. Ullian, Bland, and Simpson[5] summarized the survey literature as identifying four major roles of the clinical teacher: physician (role model), supervisor (provides opportunity for performance and gives feedback), teacher (selects, organizes, and gives information), and person (interpersonal/humanistic qualities).

Studies have focused primarily on clinical teaching in the ward setting. With changes in health care delivery, emphasis on ward teaching has diminished because patients are often not admitted preoperatively and are in the hospital for shorter periods of time. For surgical teaching, this has led to an increased importance of other teaching locales, including ambulatory clinics and the operating room. Only one study has specifically addressed teaching behaviors in the operating room.[6] This study found differences between resident and student preferences for teaching behaviors, with very specific items, such as letting the learner feel the pathology emerging, being important in operating room teaching.

Observational studies of clinical teaching have focused on teaching internal medicine in the ward setting, with Mattern and coworkers[7] and Irby[8,9] using observations of teachers and interviews to determine which behaviors were most effective. Mattern and colleagues found that listening to case presentations, managing a case discussion, presenting didactic talks, making bedside visits, and approaching psychosocial issues were all important in ward teaching. Irby focused on planning, interactive thinking within rounds, and reflecting on rounds as behaviors used by effective teachers. Preplanned curriculum scripts were also seen as an important component of ward teaching. Irby characterized the forms of knowledge used by expert teachers, which were felt to be context specific. Although these two studies have many implications for surgical teaching, they occurred in the context of ward rounds, in which considerable time was purposely set aside for case discussion and didactic presentations. This setting varies substantially from the typically rapid ward rounds that occur before work in the operating

room on a busy surgical service, in the operating room setting, and in the busy surgical clinic with patients scheduled every 15 minutes. The teaching effectiveness literature in education has found that teacher characteristics or attributes successful in one setting may be very different from those required in another setting.[10] Teacher effectiveness is likely very context and subject specific. A replication of the research of Irby and Mattern and colleagues done in surgical settings would be useful in outlining effective surgical teaching.

Research on clinical teaching has yielded information on valuable teaching behaviors, and many research opportunities exist for similar research specific to surgical settings. The way in which effective clinical teachers, and especially effective surgical teachers, incorporate teaching behaviors into their everyday activities has not been well established. Pressures such as the shift toward outpatient care have necessitated a change in the locale and focus of clinical teaching. Research with a focus on how to enable the surgical teacher to maximize the learning resources available would be invaluable.

Faculty Development

Faculty development can take several different forms, with the short workshop being the most widely used method. The focus of studies in the faculty-development literature has been descriptive, with the intent of aiding others in their own efforts.

Despite the widespread use of faculty-development interventions, outcome measures of their efficacy in changing teaching behaviors are limited. Evaluation of faculty-development efforts in the medical education literature has relied primarily on ratings by the workshop participants or knowledge gain of participants. Studies measuring changes in performance by either observations of teachers or by student evaluations of teaching before and after faculty-development efforts would be very useful.

For the surgeon with an interest in faculty development, many research opportunities exist. More information is needed on how to assess the learning needs of faculty before designing workshops. Descriptive studies of interventions that have been successful also have a role to play. The development of outcome measures to assess the impact of interventions on participants has wide applicability, not only in the area of faculty development for teaching but also for more general continuing medical education.

Continuing Medical Education

In an address entitled "The Importance of Post-Graduate Study," Osler stated: "More clearly than any other, the physician should illustrate the truth of Plato's saying . . . education is a lifelong process. Undergraduate education can provide direction, but is not enough, furnishing an incomplete chart for the professional voyage, and little more."[11] The need for professionals to engage in continuing education to maintain or enhance their knowledge, skills, and attitudes is self-evident; however, the optimal systems to encourage or enforce physician involvement in continuing medical education and the best methods to deliver and to monitor its outcome have not been established. The explosion of medical information over the last 50 years has meant that much of what one learns in medical training is out of date within a decade of leaving formal education programs. Thus, the pace of change dictates that lifelong learning will be the most important part of the education continuum.

In surgery, continuing education is particularly important, with new tools such as video technology and robotic surgery requiring skills that may not have been taught during residency. The challenge for surgeons and surgical educators is to develop, implement, and evaluate programs to aid in the transfer of new knowledge and new skills. Research in the efficacy of these programs is vital, as is research on how well skills transfer from the laboratory to the clinical setting. At this time, research programs with this focus are in their infancy. Researchers with an interest in this area could have a major impact on the development of programs to assist in the transfer of new skills in the future.

In a study of the change and learning in medical practice, Fox and coworkers[12] showed that the majority of physicians regularly engage in systematic processes to change their practice. Forces for change included personal (curiosity, desire for well-being) and social (regulations, peer relationships) issues; however, most changes in practice were driven by the desire to deliver health care more competently. This study found that learning varied, depending on the force for change. When change was prompted by the desire to provide better patient care, learning was more likely to be directed at solving clinical problems than if the force for change was either personal or social. These findings often have not been considered when designing continuing education experiences.

Reviews of the literature on results of continuing medical education programs have found that voluntary formal programs have an effect on the physician's ability to perform well on cognitive tests that follow the course, but the evidence for changes in actual clinical performance or health care outcomes has been relatively weak.[13] Traditional courses that rely on the dissemination of information only are the least likely to result in performance changes and have little or no effect on health care outcomes. Programs that function in the practice site of the physician, providing enabling features such as patient information, are more likely to lead to changes in clinical performance, as are programs that provide specific feedback to the clinician on his or her practice patterns. Multifaceted programs providing all of these elements, especially those that include a chart or performance review, are the most likely to lead to changes in both physician behaviors and health care outcomes.

In view of the energy and resources allocated to continuing medical education, further research is needed on the learning of physicians in practice, how to identify the learning needs of practitioners, the types of interventions most beneficial, and the outcome of continuing education programs. Despite rapid advances in surgical knowledge and technology, continuing education in surgery has received little attention. Research in areas such as how to maintain competence, how to implement new technology safely on a broad scale (e.g., laparoscopic surgery), and how to measure the impact of journals, meetings, or courses is needed.

Formal Training in Medical Education

Increasingly, departments of surgery are recognizing the need for surgeons with training in education and recruiting surgeons with specific skills in this area. Surgeons can increase their knowledge base in education through many forums, ranging from 2-hour workshops to formal fellowship training leading to a master's degree in education.

For the academic surgeon who has teaching responsibilities, but whose primary research interest is in the basic or clinical sciences, short workshops or courses aimed at developing basic teaching skills may be most appropriate. As an introduction, 2-hour to full-day workshops on issues in education are offered at the annual meeting of the Association for Surgical Education. The American College of Surgeons also offers a week-long postgraduate course on issues in education designed for the academic surgeon. The Association for Surgical Education has recently begun a Surgical Education Research Fellowship. Fellows attend a short course on research methodology given in conjunction with the annual meeting. They are then assigned a mentor and, with the mentor's assistance, develop and implement a research project in education. The fellowship is intended to provide encouragement and assistance to those isolated from other surgical education researchers.

For the surgeon whose primary academic interest is education, a formal fellowship program leading to a master's degree is recommended (Table 53-1). Most master's degree programs provide a broad foundation of knowledge in medical education and emphasize the skills required to develop and implement educational research projects. A typical program will include courses in cognitive psychology, research design and methodology, statistics, curriculum design, and adult learning, assessment (including psychometrics), and evaluation.

For the practicing surgeon who is unable to pursue a master's degree on a full-time basis, the University of Illinois program in Chicago may be most appropriate. This program allows for short periods of full-time attendance, followed by research in the home institution. For surgeons interested in pursuing a master's degree on a full-time basis, the University of Toronto has a fellowship in conjunction with the department of surgery.

Table 53-1. Master's degree in medical/health professional education.

Medical school	Contact person
Laval (Quebec)	Dr. Helene Leclere
Toronto	Dr. Richard Reznick
Michigan State University (Ann Arbor)	Dr. Robert Bridgham
Southern Illinois/ Sangamon State (Springfield)	Dr. Linda Distlehorst
University of Illinois (Chicago)	Dr. Georges Bordage
University of Washington (Seattle)	Dr. Charles Dohner
Bobigny (Paris)	
Centre for Medical Education (Dundee)	Dr. R. Harden
University of Limburg (Maastricht)	Dr. H. Schmit
University of New South Wales (Sidney)	Dr. Ari Rotem

References

1. Boyer E. The scholarship of teaching from scholarship reconsidered: priorities of the professoriate. College Teaching 1991;39:11–13.
2. Antman EM, Lau J, Kupelnick B, Mosteller F, Chalmers TC. A comparison of results of meta-analyses of randomized controlled trials and recommendations of clinical experts: treatments for myocardial infarction. JAMA 1992;268:240–248.
3. Cohen AH. Preparation for practice: an evaluation of residency education in general surgery. Unpublished thesis. Ontario Institute for Studies in Education, 1991.
4. Irby DM. Clinical teacher effectiveness in medicine. J Med Educ 1978;53:808–815.
5. Ullian JA, Bland CJ, Simpson DE. An alternative approach to defining the role of the clinical teacher. Acad Med 1994;69:832–838.

6. Dunnington G, Darosa D, Kolm P. Development of a model for evaluating teaching in the operating room. Curr Surg 1993;50:523–527.

7. Mattern WD, Weinholtz D, Friedman CP. The attending physician as teacher. New Engl J Med 1983;308:1129–1132.

8. Irby DM. How attending physicians make instructional decisions when conducting teaching rounds. Acad Med 1992;67:630–638.

9. Irby DM. What clinical teachers in medicine need to know. Acad Med 1994;69:333–342.

10. Anderson LW, Burns RB. Reviewing the research reviews. In: Anderson LW, ed. Research in Classrooms: The Study of Teachers, Teaching, and Instruction. Toronto: Pergamon, 1989.

11. McGovern JP, Roland CG. William Osler: The Continuing Education. Springfield, Ill.: Thomas, 1969.

12. Fox R, Mazmanian P, Putnam W, eds. Changing and Learning in the Lives of Physicians. New York: Praeger, 1989.

13. Davis DA, Thomson MA, Oxman AD, Haynes RB. Evidence for the effectiveness of CME: a review of 50 randomized controlled trials. JAMA 1992;268:1111–1117.

Commentary

This provocative chapter serves as a primer in an emerging field of surgical research. Many universities have recently established promotion and tenure tracks that recognize education that is valued equally with the traditional research pathway. Evaluating and rewarding faculty for teaching requires assessment of their teaching skills and the extent of learning by residents and students. The current objective examinations leave much to be desired. The development of new tools for knowledge assessment will bring a more structured approach to surgical education. It is not yet clear which techniques are effective in promoting lifelong inquisitiveness, surgical expertise, and the synthesis of the many skills required to be a safe and effective surgeon. As economic constraints diminish the time allowed for residency training, traditional methods that have been set more by dogma or belief are being challenged. The development of credible research methodology in surgical education, especially in the evaluation of inanimate models for teaching and testing technical skills, is timely and welcome.

A.S.W.

CHAPTER 54

The Nature of Surgical Research: Phenomenology to Molecular Biology and Back

A.S. Wechsler, with M.F. McKneally

Most research is stimulated by observation of an interesting phenomenon. The task of the investigator is to discover the root causes of important phenomena by developing a series of testable hypotheses. Fragmentation of the phenomenon into definable, separately analyzable components is part of the scientific process. However, as this process unfolds, the new phenomena encountered in turn become the focus of further inquiry.

Research proposals submitted by surgeons are frequently criticized as "mere phenomenology." Phenomena are objects or events, not root causes. They frequently occur in isolation from surrounding events; they are not necessarily the logical consequence of antecedent constructs, nor do they necessarily produce easily predictable, definable, or logic-based consequences. They are things unto themselves.

"What if . . . ?"

By nature, surgeons enjoy tinkering to alter the status quo; they are action oriented and attracted to inquiry based on permutations of reality, particularly those they can introduce using surgical interventions. Many surgical investigations are little more than "projects" stimulated by a particularly vexing clinical problem. The problem may be reproduced in the laboratory to allow a super-

ficial permutation frequently preceded by the question "what if" rather than an analytic one. Phenomenologic research is often the consequence of having a research tool or technique in search of a use: What if we try this technique for that problem? Phenomenologic research is clearly distinct from hypothesis-driven research. Following are some examples:

1. An investigator develops a microsampling technique for assessing catecholamine levels in tissue. The investigator wonders about the catecholamine content in a variety of tissues and generates a proposal to biopsy muscle, liver, and parathyroid gland to determine catecholamine content. This study would yield results that may be quite precise and accurate, and someone may even publish it. But it sorely lacks a purpose other than to utilize the technique.

2. Another surgeon-investigator observes that manipulation of the parathyroid gland is associated with an increase in blood pressure. Hypothesizing that catecholamines may be released from the gland during manual compression, he or she designs an experiment that tests this hypothesis by measuring catecholamine content in the gland and in the venous effluent from the gland before and after manipulation. This experiment is appropriate and hypothesis driven and may advance us toward

understanding the root cause of the phenomenon observed.

3. A surgeon who is curious about gastrointestinal (GI) function wonders about the impact of reversing a segment of ileum in situ. Several tests will be performed to support this observational experiment. It is not likely that anything useful will come from these studies because there is no clear rationale to explain why the experiment is to be performed. Alternately, another surgeon-investigator interested in slowing the rate of peristaltic transit in the GI tract reasons that reversing a segment of bowel may accomplish this purpose. An experiment designed to test this hypothesis, with appropriate tools that focus on assessing this particular outcome (i.e., transit time), is a more reasonable experiment.

4. A surgical investigator proposes to transplant a liver to the neck of an experimental animal to see whether the liver will work. This experiment is an interesting technical challenge but lacks a clear purpose. Another investigator may wish to perform the same experiment to see whether the innervation of the liver influences its function. The latter investigator is more likely to make a meaningful contribution toward the understanding of liver function.

The Hypothesis and the Link to Reason

In each of these examples, there is a probability of meaningful information being generated. However, research grants come from a limited pool of resources, and reviewers believe there is a far higher probability for scientific advancement when experiments have defined purposes that test clearly formulated hypotheses. The probability is increased if the investigator can articulate a clear vision of how the proof or refutation of the hypothesis can be linked to current reasoning about the problem. This logical connection is analogous to recognition of pieces of a puzzle that will advance the task of completing the picture, "linking facts to reason, and creating the opportunity to advance knowledge."[1]

Defining a specific hypothesis to test does not

necessarily make the research important. Investigations that are not phenomenologic should lead to an appropriate conclusion that would define a logical continuation of the study or provide an answer that will terminate a line of inquiry.

Layers of Phenomena

Confounding this approach is the parallel development of knowledge and technology that makes what seemed to be very basic root causes into phenomenological observations when they are viewed in the light of new information. It is humbling to look back over a career of investigation and to realize seemingly analytic experiments based on thoughtful hypotheses frequently did not yield results that defined root causes. How should we think about this inescapable aspect of long-term investigations? The following examples may help to analyze the problem.

Root Causes

More than 20 years ago my colleagues and I were committed to developing an understanding of the pathogenesis of ischemic injury to the myocardium during cardiopulmonary bypass and during periods of induced arrest of blood flow to the heart without cardioplegia. We pursued the fundamental hypothesis that alterations in blood flow to the myocardium during cardiopulmonary bypass were instrumental in causing subsequent impairment of myocardial performance. We argued that intracellular levels of high-energy phosphates and their intermediates were important determinants, as well as markers of cell injury, and that alterations in myocardial energetics and blood flow would ultimately be reflected in cardiac performance. Using a series of animal models, we created anatomic collaterals for occluded coronary arteries. We assessed coronary blood flow and measured intracellular high-energy phosphate levels and cardiac function. We utilized cardiopulmonary bypass as an intervention and manipulated perfusion pressure and the state of the heart (asystole, empty, beating, ventricular fibrillation). We produced brief periods of ischemia and reperfusion. We tested the hypothesis that pharmacologic agents used to support central nervous system and renal performance during cardiopulmonary bypass adversely affected coronary blood flow.

In a series of manuscripts, we presented our findings confirming the adverse effect of α-adrenergic agonists on coronary blood flow during cardiopulmonary bypass, the deleterious impact of low perfusion pressures on distribution to subendocardial heart regions supplied by collateral blood flow, the maldistribution of blood flow that occurred in hypertrophied hearts subjected to cardiopulmonary bypass, the absence of appropriate reactive hyperemia in the subendocardium of myocardium supplied by collateral coronary arteries, and the energetic and functional impairment associated with each of these phenomena.[2-12] Our research appeared targeted and hypothesis driven and led to modifications in the way clinical cardiopulmonary bypass was practiced. It sounds quite analytic now and seemed even more so at that time (the early 1980s). However, one could argue that our observations were also phenomenological in that we had not fully identified root causes. We did not know about the root causes of the 1990s, such as endothelin and nitric oxide; their roles had not yet been discovered.

Changes in Technology and Practice

As these early works were being completed, the clinical conduct of cardiac operations was changing. The model we had chosen appeared less relevant because cardioplegia was reintroduced, lengthening the duration of ischemic intervals to periods of 1 to 2 hours. We had been measuring the effects of ischemic periods of only several minutes. Reperfusion of the heart was occurring in an environment of corrected coronary anatomy, and the dangers of ventricular fibrillation in poorly controlled physiologic settings that had led to myonecrosis (lack of venting of the heart, low perfusion pressures) were now understood. Myonecrosis had been replaced with myocardial stunning as the primary deleterious consequence of ischemia and reperfusion. Myocardial stunning is a form of postischemic damage to the heart that

may be very severe but is completely reversible. It was associated with both systolic and diastolic dysfunction; the exact mechanisms were elusive. Free oxygen radicals had been implicated, as had abnormalities of calcium flux. The role of high-energy phosphate degradation was uncertain.

Stunned Cells

To study stunned but viable myocardial cells, our next period of investigation utilized models of global ischemia. We occasionally induced myocardial injury by a brief period of ischemia followed by a much more sustained period of ischemia "protected" by cold or by various cardioplegic admixtures. Because we were working more and more at the cellular level, it was necessary to develop expertise that would complement our well-established techniques for assessing myocardial function. I was fortunate to formalize my collaboration with Dr. Anwar Abd-Elfattah, a superb myocardial biochemist who understood clinical problems and who remains a close collaborator today. Dr. Abd-Elfattah developed techniques for analyzing minuscule samples of myocardial tissue, allowing us to study patient hearts and to do repeated sampling of experimental animal hearts. Based on the work of others, we formulated hypotheses postulating that delayed recovery of myocardial function after ischemia is the consequence of loss of adenosine, an important precursor to high-energy phosphates. Perhaps we were getting close to a root cause.

During the next several years our research moved to the cellular level by using intracellular biochemistry to specify events in the cell that we could relate to regional and global studies of ventricular performance. We made a series of interesting observations that were the consequence of careful hypothesis testing:

1. Myocytes lost high-energy phosphates when exposed to ischemia, and recovery was correlated with the restoration of high-energy phosphate levels to about 50% of baseline.
2. Adenosine was rapidly lost from myocytes in ischemic hearts and rapidly degraded to inosine.

3. Antioxidants diminished the deleterious consequences of stunning.
4. Inhibition of adenosine nucleoside transport favored accumulation of adenosine over inosine and greatly diminished myocardial stunning after ischemia, while accelerating recovery during reperfusion.[13-25]

In reviewing the results of this period of investigation, I was disappointed to recognize that many of these studies were still descriptive rather than analytic. Although the data were derived from experiments focused on the testing of hypotheses, the studies were still pragmatic observations of related phenomena; however, they did not provide an adequate enough fundamental understanding of the processes involved. This was frustrating because the laboratory had made the transition over a 10-year period from whole animal work to experiments designed to understand events at the tissue and cellular level. Moreover, our continuing referral back to the clinical environment was frustrating in that we knew the problems we were trying to understand, on the surface at least, were getting solved by approaches that short-circuited full understanding of the physiology. We did not fully understand the injury induced by ischemia and reperfusion, but we knew that the addition of certain substrates and the use of certain methods of reperfusing hearts after a long period of ischemia ameliorated the injury. In a sense, tinkering and phenomenology were working. What, then, was the motivation to further our fundamental studies? Some fundamental studies showed free oxygen radicals to be root causes of injury, and many laboratory investigations suggested a therapeutic role of free oxygen radical scavengers, but clinical studies were not supporting their use.

In the research arena, amelioration of ischemic injury by attempts to capitalize on endogenous cardioprotection was becoming more prevalent in the literature. Specifically, heat shock proteins were shown to be highly protective against ischemic injury. The new phenomenon was identified as *ischemic preconditioning*. In ischemic preconditioning a brief period of ischemia and reperfusion that did not produce significant myocardial injury gave experimental hearts enhanced tolerance to a much longer period of ischemia and reperfusion.

In hearts that were ischemically preconditioned, myonecrosis was drastically reduced and cardiac function was preserved. The chemical basis for ischemic preconditioning was unknown, and the way in which this phenomenon might relate to our own studies for ischemia and reperfusion was unclear.

As our studies continued, we observed that ischemia and reperfusion were associated with specific abnormalities of calcium uptake by the sarcoplasmic reticulum and that mitochondrial function was impaired after ischemia and reperfusion. The documentation of specific abnormalities in myocardial subcellular function led us to the conclusion that we would have to develop the techniques necessary to explore alterations in myocardial performance at the molecular level in order to exit the realm of observational science and phenomenology. To achieve our goal of developing hypotheses that would lead to experiments that would provide "root" understanding of the etiology of global ischemic dysfunction, we needed to go to the next level.

Molecular Biology

Dr. Mimi Jakoi became an additional collaborator who shared her expertise in the tools of molecular biology as we approached solving this problem together. We focused heavily on highly controlled models utilizing isolated organ techniques described in Chapter 49 of this textbook. Drs. Yeh and Entwistle brought to the laboratory their expertise acquired in the course of doctoral studies in physiology with a heavy focus on molecular mechanisms of myocardial dysfunction. Certainly bringing our studies to the level accessible with the tools of molecular biology (such as Northern blotting and differential displays) should allow elucidation of the most fundamental aspects of our queries. Moreover, such an approach appeared logical. The time course of stunning suggested that the delay in functional recovery might be the consequence of altered gene programs responsible for subcellular elements necessary for cardiac contraction.

These studies required an unusual approach. Studies performed by molecular biologists frequently focus on the single occurrence of an event or the isolation of a single nucleic acid sequence or gene product—a deterministic, reductionist approach. In our unique experimental environment the hypotheses that we wished to test required interventions that had functional consequences of varying predictability in experimental models of varying stability. We were dealing with a complex system. To minimize variability we kept our approach simple. We used an isolated blood-perfused rabbit heart with an isovolumic balloon as our model. We created a period of ischemia until a specific physiologic endpoint (10 mm Hg of contracture pressure) had been achieved and then reperfused the hearts. Experiments were terminated after 2 hours of reperfusion, and functional data were recorded. Hearts underwent RNA isolation and were probed with specific nucleic acid sequences from specific target genes. Using this approach we had to make best-guess hypotheses concerning the genes that might be affected, but we did so based on studies of sarcoplasmic reticulum that suggested disorders in the function of this cellular substructure.

Our studies demonstrated abnormalities in the messenger RNAs that controlled coding for proteins involved in three aspects of sarcoplasmic reticular function. These aspects included the gene responsible for releasing calcium, a regulatory protein that influenced the calcium uptake channel, and the gene controlling the system responsible for calcium uptake. Remarkably, some genes expressed more messenger RNA while others decreased it, providing what we chose to label "discoordinate gene expression" as a consequence of stunning. We observed the sharp rises in heat shock genes induced by myocardial injury and saw alterations in proto-oncogenes that served as important nuclear transcription factors.[26–39]

Did we achieve our goal? In the beginning of this chapter I addressed the criticism of surgical research as being phenomenological rather than analytic. I defined two common errors. The first was failure to generate a testable hypothesis. The other route to phenomenology was to ask questions of too superficial a nature and by doing so fail to achieve a sense of the root cause of physiologic events. It is an interesting and humbling experience to review one's own work. At each stage the investigations were based on reasonable

hypotheses and employed valid scientific methods for testing. Changing elements in the clinical environment were a frequent cause for shifts in direction. With the evolution of new laboratory tools, scientific information once identified as endpoints became new starting points.

In the small dimensions of information achieved through the tools of molecular biology, testable hypotheses once again yielded information that requires further understanding and probing through the generation of new hypotheses. Confirming the hypothesis that ischemia and reperfusion produce changes in fundamental gene expression now requires alteration in the conditions of ischemia and reperfusion to further determine those events most responsible for influencing the gene changes. The finding that important proto-oncogenes are increased by the process of ischemia and reperfusion generates an entirely new series of hypotheses focused on the meaning of this observation. Perhaps these newly uncovered phenomena represent potentially reparative cellular changes. The trick will be to design hypotheses and experiments that can prove a root-cause linkage to repair.

Conclusion: "What if . . . ?"

Back to surgical tinkering with phenomena: Could trophic hormones accelerate the rate of recovery based on this scientific information? What would the effects of triodothyronine or growth hormone be in facilitating recovery from stunning injury? Some could argue that it was not necessary to pursue such an arduous route to test that hypothesis. One might simply have asked the same question without knowing the specifics of the gene changes induced by ischemia and reperfusion. Although the justification for administration of triodothyronine or growth hormone to accelerate recovery after stunning might have been less well developed, the hypothesis was certainly testable. We are hoping that we can bring some of the knowledge and skills we gained on our subcellular quest to bear on the new information we are gathering from our somewhat phenomenological hormonal studies.

In the account of this scientific journey, a truism of investigation becomes apparent. The search for ultimate answers is ambitious and the goal may never be achieved, but be certain to take advantage of the information uncovered in the course of the quest. Good research identifies layer upon layer of phenomena that provide the impetus to generate new hypotheses, deepening our understanding, enriching our experience with new colleagues and technology, and increasing our intellectual humility.

References

1. Bernard C. An Introduction to the Study of Experimental Medicine. New York: Macmillan, 1927.

2. Wechsler AS, Gill C, Rosenfeldt FL, Oldham HN Jr, Sabiston DC Jr. Augmentation of myocardial contractility by aortocoronary bypass grafts in patients and experimental animals. J Thorac Cardiovasc Surg 1972;64:861.

3. Wechsler AS, Sabiston DC Jr. Effects of aortocoronary bypass grafts on myocardial contractile state: response to catecholamine stress. In: Bloor CB, Glisson RA, eds. Current Topics in Coronary Research. New York: Plenum, 1973, pp. 263–278.

4. Cox JL, Pass HI, Wechsler AS, Oldham HN Jr, Sabiston DC Jr. Evaluation and transmural distribution of collateral blood flow in acute myocardial infarction. Surg Forum 1973;24:154.

5. Pass HI, Cox JL, Wechsler AS, Oldham HN Jr, Sabiston DC Jr. Response to coronary collateral circulation to increased myocardial demands. Circulation 1973;48(suppl. IIV):92.

6. Cox JL, Anderson RW, Currie WD, Wechsler AS, Sealy WC, Sabiston DC Jr. Effects of sustained ventricular fibrillation on non-hypertrophied heart. Surg Forum 1974;35:189–191.

7. Cox JL, Pass HI, Wechsler AS, Oldham HN Jr, Sabiston DC Jr. Coronary collateral circulation during stress and the effects of aortocoronary bypass grafts. J Thorac Cardiovasc Surg 1976;71:540–549.

8. Cox JL, Anderson RW, Pass HI, Currie WD, Roe CR, Mikat E, Wechsler AS, Sabiston DC Jr. The safety of induced ventricular fibrillation during cardiopulmonary bypass in non hypertrophied hearts. J Thorac Cardiovasc Surg 1977;74:423–433.

9. Symmonds JB, Kleinman LH, Wechsler AS. Effects of methoxamine on the coronary circulation during cardiopulmonary bypass. Circulation 1976; 2(suppl.):213. Abstract. J Thorac Cardiovasc Surg 1977;74:577–585.

10. Hill R, Chitwood WR, Kleinman LH, Wechsler AS. Compressive effects of ventricular fibrillation in normal hearts during maximal coronary dilatation by adenosine. Surg Forum 1977;28:257–259.

11. Chitwood WR, Hill R, Kleinman LH, Wechsler AS. Pressure-flow characteristics of the coronary collateral circulation during cardiopulmonary bypass: effects of hypothermic perfusion. Surg Forum 1977;27:268–270.

12. Kleinman LH, Yarbrough JW, Wechsler AS. Pressure-flow characteristics of the coronary collateral circulation during cardiopulmonary bypass: effects of hemodilution. J Thorac Cardiovasc Surg 1978;75:17–27.

13. Peyton RB, Pellom GL, Currie WD, Jones RN, Olsen CO, Van Trigt P, Sink JD, Wechsler AS. Improved tolerance to ischemia in hypertrophied myocardium by preischemic ATP enhancement. Surg Forum 1980;31:315–317.

14. Jones RN, Attarian DE, Currie WD, Olsen CO, Hill RC, Sink JD, Wechsler AS. Metabolic deterioration during global ischemia as a function of time in the intact normal dog heart. J Thorac Cardiovasc Surg 1981;81:264–273.

15. Sink JD, Pellom GL, Currie WD, Hill RC, Olsen CO, Jones RN, Wechsler AS. Relationship of ischemic contracture to high energy phosphate content and mitochondrial function in hypertrophied myocardium. J Thorac Cardiovasc Surg 1981;81:865–873.

16. Attarian DE, Jones RN, Currie WD, Hill RC, Sink JD, Olsen CO, Chitwood WR Jr, Wechsler AS. Characteristics of chronic left ventricular hypertrophy induced by subcoronary valvular aortic stenosis. I. Myocardial blood flow and metabolism. J Thoracic Cardiovasc Surg 1981;81:383–388.

17. Attarian DE, Jones RN, Currie WD, Hill RC, Sink JC, Olsen CO, Chitwood WR Jr, Wechsler AS. Characteristics of chronic left ventricular hypertrophy induced by subcoronary valvular aortic stenosis. II. Response to ischemia. J Thorac Cardiovasc Surg 1981;81:389–395.

18. Jones RN, Hill ML, Reimer KA, Wechsler AS, Jennings RB. Effect of hypothermia on the relationship between ATP depletion and membrane damage in total myocardial ischemia. Surg Forum 1981;32:250–253.

19. Peyton RB, Jones RN, Sabina R, Swain JL, Van Trigt P, Spray TL, Holmes EW, Wechsler AS. Transmural high energy phosphate gradients in patients with ventricular hypertrophy. Surg Forum 1981;32:268–279.

20. Jones RN, Payton RB, Samina R, Swain JL, Holmes EW, Spray TL, Van Trigt P, Wechsler AS. Transmural gradient in high energy phosphate content in patients with coronary artery disease. Ann Thorac Surg 1981;32:546–553.

21. Swain JL, Sabina RL, Payton RB, Jones RN, Wechsler AS, Holmes EW. Derangements in myocardial purine and pyrimidine nucleotide metabolism in patients with coronary artery disease and left ventricular hypertrophy. Proc Natl Acad Sci USA 1982;79:655–659.

22. Wechsler AS, Payton RB, Jones RN, Attarian DE, Sink JD, Van Trigt P, Currie WD. Depressed high energy phosphate content in hypertrophied ventricles of animals and man: the biologic basis for increased sensitivity to ischemic injury. Ann Surg 1983;196:278–284.

23. Abd-Elfattah AS, Wechsler AS. Superiority of HPLC to assay for enzymes regulating metabolism of adenine nucleotide intermediates: 5′-nucleotidase, adenylate deaminase, adenosine deaminase, and adenylosuccinate lyase. J Liquid Chromatography 1987;10:2653–2694.

24. Rosen GM, Halpern HJ, Brunsting LA, Spencer DP, Strauss KE, Bowman MK, Wechsler AS. Direct measurement of nitroxide pharmacokinetics in isolated hearts situated in a low-frequency electron spin resonance spectrometer: implications for spin trapping and in vivo oxymetry. Proc Natl Acad Sci USA 1988;85:7772–7776.

25. Abd-Elfattah AS, Jessen ME, Lekven J, Doherty NE III, Brunstig LA, Wechsler AS. Myocardial reperfusion injury: role of myocardial hypoxanthine and xanthine in free radical mediated reperfusion injury. Circulation 1988;78:224–235.

26. Wechsler AS. Free radicals: the reperfusion ninja. Ann Thorac Surg 1989;47:798.

27. Dworkin GH, Abd-Elfattah AS, Yeh T Jr, Wechsler AS. Efficacy of recombinant derived human superoxide dismutase on porcine left ventricular contractility following normothermic global myocardial ischemia and hypothermic cardioplegic arrest. Circulation 1990;82:359–366.

28. Abd-Elfattah AS, Jessen ME, Hanan SA, Tuchy G, Wechsler AS. Is adenosine-5′-triphosphate de-

29. rangement or free-radical-mediated injury the major cause of ventricular dysfunction during reperfusion? Role of adenine nucleoside transport in myocardial reperfusion injury. Circulation 1990; 81(suppl. 82):341–350.

29. Lehman JD, Dyke CM, Abd-Elfattah AS, Yeh T Jr, Ding M, Ezrin A, Wechsler AS. Polyethylene glycol-conjugated superoxide dismutase (PEG-SOD) attenuates reperfusion injury when administered 24 hours before ischemia. J Thorac Cardiovasc Surg 1991;102:124–131.

30. Abd-Elfattah AS, Wechsler AS. Myocardial protection in cardiac surgery: subcellular basis for myocardial injury and protection. Adv Card Surg 1992;3:73–112.

31. Greenfield DT, Greenfield LT, Hess ML. Enhancement of crystalloid cardioplegic protection against global normothermic ischemia by superoxide dismutase plus catalase but not diltiazem in the isolated, working rat heart. J Thorac Cardiovasc Surg 1988;95:799–813.

32. Ding M, Dyke CM, Abd-Elfattah AS, Lehman JD, Dignan RJ, Wechsler AS. Efficacy of a hydroxyl radical scavenger (VF233) in preventing reperfusion injury in the isolated rabbit heart. Ann Thorac Surg 1992;53:1091–1095.

33. Wechsler AS, Mangano DT. Introduction to a report from the second meeting of the Working Group on Management of Perioperative Myocardial Ischemia: myocardial stunning. J Card Surg 1993;8:201–203.

34. Walsh RS, Abd-Elfattah AS, Daly JJ, Wechsler AS, Downey JM. Selective blockade of nucleoside transport channels prevents preconditioning of rabbit myocardium. Surg Forum 1993;44:234–236.

35. Wechsler AS, Entwistle JWC III, Ding M, Yeh T Jr, Jakoi ER. Myocardial stunning: association with altered gene expression. J Card Surg 1994;9 (suppl.):537–542.

36. Yeh T Jr, Entwistle J III, Graham L, Wechsler AS, Jakoi ER. Carotid ligation alters myocardial gene expression. Surg Forum 1994;45:320–322.

37. Wechsler AS, Entwistle JWC III, Yeh T Jr, Ding M, Jakoi ER: Early gene changes in myocardial ischemia. Ann Thorac Surg 1994;58:1282–1284.

38. Abd-Elfattah AS, Wechsler AS. Myocardial preconditioning: a model or a phenomenon? J Card Surg 1995;10:381–388.

39. Entwistle JWC, Graham LJ, Jakoi ER, Wechsler AS. Myocardial stunning: changes in cardiac gene

expression after global ischemia and reperfusion. Surg Forum 1995;46:209–211.

Commentary

This fascinating account takes us step-by-step with Dr. Wechsler and his research team as they explore below the surface of the clinical phenomenon of ischemic myocardial injury. The quest for root causes takes them to the level of cellular genetic control of myocardial repair mechanisms. Curiously, each layer of exploration seems to lead to subsurface phenomena; the paradigmatic disjunction between phenomenology and root causes does not fit reality as they illuminate its deeper layers. Though the goal continues to elude them, they begin to mine a different phenomenon, the effect of certain hormones on myocardial recovery.

Changes in clinical practice of myocardial protection outside their control changed the research questions. The laboratory confrontation of the frightening, irreversible clinical complication of myonecrosis from ischemic contracture ("stone heart") became irrelevant as surgeons learned to avoid this dreaded complication by using cardioplegic solutions. The focus shifted to the reversible clinical phenomenon of "myocardial stun-ning." The ultimate goal of understanding the mechanism of ischemic myocardial injury seems elusive. The therapeutic question implied in the quest is "How can we extend the period of ischemia long enough to allow us to perform the surgery necessary to ameliorate the mechanical or physiologic condition of the patient's underlying heart disease?" In the closing paragraphs, the voice of the surgeon, who likes to tinker with mechanisms and phenomena encountered in daily practice in the operating room, asks a question from outside the logical sequence of molecular genetic analysis: "but *what if* we add growth factors or trophic hormones, like thyroxine?" A new mine shaft is begun, starting at a different place on the phenomenological terrain but inevitably using the tools and techniques developed as the first was built. When they meet, the shifting ground of clinical practice will inevitably have rendered some of what they will discover less relevant for immediate application to heart surgery. It will nevertheless add generalizable knowledge that will advance science by illuminating causal mechanisms lurking elusively beneath the phenomenological surface of an important clinical problem. Though Dr. Wechsler found it humbling to review this work, it is an inspiring story.

M.F.M.

Analyzing Outcomes

CHAPTER 55

Outcome: Definition and Methods of Evaluation

W. Lorenz

Introduction

Why do we need concepts and assessment of outcome? An alternative to cell and molecular biology as a means of modeling reality in medicine is found in the outcome movement. The role of the scientist is no longer simply the precise methodologist or the sophisticated thinker but also the provider, a person whose primary concerns reflect the needs of the individual and of society. Relman proposed the concept of three revolutions in medical care: 1950–1970 was the era of expansion, 1971–1985 was the revolt of payers, and 1986 to present day is the outcome movement.[1] This classification seems to go against the classical definition of science, per se, but is in fact not a new concept; indeed, Francis Bacon in the seventeenth century defined science as a service for welfare.[2] Now critical questions arise when concepts of outcome are implemented after some modeling and experimentation: Is the outcome movement the right direction for medicine to be headed? As Epstein asks: Will it get us where we want to go?[3]

In his article, Epstein addresses "new directions in assessing outcomes" (Table 55-1). None of them are really new; the paper is a critical review. But his statements are healing oil in the wounds of researchers who have always considered concepts and assessment of outcome as science, not

just as medical routine that is somehow less valuable than basic science. Note that the new directions listed in Table 55-1 are in addition to the former means of analyzing outcome; mortality and complication rates are still considered, but their value is generally limited to scenarios involving high mortality rates. The table suggests that new factors have to be taken into account to improve the scope of outcome analysis.

Absence or relief of pain should be added as one additional important dimension of outcome. Its influence is evident in the development of minimally invasive surgery, and it is an important concern for patients in the final stages of life.[4] It would seem that, in fact, very little is known about improving the state of patients approaching death. Surprisingly, in his report, Allen revealed that religion, spirituality, or concern for one's afterlife play a remarkably insignificant role in the process of dying well, when compared with fear of pain, shortness of breath, depression, and loss of cognitive function. Death is not the worst outcome; dying badly is worse.[5] This is a relevant study in a society with increasing numbers of aged patients, but it is also relevant in surgical illness scenarios, including cancer, coronary artery disease, polytrauma, and sepsis.

Epstein has formulated a statement that is a good summary for concepts and assessment of outcome:

Table 55-1. New directions in assessing outcomes.

Formerly:	Mortality
	Readmission
	Complications
	Other traditional measures of clinical outcome
Now	Functional status
(in	Emotional health
addition	Social interactions
to former	Cognitive function
assessments)	Degree of disability
	Other valid indicators of health

Data from Epstein[3]

Table 55-2. Criteria for good measurement of outcomes: a problem between different disciplines.

- Reliability
  (precision, representativeness, dependability)
- Responsiveness (sensitivity)
- Practicality (usefulness, costs)
- Validity (accuracy, clinical relevance)

Items integrated from Wood-Dauphinee and Troidl[6] and Lorenz et al.[7]

instruments based on subjective data from patients can provide important information that may not be evident from physiologic measurements and may be as reliable as—or more reliable than—many of the clinical, biochemical, or physiologic indexes on which doctors have traditionally relied.

This statement is significant, considering the conflicting attitudes of the Western world to clinical research: molecular biology or clinimetrics? In theory, they complement each other, but in reality they are entirely unrelated or are even in opposition.

Criteria for Good Measurement of Outcome: Do We Really Get What We Want?

Deciding on criteria for good measurement of outcomes is not so much a problem in basic research, but it is a considerable challenge to formulate criteria that are suitable for all the various disciplines contributing to medical outcome (Table 55-2). Within a single discipline, it is not difficult to define consensus criteria. Clinical chemistry is an excellent example; a group of experts analyzed and defined the criteria over a period of several years,[8] published them regularly in the official international journals,[9] and even incorporated them into the German federal law.

Let us examine the categories listed in Table 55-2:

1. *Reliability.* According to the clinical chemists, reliability is simply concerned with whom you

trust and is an aggregate criterion—a metacriterion—for sensitivity, specificity, precision, and accuracy. However, the clinical relevance of such a definition has been questioned.[10,11] In addition, this terminology does not apply in clinimetrics,[7] where reliability means reproducibility of results and measurements with the smallest possible variance or imprecision.[6] In other words, do I get the same effects if I send patients to different places, such as Cologne, Paris, London, or New York? This issue is clinically relevant in our modern era of globalization.

An additional dimension to this criterion is found in economics and public health research (Figure 55-1) and is denoted *dependability*.[12] In Figure 55-1, *performance* means optimum provision of health care for only a few subjects (such as lung transplantation with more than $100,000 per year of life saved). Dependability, however, means medium-quality provision (such as "good" surgery for symptomatic gallstone disease), but for as many individuals as possible with this same quality. Optimum outcome, or efficient system solution, also considers the costs and is clearly a compromise between all three variables; it must be defined as a consensus of the whole society in which the system works.

2. *Responsiveness.* Otherwise known as sensitivity, responsiveness is not very complicated. It simply means, especially in a response to treatment, that the higher the score in the particular criterion's scale, the better the outcome.

3. *Practicality.* Practicality is highly important for measuring outcome. A test may work excellently in supernatants of cell cultures or in blood of nude mice but not in humans under routine conditions, or it may be too costly to be applied in a series of patients. An example

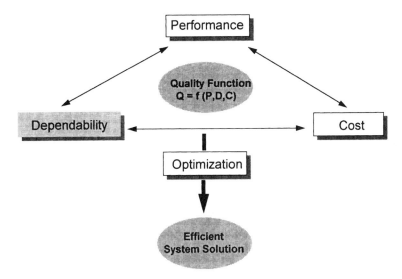

Figure 55-1.   The multiple-criteria optimization problem. Data from Specker.[12]

that highlights this problem was the measurement of HLA-DR expression on the surface of monocytes as a criterion for improvement in sepsis—clearly an outcome variable. Flow cytometry was needed for measuring this improvement, but the comparison of values between different centers with different instruments revealed that it was impossible to use it as a general indicator for an improved outcome in sepsis. In addition, the instruments were too expensive to be implemented in facilities other than those of universities.

4. *Validity.* Validity is deliberately placed at the end of the list, since it is the criterion for good measurement that produces the most controversy in the assessment of the quality of medical care. This criterion is—according to Wood-Dauphinee and Troidl—the degree to which an instrument measures what it claims to measure.[6]

Again, in clinical chemistry, validity is relatively easy to measure. A sample has a given amount or concentration. This analyte is measured by a technician or an autoanalyzer. The two values—given versus measured—are compared, and the deviation of the two values is the accuracy. Minimization of the difference means "good" accuracy, and a standard of acceptable deviation has to be defined by the consensus of a society.

But in the analysis of the health of a patient, or in the measurement of his or her quality of life, do we really "know" what we claim to measure? Is the positive change of a biochemical parameter an improvement of a patient's health status or is it clinically irrelevant? Clinical relevance is part of the validity of measurement in outcome research and it explains why molecular biology and biophysics can be extremely precise but also precisely wrong. Again, the failure of all sepsis trials to date[13] is an example of the present invalidity in the application of principles of basic research to the improvement of patient outcome.

However, are the methods of clinimetrics any better than biomedical assays? Instruments for measuring quality of life can fail in the same way as cytokine assays in sepsis trials. An example of this issue has been found recently in patients with solid cancer of the abdominal and respiratory tract.[14] In these patients, quality of life, as a subjective outcome measurement after operation, was assessed by an established tool that had found consensus in Europe and in other countries: "The European Organisation for Research and Treatment of Cancer (EORTC) Quality of Life Questionnaire."[15] The questionnaire contains 30 Likert-scaled items, structured in four domains: somatic symptoms, functional status, emotional function-

Table 55-3. Experienced social stigma scale

My relatives and friends . . .	Never	Sometimes	Often
1. Are too worried about me	0	1	2
2. Give me the feeling that I am ill	0	1	2
3. Have no confidence in my abilities	0	1	2
4. Annoy me because of their consistent talking about my illness	0	1	2
5. Treat me like a baby	0	1	2
6. Make a lot of fuss about my illness	0	1	2
7. Are tiring because of their overprotection	0	1	2
8. Are nice, but are not able to understand my real problems	0	1	2

Data from Koller et al.[14]

ing, and social functioning. It deliberately avoids any hierarchical structuring of mind and body but includes a universal assessment of quality of life, essentially an expansion of the classic "How do you feel?" Lastly, the index is restricted to a well-defined target group: cancer patients.

This EORTC questionnaire had been rigorously evaluated using psychometric statistical methods. Reliability was studied by a test called Cronbach's Alpha,[16] sensitivity by changes after treatment, and construct validity by item-subscale correlations and group differences. Using this multiaspect-multimethod approach,[17] an accuracy of 96% for the questionnaire's outcome analysis was obtained.[18] This type of formal, almost mechanical evaluation of tests on outcome is now fashionable worldwide. It is the adaptation to the popular ideal in biomedicine: to be able to say "my biochemical test is highly sensitive and specific and has a coefficient of variation of only 1%."

But are we really measuring what we are looking for? To test that, we correlate the measurement of quality of life in existing patients (not volunteers) with measurements in the same patients of psychological or social conditions that we consider unrelated to health-related quality of life, for example, how their relatives or friends judge and treat them (so-called social "stigmatization") and how their doctors judge and treat them (so-called "objective health status"). For our regression analysis we again use a clinimetric index,[19] the Experienced Social Stigma Scale, which was also evaluated using the same psychometric-statistical methods as for the EORTC questionnaire.[14]

What results do we expect? Firstly, the health-related quality of life index should measure what the patient experiences about himself or herself by observation, introspection, and interpretation—termed a *hermeneutic* approach[20]—not what others, for whatever reasons, think about the patient. Table 55-3, illustrating social stigmatization, contains a number of items that highlight the relationship of humans to each other, not only those related to the

Table 55-4. Regression analysis: quality of life, experienced social stigma, and objective health status.[a]

Domain or paradigm	Emotional dysfunctioning	Global QL[b]	Somatic symptoms
Experienced social stigma	0.58**	0.33*	0.51**
Objective health status			
Physician (follow-up)	0.40**	0.24	0.31*
Consultant (medical record)	0.04	0.07	0.19
Emotional dysfunctioning	—	0.50**	0.75**
Global QL	0.50**	—	0.67**

[a]Pearson correlation coefficient: **$p < 0.01$, *$p < 0.05$

[b]QL, quality of life. Cronbach's alpha (scale and interrater reliability) always >0.80.

Data from Koller et al.[14]

Table 55-5.   Concept of outcome.

- Characterized by attributes, associations, and clusters
- Characterized by culture, religion, and philosophy of life
- Characterized by agreement with various objectives: telos of life, autonomy, satisfaction, and the mechanical model of doctor's success

Table 55-6.   A dialogue between two philosophically minded clinicians.

Dr. B: Disease is a fault in the biological machine

Dr. C: You are a biological reductionist; you reduce human beings to biological organisms

Dr. B: Disease is regarded as a deviation from the species design

Dr. C: The primary concern of clinical medicine is a subjective disease and subjective health

Constructed and abbreviated from Wulff et al.[20]

disease state. Secondly, the health-related index should show some correlations to the doctor's assessment of the objective health status, since we are strong believers in the accuracy of the biomedical or "mechanical" model of the disease.[20]

What do we observe? First, regression analysis in Table 55-4 demonstrates a strong correlation between health-related quality of life (global and subscale) and social stigma. In other words, by the EORTC index we expect to be able to measure mainly social stigma and not the health-related or surgery-related quality of life. Second, the results demonstrate further that the doctor's rating about the "objective" health status related poorly to the patient's own assessment of his or her quality of life, especially if the consultant knew the patient from the operation and visits, but not from a systematic tumor follow-up, and developed his or her statement from data found in the medical record.[21]

What do we conclude? We measured quality of life as a postoperative outcome and the health status objectively (biochemically), but these two outcomes did not correspond. We do not know whether we should use neither method or whether we should treat the patient more or less according to his or her personal environment (social stigma) after the operation. This issue is an example of the problems we face in testing validity or clinical relevance.

Concepts of Outcome: The Mechanical, Hermeneutic, or Critical Approach?

We are still far away from an explicit definition of medical outcome. Following Popper's recommendation (see chapter 1), we should avoid giving a definition of outcome in a way that is traditional in physics and chemistry. In mathematics or in formal logic, you may find on the left side of the equation the term "outcome equals," and on right side the explicit, all-encompassing classification. The application of this type of definition to human biology reduces medicine to the mechanical. Similarly, we should not simply translate outcome into result since it is far more complex than an elementary number.

As in Table 55-5, we should characterize outcome by attributes, associations, and clusters, as we have already proposed in Table 55-1 and in the regression analysis for demonstrating validity (Table 55-4). In addition, however, outcome has to be characterized according to the influences of culture, religion, and philosophy of life. This area is somewhat profound but essential in assessing the validity of outcome measurement. We characterize outcome in relation to various factors: the telos of life, autonomy of the patient, and patient's satisfaction. Additionally, objective measurements are needed, such as observing the normalization of transaminases, blood sugar range, and so forth. H. Wulff calls this objective approach the mechanical model of a doctor's success.[20]

In Wulff's book, the argument on the validity of outcome assessment is based on two examples: a dialogue between two clinicians and a comparison of the meaning of illness in several European languages. The dialogue compares—in classical Platonian style—two models of disease and two approaches to assess outcome (success) of a doctor's treatment (Table 55-6).

Doctor B and Doctor C

Doctor B believes in the biological model of disease—in our day, most likely he is a cell and mo-

Table 55-7. Etymology of words for *illness* and *ill*.

Language	Term	Semantics
English	*Disease*	Dis-ease (not free from discomfort)
Greek	*Pathos*	Suffering
Russian	*Boljezn*	Pain
French	*Maladie*	In bad state
Danish	*Syg*	Worried or sorrowful
Latin	*Patients*	One who suffers
German	*Krank*	Curved or bent (*krumm* or *gebeugt*)

Constructed from Wulff et al.[20]

lecular biologist. He believes that the causes of hypertension and cancer can be reduced to abnormalities in the structure or regulation of genes.

Doctor C believes in the hermeneutic model of disease, in a critical model developed by an intellectual and empirical interaction between both views, and finally in an integrative model. The latter is very important, since the hermeneutic approach alone is also a type of reductionism. Doctor C has most likely studied both medicine and psychology or sociology or is a particular hobbyist in these disciplines. She has also studied cultural sciences such as linguistics and history.

Doctor C believes that hypertension and cancer involve subjective dimensions such as anxiety, lack of freedom and will, and a disturbed understanding that have to be communicated and interpreted by the individual patient. Bringing these dimensions into the disease concept is called the hermeneutic approach.

In the dialogue (Table 55-6), Doctor B proposes and defends the biological concept of disease and therefore also a biological outcome. Doctor C proposes a biological and subjective concept of disease and outcome. However, it must be emphasized that Doctor B is not just a neutral observer; he acknowledges the concept of "species design." The patient should be cured by normalizing him or her according to a model that defines the characteristics of an average human subject. Doctor C's beliefs are far more complex: She wants to heal subjective disease, create well-being, restore autonomy—even if the patient is confined to a wheelchair—and normalize biological parameters. The validity criterion

for these two views is clear: Do we observe our predicted outcome?

The Meaning of *Illness* in Europe

An etymological analysis of the words for *illness* and *ill* in European languages (Table 55-7) reveals striking variation, which probably explains to some extent why German doctors and doctors of some other nationalities have such problems with outcome research, as well as understanding clinical research in other European countries. In stark comparison to most other European languages, the German word for *ill*, *krank*, means "curved" or "bent," suggesting the purpose of medicine is to "straighten up" the patient, *ihn gerade machen*. This concept of disease, which has developed in German society over several centuries, is quite mechanical.

Aggregate Variables for Measuring Surgical Outcome: How Do the Indices Fit the Concept?

It is obvious from the critical concept of disease that if this concept is transformed into a clinical measurement of outcome, the decisive criteria must be an aggregation of variables with several dimensions. There are, at present, a series of constructs, surveys, indices, and scores available. Ware[22] has summarized them in an excellent review. However, they were mostly developed for nonsurgical fields, although one of them is used in ongoing clinical trials:[28] the quality of well-being scale, or QWB.[23]

At present, we are working with three indices and will mention them briefly:

QWB scale. The QWB scale is an evaluated index, used especially in rheumatology. Its application in surgery is fairly new.[24]

McPeek index. The McPeek index has been developed for anesthesiology and surgery[25] and has been evaluated and modified in three different trials.[26] It is a recovery index and analyzes a time period of up to 30 days postoperative.

Calculus of clinical benefit.[27] The calculus of clinical benefit has the strongest theoretical basis of all systems mentioned. To our knowledge, however, it has not yet been applied in clinical routine or clinical trials.

Hence, at this moment, we do not know exactly how the available indices pertain to the concept of outcome developed in this introductory chapter. Clinical studies are now required, since we have learned about and emotionally accepted the presence and necessity of the outcome movement.

Conclusion: A Change of Paradigms?

Outcome research and outcome analysis redefine the role of scientists in medicine. This role is committed to the survival and well-being of individuals and societies. It extends the domains of interest for outcome and provides refined criteria for good measurement.

Great emphasis has to be given to the criterion of validity; it has much greater value than its mere accordance with certain test criteria.

Outcome is a concept, not just a term with a mechanical definition. It is characterized by attributes, associations, and clusters on several levels of epistemology and is intrinsically related to the concepts of disease and health. Outcome scales are therefore always aggregate variables rather than individual variables such as the mortality rate. These variables have to be determined through consensus among patients, doctors, and society.

References

1. Relman S. Assessment and accountability. The third revolution in medical care. New Engl J Med 1988;319:1220–1222.
2. Fisher EP. Francis Bacon oder Von der Wissenschaft im Dienst der Wohlfahrt. In: Aristoteles, Einstein, & Co. Eine kleine Geschichte der Wissenschaft in Porträts. München and Zürich: Piper, 1995, pp. 86–100.
3. Epstein AM. Sounding board. The outcomes movement—will it get us where we want to go? New Engl J Med 1990;323:266–269.
4. Allen JR. Good care of the dying patient. JAMA 1996;275:474–478.
5. Patrick DL, Starks HE, Cain KC, Uhlmann RF, Pearlman RA. Measuring preferences for health states worse than death. Med Decis Making 1994; 14:9–18.
6. Wood-Dauphinee SL, Troidl H. Assessing quality of life in surgical studies. Theor Surg 1989;4: 35–44.
7. Lorenz W, Neugebauer E, Uvnäs B, Beaven MA, Ennis E, Granerus G, Green JP, Keyzer I, McBride PT, Mannaioni PF, Pearce FL, Watkins J. Munich consensus development conference on histamine determination. In: Uvnäs B, ed. Histamine and Histamine Antagonists. Handbook of Experimental Pharmacology, vol. 97. Berlin and Heidelberg: Springer-Verlag, 1991, pp. 81–92.
8. Greiling H, Gressner AM. Lehrbuch der Klinischen Chemie und Pathobiochemie. Allgemeine Klinische Chemie. Stuttgart: Schattauer Verlagsgesellschaft, 1989, pp. 1–82.
9. Büttner J, Borth R, Boutwell JH, Broughton PM, Bowyer RC. Approved recommendation (1979) on quality control in clinical chemistry. Part 6. Quality requirements from the point of view of health care. J Clin Chem Clin Biochem 1980;18:861–866.
10. Feinstein AR. Clinical biostatistics. XXXI. On the sensitivity, specificity, and discrimination of diagnostic test. Clin Pharmacol Ther 1975;17: 104–116.
11. Hilden J. The concept of medical usefulness in clinical chemistry and the difficulty of applying it to questions of research policy. In: Horder M, ed. Assessing Quality Requirements in Clinical Chemistry. Helsinki: Finnish Government Printing Center, 1980, pp. 31–46.
12. Specker B. Modeling and optimization of complex

systems using generalized stochastic petri nets. Thesis. University of Haute Alsace, 1995.

13. Bone RC. Why sepsis trials fail. JAMA 1996; 276:565–566.

14. Koller M, Kussmann J, Lorenz W, Jenkins M, Voss M, Arens E, Richter E, Rothmund M. Symptom reporting in cancer patients. Cancer 1996;77: 983–995.

15. Aaronson NK, Beckman J. The Quality of Life of Cancer Patients. New York: Raven, 1987.

16. Cronbach LJ. Coefficient alpha and the internal structure of tests. Psychometrika 1951;16: 297–334.

17. Cronbach LJ, Meehl PE. Construct validity in psychological tests. Psychol Bull 1955;52:281–302.

18. Koller M, Kussmann J, Lorenz W, Rothmund M. Die Erfassung und Dokumentation der Lebensqualität nach Tumortherapie. In: Wagner G, Hermanek P, eds. Organspezifische Tumordokumentation. Berlin and Heidelberg: Springer-Verlag, 1995, pp. A 2.1–A 2.12

19. Feinstein AR. Clinimetrics. New Haven and London: Yale University, 1987.

20. Wulff HR, Andur Pedersen S, Rosenberg R. Philosophy of Medicine. Oxford and London: Blackwell Scientific, 1986.

21. Rohde H, Troidl H, Lorenz W. Systematic follow-up: a concept for evaluation of operative results in duodenal ulcer patients. Klin Wschr 1977;55: 925–932.

22. Ware JE. The status of health assessment 1994. Annu Rev Public Health 1995;16:327–354.

23. Kaplan RM, Bush JW, Berry CC. Health status: types of validity and the index of well-being. Health Serv Res 1976;11:478–507.

24. Westhoff G. Handbuch psychosozialer Meßinstrumente. Göttingen: Hogrefe, 1993, pp. 692–696.

25. McPeek B, Gasko M, Mosteller F. Measuring outcome from anesthesia and operation. Theor Surg 1986;1:2–9.

26. Lorenz W, Dick W, Junginger T, Ohmann C, Ennis M, Immich H, McPeek B, Deitz W, Weber D, members of the Trial Group Mainz/Marburg. Induction of anaesthesia and perioperative risk: influence of antihistamine H_1- + H_2-prophylaxis and volume substitution with Haemaccel-35 on cardiovascular and respiratory disturbances and histamine release. Theor Surg 1988;3:55–77.

27. Little M. Humane Medicine. Autonomy and a Calculus of Clinical Benefit. Cambridge: Cambridge University, 1995, pp. 78–88.

28. Wittmann DH, personal communcation, 1997.

Commentary

This chapter is an intellectually challenging presentation of outcomes of clinical interventions that confronts traditional measurements of success or failure. Variables other than those that are traditional and measurable have been disregarded in the past because the endpoints were "soft"; we believed they could not stand up to scientific criticism and scrutiny. As the field has matured, thoughtful scientists have been able to measure outcomes that relate to aspects and qualities of life that they previously ignored. As in traditional biologic science, a good outcome measure must be robust enough to withstand assessment from many cross-referenced approaches. Some of these approaches are explained in this chapter. Clinical research using scientifically valid tools is no better or worse than other scientific disciplines. It can have an important impact on practice and on society. Determining generally accepted values for different outcomes will make them useful in helping to determine health policy. For example, an operation that consistently prolongs life by 6 months but diminishes the quality of residual life while adding cost might be misunderstood if analyzed only by measuring endpoints such as survival. The information derived from the outcome data would be accurate, but wrong, if it led us to believe in the utility of the procedure for patients and society.

A.S.W.

CHAPTER 56

Quality Improvement: Applying Outcomes Analysis to Patient Care

S.W. Dziuban Jr.

*Once upon a time doctors had nearly complete pro-
fessional autonomy. . . .*

—J.P. Kassirer[1]

*From unquestioned God to accountable production
worker is a long way to fall in a few short years. But
with a trillion dollars in annual health care spending
on the table. . . .*

—J.D. Kleinke[2]

Introduction

The traditional surgical investigator has been "a
bridge tender, channelling knowledge from biological science to the patient's bedside and back
again."[3] The goal of pursuing both research and
surgical practice has been a challenge;[4] successful
models might have involved a split commitment
between "pure research" and "applied care" or
melding the two in a clinical trial on a defined
and controlled patient subset.

By contrast, in clinical outcomes analysis (also
called outcomes research, outcomes study, or outcomes management), scientific methods and research are applied to study the less-controlled and
more heterogeneous mainstream of patient care.
This phenomenon has emerged as a fusion product from economic and political forces, colliding
with clinical knowledge and practices, quality improvement efforts, statistical methods, and information technology.

What is the goal of outcomes analysis? The
same as the ultimate goal of other research: the
continual improvement of care and results for our
patients. Why not, then, apply research methods
directly to our mainstream care processes and results? This concept, with roots in industry, emphasizes feedback of clinical outcomes data to care
providers in a nonadversarial environment, to
identify opportunities for improvement in the
processes of care.[5] The same data can also serve
other more pragmatic purposes, such as demonstrating performance to consumers or regulatory
agencies or as a negotiating or contracting tool.[6]

Although outcomes analysis is still in its infancy[7] and is fraught with difficulties,[8] there is a
widespread demand from payers, regulatory agencies, and consumers for outcomes data, often with
little concern for the rigors of scientific accuracy.
A rapidly growing industry catering to this demand ventures to "collect data from diverse
sources, develop confidential algorithms to judge
the performance of individual practitioners, and
sell the profiles to third-party payers and employers . . . despite well-documented flaws in their
data bases."[1]

Surgeons are lead players in this scenario, because operative procedures are easily identified
and attributable to a specific surgeon. It is important that surgeons not only learn about outcomes
analysis but also assert leadership in the effective
use (and avoiding abuse) of outcomes data.[1] The

challenge is to move away from being targets or victims of the flawed data of others toward ownership and expertise in the productive use and limitations of our own data.

Historical Perspective

The evolution of surgical audit, from ancient practices of census statistics, has been thoroughly reviewed in an excellent monograph by Pollock and Evans.[9] Pollock and Evans point out that clinical research is largely a product of the last century, because of past emphasis on the idealized doctor-patient relationship, reverence for scholastic authority over logical thinking, and lack of progress in statistical methods.[10] Even in recent decades, with the explosion of medical research, clinical teaching and practice have maintained a strong emphasis on the necessity of knowing and treating each patient as an individual. This attitude is reflected in the traditional tool of surgical review, the mortality and morbidity case conference. Early models of quality assurance were similarly characterized by case inspection, focusing on exceptions and outliers at the tails of the bell curve.[11]

Meanwhile exponentially increasing health costs have stimulated a massive health care reform effort, seeking not only cost containment but also clearer evidence of quality, good results, and proven value for cost.[12] In this "era of assessment and accountability"[13] many regulatory agencies, purchasers, consumer interest groups, and patients themselves now seek to evaluate the quality and value of clinical care. This broadened scrutiny has created the "industrialization of medicine, ushered in by the appearance of tools and methods for measuring and managing its practitioners, [that] echoes what every major U.S. industry experienced several decades ago."[2]

From this industry experience, both in the United States and in Japan, comes a well-developed science of continuous improvement that is now being applied to health care.[11,14,15] This new approach departs from traditional medical quality review, which sought to identify nonconforming individuals (the "bad apples" theory); instead, it views patient care as a complex process with measurable outcomes that can be optimized by tech-

niques proven valuable in industry. Several refreshingly different principles characterize this newer perspective:

1. Recognize that all members of the care process (i.e., not just physicians) exert important influence on outcomes.
2. Reduce fear and the disciplinary approach—assume that most people are already trying hard to produce good quality.
3. Focus on improving care processes rather than individuals, with an open attitude that values the identification of problems as a necessary step for improvement.
4. Address efforts at the mainstream of care, the large body of the bell curve, not just the small area under the tails of the curve.
5. Eliminate unnecessary variation by sharing practice information and modeling "best practices."

Outcomes analysis is an essential component of this new improvement approach: it provides us with the information that helps guide our improvement efforts. But does this industrial analogy translate well to patient care? How might it work?

Applying Outcomes Analysis to Clinical Care

The most extensive clinical experience with outcomes analysis has been in the area of cardiac surgery, particularly coronary artery bypass graft (CABG). CABG surgery has high volume, homogeneity, and relatively well-defined risk factors that provide an ideal opportunity for statistical analysis. Efforts are being made to extend the knowledge gained from using these techniques in CABG surgery into other areas, though there will likely need to be different adaptations of the basic principles. However, CABG surgery serves as an excellent example illustrating the principles, methods, and techniques of this work.

Obtaining Outcomes and Process Data

Getting data is the first step toward analysis. Obtaining standardized, clinically relevant data usually requires a dedicated and relatively expensive process of data collection. This data collection is best performed by trained staff who are closely in touch but not identical with the clinical care teams. Data designed for administrative or reimbursement purposes such as DRGs, although readily and inexpensively available, do not accurately reflect the necessary clinical information. Typical useful types of data include patient identification and demographics, risk factors, details of the care process, and outcomes. Having a database format that allows linking to other patient information—for example, costs or resources used—is a potential advantage because it allows exploration into other related questions that inevitably arise.[6]

Outcomes data would ideally reflect any or all components of health status influenced by patient care. Examples are longevity or death, complications of disease, complications of care, physiologic stability or reserve, functional status, role function (e.g., return to work), and quality of life.[8] In reality the complexity of such measurements and the cost of chronic follow-up have often led to the use of a simple, short-term indicator such as acute postoperative mortality and complications. Although this is reasonable and useful as a starting point, we must recognize its limitations as a proxy for overall outcome benefit.

Although process data might not be the initial goal, it quickly becomes important when questions about different outcomes arise. It is therefore an advantage to have process data included as early as possible; the problem is that it is not always easy to predict which process variables will be needed, since the questions that will be raised by the data are not known in advance. Examples of process data elements might be any details of the surgical procedure, anesthesia, or postoperative care that are of particular interest. Examples for CABG surgery might be surgeon name, type of procedure, type of cardioplegia, and operative time.

In designing a new database, it is best to be conservative about the number of data variables collected and resist any temptation to collect "the most complete" data set possible. Smaller is often better when it comes to data forms: completion will be better, cost and effort will be more maintainable, and fewer resources will be wasted on collecting data that may not be useful. The value

of each data element should be carefully weighed against the overall negative impact of too many data elements. Consider the number of patients involved and the fact that each data element has to be analyzed, often in several different ways, to be useful. Among the different CABG study systems, one side of one sheet of paper is the minimum, two sides of one sheet is tolerable, and four sides (two sheets) is the upper limit.

Risk Adjustment to Compensate for Patient Differences

Industrial quality experts have long recognized that variations in input material will lead to wider variations in output. Patients clearly have inherently uncontrollable variations at presentation, described by various terms such as risk factors, case mix, severity of illness, and comorbidities.[8] Clinicians are quick to recognize and even expect that outcome variations may be due to differences in patient characteristics and not necessarily due to differences in care processes. Can one even make fair comparisons of outcomes among uncontrolled groups?

Risk adjustment is the process of quantifying patient variations using a mathematical model, for the purpose of making outcomes more comparable. If outcomes could be perfectly risk adjusted, they would then be comparable because the risk model would compensate for differences among patients. In reality, risk adjustment is an imperfect approximation. No model is perfect; it has been said that "All models are wrong; some are useful."[16] There are different risk-adjustment models even for CABG surgery; five major national or regional risk-adjusted CABG models have recently been compared, along with a thorough discussion of the difficulties and limitations of modeling.[8,17]

The practical effect of using a risk-adjustment model is the ability to calculate the theoretical risk of mortality for each patient. The sum of risks for a group of patients gives the theoretical risk of mortality for that group. This value is called the predicted or expected mortality. The ratio of the actual or observed mortality to the expected mortality (O/E ratio) indicates how many deaths occurred in comparison to the number expected from the model. An O/E ratio greater than 1 indicates more deaths than expected (implying poorer results and performance), and a ratio less than 1 indicates fewer deaths (implying better results and performance).

External Comparison Gives Meaning to Outcomes Data

Even risk-adjusted outcomes data have limited utility in isolation. Some comparison to a standard is necessary to give meaning to the results. In industry, the standard might be the purchaser's tolerance specifications. In medicine we generally seek to optimize results; but how do we know the optimal potential result? Comparison to external data or standards gives guidance and meaning to our results.

Exactly comparable data are often limited or unavailable, and different approximations must often suffice. Historical data, available after time for one institution or for one practitioner, are important for evaluating internal consistency but provide no comparative standard. Results of controlled studies published in the literature usually do not match the characteristics of an outcomes analysis population but can provide some relative guidelines. The two most useful types of comparative standards are

1. Multiple centers or providers participating with the same outcomes data system.
2. A best-practices model that can be used as a benchmark or optimal results target.

External comparative data are so important that they might well dictate which data system should be selected for outcomes monitoring needs. The most sophisticated and ideally structured private database, used in isolation by one care provider, may not yield as much useful information as a less ideal data system that has the benefit of multiple participating providers. Sharing data is obviously necessary to receive the benefits of comparison. Commonly there are some hurdles to openly sharing data, and some arrangements respecting confidentiality are usually necessary. An additional obstacle to sharing comparative data among peers occurs if they are in a competitive situation.

Even with good external comparisons, risk-adjusted outcomes data serve only to raise questions, not to provide answers. For example, if an institution identifies a higher average postoperative mortality than its peers, the reason is unlikely to be immediately obvious. Where or why did the higher mortality occur? What processes could be changed to reduce the operative mortality? Risk-adjusted comparative outcomes data are just the starting point of analysis; the next steps are to identify underlying causes in the processes of care and to evaluate where and how change might be needed.

Using Outcomes Data to Evaluate and Change Care Processes

A risk-adjusted outcome number is a simplified summation or average figure that represents many different categories of patients, care techniques, care providers, and the interactions among them all. It is like the bottom line of a financial statement indicating a red or black figure: a useful summary but, like any summary, concealing the underlying realities and details that produce the bottom line. Does a poorer (or better) summary figure indicate that all patients have poorer (or better) results? Or, more likely, is there a mix of poorer and better results in different categories of patients? Just as managing finances requires delving into the inner details that combine to form the bottom line, likewise managing risk-adjusted outcome figures requires the same kind of exploration into the underlying details of the patients and the processes of care.

The complexity of this reality is unappealing to some who would prefer to think that patient care can be evaluated like toasters in a consumers guide. Such oversimplification leads to the kind of "scorecard" thinking[18] that reflects the punitive and less productive bad-apples approach.[14] This perceptual problem is not likely to disappear given the current atmosphere of external scrutiny over health care.

The underlying processes of care can only be effectively researched and understood by the very care providers who use and understand these processes. To succeed, this effort requires some cultural and organizational factors, including leadership; investments of time, capital, and expertise;

respect for health care workers; and individual physician involvement.[14] But given the motivation and effort, how might we actually use outcomes data?

Exploring the Data: Subset or Strata Analysis?

Facing a summary or bottom line outcomes figure is like looking at a question; the answer may not be obvious in terms of the underlying problems or opportunities. The ability to explore the underlying data is the key to finding answers to the question. Unlike traditional research directed at a defined hypothesis, this data exploration resembles an exploratory operation, where the findings cannot be fully anticipated.

Dissection of the data to isolate and compare different subsets or strata is the basic approach. The process is multidimensional: It may be necessary to look from many different angles, at different cross sections, to find a useful perspective. Breakdowns that might be helpful include patient age, condition, types of operations, surgeon, or any other available data factors.

Naturally, different subsets of the data under study will have different outcomes; for this reason, access to the corresponding internal details of the comparative data set is essential. It would be ideal to get comparative risk-adjusted outcomes that match each subset of each breakdown stratification under study. For example, one might ask how patients over age 70 having emergency surgery in one group compared to the external group.

As the number of patients in any subset gets smaller, the risk-adjustment mathematics tend to become less precise and perhaps less useful. But to the extent that two subsets of patients under comparison are more closely similar, even unadjusted outcomes differences begin to convey information—or at least suggest possibilities.

Unfortunately the internal details of comparative databases are not always available. A useful compromise is to know the prevalence and outcomes figure (e.g., mortality) associated with each data element in both data sets. This information can provide an idea of the population characteristics and outcomes in relation to the comparison population. Data elements that report mutually exclusive and exhaustive categorizations (e.g.,

elective versus urgent versus emergency) may be particularly useful. A case example using data explored in this way is given in a later section.

Evaluating and Changing Care Processes

Once a problem or an area for desired improvement is identified, the care processes involved must be evaluated for potential changes. This evaluation is an essential component and probably the greatest challenge in carrying outcomes analysis through to improvements in care. If relevant process variables are included in the data set, then some association of a process variable with the outcome under evaluation may occur. More likely, the process issue may be too complicated to be completely described in terms of simple data elements.

It is possible that no obvious problem or limitation of care is immediately perceived, since obvious flaws are usually recognized and changed. Invisible or even accepted patterns of care may be at issue; there may be subtle or powerful resistance to change, especially if the current process is perceived as being necessary or the best available.

On the other hand, outcomes data may direct attention at a care problem that has been known but not changed, perhaps because of its underestimated impact, its high cost factors, or the priority of other conflicting needs. Thus outcomes data can help clinicians to recognize unseen limitations or to persuade them of the need for changing things that previously resisted change because of cost or other trade-offs.

The Northern New England Cardiovascular Disease Study Group has used a technique of comparative process analysis among five different centers performing cardiac surgery. In this approach, a group of representative specialists traveled around to other centers, focusing on observing process of care in their own specialty.[19] This direct process comparison emphasized the full scope of care before, during, and after the surgical procedure and was facilitated by a broad commitment to allow observation and openly share information.

There are many challenges in using outcomes data to evaluate and change care processes: identifying targets for change, developing agreement among involved parties, knowing the direction of desired change, and effecting that change. The essentials to success, in our experience, are communication and teamwork.

Case Example: Using Outcomes Analysis for Improvement

The experience of one hospital illustrates the use of outcomes analysis to improve results even when traditional patient case review had failed. A more detailed description has been published.[20]

OUTCOME DATA ANALYSIS FOR CASE IMPROVEMENT

- Acquire outcome data.
- Risk adjust data.
- Perform external comparisons.
- Use data to
  — evaluate subset analysis,
  — evaluate case process,
  — change case process.
- Reevaluate new outcome.

The Risk-Adjusted Comparative Data

Since 1989 the New York State Department of Health (DOH), with a cardiac advisory committee, has monitored CABG surgery with case-specific data. Annual public releases of hospital- and surgeon-specific risk-adjusted CABG mortality rates have been made since 1992.[21-23]

The New York State Cardiac Surgery Reporting System (CSRS) was perceived as externally imposed and, in the early phases, was regarded with little enthusiasm or understanding of its potential. It was a shock and disappointment in late 1992 when the DOH public data release showed that the hospital's actual CABG mortality of 4.6%, against an expected (risk-model predicted) mortality of 2.1%, resulted in a risk-adjusted mortality of 6.6%, which was statistically significantly higher than the statewide average of 3.1%.[21]

Immediately in January 1993 a multidisciplinary group was established to analyze the situation. Initially skeptical, the group criticized the risk adjustment as inadequate ("our patients are sicker than it indicates"); however, they resolved to thoroughly evaluate patient care.

Exploring the Data by Subset Analysis

Three investigations were begun: repeat abstraction of all CABG patient records to check risk-factor accuracy, repeated reviews of all cases of CABG patient death, and an exploration of the detailed case-specific data contained in the CSRS database.

The first two investigations yielded limited benefit. It was found that the patients' records had been abstracted accurately for the risk factors documented, but the records themselves did not contain optimal documentation about the presence or absence of all risk factors. This omission served to emphasize the importance of better attention to communication and chart documentation. Multiple mortality reviews failed to find evidence of errors or problems in care, although it was noted that most deaths occurred in very sick and high-risk patients.

The third investigation explored the detailed outcomes data in the CSRS database, breaking down the whole patient population into different cross sections, looking for patterns of excess mortality. This investigation succeeded in finding some meaningful patterns within a small subset of the patients:

1. There was a higher-than-average proportion of emergency CABG patients having a high patient acuity profile: those within 24 hours after an acute myocardial infarction, in shock, or hemodynamically unstable (referred to herein as AMISHU).
2. The majority of all patients (90%) had non-emergency CABG with mortality rates equal to or lower than statewide average. The emergency patients (10% of all) had a higher mortality (11–26%) than the statewide average (7.7%).
3. Among the emergency patients, half had the high-acuity (AMISHU) profile and a higher mortality rate of 31%; the other half of the emergency patients had a mortality of 6.8%.

Evaluating and Changing Care Processes

Once these facts were recognized, attention focused on reviewing the care processes for the high-acuity (AMISHU) subgroup. Lacking specific errors to correct, the approach was to consider new ways to optimize every possible aspect of their care. Importantly, because this approach was multidisciplinary, it covered not only each specialty's care but also the interactions and transitions among them. It was in those intersections or transfers of care that some of the most important changes occurred.

Available data on process variables were limited but somewhat useful. For example, we found that only about one-fourth of the high-acuity (AMISHU) group had received an intraaortic balloon assist device preoperatively, a smaller number than one might expect in such unstable patients.

Most of the care process changes occurred through debate and consensus. The general focus was to increase the stability of emergency patients and reduce any ongoing ischemia. Changes involved all aspects of care, including cardiology, surgery, anesthesia, nursing, emergency department, and even administration. Often there was concern about making changes for the worse. For example, there was concern that increasing the use of the intraaortic balloon might cause more complications of limb ischemia; this was followed and is discussed in a later section.

Improved Outcomes Resulted

By the end of that year (1993) it was clear that a dramatic improvement in survival had occurred: The CABG mortality in high-acuity (AMISHU) patients dropped from 31% to 5%, despite a doubling increase in the number of high-acuity (AMISHU) cases performed. The overall program CABG mortality dropped by nearly half from 4.6% to 2.6%, and the risk-adjusted mortality dropped from 6.6% to 2.46%.[23] Improvements have persisted; the overall actual CABG mortality was 1.3% in 1994 and 2.0% in 1995; the risk-adjusted figures are not yet available for those years.

Benefits have accrued across the program, beyond the outcomes of CABG mortality. Of greatest significance is the pattern of multispecialty teamwork and communication that has evolved. In addition, the approach of using outcomes data

to track and offer feedback for care processes has been extended to other areas.

An example of this spin-off is a separate project that arose from the concerns we had about causing more limb ischemia complications due to increased use of the intraaortic balloon. The critical care nurses started monitoring practice processes and outcomes of balloon patients. By following the occurrence of complications and reviewing the associated placement techniques, we have evolved guidelines suggesting use of smaller balloons in patients below a threshold physical size and also recommended more use of sheathless balloons. In addition we have agreed on a policy that once there are even early findings of vascular compromise, balloon removal will be done by vascular surgeons in the operating room, to manage arterial closure or repair with the goal of maintaining vascularity of the extremity. The incidence of leg ischemia has dropped, despite higher levels of balloon use.

Controversies, Benefits, and Limitations of Clinical Outcomes Data

Several specific issues remain problematic in using outcomes data.

Clinician Confidence in Risk-Adjustment Models

One of the problems in accepting outcomes data has been the lack of confidence that clinicians place in the risk-adjustment models and the mathematical compensation for individual patient risk. Overall statistical validity in a large population has not completely translated to make surgeons believe in the accuracy for their smaller populations or for individual patients. In the state of New York, surgeons' cases are combined in a rolling 3-year sample to accumulate a more significant volume of cases. However, this procedure forces them to carry a historical "tail," so that recent changes might not be reflected accurately.

Another concern surrounds the issue of small rates of negative outcomes; for example, in CABG surgery, mortality might be 2% or 3%, and in percutaneous transluminal coronary angioplasty (PTCA) mortality might be less than 1%. Clinicians performing these procedures often fear that a small number of "bad cases" could exert a disproportionate impact on their results. The argument that statistical testing proves that a model corrects for high-risk cases, and will not penalize for accepting high-risk cases, does not always hold sway in the clinician's mind.

These doubts induce another concern: that clinicians' decision making, traditionally guided primarily by the patient's best interests, will become contaminated with other conflicting interests such as self-protection. As one physician put it, "Now I not only have to worry about what's best for my patient, I also worry about what's best for my numbers." The issue of confidence remains an important one even aside from the statistical validity of risk models.

Using Administrative Data for Risk Adjustment

Faced with the cost and complexity of collecting specialized clinical data for risk adjustment, many agencies and managed care entities are increasingly using an alternative in the form of secondary or administrative data: that data developed for reimbursement or regulatory purposes (e.g., DRGs, ICD-9-CM, or UB-92). In these cases the risk adjustment may be based on either costs, length of stay, or extent of comorbidity documented for financial purposes. Although such data have the appeal of being standardized and readily available at considerably less cost, they are not really based on clinical risk factors and are, appropriately, even less credible to clinicians.[8]

When data are presented as risk adjusted, care must be taken to ascertain the risk basis and to recognize its limitations. Perhaps there is a legitimate role for administrative data as a first step in the examination of diversely mixed populations, to identify where potential questions may occur. However, such potential questions will inevitably need more focused and specific clinical analysis to clarify their significance and their underlying causes.

Public Disclosure of Clinical Outcomes Data

Public disclosure of provider profiles, with physician- or hospital-specific outcome results, is highly controversial. In New York State, surgeon-specific results have been published since the press won a freedom-of-information lawsuit. The DOH asserts that monitoring and release of risk-adjusted CABG data are beneficial for consumers and have helped reduce the associated mortality across the state.[24] Concerns have been expressed about other potential negative impacts of public disclosure: increased reporting of risk factors,[25] unfair damage to the reputation of good surgeons caught in bad situations,[26] and the possible referral of high-risk patients out of state.[27] These benefits and hazards have been discussed, with emphasis on the importance of measures such as oversight by a clinical advisory committee, external audits, and evaluation of the risk-adjustment model.[28]

Other interesting insights are provided into the statewide effects of the New York system.[28,29] Between 1989 and 1992, 27 surgeons in New York State doing low volumes of CABG (less than 50 cases per year) stopped performing this procedure. All of the surgeons who stopped performing CABG had mortality rates 2.5 to 5 times the statewide average and more than twice the average rate for all low-volume surgeons. Their combined risk-adjusted CABG mortality rate was 11.9%, as opposed to the statewide average of 3.1%.

Despite the limitations and controversies, some definite improvements have been associated with the New York system. It remains speculative whether these changes would have occurred from feedback of detailed comparative outcomes information to providers alone. Although such feedback is probably the most important factor in accomplishing improvement, it seems likely that the external pressure of public release "played an important part in galvanizing physicians and hospitals to seize these opportunities to improve."[12] While the improvement process may have been accelerated, there have been detrimental effects and adversarial reactions among providers induced by the scorecard approach. The collection and public disclosure of outcomes data by an external agency put caregivers on a collision course with each other and with public health authorities. The intellectual honesty of scientific research, and reflective collaboration, provided an enlightened course correction. Our challenge is to integrate these elements and the best principles and practices of patient care into the pragmatic and turbulent mainstream of health care delivery.

References

1. Kassirer JP. The use and abuse of practice profiles. New Engl J Med 1994;330:634–635.
2. Kleinke JD. Medicine's industrial revolution. *Wall Street Journal,* August 21, 1995.
3. Moore FD. The university in American surgery. Surgery 1958;44:1–10.
4. Chiu RCJ, Mulder DS. Roles for the surgical investigator. In: Troidl H, Spitzer WO, McPeek B, Mulder DS, McKneally MF, Wechsler AS, Balch CM, eds. Principles and Practice of Research. New York: Springer-Verlag, 1991, pp. 10–15.
5. Hammermeister KE, Daley J, Grover FL. Using outcomes data to improve clinical practice: what we have learned. Ann Thorac Surg 1994;58: 1809–1811.
6. Denton TA, Chaux A, Matloff JM. A cardiothoracic surgery information system for the next century: implications for managed care. Ann Thorac Surg 1995;59:486–493.
7. Ebert PA. The importance of data in improving practice: effective clinical use of outcomes data. Ann Thorac Surg 1994;58:1812–1814.
8. Iezzoni LI. Using risk-adjusted outcomes to assess clinical practice: an overview of issues pertaining to risk adjustment. Ann Thorac Surg 1994;58:1822–1826.
9. Pollock A, Evans M. Surgical Audit. London: Butterworth, 1989.
10. Pollock AV. Historical evolution: methods, attitudes, and goals. In: Troidl H, Spitzer WO, McPeek B, Mulder DS, McKneally MF, Wechsler AS, Balch CM, eds. Principles and Practice of Research. New York: Springer-Verlag, 1991, pp. 3–9.
11. O'Connor GT, Plume SK, Wennberg JE. Regional organization for outcomes research. Ann N Y Acad Sci 1993;703:44–51.
12. Barbour G. The role of outcomes data in health care reform. Ann Thorac Surg 1994;58:1881–1884.
13. Relman AS. Assessment and accountability—the third revolution in medical care. New Engl J Med 1988;319:1220–1222.
14. Berwick DM. Continuous improvement as an ideal in health care. New Engl J Med 1989;320:53–56.
15. Laffel G, Blumenthal D. The case for using industrial quality management science in health care organizations. JAMA 1989;262:2869–2873.
16. Box G, quoted by Berwick DM. Commentary in: Batalden PB, Stoltz PK. A framework for the continual improvement of health care. Journal on Quality Improvement 1993;19:425–452.
17. Daley J. Criteria by which to evaluate risk-adjusted outcomes programs in cardiac surgery. Ann Thorac Surg 1994;58:1827–1835.
18. Topol EJ, Califf RM. Scorecard cardiovascular medicine—its impact and future directions. Ann Intern Med 1994;120:65–70.
19. Kasper JF, Plume SK, O'Connor GT. A methodology for QI in the coronary artery bypass grafting procedure involving comparative process analysis. Qual Rev Bull 1992;18:128–133.
20. Dziuban SW, McIlduff JB, Miller SJ, DalCol RH. How a New York cardiac surgery program uses outcomes data. Ann Thorac Surg 1994;58:1871–1876.
21. Coronary Artery Bypass Surgery in New York State: 1989–1991. Albany: New York State Department of Health, December 1992.
22. Coronary Artery Bypass Surgery in New York State: 1990–1992. Albany: New York State Department of Health, December 1993.
23. Coronary Artery Bypass Surgery in New York State: 1991–1993. Albany: New York State Department of Health, June 1995.
24. Hannan EL, Kilbum H, Racz M, Shields E, Chassin MR. Improving the outcomes of coronary artery bypass surgery in New York State. JAMA 1994;271:761–766.
25. Green J, Wintfeld N. Report cards on cardiac surgeons—assessing New York State's approach. New Engl J Med 1995;332:1229–1232.
26. Bumiller E. Death rate rankings shake New York cardiac surgeons. *New York Times,* September 6, 1995.
27. Omoigui NA, Miller DP, Brown KJ, Annan K, Cosgrove D 3rd, Lytle B, Loop F, Topol EJ. Outmigration for coronary bypass surgery in an era of public dissemination of clinical outcomes. Circulation 1996;93:27–33.

28. Chassin MR, Hannan EL, DeBuono BA. Benefits and hazards of reporting medical outcomes publicly. New Engl J Med 1996;334:394–398.

29. Hannan EL, Siu AL, Kumar D, Kilburn H Jr, Chassin MR. The decline in coronary artery bypass graft surgery mortality in New York State. JAMA 1995;273:209–213.

Commentary

This chapter is centered around a case study demonstrating how outcome analysis may be used to improve patient care. In contrast to the more extensive outcome analyses suggested by Lorenz in chapter 55, the endpoints in this study are simple—primarily risk-adjusted mortality. This focus is appropriate because mortality has a high enough occurrence in this patient population to be a highly meaningful endpoint. Other interesting issues are raised within the chapter. For example, who owns outcome data? Are there adverse effects to putting too much pressure on institutions to alter outcomes that might force institutions to stop treating high-risk patients—particularly when these are the patients who potentially derive the greatest benefit from a given intervention? How does one overcome the most fundamental element that is not measured in these analyses? Specifically, every patient enrolled in the study had the decision made by a surgeon that the patient would potentially benefit from operation. Do the risk-adjustment protocols adequately compensate for those elements of decision making that may incorporate other undefined outcome measures that are of great importance (as emphasized by Lorenz)? The chapter is highly pragmatic; it makes the important point that all surgeons should be involved in a continuing research process whose goal is the improvement of patient care.

A.S.W.

Commentary

Dr. Dziuban has written a very interesting chapter on outcomes research, drawing our attention to the need to take both the professional and con-

sumerist perspective on the various outcomes of treatment. It is the collision of the view of the consumer with the known prejudice of the biologist toward hard data that has brought onto the scene this new frame of research into outcomes. The taxonomy of research into outcomes is not completely defined. A good overview of it is found in Orchard.[1] Briefly, outcomes can be divided into *professional* outcomes (e.g., sepsis, recurrence after surgery), *patient* outcomes (the relief from pain and symptoms afforded by surgery), and *population*-based outcomes (the effect of outcomes on the political economy of the country, in particular return to work or return to normal functioning in society).

Politicians and consumer groups want outcomes to be presented as competitive league tables to allow them to compare good with bad. Although this idea is attractive, life is not that simple. Outcomes are determined by factors, such as age, gender, pathology, and so forth, beyond the control of clinicians.

Outcomes research is made difficult by problems of case mix. We have looked very carefully at outcomes after upper gastrointestinal surgery in a fairly large series. The effect of case mix on the outcomes after surgery was demonstrated quite clearly.[2] Unfortunately, despite the difficulties, people still hanker for simple competitive tables and are unconvinced by the difficulties and pitfalls of using routine outcome data in this way.

So, outcomes research is here to stay, as Dr. Dziuban points out. However, it is a form of research that requires the same meticulous attention to detail that Dr. Dziuban and other surgeons have shown when looking at coronary artery bypass surgery. This excellent chapter, setting out what can and cannot be done in this field, describes a new challenge that surgical researchers ought to take up with their customary enthusiasm and precision.

1. Orchard C. Comparing healthcare outcomes. Br Med J 1994;308:1496–1499.

2. Devlin HB, Rockall RA, Logan RFA, Northfield TC. Variation in outcome after acute upper gastrointestinal haemorrhage. Lancet 1995;346:346–350.

H.B. Devlin

Commentary

In 1983 Professor J.R. Hampton wrote that "Clinical freedom should have been strangled long ago, for at best it was a cloak for ignorance and at worst an excuse for quackery."

Outcome analysis is essential if we are going to apply the results of research to the treatment of patients. We must know what happens to our patients, not only in terms of 30-day mortality but also of long-term morbidity and mortality and quality of life.

We have all been fascinated by the New York State Department of Health's reporting of deaths after coronary artery bypass grafting classified by hospitals and individual surgeons. The publication of above-average death rates stimulated hospitals to conduct closer examinations of the processes of surgical, anesthetic, and postoperative care. By the end of 1993 there had been a dramatic improvement in survival, and the mortality in high-risk (AMISHU) patients had fallen from 31% to 5% and the risk-adjusted mortality from 6.6% to 2.5%. These are remarkable figures. Can we emulate them? Can we improve the results of other interventions? We will not know until we audit the outcome of every patient who comes under our care.

A.V. Pollock

CHAPTER 57

Health Services Research

J.I. Williams, J. Höher, and K.W. Lauterbach

An Introduction to Health Services Research

The goal of health services is to provide opportunities for effective care to persons who can benefit from it in a manner that is acceptable to the consumer and the provider, at a cost that is acceptable to the public at large. Health services research strives to determine whether that goal has been achieved, in whole or in part, and to identify factors that enhance or diminish the possibility of achieving that goal.

Health services research is a field of study rather than a discipline. Investigators come from the health sciences, social sciences, management sciences, and information sciences, as outlined in Figure 57-1. The banners under which individuals come together to undertake health services research include health systems research, clinical epidemiology, technology assessment, clinical decision analysis, operations research, health economics, medical sociology, and medical anthropology.

Scientists and clinicians have questioned the benefits of medical interventions in relation to their hazards and costs for centuries, but it has only been over the past 50 years that the principles, concepts, methods, and statistics for health services research have been developed. Through the development of social medicine in Great Britain, epidemiological concepts and methods were applied to the broad spectrum of health problems and behaviors. The randomized trial was introduced for the study of the efficacy of drugs and extended to other interventions. Sociologists, economists, demographers, and political scientists brought their concepts, methods, and statistics, and clinical psychologists and anthropologists contributed observational methods for use in health services research.

Reasons for Health Services Research

The reasons for health services research come from the challenges and problems countries face in the organization, financing, and provision of health services. At the risk of oversimplification, one can differentiate between challenges in the industrialized and developed countries with high income, and those in developing countries with low and middle levels of income.

The World Bank[1] estimated that in 1990 the world expenditures on health care, public and private, were about $1,700 billion, or 8% of the total world product. High-income countries expended about 90% of this amount, or about $1,500 per person. Developing countries spent about $170 billion, which was 4% of their gross national product, or about $41 per person. Among the prob-

Figure 57-1. Disciplines in health services research.

• **Social Sciences**	• **Health Sciences**
Anthropology	Biostatistics
Demography	Epidemiology
Economics	• **Business**
History	Decision theory
Political science	Finance
Psychology	Management
Sociology	Organizational theory
• **Other**	Operations research
Informatics	

lems that health services research addresses in developing countries is misallocation of monies to expensive clinical and hospital interventions of low cost-effectiveness at a time when highly cost-effective interventions such as the treatment of tuberculosis and sexually transmitted diseases are underfunded. While the poor lack access to basic health services, government spending goes disproportionately to the affluent in the form of subsidies to private and public health insurance and subsidized care in tertiary hospitals. The *World Development Report,* issued by the World Bank,[1] set forth a plan for investing in health and addressing these problems.

In developed countries there is little evidence concerning the effectiveness and efficiency of the treatment of many routinely administered treatments and diagnostic tests. Additionally a number of new problems for the provision of health care are arising that alone would provide enough reason for investing more into health services studies. Among them are demographic changes. These are most pronounced in Europe where we can expect an increase of 20–50% in the number of people age 65 and older in the next 30 years, and a dwindling number of young people who can support the publicly financed health care systems.[2]

For these reasons, in 1990 the Commission on Health Research for Development,[3] an independent international initiative, called for an international program of research for enabling people in diverse circumstances to apply health care solutions that are presently available and to generate new knowledge to tackle health care problems without solutions. Not only does research provide

the basis for effective planning and the best use of scarce resources, it is a critical part of social and human development. The Commission stated that without health research, countries would often fly blind in their attempts to improve the health of their citizens. It proposed a program of internal collaboration in funding from public and private sources, and international and national governments and agencies for building and sustaining research capacity within developing countries. The demand for research that addresses issues and problems in health care and policy is universal.[3]

Defining Health Services Research

There is no one widely accepted definition of health services research. After reviewing various definitions, the Committee on Health Services Research of the Institute of Medicine,[4] provided the following definition:

> Health services research is a multidisciplinary field of inquiry, both basic and applied, that examines the uses, costs, quality, accessibility, delivery, organization, financing, and outcomes of health care services to increase knowledge and understanding of the structure, processes, and effects of health services for individuals and populations.

Basic research that generates new knowledge about fundamental individual and institutional behaviors that may not be useful in the short term is important. However, the primary demand is for research that can be applied to problems and issues of more immediate interest to the public, and the providers and agencies responsible for governing health care. The key areas of health services research are displayed in Figure 57-2.

Another way to define health services research is to look at the work of those who do the research. The Committee on Health Services Research[4] identified about 5,000 health service researchers in the United States. They found that this workforce has three broad components: researchers who create, design, supervise, and report on basic and applied projects; individuals who as-

Figure 57-2.   Key areas for health services research.

- Organization and financing
- Access to practitioners
- Patient and consumer behaviors
- Quality of care
- Clinical evaluation and outcomes
- Informatics
- Clinical decision making
- Health professions workforce
- Equity and health care
- Economic evaluation of interventions
- Pharmacoeconomics
- Technology assessments

sist in the research under the direction of others; and those who analyze health services information and apply tools of health services research in management and policy settings. Most of the researchers were employed in academic institutions, private research organizations, and consulting groups. There are rapidly growing opportunities for research in health plans, insurance companies, and similar organizations.

Two Examples of Health Services Research

There have been two large studies that have tied the organization and financing of health services to the health needs of the individuals and their satisfaction with the care they received. The studies are summarized in structured abstracts. These studies can give only a very limited introduction into the wide array of studies concerning health services research. Still, they are exemplary because they combine data about patients, delivery systems, and socioeconomic factors in a way that can have immediate policy consequences. These studies are also important beyond their immediate results in that they overcame important methodological problems such as the management of large data sets that were subsequently confronted in other studies. Finally, they helped to train a number of young researchers who later became leaders in health services research.

ABSTRACT No. 1

Study

Health Care: An International Study. World Health Organization/bInternational Collaborative Study of Medical Care Utilization, 1964–1974. Kerr White and others.[5,6]

Objectives

To study the extent to which personal determinants of health and health behavior affect the uses of health services, and to compare the impact of health service systems on these relationships.

Design

Cross-sectional comparisons of surveys and health service systems.

Settings

Twelve study areas in seven countries: four in Canada (Grand Prairie, Alberta; Saskatchewan; Fraser, British Columbia; and Jersey, British Columbia); two each in Yugoslavia (Banat, Serbia and Rijeka, Croatia) and the United States (Baltimore, Maryland and northwestern Vermont); one in each in Argentina (Buenos Aires), Finland (Helsinki), Poland (Lodz), and the United Kingdom (Liverpool).

Subjects

A total of 48,000 persons in probability samples from the 12 areas.

Measurements

Standard measures of perceived need, resources, and uses of health service systems in the 12 areas. Survey of health services resources and organizational factors in the systems.

Results

Mortality. Area standard mortality ratios were relatively close to a median of 8.4 deaths per 1,000. Infant mortality rates were higher for Buenos Aires, Lodz, and Banant.

Perceived health. There were minimal variations in self-reported health: 40% saw themselves as functionally healthy; 10% of subjects in North America, Buenos Aires, and Liverpool reported chronic and disabling conditions; rates in Yugoslavia, Helsinki, and Lodz were two to three times as high. Reported rates for sickness and bed days followed a similar pattern.

Health services utilization. There were marked variations in rates of physician visits, volume of physician use, volume of hospital nights, and uses of prescribed and nonprescribed medications. Utilization rates did not correspond to areas' variations in sickness, chronicity, and disability.

Systems. Uses of physicians and hospitals for healthy and unhealthy persons were not related to resources or financial barriers across areas. Use of hospitals was related to availability of hospital beds. Volume of ambulatory care physicians was inversely related to supply of short-term beds. The balance between physicians (generalists and specialists) and hospital beds may be an important determinant of hospital use.

Conclusion

Perceived need is the major prerequisite for the demand for health care. Predisposing and enabling factors influence use. The supply and distribution of resources are critical factors in access to and demand for health services. Physicians largely determine point of entry and uses of health services system. The process is influenced by a number of factors including the local structure of health services and financing and payment mechanisms. Epidemiology and health services research is a means for assisting politicians, planners, professionals, and the public in allocating resources rationally and compassionately.

Abstract No. 2

Study

RAND Health Insurance Experiment: Controlled Experimentation as Research Policy, 1971–1986. Joseph Newhouse and Insurance Experiment Group.[7-10]

Background

Five health insurance plans were designed from the study: four had varying levels of cost sharing by enrollees (25%, 50%, 95%, and individual deductible), and one offered free care. There was a maximum dollar expenditure per year of 5%, 10%, or 15% of income, or $1,000, whichever

was less. A health maintenance organization (HMO) provided free care.

Objectives

To determine the effects of cost sharing on uses of services and health outcomes, determine if these effects varied by income group; determine the effects of covering outpatient as well as inpatient services, and estimate the reduction in use and resulting health effects in a HMO.

Design

Randomized controlled experiment.

Settings

Six sites: Dayton, Ohio; Seattle, Washington; Fitchburg/Leominister, Massachusetts; and, Georgetown County, South Carolina.

Patients

A total of 7,700 individuals were enrolled. About 2,000 of the enrollees received their care through the HMO. The enrollees in the study participated for either 3 or 5 years. Persons eligible for Medicare because of age or disability were excluded.

Measurements

Uses and costs of inpatient and outpatient services, appropriateness of care for conditions and indications, self-reports of health status, and consumer satisfaction.

Results

Uses and costs of services. The main comparisons were between free care (FC) and fee-for-service (FFS) care. The dollars spent per person per year were about 50% higher for FC than FFS. Participants in the FC plan averaged 2 more physician visits per year, and their hospital admission rate was 25% higher than for those in FFS plans.

Health outcomes. FC had no effect on habits associated with cardiovascular diseases and some types of cancer. There were no effects of FC on any of five measures of health status. The effects of FC were evident in improved levels of dental care. FC patients with visual problems or hypertension received better care, and improvements appeared to be greater among the poor. The investigators estimated the reductions in mortality that could result from the differences in outcomes and concluded they were not sufficient to justify FC for all adults.

HMO. Hospital admissions were 40% less for the HMO than the FFS plan. For the average participant, there were no differences in outcome. The poor and sick in the HMOs may have had more bed days and serious symptoms than the poor and the sick in FFS.

Satisfaction. HMO enrollees had either been subscribers or they joined the HMO at the time of randomization. Prior HMO enrollees were as satisfied with their care and services as FFS participants. Enrollees new to the HMO were less satisfied with waiting times and the availability of specialists and hospitals. Some preferred FFS care and were willing to pay for it.

Conclusion

The Rand Health Insurance Experiment (RHIE) is a hallmark, randomized controlled experiment in health services research. Innovative methods for assessing health outcomes and quality of care were developed for the project. The implications of the RHIE for the organization and financing of health services continue to be debated.

Research Methods in Health Services

For the most part, health services research is population based. It involves studies of the needs and determinants of the health of the population, the appropriateness and efficiency with which the population is provided services, and the resulting health outcomes for the population served. The key methods for health services research include: health surveys of individuals and households, analysis of health administrative data, methods for defining appropriateness of care, benchmarks and performance indicators, measures of health outcomes, and the methods for economic analysis. Brief descriptions of the methods are presented in Figure 57-3.

Population Health Surveys

Population surveys are routinely conducted in the European and North American countries. The

Figure 57-3.   Methods for health services research.

- Health surveys of individuals and households
- Analysis of health administrative data
- Defining appropriateness of care
- Benchmarks and performance indicators
- Assessing health outcomes
- Economic evaluations

surveys typically include questions on the demographic characteristics of the individuals and households, work and socioeconomic characteristics, acute and chronic health problems, limitations of activities and disabilities stemming from health problems, health knowledge, beliefs and attitudes, health behaviors concerning health promotion and disease prevention (e.g., smoking, drinking, exercise, nutrition, and participation in screening programs), utilization of health professional and hospital services.

The results are used to draw health profiles of the communities surveyed, construct indicators of population, define health needs, monitor behaviors related to health promotion and disease prevention, and indicate the access to, use of, and satisfaction with health care and services. Ideally the questionnaires and interview schedules would be standardized over time and across nations, states, and provinces.[11] The reality is that the methods vary enough across surveys that it is difficult to make cross-national comparisons such as those provided by Kerr White and his colleagues.[12]

Health Administrative Data

The revolution in computing systems, combined with the development of information technologies, has resulted in data that was gathered for financial and administrative purposes being accessible for health services research. Canada has universal public health insurance. Provinces decide on the health services they will fund, and they administer the programs.

The Institute for Clinical Evaluative Sciences (ICES) in Ontario is funded by the Ministry of Health to study access to and efficiency and effectiveness of medical services in the province.

Much of the research is based on one or more of the following: hospital discharge summaries, physician claims, the drug benefit plan for the elderly, and home care. As almost all hospital and physician services are covered by public insurance, the coverage of the services provided is nearly universal. The drug benefit plan covers the elderly, and until this year all drug costs were covered by the plan. There are home care programs throughout the provinces, but the services are organized at the municipal levels, and the coverage varies accordingly.[13,14]

Researchers at ICES have assessed the quality of the demographic, diagnostic, and intervention data in the databases.[15] The reliability and validity of the demographic data and the primary services provided are very high in all four databases. The quality of the data on primary diagnosis is high for hospital discharge summaries. Diagnosis is an optional field on physician claims, is not recorded on drug claims, and may not be included on home care data. Data on secondary diagnoses and complications on the hospital discharge summary generally are not reliable except for the most salient conditions.

The methods for the analysis of administrative databases have been well established by Wennberg,[16] Roos and Roos,[17] and McPherson and co-workers.[18,19] They are summarized in a series of articles included in a book edited by Anderson and Mooney.[20] Explaining variations in the rates of health care utilization and finding strategies for reducing them continue as major tasks of health services. Generally speaking, rates for surgical procedures are higher in the United States than in most European countries, and the rates for Canada fall somewhere in the middle, depending on the procedure. There variations among areas within a country can be greater than the variations between countries.[21] Obviously, if the variations could be reduced by lowering utilization, particularly in areas with high rates, there would be a potential for reducing the overall costs of health services. There is also a concern that variations indicate that utilization may not be related to appropriateness of care. Low utilization could imply that needs were not being met, and high utilization may indicate that services are provided inappropriately.[22] The source of the variations can be determined by assessing the availability of services, the rationalization of care, and the characteristics of the population serviced. Variations in procedures are minimal when physicians agree on treatment procedures, as they do for fractured hips and inguinal hernia. Variations are marked for conditions for which there is less consensus concerning treatment, such as for the management of back problems, dental extractions, and asthma in adults.[23] Marked variations in rates are a screening test for the access, efficiency, and effectiveness of medical practice. Variations may identify possible problems, but additional investigations are required to identify patterns of practice that are contrary to evidence and guidelines.

Variations over time mark the changes in practice, such as reclassifying procedures as suitable for same-day surgery instead of requiring inpatient stays, and the introductions of new technologies, such as the use of laparoscopic procedures in general surgery. Trends over time also indicate the rate at which practices change in response to the dissemination of knowledge. By linking services to indications, the appropriateness of services can be assessed, and variations in rates can be related to the criteria for appropriateness.

Appropriateness of Care

Figure 57-4 gives an indication as to how evidence can be derived for relating guidelines for practice to patterns of practice. The Cochrane Collaborative Project based at Oxford University is designed to collate the results from all randomized trials and synthesize the evidence into guidelines for practice. The publications on effective care in pregnancy and childbirth and the effective care of the newborn were the first major books to come from the project.[24] However, there is "black and white" evidence from clinical trials for only a minority of medical decisions and interventions. The efficacy results obtained in well-designed, randomized trials, based on standardized protocols may not translate into effectiveness in everyday practice.

The task is to develop guidelines for the gray zones of practices. Also, there is the need do research on the guidelines that are derived from the evidence, asking the question whether they are

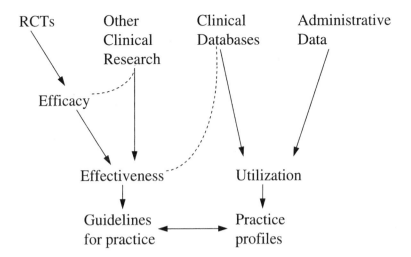

Figure 57-4.   Building evidence for evaluating health care.

valid, reproducible, unambiguous, and helpful in clinical practice.[25] Evidence itself may be taken from other clinical research, clinical databases, and case registries. Consensus conferences are used to bring experts together to render guidelines for care based on implicit criteria for assessing the broad array of clinical research and evidence. RAND researchers have developed methods for synthesizing the knowledge and experience of experts and deriving detailed assessments of appropriateness of care based on explicit criteria.[26] Researchers review the literature for a particular procedure and define the indications for the procedure in terms of symptoms, medical history, and diagnostic tests. The indications for procedures are combined into clinical scenarios. The panel members initially are to make their ratings on a nine-point scale, with 1 being extremely inappropriate and 9 being extremely appropriate. After considering the ratings and indications from the first round, the indications for conditions are modified, scenarios are altered or dropped, and the ratings are repeated.

Using the data from the study of Medicare patients, Leape and his colleagues[27] studied variations in use of coronary angiography, carotid endarterectomy, and upper gastrointestinal tract endoscopy across 23 adjacent counties in one state. Taking appropriateness criteria derived from the RAND methods, they audited the hospital charts and rated the appropriateness of the procedures. The variations in county rates per 10,000 Medicare enrollees ranged from 13 to 158 for coronary angiography, from 5 to 41 for carotid endarterectomy, and from 42 to 164 for upper gastrointestinal tract endoscopy. The rates of inappropriate use by county ranged from 8% to 75% for coronary angiography, from 0% to 67% for carotid endarterectomy, and from 0% to 25% for endoscopy. The variations in utilization rates could not be explained by variations in appropriateness of care for the procedures studied.

In Ontario, nine centers provide coronary artery bypass surgery, and they are joined within the Provincial Adult Cardiac Care Network of Ontario (PACCN). Researchers at ICES and clinicians in the network employed the RAND procedures with an expert panel to create an urgency rating for prioritizing patients in the queue for surgery.[28] Results of the rating exercise were used to create triage guidelines. Patients with urgent priority scores should have surgery within 3 days, and the recommended waiting times extend to 6 months for patients with elective priority scores. Since there have been criticisms of the deaths and delays in queues for coronary surgery in Canada by American groups opposed to "socialized medicine," researchers from ICES and PACCN examined the experience of 8,517 patients leaving the registry between October 1991 and July 1993. Among the 8,213 patients receiving surgery, the median wait was 17 days, and the median waiting times ranged from one day for urgent cases to 40 days for those with low priority scores. Waiting times did vary inequitably among the nine centers but the patients rarely suffered critical events or extreme delays.[29] The result of this study has been to transfer patients across centers and convince the government to expand the programs in hospitals with the longer waiting times. A subsequent study has shown that referring specialists in Ontario have accepted the priority scores, and this facilitates the managing of the waiting lists.[30]

Based on an overview of randomized trials, the Coronary Artery Bypass Graft Surgery Trialists Collaboration developed a score to indicate the risk of death if surgery is not performed, based on clinical indications of severity of disease.[31] Hux and her colleagues[32] used the score to define three levels of survival benefit from surgery (high, moderate, and low), and they applied to the PACCN for data on 5,058 patients in Ontario undergoing CABG surgery in 1992. About 95% of the cases from across the nine centers were judged to have been managed in a clinically appropriate manner. However, there is a threefold variation in surgical rates across the counties of Ontario. As the rates increased, the proportion of high-benefit cases in the counties declined, and the proportion of low-benefit cases increased. These results suggest that while the ratings of appropriateness are high across areas, there may be diminishing marginal returns for specific outcomes with rising local use of procedures. This is consistent with the findings by Black and his colleagues who concluded that areas with high rates of elective surgery for benign prostatic hyperplasia provided surgery to higher proportions of men with low levels of need and limited potential benefit.[33] Variations in rates may suggest variations in patient selection.

Benchmarks and Performance Indicators

Basinski[34,35] established three benchmarks for judging hospital performance during this era of restructuring: average length of stay, day-surgery rates, and readmissions. While there are variations, across the board hospital efficiency continues to improve, with declines in lengths of stay

for a wide range of conditions. For the years that the data have been collected, the age-sex-adjusted day-surgery rate per 1,000 patients has increased from 57.6 to 68.8.[35] Concern has been expressed by providers and consumers that patients are being discharged "quicker and sicker." The analysis of readmission rates for selected medical and surgical conditions and for newborns indicates that the readmission rates have remained constant.[35]

Methods for Assessing Outcomes

The quest for measures of outcome that can be used in shaping health policy is perpetual. In this section we briefly review hospital mortality rates as outcomes, procedures that serve as proxy indicators of outcome, and measures of health status and quality of life.

Starting in 1986, the Health Care Financing Administration (HCFA) in the United States began publishing the inpatient mortality rates for Medicare patients. The listings of inpatient mortality rates released to the public included the names of the hospitals. According to HCFA's calculations, 142 hospitals had significantly higher death rates than was predicted, and 127 hospitals had significantly lower rates. The first prediction model developed by HCFA had adjustments for case mix, but this did not accurately capture the severity of illness. There were other methodological flaws as well. The model has been refined over the years, but the question remains whether the data on comorbidity, complications, and severity available on hospital discharge abstracts are sufficiently good to adequately adjust for hospital variations in case mix.[36]

At the beginning of this decade, the New York State Department of Health[37] began publishing in-hospital, case mortality rates for the 30 hospitals that provide coronary artery bypass graft (CABG) surgery. Each of the hospitals performing this procedure submits data to the Health Department on the clinical characteristics of CABG patients and their status at discharge. This information is entered into a database along with information about the hospital and surgeon. The Health Department developed a multivariate risk factor equation for predicting deaths based on the demographic characteristics and clinical data on ventricular function, hemodynamic state, comorbidities, ischemia, severity of disease, and prior open-heart operations.

For each hospital and surgeon, the report lists the cases, deaths, observed mortality rate, expected mortality rate, and risk-adjusted mortality rate, along with the 95% confidence intervals for the risk-adjusted mortality rate as an indicator of rates that are significantly high or low. Only surgeons performing 200 or more CABG operations during the time period are listed by name.

Hannan and others[38] have observed the changes in rates for CABG surgery performed in New York State from 1989 through 1992. The overall in-hospital death rates declined from 3.52% to 2.78%. They attributed the decline in the exodus of low-volume surgeons with poor performance, the better performance of surgeons who entered the system, and the performance of surgeons who did not have consistently low volumes.

There is another explanation as well. Omoigui and his colleagues[39] reviewed 9,442 isolated coronary bypass operations performed at the Cleveland Clinic from 1989 through 1993. They compared the mortality experiences of patients from New York, Ohio, other states, and other countries. The observed mortality rate for patients from New York (5.2%) was greater than the rates for patients from Ohio (2.9%), other states (3.1%), and other countries (1.4%). Compared to other patients, patients from New York were more likely to have had prior heart surgery and more severe disease. The expected mortality rate was thus higher than for the other patient cohorts. Omoigui and his colleagues also compared mortality outcomes by state of referral for the 1980 to 1988 time periods, and these patterns were not evident in that data. They concluded that the public dissemination of outcome data in New York resulted in a referral of high-risk patients to an out-of-state clinic.

It can be noted that ICES researchers worked with the Provincial Adult Cardiac Care Network of Ontario (PACCN) to create a six-variable risk index (age, sex, left ventricular function, type of surgery, and repeat operation) for predicting in-hospital mortality, intensive care unit stay, and overall hospital length of stay following cardiac surgery.[40] The overall mortality rate following CABG surgery was 3.01%, and the risk-adjusted mortality rate declined from 3.17% in 1991 to 2.93% in 1993. The risk-adjusted mortality rates for the nine hospitals were within the expected range during the study period, except that one hospital had a significantly lower rate in 1991. All hospitals performed over 300 CABG procedures in 1992 and 1993, and only 2 of 42 cardiac surgeons performed less than 50 CABG procedures in 1993.[41] The members of the PACCN are using the results as feedback for the quality assurance program, but they have decided not to publish reports such as those concerning New York or Pennsylvania.

There are at least three major limitations to mortality as an indicator in outcome studies. There is still little consensus as to how well various measures of severity and comorbidity adequately adjust for case mix.[42] Secondly, less than 3% of admissions to acute care hospitals end in death, so mortality reviews, at best, provided a narrow view of the quality of care. Thirdly, mortality as the primary indicator for the quality of care of a hospital can produce the incentive of not admitting or of transferring high-risk patients, particularly if adjustment for severity of illness and comorbidity is incomplete in the reporting.

There are indicators that serve as proxies to outcomes. For example, mammography, pap smears, and blood pressure monitoring are screening tests that serve as proxy indicators for outcomes, since there is ample evidence that early detection of breast cancer, cervical cancer, and heart disease can lead to prolongation of life and enhanced quality of life. Data on these indicators are available through population health surveys and administrative databases.

Guidelines regarding caesarean section[43] have been disseminated and discussed widely with physicians in the United States and Canada, but initially there was little response in terms in caesarean section rates.[44] The rates in Ontario peaked in the mid-1980s at 20% of deliveries and have fallen to 17% of deliveries in 1994, primarily because of the decrease in the number of repeat caesarean sections.[45] This shift is consistent with guidelines. However there are marked variations in caesarean rates by hospital, ranging from a low of 10% to a high of 25%, and the rates serve as benchmarks for the hospitals. The Society of Obstetricians and Gynaecologists of Canada issued guidelines in 1995 for the diagnosis and management of dystocia and fetal distress.[46] Researchers at ICES continue to monitor caesarean sections by indication, to estimate the impact of the guidelines.

Experimental studies established that primary tumors of the breast are managed effectively with breast-conserving surgery and radiotherapy.[47] In Ontario, the overall rates of breast-conserving surgery increased from 57% in 1991 to 64% in 1994, and variation in rates by hospital declined.[48] With the introduction of mammography screening and articulation of the consumer choices in management at the National Forum on Breast Cancer, women are becoming aware of treatment options and outcomes. While health administrative data do not indicate the reasons for the treatment, one can follow the data from surveys and hospitals to determine if trends in mammography screening and breast-conserving surgery continue to move in the expected directions with further reductions in variations.

Groups in the United States have classified various medical conditions as markers of appropriate primary care.[49,50] The conditions are classified as ambulatory care sensitive, and hospital admissions for these conditions are referred to as preventable hospitalizations. The basic idea is that appropriate ambulatory care can make many hospitalizations for these conditions unnecessary. Examples of these marker medical conditions are asthma, congestive heart failure, diabetes, and depression. In Ontario, the rates of hospitalization for asthma and congestive heart failure were found to be higher in rural areas, where access to primary care can be a problem, than in urban areas.[51]

In a comparative study of cities in Ontario and United States cities, Billings and others[52] examined hospitalization rates for ambulatory care–sensitive conditions with respect to income levels of where individuals lived. On average, persons in low-income areas had hospitalization rates that were higher than for persons living in high-income areas. However the variations in rates of preventable hospitalizations in Ontario were not as dramatic as those found in the U.S. cities. In

Toronto, with universal coverage and reduced barriers to primary care, low-income areas had 39% higher hospitalization rates than the more affluent areas. Overall in the United States, where there are problems with lack of access to health insurance and primary care, low-income areas had hospitalization rates that were 340% higher than those in high-income areas.[52]

Outcome Measures for Health Status and Quality of Life

There are extensive reviews and critiques for measures of physical, emotional, and social health functioning and health-related quality of life. The works by Bowling,[53,54] McDowell and Newell,[55] and Spilker[56] provide the excellent coverage of the measures. There are basically three types of measures that have been developed: measures of general health status or functioning, measures that are disease specific, and utility measures for assessing preferences for health states. Examples of coding measures are listed in Figure 57-5. Researchers are encouraged to include at least one measure of each type in clinical research and the evaluations of interventions and health technologies in order to obtain patient perspectives on outcomes.[57]

The four leading measures for assessing general health functioning or status are the Sickness Impact Profile (SIP),[58] Nottingham Health Profile

Figure 57-5. Measures for health status and quality of life.

- **General health status/quality of life**
  Dartmouth COOP Charts
  Nottingham Health Profile
  Sickness Impact Profile
  Short Form Health Survey–36 Items
- **Disease-specific measures**
  Barthel Index
  Karnofsky Performance Index
- **Utilities and patient preferences**
  Standard gamble method
  Time trade-off method
  Disability and Distress Scale
  EuroQol Quality of Life Scale
  Health Utility Index
  Quality of Well-Being Scale

(NHP),[59] Short Form Health Survey–36 Items (SF-36),[60,61] and Dartmouth COOP Charts for Primary Care Practice.[62] The measures reflect the World Health Organization[63] definition of health in terms of physical, mental, and social well-being. Each measure creates separate scores for several dimensions of health. All four measures have been used extensively in population surveys, clinical research, and health services researchers, and they have been translated into a number of languages for use in international studies.

The generic measures are broadly applicable across diseases, conditions, populations and concepts. The measures are better at describing general health status than detecting clinically important changes in functioning. The measures provide profiles of dimension scores rather than a unitary value, so the health states and effects of interventions may be difficult to interpret. The length of the instruments can be a problem in usage as well.[64] Comparative research has demonstrated reasonably well that the measures are suitable for detecting group differences in health, but they generally are not appropriate for comparing individuals, or monitoring changes within individuals over time.[65] This is why these measures are often of limited importance for individual patients. They can rarely be used to monitor treatment progress.

Disease-specific measures are designed to assess the impact of disease and the treatment of it on symptoms and impairments in functioning considered important to patients and clinicians. The measures are usually designed so that they are responsive to significant clinical changes, particularly in response to therapeutic interventions. The measures may produce single scores or they can be multidimensional. Of the hundreds of measures that are in use, the Karnofsky Performance Index[66] for cancer patients and the Barthel Index[67] for assessing stroke patients are older measures that continue to be used widely. The main strength of this class of measures is also their main limitation, the results are specific to the condition so there is no way to make comparisons across conditions or populations. Also, it is difficult to assess the impact of a treatment on the general quality of life of a patient, leaving unanswered the question of whether the improvement is, all things considered, meaningful.

The general impact of a treatment on survival and quality of life is best determined by so-called utility measures. Utility measures are designed to assess patients' preferences for health states, usually on a scale that ranges from 0, indicating death, to 1, the score for perfect health. The standard gamble is a method that has been used extensively in the field of decision analysis, and it is based on the fundamental axioms of von Neumann and Morgenstern.[68] Persons in a chronic health state of ill health (e.g., end-stage renal disease) are presented with the gamble of a treatment (e.g., transplantation) that could either return the ill to health or result in death. The probability of health following the treatment is altered until the subject is uncertain as to which treatment to choose, and that probability becomes the utility value.

The time trade-off method was developed by Torrance and his colleagues[69] as an alternative to the standard gamble. With this method, the utility value reflects the trade-off between the time the person would spend in a chronic state (e.g., time spent on dialysis), as opposed to the time he or she would have in a healthy state if a treatment alternative (e.g., successful kidney transplant) were chosen. Both of these measures are based on the theory of decision making under conditions of uncertainty, but there is debate as to how the theory applies to choices in health policy. Making choices with the standard gamble and time trade-offs is a conceptually demanding task, and the subjects can be reluctant to gamble with health. The utility values are developed one condition at a time, and they are available for a limited selection of health states. The principal advantage of using utility scales is the possibility of comparing health programs that improve only the quality of life, with those that improve either survival or the quality of life and survival at the same time. A program that, for example, saves a given number of utility units is equally as beneficial as any other program with the same score, independent of the question of how this impact was achieved.

Additionally there are a number of multidimensional utility scores such as the Quality of Well-Being Scale,[70] Rosser's Disability and Distress Scale,[71] the Health Utility Index3,[72] and the EuroQol Quality of Life Scale.[73] The Quality of Well-Being Scale is used widely in the United

States, EuroQol was developed for use in European countries, and the Health Utilities Index, developed for use in clinical research, has been incorporated into population health surveys in Canada. There is collaboration between the researchers in Canada and Europe, with the hope of comparable scores, if not methods, for the EuroQol and Health Utilities Index. The four measures provide preference weights for general health states. The information they provide is different from the utility scores produced by the standard gamble and time trade-off methods because they do not provide an opportunity to translate quality of life gains into survival gains. This makes them less useful for economic evaluations.

In 1988, Ellwood,[74] the godfather of the Health Maintenance Organization, and Relman[75] independently called for the use of the measures for a new kind of accountability in health care that would take the consumers' perspective into account. Since that time there has been a proliferation of new measures, and refinements of existing ones. There are debates about the desired properties of the measures[65,76,77] and the standards for their development[78] and use.[79]

There is little standardization and consensus about measures to be used and the properties they should possess. Physicians, nurses, and other providers infrequently use measures for assessing the effects of clinical encounters. Lastly, the design of care has to be coordinated with the assessment of outcomes. It is neither clear that the measures work in the real world, nor that the information gleaned from them can be used to make real changes.

Methods for Economic Evaluations

Health economists have been developing and promoting models for comparative cost analyses of alternative health interventions.[64,80] Four types of analyses have been proposed: cost-minimization analysis, cost-effectiveness analysis, cost-benefit analysis, and cost-utility analysis. On the cost side of the equation, most studies include the costs of provider time, supplies, equipment, and related services. Appropriate portions of administrative, overhead, and capital cost should be allocated to the costs as well. Researchers may or may not include out-of-pocket expenses of the patient and the family. It is relatively uncommon for researchers to attach dollar values to the time patients and family members contribute to care, or the indirect costs of time lost from work, and the psychic costs of pain and suffering. If the cost implications and consequences are realized over time or in the future, they are discounted and expressed in current dollars. (See Figure 57-6.)

In *cost-minimization analysis,* one assumes that the effects of the alternative interventions or programs are equal, and the task is to determine if one intervention or program is less costly than the other.

Cost-effectiveness analysis is predicated on the assumption that the alternative interventions produce clinically important differences in outcomes for a given health problem, with respect to mortality, morbidity, function status, and/or quality of life. If there are significant reductions in mortality, the effects can be expressed in survival time and years of life gained.

Cost-benefit analysis involves assigning dollar values to the effects. By quantifying the effects of programs and interventions in dollar values, it would be possible to compare the costs and benefits of different interventions such as hypertension screening, hip replacements, and kidney transplants. Monetary values have to be placed on the benefits as well: life years gained, disability days avoided, complications avoided, and reduced dis-

Figure 57-6. Health economic evaluations.

- **Cost minimization:** Two or more interventions for the same problem produce same effects. Choose the least costly intervention.

- **Cost-effectiveness analysis:** Two or more interventions for the same problem produce important differences in outcomes. Choose after weighting costs against difference in effects.

- **Cost-benefit analysis:** Two interventions for the same or different problems produce different effects, and all costs and benefits are expressed in dollars. Choose intervention with best cost-benefit ratio.

- **Cost-utility analysis:** Two or more interventions for the same or different problems produce effects quantified as utility values or quality-adjusted life years. Choose intervention with best cost-utility ratio.

ruptions to work, family, and social activities. The methods for quantifying benefits in dollar values are sufficiently difficult and so highly controversial that one seldom sees such studies.

Cost-utility analysis starts with the assignment of a utility or preference values to the health states resulting from disease and management. The utility measures described in the previous section are used for this purpose. By multiplying the life years gained by the utility value, the outcomes are expressed in terms of quality-adjusted life years (QALYs).[98]

Economics methods build directly on the other methods for health services research. They are designed to provide summary statements about the worth of health programs and interventions. The summary statements carry the advantages and limitations of the data and methods on which they are based.

Challenges for Health Services Research

Health services research in the future has to meet a number of challenges if it is to deliver on the task of assessing equity, efficiency, and effectiveness: establishing a perspective on the population; relating the associations and trade-offs between access and equity, efficiency, and effectiveness; and providing economic evaluations of interventions and connecting the evidence to decisions in health policy.[82]

Setting the Population Perspective

We have recently been reminded by Mckeown's[100] treatise that medicine is only one of the determinants of health, and that health services may play only a minor role in improving the health of the populations.[84,85] One challenge is to relate health services to well-defined populations. Ideally, researchers would be able to assess all health services provided to a population, taking into account the social, economic, and ethnic determinants of health status in addition to the characteristics of the individuals.[86]

One approach is to combine data from population health surveys and health administrative databases so that the health information about the

participants can be linked to their subsequent uses of medical and social services. Longitudinal surveys are complex and expensive. Researchers will be able to study trends at the level of the nation and province, but the sample sizes will not be adequate to relate health and health services for regions or districts, or to estimate the impacts of specific interventions for specific diseases and conditions.

Regionalization of health services affords another opportunity for establishing a population perspective. For example, in England, Sweden, and some provinces in Canada, regional health authorities are responsible for allocating funds to services and ensuring that the health needs of the population are met. Regional data on the uses of health services and vital statistics can be linked to estimate the impact of health services on the population served.[86]

A third approach is to define populations in terms of subscribers to health insurance plans, or persons rostered to providers who are funded on a per capita basis. It may be difficult to accurately define the populations served by various plans with respect to salient demographics such as socioeconomic, ethnic, and health characteristics. Competition and managed care dominate health services in the United States. Health insurance firms and providers are striving to control costs and services as they compete for contracts with employers and consumers who buy the insurance plans or pay for the services. As they compete for buyers and enrollees, it will be interesting to see how they will provide data on costs, services, and outcomes. One promising benchmarking approach is the Health Employer Data and Information Set (HEDIS) in which managed care organizations voluntarily report on several outcomes indicators and proxies, which allows competition not only with respect to volume and price of coverage, but also with respect to quality of care.[87]

In England, general practitioners with large practices can contract with the National Health Service to be fund holders. They receive budgets to purchase some hospital services, diagnostic tests, drugs, and some community health services for the patients registered in their practices. In addition, they receive management allowances and additional funding for the required information systems. The flexibility in purchasing services provides incentives for efficiency and improvements in quality of care. There is a cost for the added layer of management, and a two-tier system of primary care may emerge. While there is a potential for relating the efficiency and effectiveness to the needs of the "populations" served, providers, managers, and researchers have some distance to travel before the potential is realized.[88] In Germany, several pilot projects with national sickness funds are currently starting. These sickness funds and regional physician's offices contract in such a way that, through the implementation of health services research data, hospitalization rates can be reduced.[89]

A fourth approach is to break the population down into service areas by defining the markets for hospitals and other services. Wennberg and others[90] took the Medicare data for the United States, and divided the postal codes of the enrollees to 3,436 hospital service areas. In each area, more Medicare patients were hospitalized locally than in any one other area. Originally the goal was to define the areas to allow for the possibility of competition at the level of secondary care. However, given the distribution of the American population, 82% of the hospital areas with 39% of the population had only one hospital. Twelve percent of the areas with 23% of the population had either two or three hospitals, and the remaining 5% of the areas had four or more local hospitals and 37% of the population. The average population size of the areas was 180,000 people, with half of the areas having fewer than 30,000 residents.

Secondary care facilities refer patients to regional hospitals. Wennberg and others[90] grouped the hospital service areas into 306 hospital referral regions. The hospital referral regions overlap city and state boundaries. Even so, about half of the regions had populations of fewer than 500,000 residents. One-quarter of the regions served a large population of one million residents or more. Working with a number of health administrative databases, Wennberg and others[90] displayed the variations of health resources and the utilization rates of Medicare patients across the hospital referral regions. It is unclear how the areas defined in the Dartmouth Atlas can be linked to current and future patterns of managed care and competition in the United States.

Hospital service areas are an important concept for populations that are defined regionally or by service plans. It is not uncommon for secondary and tertiary hospitals to serve as referral centers for a number of regions or plans. For a given population, knowledge of hospital service areas may define opportunities for restructuring or reorganizing the service delivery system.[91]

Access and Equity

In the United States, where an estimated 37 million citizens are without health insurance, and the number of underinsured is about 48 million, there is a continuing research emphasis on access to care.[82] Insurers and providers attempt to limit liabilities and control costs through restricting access to specialists and hospital beds, and major problems have arisen with respect to access and equity for those with insurance coverage. While HMOs have been targeted for criticism, other providers of managed care have been criticized as well.[92]

In countries where universal access to medical care is a right guaranteed by public programs, inequities in health have been key issues.[93] The Black Report[94] and the Health Divide Report[95] have demonstrated that while there have been reductions in mortality and improvements in access to care since the introduction of the National Health Services, inequities in health by region and social groups, defined in terms of employment, socioeconomic status, and other characteristics, have either persisted or increased since World War II. England has addressed the issue by allocating resources geographically by level of need. Following the report of the Resource Allocation Working Party in 1978, the formula for the allocation of funds was based on sex- and disease-specific standard mortality ratios (SMRs) and bed occupancy rates for the regions. With the growing criticisms of the use of the SMRs to define health, social, and economic needs, the formula was revised to include all-cause SMRs for deaths before the age of 75 years, and the weight given to the SMR was reduced; bed utilization was replaced by a measure of demand for all hospital and community services and an adjustment for regional variations for the costs of those services.[96]

As Whitehead[95] noted, not only are there criticisms of the model and the indicators, the inequities among social groups within a region are not taken into account. To the extent that investments in education, social programs, and employment can reduce inequities in health, it can be reasonably argued that resources from the health budget should be reallocated to those sectors of the public economy.

The last step to consider for addressing inequities would be to introduce health interventions aimed at specific problems contributing to the inequities. In a review of experimental studies of interventions directed toward accidents, cancer risk factors, coronary artery disease and stroke, sexual health; HIV/AIDS; preventing teenage pregnancy, pregnancy and childbirth, and mental health, Arblaster and others[97] found an absence of comprehensive empirical evidence to support the potential benefits of such community-based programs.

Effectiveness AND Efficiency: The Outcomes Movement

Bunker, Frazier, and Mosteller[98] listed the medical interventions in this century that have had the greatest impact on improving survival and quality of life for patients whose conditions were such that mortality was not an issue. They identified interventions that have been unquestionably effective in improving quantity of life (e.g., immunization for diphtheria, and the collection of technologies for the treatment of ischemic heart disease and hypertension) and quality of life (e.g., the collection of technologies for correcting vision problems, hip and knee replacements). However, the costs and effects of most medical interventions are not known. Researchers are working on strategies for directly relating the costs of medical care to the benefits produced.[99]

The major initiatives in the outcomes movement are found in England and the United States. In England, the Department of Health has established the Central Health Outcomes Unit to encourage and coordinate the development of methods, data collection systems, analysis, and expertise. The Department of Health also established the United Kingdom Clearing House for the Assessment of Health Outcomes at the University of Leeds. There are a number of research

units, including the one at the Royal College of Physicians, that have had held workshops for physicians on the uses of outcome measures.[100]

In the United States there are a number of governmental agencies, proprietary groups, foundations, and independent associations involved in developing outcomes that can be related to management.[101] Two such undertakings are the U.S. Agency for Health Care Policy and Research and the Medical Outcomes Study.

In 1989 the U.S. government created the Agency for Health Care Policy and Research (AHCPR) to fund research on the costs and effectiveness of services delivered to Medicare beneficiaries. Under its Medical Treatment Effectiveness Program, the AHCPR funds patient outcomes research, clinical practice guideline development, scientific data development, and research dissemination. The AHCPR has funded multicenter interdisciplinary programs of research on the effectiveness of alternative strategies for the prevention, diagnosis, treatment, and management of a wide variety of acute and chronic conditions. There are 19 Patient Outcome Research Teams to study hip fracture repairs and osteoarthritis, total knee replacement, benign prostatic hypertrophy and localized prostate cancer, pneumonia, cardiac arrhythmias, local breast cancer, acute myocardial infarction, dialysis care, low-back pain, low birth weight in children of minority and high-risk women, childbirth, biliary tract disease, ischemic heart disease, prostatic diseases, stroke, testing prior to cataract surgery, cataract management, and diabetes. The first contracts were set in 1989, and they have been of 5 to 10 years in duration. Publications based on the studies are now appearing in the literature.[101]

The Medical Outcomes Study conducted by the Health Institute, New England Medical Center, and RAND was designed to determine if variations in patient outcomes can be related to systems of care, clinician specialty, and clinicians' technical and interpersonal styles. The study started with 28,257 adults treated by 345 clinicians in Boston, Chicago, and Los Angeles for hypertension, congestive heart failure, myocardial infarction, depression, or type II diabetes. Greenfield and his colleagues[102] reported that the outcomes for type II diabetes were not related to specialty or variations in management. Ware and his colleagues[103] followed a random sample 2,235 patients for 4 years, and found no differences in physical and mental outcomes for the average patient. They did find that the elderly, poor, and chronically ill had worse physical health outcomes in HMOs than in the fee-for-service systems, but the mental health outcomes were not related to type of managed care. However, in a randomized trial of Medicare patients assigned to HMOs and fee-for-service plans, Lurie and others[104] found the outcomes for the two types of care to be equal.

Disease management systems are a variation on the theme. Drug companies and other contractors target diseases with high prevalence rates, whose outcomes should be sensitive to variations in management in the community and hospital. Diabetes and asthma are two diseases for which management systems are being marketed to hospitals. Targeting of specific diseases and the marketing management systems for them can lead to segmentation of health services. From the perspective of population health, the impacts have yet to be determined.[105]

The outcomes management systems have been underway for a decade, and the world is waiting for the verdict on whether or not they will work. Companies are marketing disease management programs to hospitals and other providers on the premise that they can improve outcomes at reduced costs, but it is too early to tell if they will be successful.

Economic Evaluation of Interventions

Laupacis and his colleagues[106] proposed setting guidelines for the funding of technologies that would take into account cost per quality-adjusted life year (QALY) and the quality of the evidence of the effectiveness of the technology. If a new technology had grade A (best) evidence and cost less than existing technology, it would be accepted. Conversely, a technology with grade E (worst) evidence that cost more would receive no funding. A grade B technology is to cost less than $20,000 per QALY, a grade C technology is to cost between $20,000 and $100,000, and a grade D technology is to cost more than $100,000 per QALY.

Maynard[107] produced a "league table" in which he ranked a number of interventions in terms of costs per QALY gained from a number of studies to demonstrate the relative cost-utility ratios for a number of interventions. For example, the costs per QALY, expressed in 1990 pounds British sterling, were 220 for cholesterol testing and diet therapy, alone; 1,100 for pacemaker implantation; 1,180 for hip replacement; 2,090 for CABG surgery of the left main vessel; 21,970 for hospital dialysis; and 107,780 for neurosurgical intervention for malignant intracranial tumors.

Drummond, Torrance, and Mason[108] critically appraised the studies that produced the costs per QALY. They assessed the discount rate, method for estimating the utility values, range of costs and consequences included, and choice of intervention or program for the comparison. The methods varied across the studies, and the discrepancies could have biased the results. Information on key components was frequently missing. Had the information been available for all costs and consequences, the biases would likely have been more marked.

Further, it can be noted that the concept of quality-adjusted life year is a controversial concept in and of itself.[109] For most interventions, we do not have long-term follow up data for patients that tracks changes in health status over time. Even if the data and concepts were sound, one would wonder whether the allocation of health resources could rest on such narrow utilitarian principles.[110]

Groups such as Drummond and colleagues[80] and the Task Force on Principles for Economic Analysis for Health Care Technology[111] have proposed new standards for conducting economic analyses of interventions. The challenges for comparing and economically evaluating management systems continue for health service researchers.

Evidence and Health Policy Decisions

The reasons for health services research and the potential uses of the results in making health policy decisions are clear and demanding. In his Rock Carling Fellowship address, Cochrane[112] noted that expenditures and development of the National Health Services in England took place without regard to information on efficiency and effectiveness. If decisions can be made to expand

and develop health services without regard to evidence, so can the decisions about restructuring and rationalization of health services and the constraints of costs for health care.

Health service research often has to rely upon observational studies based on quantitative epidemiological research, to evaluate the effectiveness of health care.[113,114] Black[113] pointed out that when evaluating the effects of services, a randomized trial may be unnecessary, inappropriate, impossible, or inadequate, particularly when the external validity of the findings is required to define its impact on the population. As Naylor and Guyatt[114] note, for observational studies to be credible, the outcome measures must be accurate and comprehensive, the comparison groups must be clearly identified and sensible, and either the comparison groups must be similar with respect to important determinants of outcome, or the differences have to be adjusted for in the analysis. Researchers have to meet these demands if the evidence is to be a credible basis for health policy decisions.

Some health policy decisions are purely political and are beyond the reach of research evidence. Other decisions are within the reach of research. Decisions are made that do take evidence into account, but for some decisions the evidence may not exist, or it may not be effectively transferred to those making decisions. All of the players involved in making decisions about health care—policy makers, planners, managers, health professionals, and consumers—are looking for high-quality information that is relevant, made public, and disseminated for use. The interest in health services research is matched with monies to support the research programs and projects. Health services research will remain an active and vital field of activity for the foreseeable future. All interest parties are invited to participate.

References

1. World Bank. World Development Report 1993: Investing in Health. New York: Oxford University, 1993.
2. Breyer F. Cost dynamics, demographic development, and medical progress. Zentralbl Chirur 1995;120(7):496–501.
3. Commission on Health Research for Development. Health Research: Essential Link to Equity in Development. New York: Oxford University, 1990.
4. Institute of Medicine. Health Services Research. Workforce and Educational Issues. National Academy, Washington, DC, 1996, pp. 1–8.
5. Kohn R, White KL, eds. Health Care: An International Study. New York: Oxford University, 1976.
6. White KL. Health care organization: an epidemiologic perspective. In: White KL, Frenk J, Ordóñez C, Paganini JM, Startfield B, eds. Health Services Research: An Anthology. Washington, DC: Pan American Health Organization; 1992, pp. 657–673.
7. Newhouse JP, Insurance Experiment Group. Free for All? Lessons from the RAND Health Insurance Experiment. Cambridge, MA: Harvard University, 1993.
8. Newhouse JP. Controlled experimentation as research policy. In: Ginzberg E, ed. Health Services Research. Key to Health Policy. Cambridge, MA: Harvard University; 1991, pp. 161–194.
9. Brook RH, Ware JE Jr, Rogers WH, Keeler EB, Davies AR, Donald CA, Goldberg GA, Lohr KN, Masthay PC, Newhouse JP. Does free care improve adults' health? Results from a randomized controlled trial. New Engl J Med 1983;309: 1426–1434.
10. Ware JE Jr, Brook RH, Rogers WH, Keeler EB, Davies AR, Sherbourne CD, Goldberg GA, Camp P, Newhouse JP. Comparisons of health outcomes at a health maintenance organization with those of fee-for-service care. Lancet 1986; 1:1017–1022.
11. Anderson GF, Alonso J, Kohn LT, Black C. Analyzing health outcomes through international comparisons. Med Care 1994;32(5):526–534.
12. Kunst AE, Guerts JJM, van den Berg J. International variation in socioeconomic inequalities in self reported health. J Epidemiol Commun Health 1995;49:117–123.
13. Naylor CD, Anderson GM, Goel V, eds. Patterns of Health Care in Ontario: The ICES Practice Atlas, 1st edn. Ottawa: Canadian Medical Association, 1994.
14. Goel V, Williams JI, Anderson GM, Blackstein-Hirsch P, Fooks C, Haylor CD, eds. Patterns of Health Care in Ontario: The ICES Practice At-

las, 2nd edn. Ottawa: Canadian Medical Association, 1996.

15. Williams JI, Young W. A summary of studies on the quality of health care administrative databases in Canada. In: Goel V, Williams JI, Anderson GM, Backstein-Hirsch P, Fooks C, Naylor CD, eds. Patterns of Health Care in Ontario: The ICES Practice Atlas, 2nd edn. Ottawa: Canadian Medical Association, 1996, pp. 339–346.

16. Wennberg JE, Gittlesohn A. Variations in medical care among small areas. Sci Am 1982;246(4) 120–134.

17. Roos NP, Roos LL Jr. Surgical rate variations: do they reflect health or socioeconomic characteristics of the population. Med Care 1982;20:945–958.

18. McPherson K, Strong PM, Epstein A, Jones L. Regional variations in the use of common surgical procedures: within and between England and Wales, Canada, and the United States of America. Soc Sci Med 1981;15:273–288.

19. McPherson K, Wennberg JE, Hovind OB, Clifford P. Small area variations in use of common surgical procedures. An interaction comparison of New England, England, and Norway. New Engl J Med 1982;307:1310–1314.

20. Andersen TF, Mooney G, eds. The Challenge of Medical Practice Variations. London: Macmillan, 1990.

21. McPherson, K. Why do variations occur? In: Andersen TF, Mooney G, eds. The Challenge of Medical Practice Variations. London: Macmillan, 1990, pp. 16–35.

22. Cohen MM, Naylor CD, Basinski ASH, Ferris LE, Llewellyn-Thomas HA, Williams JI. Small-area variations: what are they and what do they mean? Can Med Assoc J 1992;146:467–470.

23. Roos NP, Wennberg JE, McPherson K. Using diagnosis-related groups for studying variations in hospital admissions. Health Care Financ Rev 1988;9:53–61.

24. Ward, JE, Grieco V. Why we need guidelines for guidelines: a study on the quality of clinical practice guidelines in Australia. Med J Aust 1996; 165(10):574–576.

25. Chalmers I, Enkin M, Keirse MJNC, eds. Effective Care in Pregnancy and Childbirth. London: Oxford University, 1990.

26. Brook RH, Chassin MR, Fink A, Solomon DH, Kosecoff J, Park RE. A method for the detailed

assessment of the appropriateness of medical technologies. Int J Technol Assess Health Care 1987;2:53–63.

27. Leape LL, Park RE, Solomon DH, Chassin MR, Kosecoff J, Brook RH. Does inappropriate use explain small-area variations in the use of health care services? JAMA 1990;263:669–672.

28. Naylor CD, Baigrie RS, Goldman BS, Basinski A. Clinical practice assessment of priority for coronary revascularization procedures. Lancet 1990;335:1070–1073.

29. Naylor CD, Skyora K, Jaglal SB, Jefferson S, Steering Committee of the Adult Cardiac Care Network of Ontario. Waiting for coronary artery bypass surgery: population-based study of 8517 consecutive patients in Ontario, Canada. Lancet 1995;346(8990):1605–1609.

30. Naylor CD, Levinton CM, Baigrie RS. Adapting to waiting lists for coronary revascularization: do Canadian specialists agree on which patients come first? Chest 1992;101:715–722.

31. Yusuf S, Zucker D, Peduzzi P, Fisher LD, Takaro T, Kennedy JW, Davis K, Killip T, Passamani E, Norris R, et al. Effect of coronary artery bypass graft surgery: overview of 10 year results from randomized trials by the Coronary Artery Bypass Graft Surgery Trialists Collaboration Group. Lancet 1994;344:563–570.

32. Hux JE, Naylor CD, Steering Committee of the Provincial Adult Cardiac Care Network of Ontario. Are the marginal returns of coronary artery surgery smaller in high-rate areas? Lancet 1996; 348:1202–1207.

33. Black N, Glickman ME, Ding J, Flood AB. International variations in intervention rates: what are the implications for patient selection? Int J Technol Assess Health Care 1995;11:719–732.

34. Basinski AS. Use of hospital resources. In: Naylor CD, Anderson GM, Goel V, eds. Patterns of Health Care in Ontario: The ICES Practice Atlas, 1st edn. Ottawa: Canadian Medical Association, 1994, pp. 165–306.

35. Basinski AS, Thériault M-E. Patterns of hospitalization. In: Goel V, Williams JI, Anderson GM, Blackstein-Hirsch P, Fooks C, Naylor CD, eds. Patterns of Health Care in Ontario: The ICES Practice Atlas, 2nd edn. Ottawa: Canadian Medical Association, 1996, pp. 196–246.

36. Iezzoni LI, Greenberg LG. Risk adjustment and current health policy debates. In: Iezzoni LI, ed.

Risk Adjustment for Measuring Health Care Outcomes. Ann Arbor, MI: Health Administration; 1994, pp. 347–403.

37. New York State Department of Health. Coronary artery bypass surgery in New York state 1990–1992. In: Vibbert S, Migdail KJ, Strickland D, Youngs MT, eds. The 1995 Medical Outcomes & Guidelines Sourcebook. Washington, DC: Faulkner & Gray, 1994, pp. 466–480.

38. Hannan EL, Siu AL, Kumar D, Kilburn H, Chassin MR. The decline in coronary artery bypass graft surgery mortality in New York state. JAMA 1995;273(3):209–213.

39. Omoigui NA, Miller DP, Brown KJ, Annan K, Cosgrove D 3rd, Lytle B, Loop F, Topol EJ. Outmigration for coronary bypass surgery in an era of public dissemination of clinical outcomes. Circulation 1996;93:27–33.

40. Tu JV, Jaglal SB, Naylor CD, Steering Committee of the Provincial Adult Cardiac Care Network of Ontario. Multicentre validation of a risk index for mortality, intensive care unit stay, and overall hospital length of stay after cardiac surgery. Circulation 1995;95:677–684.

41. Tu JV, Naylor CD, Steering Committee of the Provincial Audit Cardiac Care Network of Ontario. Coronary artery bypass mortality rates in Ontario. A Canadian approach to quality assurance in cardiac surgery. Circulation 1996;94:2429–2433.

42. Iezzoni LI, Ash AS, Shwartz M, Daley J, Hughes JS, Mackierman YD. Predicting who dies depends on how severity is measured: implications for evaluating patient outcomes. Ann Intern Med 1995;123:763–770.

43. Indications for cesarean section: final statement of the Panel of the National Consensus Conference on Aspects of Cesarean Birth. Can Med Assoc J 1986;134:1348–1352.

44. Lomas, J, Anderson GM, Domnick-Pierre K, Vayda E, Enkin MW, Hannah WJ. Do practice guidelines guide practice? New Eng J M 1989;321:1306–1311.

45. Anderson GM, Axcell T. Cesarean section: provincial trends and hospital-specific rates. In: Goel V, Williams JI, Anderson GM, Blackstein-Hirsch P, Fooks C, Naylor CD, eds. Patterns of Health Care in Ontario: The ICES Practice Atlas, 2nd edn. Ottawa: Canadian Medical Association, 1996, pp. 170–177.

46. Society of Obstetricians and Gynaecologists of Canada. Dystocia. (Policy Statement No. 40) Ottawa: Society of Obstetricians and Gynaecologists of Canada, 1995.

47. Early Breast Cancer Trialists' Collaborative Group. Effects of radiotherapy and surgery in early breast cancer. New Engl J Med 1995;333:1444–1445.

48. Goel V, Iscoe NA, Sawka C. Breast cancer surgery. In: Goel V, Williams JI, Anderson GM, Blackstein-Hirsch P, Fook C, Naylor CD, eds. Patterns of Health Care in Ontario: The ICES Practice Atlas, 2nd edn. Ottawa: Canadian Medical Association, 1996, pp. 183–186.

49. Billings J, Zeitel I, Lukomnik J, Carey TS, Blank AE, Newman L. Impact on socioeconomic status on hospital use in New York City. Health Aff 1993;12:162–173.

50. Weissman JS, Gatsonis C, Epstein M. Rates of avoidable hospitalization by insurance status in Massachusetts and Maryland. JAMA 1992;268:2388–2394.

51. Anderson GM. Common conditions sensitive to ambulatory care (asthma and congestive heart failure). In: Goel V, Williams JI, Anderson GM, Blackstein-Hirsch P, Fook C, Naylor CD, eds. Patterns of Health Care in Ontario: The ICES Practice Atlas, 2nd edn. Ottawa: Canadian Medical Association, 1996, pp. 104–110.

52. Billings J, Anderson GM, Newman LS. Recent findings on preventable hospitalizations. Health Aff 1996;15:239–249.

53. Bowling A. Measuring Disease: A Review of Disease-Specific Quality of Life Measurement Scales. Philadelphia: Open University, 1995.

54. Bowling A. Measuring Health: Review of Quality of Life Measurement Scales. Philadelphia: Open University, 1991.

55. McDowell I, Newell C. Measuring Health: A Guide to Rating Scales and Questionnaires, 2nd edn. New York: Oxford University, 1996.

56. Spilker B, ed. Quality of Life and Pharmacoeconomics in Clinical Trials. New York: Lippincott-Raven, 1996.

57. Williams JI, Wood-Dauphinee S. Assessing quality of life: measures and utility. In: Mosteller F, Falotico-Taylor J, eds. Quality of Life and Technology Assessment. Washington, DC: National Academy, 1989, pp. 65–115.

58. Bergner M. Bobbit RA, Carter WB, Gilson BS. The Sickness Impact Profile: development and final revision of a health status measure. Med Care 1981;19:787–805.

59. Hunt SM, McEwen J, McKenna SP. Measuring Health Status. London: Croom Helm, 1986.

60. Ware JE Jr, Snow KK, Kosinski M, Gandek B. SF-36 Health Survey: Manual and Interpretation Guide. Boston, MA: The Health Institute, New England Medical Center, 1993.

61. Ware JE Jr, Kosinski M, Keller SD. SF-36 Physical and Mental Health Summary Scores: A New Users Manual. Boston, MA: The Health Institute, New England Medical Center, 1996.

62. Nelson EC, Landgraf JM, Hays RD, Wasson JH, Kirk JW. The functional status of patients: how can it be measured in physicians' offices? Med Care 1990;28:1111–1126.

63. World Health Organization. The First Ten Years of the World Health Organization. Geneva: World Health Organization, 1958.

64. Patrick DL, Erickson P. Health Status and Health Policy: Allocating Resources to Health Care. New York: Oxford University, 1993.

65. McHorney CA, Tarlov AR. Individual-patient monitoring in clinical practice: are available health status surveys adequate? Qual Life Res 1995;4:293–307.

66. Karnofsky DA, Abelmann WH, Craver LF, Burchenal JH. The use of nitrogen mustards in the palliative treatment of carcinoma. Cancer 1948; I:634–656.

67. Mahoney FI, Barthel DW. Functional evaluation: the Barthel Index. Maryland State Med J 1965; 14:61–65.

68. Drummond MF, Stoddart GL, Torrance GW. Methods for the Economic Evaluation of Health Care Programs. New York: Oxford University, 1987.

69. Torrance GW, Thomas WH, Sackett DL. A utility maximization model for the evaluation of health care programmes. Health Serv Res 1972; 7:118–133.

70. Kaplan RM, Bush JW, Berry CC. Health status: types of validity and the Index of Well-Being. Health Psychol 1982;1:61–80.

71. Rosser RM. A health index and output measure. In: Walker SR, Rosser, eds. Quality of Life: Assessment and Application. Lancaster, England: MTP, 1987:133–160.

72. Torrance GW, Feeny DH, Furlong WJ, Barr RD, Zhang Y, Wang Q. Multiattribute utility function for a comprehensive health status classification system. Med Care 1996;34(7):702–722.

73. EuroQol Group. EuroQol: a new facility for the measurement of health-related quality of life. Health Policy 1990;16:199–208.

74. Ellwood PM. Shattuck lecture—outcomes management: a technology of patient experience. New Engl J Med 1988;318:1549–1556.

75. Relman AS. Assessment and accountability: the third revolution in medical care. New Engl J Med 1988;319:1220–1222.

76. Guyatt GH, Kirshner B, Jaeschke R. Measuring health status: what are the necessary measurement properties? J Clin Epidemiol 1992;45:1341–1345.

77. Williams JI, Naylor CD. How should health status measures be assessed? Cautionary notes on Procrustean frameworks. J Clin Epidemiol 1992; 45:1347–1351.

78. McDowell I, Jenkinson C. Development standards for health measures. J Health Serv Res Policy 1996;1:238–246.

79. Staquet M, Berzon R, Osoba, Machin D. Guidelines for reporting results of quality of life assessments in clinical trials. Qual Life Res 1996;5: 496–502.

80. Drummond MF, Brandt A, Luce B, Rovira J. Standardizing methodologies for economic evaluation in health care. Int J Technol Assess Health Care 1993;9(1):26–36.

81. Richardson J. Cost-utility analysis in health care: present status and future issues. In: Daly J, McDonald I, Willis E, eds. Researching Health Care: Designs, Dilemmas, Disciplines. London: Tavistock/Routledge, 1992.

82. Aday LA, Begley CE, Lairson DR, Slater CH. Evaluating the Medical Care System. Effectiveness, Efficiency, and Equity. Ann Arbor, MI: Health Administration, 1993.

83. McKeown T. The Role of Medicine: Dream, Mirage, or Nemesis? Princeton, NJ: Princeton University, 1976.

84. Amick BC, Levine S, Tarlov AR, Walsh DC, eds. Society and Health. New York: Oxford University, 1995.

85. Evans RG, Barer ML, Marmor TR, eds. Why Are Some People Healthy and Others Not? New York: Aldine de Gruter, 1994.

86. Roos NP, Black C, Frohlich N, DeCoster C, Cohen M, Tataryn DJ, Mustard CA, Roos LL, Toll F, Carriere KC, Burchill CA, MacWilliam L, Bogdanovic B. Population health and health care use: an information system for policy makers. Milbank Q 1996;74(1):3–49.

87. Schroeder J, Lamb S. Data initiatives: HEDIS and the New England Business Coalition. Am J Med Qual 1996;11(1):S58–S62.

88. Leese B, Drummond MF. General practice fund-holding: maverick or catalyst? In: Drummond MF, Maynard A, eds. Purchasing and Providing Cost-Effective Care. London: Churchill Livingstone, 1993.

89. Schunz R, Buck RA. Model project of section 275a SGBV for assessing the need for hospital treatment and implementation in Schleswig-Holstein. Gesundheitswesen 1995;57(1):8–12.

90. Wennberg JE, Cooper MMC, Dartmouth Atlas of Health Care Working Group. The Dartmouth Atlas of Health Care in the United States. Chicago: American Hospital Association, 1996.

91. Ruth A, DeBoer D. Patient origin and market share—tools to assist with hospital planning. In: Goel V, Williams JI, Anderson GM, Blackstein-Hirsch P, Fook C, Naylor CD, eds. Patterns of Health Care in Ontario: The ICES Practice Atlas, 2nd edn. Ottawa: Canadian Medical Association, 1996, pp. 147–168.

92. Bodenheimer T. The HMO backlash—righteous or reactionary? New Engl J Med 1996;335:1601–1604.

93. Wagstaff A, Paci P, Van Doorslaer E. On the measurement of inequalities in health. Soc Sci Med 1991;33(5):545–557.

94. Black D, Morris JN, Smith C, Townsend P, The Black Report. In: Townsend P, Davidson N, eds. Inequalities in Health. London: Penguin Books, 1992.

95. Whitehead M. The health divide. In: Townsend P, Davidson N, eds. Inequalities in Health. London: Penguin Books, 1992.

96. Mays N. Geographical resource allocation in the English National Health Service, 1974–1994: the tension between normative and empirical approaches. Int J Epidemiol 1995;24:S96–S102.

97. Arblaster L, Lambert M, Entwistle V, Forster M, Fullerton D, Sheldon T, Watt I. A systematic review of the effectiveness of health service interventions aimed at reducing inequalities in health. J Health Serv Res Policy 1996;1(2):93–103.

98. Bunker JP, Frazier HS, Mosteller F. Improving health: measuring effects of medical care. Milbank Q 1994;72(2):225–258.

99. Williams JI, Naylor CD, Health Services Research Group. Outcomes and the management of health care. Can Med Assoc J 1992;147:1775–1780.

100. Frater A, Sheldon TA. The outcomes movement in the USA and UK. In: Drummond MF, Maynard A, eds. Purchasing and Providing Cost-Effective Care. London: Churchill Livingstone, 1993.

101. Rosenthal MT, ed. The 1997 Medical Outcomes and Guidelines Sourcebook: A Progress Report and Resource Guide on Medical Outcomes Research and Practice Guidelines Developments, Data, and Documentation. New York: Faulkner & Gray, 1996.

102. Greenfield S, Rogers W, Mangotich M, Carney MF, Tarlov AR. Outcomes of patients with hypertension and non-insulin-dependent diabetes mellitus treated by different systems and specialties: results from the Medical Outcomes Study. JAMA 1995;274:1436–1474.

103. Ware JE Jr, Bayliss MS, Rogers WH, Kosinski M, Tarlov AR. Differences in 4-year outcomes for the elderly and poor, chronically ill patients treated in HMO and fee-for-service systems: results from the Medical Outcomes Study. JAMA 1996;276:1039–1047.

104. Lurie N, Christianson J, Finch M, Moscovice I. The effects of capitation on health and functional status of the Medicaid elderly. Ann Intern Med 1994;120:506–511.

105. Epstein RS, Sherwood LM. From outcomes research to disease management: a guide for the perplexed. Ann Intern Med 1996;124:832–837.

106. Laupacis A, Feeny D, Detsky AS, Tugwell PX. How attractive does a new technology have to be to warrant adoption and utilization? Tentative guidelines for using clinical and economic evaluations. Can Med J Assoc 1992;146:473–481.

107. Maynard A. Developing the health care market. Econ J 1991;101:1277–1286.

108. Drummond MF, Torrance G, Mason J. Cost-effectiveness league tables: more harm than good? Soc Sci Med 1993;37(1):33–40.

109. Gafni A, Birch S. Guidelines for the adoption of

new technologies: a prescription for uncontrolled growth in expenditures and how to avoid the problem. Can Med Assoc J 1993;148:913–917.

110. Naylor CD, Williams JI, Basinski A, Goel V. Technology assessment and cost-effectiveness analysis: misguided guidelines? Can Med Assoc J 1993;148:921–924.

111. Task Force on Principles for Economic Analysis for Health Care Technology. Economic analysis of health care technology. Ann Intern Med 1995; 123:61–70.

112. Cochrane AL. Effectiveness and Efficiency: Random Reflections on Health Services. London: Nuffield Provincial Hospitals Trust, 1971.

113. Black N. Why we need observational studies to evaluate the effectiveness of health care. Br Med J 1996;312:1215–1218.

114. Naylor CD, Guyatt GH, Evidence-Based Medical Working Group. Users' guide to the medical literature. X. How to use an article reporting variations in the outcomes of health services. JAMA 1996;275:554–558.

Decision Analysis, Cost-Benefit Analysis and Cost-Effectiveness Analysis in Surgical Research

J. Kievit

Introduction

The goals of health care have been defined by Lohr in 1988 as "to limit mortality, disease, disability, and discomfort, and optimize satisfaction."[1] Given such ambitious goals, described on a high level of aggregation, the value of medical interventions is evaluated in more and more complex terms. New outcome measures have evolved beside more classical ones such as morbidity, mortality and *n*-year survival. They include both one-dimensional outcomes such as quality of life, utility, and costs, but also explicitly multidimensional ones such as quality-adjusted life years (QALYs) and costs per QALY. Modern forms of research are evolving. Research on treatment has passed from the retrospective analysis of single-patient series to large-scale randomized controlled trials of surgical treatment. Research on diagnostic testing addresses questions about the value of diagnostic tests, in which "value" is expressed not only in terms of sensitivity and specificity, but also with respect to influence on medical outcome. All these research efforts are aimed at answering questions that seemed irrelevant before, but are more and more relevant today, in a time when society is confronted with rising costs and limited resources and expects value for money. Do we do things for the right reasons, and in the right way? Do our interventions have the right effects, at acceptable costs?

What evidence do we have for the choices we make?

This chapter deals with the potential and limitations of decision analysis, cost-benefit analysis, and cost-effectiveness, in helping to find answers to such questions. Clinical decision analysis is the discipline that uses an explicit quantitative method to analyze and support decision-making processes in medicine, with the goal to rationalize and improve both the decision-making processes themselves, and to improve the outcome of medical decisions. Decision analysis, cost-effectiveness analysis, and cost-benefit analysis have much in common: they all use explicit, quantitative, and probabilistic "model" representations of reality to calculate the consequences of choices. Their difference lies in the outcome measures calculated. Clinical decision analysis calculates expected medical outcomes only and ignores the issue of costs. In contrast, cost-effectiveness analysis and cost-benefit analysis compare outcomes with costs. To do this, cost-effectiveness analysis expresses medical outcomes in one general effect parameter (such as QALYs) that is then compared with costs in a two-dimensional analysis. This provides the possibility to explicitly calculate value-for-money. Cost-benefit analysis is one-dimensional; even nonmonetary outcomes are translated into monetary terms, and the result of the analysis is the net balance between monetary costs and monetary benefits. To word it differently; in cost-benefit analysis the exchange of nonmonetary effects into (negative) costs occurs before the calculation of expected outcomes and is thus hidden from view in the final result. In cost-effectiveness analysis the weighing between nonmonetary outcomes and costs is done explicitly after the calculation of expected outcomes and can be done differently by different interpreters. The choice to use one or the other method depends on many circumstances such as the question posed, and the party asking it. In the following, we will use cost-effectiveness as an example to illustrate the technical aspects of these methods.

Methods and Issues of Cost-Effectiveness Analysis

In cost-effectiveness analysis, as in decision analysis, cost-benefit analysis, and, in fact, in all research, the most essential step is an unambiguous definition of the research question. We will describe this process in four sections dealing with problem specification, problem structure, data assessment, and calculation.

Problem Specification

To get the clinical problem adequately specified, agreement must exist on at least five aspects:

1. *What is the precise medical question posed, and who is asking it with what purpose?* It does not suffice to ask whether "some intervention" is cost-effective. This question is unanswerable because it lacks specification and detail. Answerable is a question from a department of finance of a hospital about the short-term cost-effectiveness of laparoscopic cholecystectomy in comparison to open cholecystectomy, given the present reimbursement system. Likewise answerable is the question from a ministry of health, as to whether it is more cost-effective to diagnose persisting posttraumatic knee complaints using MRI than using arthroscopy, with the aim to minimize both long-term morbidity and intervention costs. Likewise answerable would be a question on the relative cost-effectiveness of spiral CT-scan in comparison to ventilation-perfusion scanning for the diagnosis and treatment of suspected pul-

monary embolism, with the aim to minimize mortality. Thus, the question needs specification and detail, one must know who asks (which of the parties involved, such as patient, hospital, health care insurance company, or society), and what the purpose of the question is (reducing the involved party's costs, improving effects for patients or society, or both).

2. *What is the intervention strategy in question, and what is the patient category and the context in which the intervention is considered?* Cost-effectiveness analysis per definition deals with interventions that are supposed to provide desirable effects, be it at a certain cost-price. Interventions in medicine come in two main categories: treatments and diagnostic tests. The aim of treatment is to cure the disease or, if this is not possible, to reduce its negative aspects. At an operational level these aims are translated into desired effects such as reducing mortality and morbidity and thereby increasing life expectancy and improving quality of life. For most treatments these desired effects come at a price, that of the complications and costs of the treatment itself. The aim of diagnostic tests is to identify the underlying disease that causes a problem. In practice, testing helps to assess disease probability in the face of uncertainty. Thereby, diagnostic testing helps in the weighing of the desired and undesired effects of treatment that necessarily underlie the treatment choice. Intervention choices, in principle, come in three types, in order of increasing aggressiveness: (a) doing nothing; (b) performing one or more diagnostic tests, followed by treatment in the case of a positive test result; and (c) giving treatment without preceding testing. Doing nothing is preferable at very low levels of disease probability, while increasing disease probability may justify testing and treatment, as is illustrated in the classical paper "The threshold approach to clinical decision making."[2]

3. *What are the alternative strategies, and what are the advantages and drawbacks of each strategy?* The question concerning the cost-effectiveness of an intervention strategy can be answered only if this strategy is compared to an alternative (such as doing things in the usual way, or doing nothing). Only on the basis of comparison may the intervention-specific costs and gains (added effects) be identified and com-

pared. Noncomparison leads to erroneous conclusions.

In an earlier publication we found that in patients who undergo colon cancer follow-up using carcinoembryonic antigen (CEA), the costs are $3,377 and the outcome is 6.41 QALYs.[3] Noncomparison would elicit the conclusion that CEA-directed follow-up is highly efficient and has a cost-effectiveness ratio of $527 per QALY ($3,377/6.41). One would need to know the costs and effects of the alternative strategy (no follow-up), which provides 6.29 QALYs at $1,839. Comparison of the two makes it clear that CEA-directed follow-up generates a mean 0.01 QALY only (6.41 − 6.39), at an added cost of $1,478 ($3,377 − $1,839), giving a marginal cost-effectiveness ratio of $86,227 per QALY ($1,478/0.02).

There are no standard rules concerning which alternative strategies should be taken into consideration, however, strong arguments exist in favor of always considering at least the extremes (doing nothing and treating everyone), since this identifies the range of potential outcomes in which the strategy investigated must be placed. It cannot be sufficiently emphasized that it is crucial to specify the arguments that are brought forward in favor of and against each strategy. Only by knowing what steers decision making and policy choices can one hope to influence them, and many decision analyses and cost-effectiveness analyses have missed their effect, precisely because they failed to identify (and thus target) the arguments that determined choices in real life.

4. *What are relevant effect parameters?* The relevant effect parameters are largely dictated by the aims of the intervention at hand, more specifically, the desired and undesirable effects. Other important considerations are the arguments that have been brought forward in favor of and concerning various strategy alternatives. Thus for laparoscopic cholecystectomy, relevant effect parameters may be mortality, severe morbidity, pain, duration of hospitalization, and duration until return to work. For colon cancer follow-up, relevant effect parameters may be lead time and detection of asymptomatic incurable disease or asymptomatic curable disease. Depending on the parties involved (both those for whom the analysis is performed, and those who will experience the effects of a policy change), these effect parameters have greater or lesser weight and may be categorized into one primary effect parameter, and one or more secondary effect parameters.

5. *What are relevant costs?* The issue of costs is as least as critical as that of relevant outcomes. Beforehand, many choices must be made about the way in which costs are brought into the cost-effectiveness equation. For these choices we refer to the later section about data on costs.

Cost-Effectiveness Analysis

- Define the medical question posed and purpose of inquiry
- Define intervention strategy and patient context for its use
- Define advantages/disadvantages of alternate strategies
- Identify effect parameters
- Identify relevant costs

Problem Structure

In the problem structure phase, two methods of structuring may be used. First, all potential actions and outcomes may be verbalized in a logically and chronologically correct order. This provides a descriptive algorithm in terms of "if . . . then . . . else . . ." sequences. Such an algorithm should be as simple as possible, while still incorporating the relevant issues brought forward in the problem specification phase. Another way of structuring the problem is by drawing a decision tree. Such a tree is graphical representation of the alternatives and of the potential events and outcomes. Tree-building convention states that a tree is drawn from left to right, with the stem splitting into branches at nodes. Nodes are divided into decision nodes (squares), chance nodes (circles), and terminal nodes (rectangles). Figures 58-1 and 58-2 illustrate these elements.

Data Assessment

A decision analysis needs data to quantify the various aspects of the problem represented in the algorithm and decision tree. In the second phase of the analysis, these data are gathered from vara.

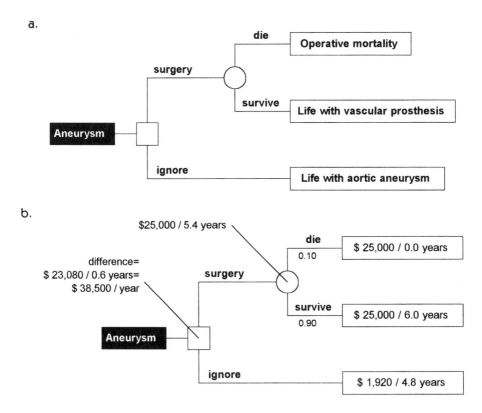

b.

Figure 58-1.   Decision tree representing the two options analyzed in example 1, concerning the cost-effectiveness of operating on an 80-year-old male patient with a 6-cm asymptomatic abdominal aortic aneurysm. In (a) the tree is drawn from left to right, the stem splitting into branches at so-called nodes. Nodes are divided into decision nodes (squares), chance nodes (circles), and terminal nodes (rectangles). At a decision node, the choice for the relevant branch can be made by the decision maker. At a chance node, the occurrence of the different branches is beyond the control of the decision maker. A terminal node represents the final outcome. In (b) includes the relevant data (probabilities below respective branches, outcomes in terminal nodes, and expected outcomes pointing toward relevant decision or chance nodes).

ious sources (such as one's own patient series, meta-analysis, or expert judgement). For the sake of clarity we will subdivide data into five basic categories: (1) data on underlying disease, (2) data on diagnostic testing, (3) data on treatment, (4) data on outcome, and (5) cost data.

Data on Underlying Disease

For a given clinical problem, the various disease categories that may be its cause, and their respective prior probabilities, should be known. Although disease prevalence is frequently used as an estimate of prior probability, this is not necessarily correct. It is better to correct this figure on the basis of

patient covariates (age, sex, signs, and symptoms) and context (primary care, hospital care, elective or acute situations, etc.). The natural course of each disease should be known, because this is the no-action standard against which the effects of medical interventions should be assessed.

Data on Diagnostic Testing

Besides the classical parameters of sensitivity and specificity, diagnostic interventions may also be characterized by their success rate and, in certain cases, even by their morbidity and mortality. Sensitivity is the potential to identify disease (i.e., the probability of a positive test in the presence of

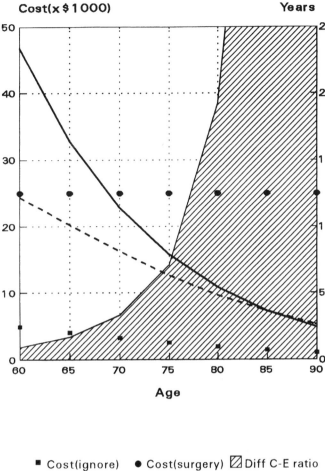

Figure 58-2.   Graph representing the results of a sensitivity analysis in example 1. The one-way seven-step sensitivity analysis illustrates the effect of age on expected outcome and cost per strategy, and on the differential cost-effectiveness of surgical treatment, versus ignoring the aneurysm.

disease), while specificity is the potential to recognize the absence of disease (i.e., the probability of a negative test in the absence of disease).

Sensitivity and specificity determine what the test result will be, given the presence or absence of disease, respectively. In clinical reality, however, the problem of test interpretation is the mirror image of this: the real-life question is how likely or unlikely the presence of disease is, given a certain test result. This question can be answered by calculating predictive values from the combination of sensitivity and specificity with prior probability in Bayes' Theorem. This theorem can easily be de-

rived from the two-by-two table (in which Se is the sensitivity, Sp is the specificity, and $p(D)$ is the prior probability of disease). (Table 58-1)

Other parameters for test performance, not limited to dichotomous tests, are the odds ratio, likelihood ratio, and ROC-curve. These fall beyond the limited scope of this chapter.

Although sensitivity and specificity are adequate parameters for test performance in the limited sense, they fail to assess the impact of a diagnostic test on health outcomes. Therefore, higher level parameters of effect have been invented. These include the potential to influence

Table 58-1.

	Disease	No disease	All
Test positive	$Se \times p(D)$	$(1 - Sp) \times (1 - p(D))$	$Se \times p(D) + (1 - Sp) \times (1 - p(D))$
Test negative	$(1 - Se) \times p(D)$	$(1 - Se) \times p(D)$	$(1 - Se) \times p(D) + Sp \times (1 - p(D))$
	$p(D)$	$1 - p(D)$	all

The positive predictive value ($PV+$) of a test is the probability that a positive test result is correct, that is, it is equal to the chance that disease is present given a positive test result, as follows:

$$PV+ \quad p(D + \mid T+) \quad \frac{Se \times p(D)}{Se \times p(D) + (1 - Sp) \times (1 - p(D))}$$

The negative predictive value ($PV-$) is the probability that a negative test result is correct, that is, it is equal to the chance that disease is absent given a negative test result, as follows:

$$PV- \quad p(D - \mid T-) \quad \frac{Sp \times (1 - p(D))}{Sp \times (1 - p(D)) + (1 - Se) \times p(D)}$$

Thus, the probability that disease is present in spite of a negative test is equal to (1 − negative predictive value):

$$p(D + \mid T-) \quad PV- \quad \frac{(1 - Se) \times p(D)}{Sp \times (1 - p(D)) + (1 - Se) \times p(D)}$$

diagnostic thinking, the potential to change the therapeutic choice, and the potential to generate better health outcome. The example of testing for HIV (the test's excellent sensitivity and specificity not justifying its routine use) or other incurable disease (such as many types of cancer recurrence) illustrates these points.

Data on Treatment

One should know the curative effect on relevant diseases, and the probability and nature of adverse outcomes (treatment-related morbidity and mortality) of the treatments under consideration. Typical parameters for the value of a treatment are safety (the absence of dangerous side effects), efficacy (the potential to generate a desired effect under optimal—trial—conditions), and effectiveness (the potential to generate a desired effect in daily practice). In the weighing of the pros and cons of treatment, it should be kept in mind that the desired effects of treatment occur mainly if the targeted disease really is the cause of the problem (i.e., in case of a correct diagnosis). On the other hand, the negative effects of treatment occur in a frequency characteristic for the treatment under consideration and are less dependent on the underlying cause of the problem. As a consequence, the balance between desired and negative effects of treatment depends on the correctness or (un)certainty of diagnosis. This again illustrates the purpose of diagnostic testing: to optimize the ratio between potential positive and negative effects of treatment by reducing uncertainty about the presence of the disease at which the treatment is aimed.

Data on Outcome

Data on medical outcome can be subdivided into data concerning quantity and quality of life, respectively. One of the most simple methods for the determination of quantity of life (i.e., life expectancy) in the presence of disease is the DEALE, which stands for *decreasing exponential approximation of life expectancy*. The DEALE is based on the (in itself incorrect) assumption that survival over time can be represented by an exponential function. Under this assumption the following formulas hold:

$$M = 1/LE$$
$$S = \mathrm{Exp}(-M*T)$$

and thus also:

$$M = -1/T * \ln(S)$$
$$LE = 1/M$$

Where

S = fractional survival

M = mortality rate (incidence density of death)

T = time of measure

LE = life expectancy

One application of the DEALE is a simple way to approximately calculate the life expectancy of a patient who has a disease with a known excess mortality. The relevant steps are as follows:

1. Determine the natural life expectancy of the patient, using available age- and sex-specific life-expectancy tables.
2. Take the inverse of the natural life expectancy to approximate the natural yearly mortality (avoid taking yearly mortality from a table to calculate life expectancy, as this will lead to an overestimation of life expectancy).
3. Add to this the yearly excess mortality rate of the disease present, to obtain the overall yearly mortality rate.
4. Take the inverse of the overall yearly mortality rate, to obtain the life expectancy with disease.

This is described in the following formula:

$$LE_{disease} = 1/(1/LE_{normal} + M_{excess})$$

Alternative techniques besides the DEALE to calculate life expectancies include Markov modeling and other forms of time-dependent survival analysis. Their use is beyond the scope of this chapter.

Besides quantity of life, the qualitative evaluation of life is more and more an important aspect of medical outcome. For qualitative assessment, three different conceptual measures are relevant: quality of life assessment, value assessment, and utility assessment.

Quality of life assessment aims at offering a descriptive inventory of a patient's function in various aspects of life, such as physical, psychological, and social function. It uses questionnaires or interviews to assess to what extent the level of function deviates from normal because of suboptimal health. Well-known general quality of life questionnaires are the Medical Outcomes Study Short Form—36 questions (MOS-SF36) and the EuroQuol.[4,5] Several questionnaires have been developed for specific diseases or disease categories. These include the Head and Neck Radiotherapy Questionnaire (HNRQ), EORTC Melanoma Module (MM), and Gastrointestinal Quality of Life Index of Troidl and Eypasch.[6–8] *Value assessment* and *utility assessment* go one step further; given the fact that the health-related level of functioning is suboptimal, they measure to what extent

dysfunction reduces the subjective value of a patient's life. If this value judgment is expressed in a figure on a ratio scale from 0 to 1, where the number obtained indicates what fractional quantity of healthy life is considered of equal value to one unit of life with disease, the value is called a *utility*.

Historically the main techniques of utility assessment that have been used in decision analysis are the standard gamble (SG), time trade-off (TTO), and visual analogue scale (VAS), although the latter is not a utility in the sense defined above.

In the *standard gamble* method, a patient is offered two options. The patient either accepts the disease or chooses some intervention that may lead to one out of two possible outcomes: the best health outcome (usually full health) with chance of p, or the worst health outcome (such as immediate death) with a chance of $(1 - p)$. At the value of p where the patient is indifferent between the two choices, p represents the utility value of the disease state. An SG utility score of 0.95 for having a permanent colostomy, using full health and death as extreme outcomes, would mean that a patient is willing to accept a mortality risk of $(1 - 0.95) = 0.05$, or 5%, to avoid disease.

In the *time trade-off* method a patient is likewise asked to choose between two options, which are, however, less dramatic. Here the choice is between a certain longer life expectancy, L, with disease, and a shorter life expectancy, S, in full health. At the point where the patient is indifferent between the two options, the utility is equal to S/L. A patient is thus asked what quantity of life he or she is willing to give up in order to improve its quality. A TTO utility of 0.9 would mean that a patient is willing to give up $(1 - 0.9) = 0.01$, or 10% of life expectancy in order to become healthy or avoid becoming diseased.

Finally, in the *visual analogue scale* method a patient is asked to indicate on a 10-cm-long horizontal line, labeled from 0 (worst health outcome) to 1 (full health), where he or she judges the health state at stake should be scaled. The utility is then equal to this number; a mark on the line at 0.8 would indicate a VAS utility of 0.8.

If the results of these methods are used for cost-effectiveness analysis or decision analysis, it must be realized that only the SG and TTO explicitly weigh quantity and quality of life (the standard gamble using risk of immediate loss as its basic issue, and the time trade-off using potential reduction in length of life). The visual analogue scaling method may well offer a number between 0 and 1, but this number does not indicate which consequences a patient is willing to take to get rid of the disease state. A patient with hemorrhoids might put a cross on the line at 0.8 to indicate that his hemorrhoid complaints are really distressing. Interpreting this as a utility figure and assuming that the patient is willing to offer 20% of his life expectancy or even to accept a 20% immediate mortality risk in order to get rid of his hemorrhoids, would almost certainly be a misunderstanding.

In spite of this, VAS values are frequently but wrongly used as utility measures because of the ease with which patients are willing to put crosses on VAS lines. This "use by availability" may severely overestimate the impact of quality of life considerations on medical decisions and will thereby underestimate the value that patients attach to their life (expectancy).

Data on Costs

Like data on outcome, data on costs are not easily gathered. The most basic problem is that the cost of medical interventions is not equal to the fee for services (be it a doctor visit, a day in hospital, or a hernia operation) that exists under the prevailing health care financing system; such fees only are the result of historical wheeling and dealing in the medical market place. Real costs are less easily obtained. Drummond, in his classical book on economic evaluation in health care, has even helped us with a 10-point checklist.[9] Five of these points specifically address issues of cost assessment: identification of all relevant costs, cost measurement (the issue of volumes), cost valuation (the issue of unit costs), cost discounting, and cost comparison (the issue of the alternative strategy). Within and besides these five points, many specific issues must be discussed and settled. These include the following:

- The health care boundary (costs within or outside health care).
- The type of cost parameters used (charges or real costs).

- The directness of costs (costs directly related to the intervention, versus indirect costs induced by increased survival).
- The variability of costs in relation to the time horizon chosen. (Depending on the extent to which their height changes in relation to production, capacity costs may on the short run be considered as fixed, and material costs as variable, while personnel costs occupy an intermediate position and may be considered semivariable.)
- The method of assessment of unit costs—costs per unit of product (such as the top-down cost-place method, in which the overall costs of a relevant production unit are divided by its overall production, or the bottom-up direct measurement of various material costs, costs of personnel time, and overhead).
- The appropriate level of detail (a detailed, accurate, assessment of costs the results of which will become invalid as soon as the circumstances change, versus a more global, best-estimate approach, the results of which may be less precise, but may remain valid for a wider range of circumstances or time period).
- Differences in costs between countries (determined by many factors such as exchange rates, the proportion of gross national product spent on health care, wages, health care accounting methods, etc.)

It is beyond the scope of this chapter to discuss these issues in more detail, and so we refer the reader to the literature list provided at the end of this chapter.

Calculation

After the problem has been specified, structured, and quantified in phases one through three, the fourth and final phase of a cost-effectiveness assessment is entered. In this phase, the results of the decision analysis may be obtained in various ways:

- *Calculating expected costs and effects.* The expected costs and effects of each branch of a decision tree are first calculated separately.
- *Calculating differential cost-effectiveness ratios (also called marginal or incremental cost-*

effectiveness ratios). The ratios of differences in costs and effects between strategies are determined, to analyze whether higher costs are justified by sufficiently higher effects.

- *Performing sensitivity analysis and threshold analysis.* Sensitivity analysis is the technique that demonstrates how sensitive the conclusion of the analysis is for a change in one or more of the variables used. The value of one or more independent variables is varied over a range, and the extent to which the expected outcomes change is determined. Threshold analysis is a special application of sensitivity analysis that indicates at what threshold level of the independent parameter the preferred choice changes.

- *Interpreting the quantitative results and drawing conclusions.* The importance of transforming the quantitative results, sometimes of a complex nature, to clear and unambiguous conclusions that are understandable to a party or parties who asked the original cost-effectiveness question, cannot be overemphasized. Only after this has been completed to the satisfaction of the party or parties asking the original question, is the analysis completed.

Some Examples

In this section some very simple examples of cost-effectiveness are given. They are deliberate simplifications of the real problems, meant to illustrate the various steps of cost-effectiveness analysis.

Example 1

Question: Is it cost-effective from a health care perspective to operate on an 80-year-old male patient with a 6-cm asymptomatic abdominal aortic aneurysm, if the accepted differential cost-effective ratio for medical interventions (defined by the Ministry of Health) is around $50,000/QALY?

Answer: Given the schedule presented above the following steps are taken.

1. Problem identification
   (a) The question relates to the costs and effects of surgical treatment of asymptomatic an-

eurysms in elderly patients. (b) The intervention in question replaces the aneurysm with a vascular prosthesis. (c) The alternative strategy is to ignore the aneurysm (frequently called the "wait-and-see" policy). (d) The relevant effect parameter is life expectancy, as it concerns an asymptomatic aneurysm. (e) The relevant costs are those of the elective operation, versus those of a wait-and-see policy, with operation only in case of rupture.

2. Problem structure
   The problem can be described in an algorithm as follows. The choice is between ignoring the aneurysm, and doing elective surgery. If the aneurysm is ignored, the patient lives his remaining life with the aneurysm until he dies of natural causes or experiences a rupture. In case of rupture, the patient may die before reaching the hospital, or may enter the hospital and be operated on. Operation may result in death, or may be successful and result in survival with vascular prosthesis until death from natural causes.

   If the patient is operated on electively, he may die from the operation or survive with a vascular prosthesis until death from natural causes.

   Alternatively, the problem can be structured in a simplified decision tree, shown in Figure 58-2.

3. The necessary data are obtained from the literature and are as follows:

   Disease   A 6-cm aneurysm has a yearly rupture rate of about 5%. In case of rupture, 60% of patients die before reaching the hospital. Of those who receive surgery, 50% die during or after the operation. This makes for an overall mortality per rupture of $(0.60 + 0.5 \times 0.40) = 0.80$, or 80%, and a yearly rupture-related mortality rate of $0.05 \times 0.80 = 0.04$, or 4%.

   Testing   Not relevant; the aneurysm has been detected by abdominal CT scanning performed for other reasons.

Treatment   Elective surgery, carrying a 10% mortality in an 80-year-old male patient, and leaving the patient with a normal life expectancy after successful operation.

Outcome   Natural life expectancy is 6 years in an 80-year-old male.

Costs   The direct health care costs of elective aneurysm surgery are $25,000, of acute surgery $20,000. Costs outside health care are irrelevant; indirect costs are not considered.

4. Calculations

The outcome of ignoring the aneurysm is as follows. Per year, $0.05 \times 0.80 = 0.04$, or 4% of patients die from the disease. Their natural life expectancy would be 6 years. Thus their life expectancy with the disease, according to the DEALE, is the following:

$$1/(1/6 + 0.04) = 4.8 \text{ years}$$

The costs of this strategy are as follows. Per life year, the rupture rate is 5%, with a surgery rate of 0.40% and a cost of $20,000. Therefore the estimated total (undiscounted) cost would be approximately as follows:

$$4.8 \times 0.05 \times 0.40 \times \$20,000 = \$1,920$$

The outcome of elective surgery is as follows. Of all patients operated on, 10% die, leaving the remaining 90% with a normal life expectancy. This makes for an overall life expectancy as follows:

$$0.10 \times 0 + 0.90 \times 6 = 5.4 \text{ years}$$

The costs are $25,000.

Thus elective surgery offers better life expectancy ($5.4 - 4.8 = 0.6$ years) at higher costs ($25,000 - \$1,920 = \$23,080$). To analyze whether improvements come at an acceptable price, we need the differential cost-effectiveness ratio of elective surgery versus leaving the aneurysm alone:

$$(\$25,000 - \$1,920)/(5.4 - 4.8)$$
$$= \$38,500/\text{QALY}.$$

Therefore, even if the maximum accepted differential cost-effectiveness ratio is $50,000/QALY, elective surgery is the preferred strategy, as it provides better outcome at acceptable costs. In conclusion, repairing a 6-cm aneurysm in 80-year-old patients is an effective and efficient intervention.

The above calculations are grave simplifications of the clinical problem. Both effects and costs are only approximations, and can be calculated better using a so-called Markov model, in which long-term effects are modeled using 1-year cycles. The differential cost-effectiveness would then come out higher, and elective surgery would thus be shown to be less efficient.

In the above example, many factors that are crucial have deliberately been left out, such as the age of the patient, the diameter of the aneurysm, and the presence or absence of specific risk factors. The influence of such factors can be analyzed using sensitivity analysis and threshold analysis. As an illustration of these techniques we will now answer the following question:

Question: What is the influence of patient age in the above example, and from what age should elective surgery not be considered, if we assume that in the 60- to 100-year age range, life expectancy halves with every 10 years, that elective surgical mortality doubles, and that other variables are not influenced?

Answer: The above relationships can be translated into the following two functions:

$$\text{life expectancy} = 6 \times 0.5^{((80-\text{AGE})/10)}$$
$$\text{elective mortality} = 0.10 \times 2^{((80-\text{AGE})/10)}$$

We can substitute these functions in the formulas we used before, and then get the following results:

Outcome of leaving the aneurysm alone:

$$1/(1/(6 \times 0.5^{((80-\text{AGE})/10)}) + 0.04) \text{ years}$$

Costs of leaving the aneurysm alone:

$$(1/(1/(6 \times 0.5^{((80-\text{AGE})/10)}) + 0.04)) \times 0.05 \times 0.40 \times \$20,000$$

Outcome of elective surgery:

$$(1 - 0.10 \times 2^{((80-\text{AGE})/10)}) \times 6 \times 0.5^{((80-\text{AGE})/10)}) \text{ years}$$

Cost of elective surgery:

Table 58-2.

Age	LE natural	LE ignore AAA	LE surgery	C-E ratio ignore AAA	C-E ratio surgery	Differential C-E ratio
60	24.0	12.2	23.4	400	1070	1800
70	12.0	8.1	11.4	400	2190	6590
80	6.0	4.8	5.4	400	4630	38470
90	3.0	2.7	2.4	400	10420	–

The required age threshold can be calculated in the following way:

$$\frac{Cost_{surgery} - Cost_{ignore}}{LE_{surgery} - LE_{ignore}} < = \$50,000/QALY$$

$$\frac{(25,000) - ((1/(1/(6 \times 0.5^{((80-AGE)/10)}) + 0.04)) \times 0.05 \times 0.40 \times 20,000)}{((1 - 0.10 \times 2^{((80-AGE)/10)}) \times 6 \times 0.5^{((80-AGE)/10)}) - (1/(1/(6 \times 0.5^{((80-AGE)/10)}) + 0.04))} < = 50,000$$

If this equation is solved for AGE, the AGE threshold can be shown to be equal to 80.8 years.

$25,000

Using these formulas we can easily construct Table 58-2 (see also Figure 58-2).

Interpretation and conclusion: This mathematical solution could, if so desired, be translated into a clinical algorithm:

> From a perspective of efficiency, 6-cm aneurysms in male patients over the age of 80 years may, in principle, be left alone, and more so as patients are progressively older.*

It goes without saying that such algorithms, aiming at optimal efficiency at an aggregate level, should be used cautiously in individual patient care. Patients not only differ strongly in health (including risk factors for surgical mortality), but also in their value assessments of various health states. It would thus be irrational to make the same choice for all patients of the same age. The even more complex ethical questions, in which case decisions should be guided by considerations of effectiveness or efficiency, however relevant, are beyond the scope of this chapter.

Example 2

Question: Is it cost-effective from a societal perspective (taking all costs to society, both within and outside health care, into consideration) to test for pheochromocytoma by urinary VMA, in

asymptomatic patients in whom an adrenal tumor is detected at abdominal CT made for other reasons?

Answer: The steps are now as follows:

1. Problem identification

   (a) The question relates to the costs and effects of diagnostic testing for pheochromocytoma, followed by treatment in case of a positive test. (b) The interventions in question are testing by urinary VMA, and treatment by adrenalectomy, in case of positive testing. (c) The alternative strategy is to ignore the adrenal tumor. (d) The relevant effect parameter again is life expectancy, as the patient is asymptomatic, but the pheochromocytoma may cause an acute hypertensive crisis with risk of death. (e) The relevant costs are those of testing, adrenalectomy and hospitalization, and being on sick leave for some time after leaving the hospital.

2. The problem can be described in an algorithm as follows:

   The choice is between leaving the adrenal tumor alone, and testing by urinary VMA. If the tumor is left alone, the patient lives his remaining life with an adrenal tumor that might be a pheochromocytoma, with the possibility of death due to hypertensive crisis. If the tumor is taken out by adrenalectomy, there is a small operative mortality risk, while in the case of successful adrenalectomy the patient leaves the hospital with a normal life expectancy.

N.B.: A more realistic Markov model developed in Leiden yields a higher age threshold of around 88 years!

The decision tree of this problem is shown in Figure 58-3.

3. The necessary parameters are as follows:

Disease	Asymptomatic adrenal tumor, found on CT scan performed for other reasons, that in 2% of cases may be a pheochromocytoma. In such cases there is a yearly 0.01 mortality rate from acute hypertensive crises.
Testing	Urinary VMA has a sensitivity for pheochromocytoma of 0.80 and a specificity of 0.90.
Treatment	Adrenalectomy, carrying a 1% mortality and leaving the patient with a normal life expectancy in case of successful operation.
Outcome	Natural life expectancy is 40 years in a 40-year-old patient.
Costs	The direct health care costs of VMA testing are $150, and of adrenalectomy are $20,000. Costs outside health care concern a 4-week sick leave after surgery, costing society a total of $2,500. Indirect costs are not considered.

4. Calculations

The outcome of ignoring the adrenal tumor is as follows: Per year, 2% of patients suffer from a yearly excessive death rate from pheochromocytoma of 1%. As their natural life expectancy would be 40 years, life expectancy with pheochromocytoma, according to the DEALE, is as follows:

$$1/(1/40 + 0.01) = 28.57 \text{ years}$$

The remaining 98% of patients do not have pheochromocytoma, and thus have a normal life expectancy of 40.0 years. Life expectancy if the adrenal tumor is not treated is the following:

$$0.02 \times 28.571 + 0.98 \times 40.0 = 39.77 \text{ years}$$

The costs of this strategy, assuming that patients that die from an acute hypertensive crisis incur no costs, are $0.

Calculating the outcome of testing by VMA is more complex. The chance of a positive test is the following:

$$sensitivity \times p(disease)$$
$$+ (1 - specificity) \times (1 - p(disease))$$
$$0.80 \times 0.02 + 0.10 \times 0.98 = 0.114$$

All patients with a positive test will undergo adrenalectomy. Since 1% of patients die from adrenalectomy, the 99% who survive have a normal life expectancy. In the case of a positive test, this makes for the following overall life expectancy:

$$0.01 \times 0 + 0.99 \times 40 = 39.6 \text{ years}$$

A negative test will occur in the remaining 88.6% (1 − 0.114) of patients.

Of these patients, the absence of pheochromocytoma can be calculated by Bayes' formula for the negative predictive value:

$$PV- = \frac{Sp \times (1 - p(D))}{SP \times (1 - p(D)) + (1 - Se) \times p(D)}$$

$$= \frac{0.90 \times 0.98}{0.90 \times 0.98 + 0.20 \times 0.02}$$

$$= 0.996$$

Thus, while 99.6% of patients with negative VMA values are disease free, 0.5% have a missed pheochromocytoma. This makes for the following overall life expectancy of in case of negative testing:

$$0.996 \times 40 + 0.005 \times 37 = 39.95 \text{ years}$$

Thus overall life expectancy in case of testing is the sum of products of probabilities and outcomes in case of positive and negative test results:

$$0.114 \times 39.6 + 0.886 \times 39.95 = 39.91 \text{ years}$$

The overall costs of the test strategy are equal to the costs of VMA for all, and costs of adrenalectomy and sick leave for those who test positively:

$$\$150 + 0.114 \times (\$20,000 + \$2500) = \$2715$$

The differential cost-effectiveness of testing versus ignoring the adrenal tumor then becomes the following:

$$(\$2,715 - \$0)/(39.91 - 39.77)$$
$$= \$19,700 \text{ QALY}$$

Note that both of the above examples are grave simplifications of the real clinical problem equivalent. They are just meant to teach cost-effectiveness methods at an elementary level.

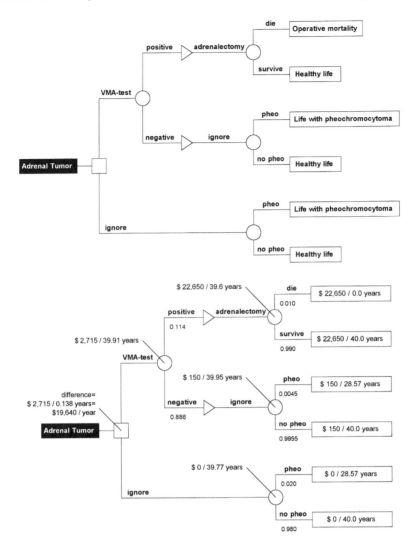

Figure 58-3. Decision tree representing the options in example 2 concerning the cost-effectiveness of testing the urine for valinyl mandelic acid in a patient with an adrenal incidentaloma. The same conventions hold as were explained for Figure 58-1. In addition, label nodes (symbolizing one event following another) are represented as triangles.

Clinical Use of Decision Analysis, Cost-Benefit Analysis, and Cost-Effectiveness Analysis

The methods of decision analysis, cost-benefit analysis, and cost-effectiveness analysis differ from the usual way of clinical decision making in that they are explicit, quantitative, based on chance, and multidisciplinary. Given these differences, these methods offer both advantages and drawbacks. Advantages are that a complex prob-lem can be dissected into smaller parts that are more easily solved. Available data can be combined and restructured in a meaningful way to help solve the smaller partial problems. Further, given that explicit and quantitative outcomes are chosen, it is clear what the goal of a choice is, and to what extent this goal may be realized. Differences of opinion can be analyzed to differences in data, or in values, and the strengths and weaknesses of the arguments brought forward can be tested.

However, drawbacks do exist. The modeling

approach used in decision analysis, cost-benefit analysis, and cost-effectiveness analysis necessitates the translation and, thereby, simplification of real-life problems into "models" such as decision trees. The answers obtained may be valid for the model, but are not necessarily equally valid for the original real-life problem. The validity of the model is determined not only by the correctness of the model itself, but may also be limited by the availability of reliable data. Finally, creating a high-quality analysis is time-consuming and requires expertise and experience.

Depending on the nature of the problem to be solved, the advantages and disadvantages are relevant to a different degree. In general, decision analysis, cost-benefit analysis, and cost-effectiveness analysis can be used most advantageously for clinical problems that have the following characteristics:

- Concern risk or uncertainty
- Are structurally complex and typically involve interactions between tests, treatment, outcome, and/or costs
- About which sufficient quantitative data are available
- In which solutions may differ for different situations and/or patients
- In which different and conflicting interests have to be considered and weighed
- Frequency of occurrence or the magnitude of the problem justifies the effort of performing a decision analysis

There is one final matter of debate. The use of decision analysis as an explicit quantitative method for decision support has become relatively accepted. The role of the other two methods, cost-benefit analysis and cost-effectiveness analysis, seems less clear. The role that cost considerations may play in clinical care, and especially in decision making between patient and doctor, is not undisputed.

Some doctors strongly object to the use of cost-effectiveness analysis. They insist that doctors should not take costs into account in choices that are in the interest of their patients, that it even is unethical to do so. They hold that it is against our professional autonomy to be concerned about costs, and that the interest of each individual patient is the sole standard by which choices should

be made. They may thus choose to strive only for the best outcome, however small the differences and however large the costs.

Others (including the author) do not agree. It is a fact of life that the health care budget in most countries is limited to a restricted fraction of the gross national product, and that this budget is far too small to use all diagnostic and therapeutic techniques to the full. In our opinion we have a responsibility toward more patients than the one that we are actually helping at a given moment in time. Therefore we should not spend all or most of our limited budget on a few patients and then find out that we do not have the funds to help those that come later. In addition we have a responsibility toward the society that pays for health care and makes it possible, for careful spending. If we do not accept this responsibility, others will almost certainly take over this role, and steer the medical profession according to their cost analyses.

In our opinion, doctors should assume collective professional responsibility for appropriate use of resources. Only with their expertise and cooperation can interventions with a too high cost-effectiveness (C-E) ratio be replaced by interventions with lower C-E ratios, leading to more health at the same or lower price. Doctors will have to guard the appropriate balance between responsibility to society, and the responsibility to the individual patient. But if doctors accept this responsibility, they should at least know the potential and limitations of the methods of cost-benefit and cost-effectiveness analysis and be able to interpret and use them judiciously.

Use of Decision Analysis, Cost-Benefit Analysis, and Cost-Effectiveness Analysis in Empirical Surgical Research

Apart from clinical application, decision analysis, cost-benefit analysis, and cost-effectiveness analysis can also be used in surgical research. They may serve as an adjunct to empirical research in roughly three ways: as a *summary* of existing medical knowledge; as *support* for past, present, or future research; and as a *substitute* for research that is not feasible for reasons of practical or financial limitations.

Applied as a summary, these methods may be used to represent the present state of medical knowledge concerning a clinical problem. As such they may have greater scope and flexibility than classical meta-analyses, but at the same time may be less lucid because of their complexity, and less reliable because of the various unproven assumptions on which they may be based. As a means of support, decision analysis, cost-benefit analysis, and cost-effectiveness analysis may be used to improve the effectiveness and efficiency of empirical clinical research in various ways. They may be used to dissect a complex problem into smaller, more manageable parts, and to assess the relative importance of these parts. They may help to identify the most relevant trial arms, and the data that should be recorded. They may be used to estimate trial size, to simulate clinical trials, and thus to predict their outcome. And they may be used to combine the results from different diagnostic and therapeutic research efforts, allow for the extrapolation of conclusions to other situations, or predict the effects of policy changes. They thus may expand the scope of empirical research, albeit at the expense of reduced robustness of the conclusions obtained. Finally, as a substitute, these methods can be used in cases where clinical trials are deemed not feasible, or inefficient. Although the Monte Carlo simulation of a model may offer important information, it is no real substitute for empirical data. The validity of conclusions depends strongly on the correctness of the structure, data, and assumptions underlying the model, that is, on the pretrial state of medical knowledge. Here, as everywhere, the classical "garbage in—garbage out" principle holds.

In conclusion, decision analysis, cost-benefit analysis and cost-effectiveness analysis are relatively new methods, that have expanded the armamentarium of surgical research. They may be used to answer questions of effectiveness and efficiency that are becoming more and more relevant.

References

1. Lohr KN. Outcome measurement: concepts and questions. Inquiry 1988;25:37–50.

2. Pauker SG, Kassirer JP: The threshold approach to clinical decision making. New Engl J Med 1980; 302:1109–1117.

3. Kievit J, van de Velde CJH. Utility and cost of carcinoembryonic antigen monitoring in colon cancer followup: a Markov analysis. Cancer 1990;65: 2580–2587.

4. Ware JE, Sherbourne CD. The MOS 36-item Short Form Health Survey (SF-36). I. Conceptual framework and item selection. Med Care 1992;30: 473–483.

5. EuroQol Group. EuroQol—a new facility for the measurement of health related quality of life. Health Policy 1990;16:199–208.

6. Browman GP, Levine MN, Hodson DI, Sathy J, Russell R, Skingley P, Cripps C, Eapen L, Girard A. The Head and Neck Radiotherapy Questionnaire: a morbidity/quality of life instrument for clinical trials of radiation therapy in locally advanced head and neck cancer. J Clin Oncol 1993;11: 863–872.

7. Sigurdardottir V, Bolund C, Brandberg Y, Sullivan M. The impact of generalized malignant melanoma on quality of life evaluated by the EORTC questionnaire technique. Qual Life Res 1993; 2:193–203.

8. Eypasch E, Wood-Dauphinee S, Williams JL, Ure B, Neugebauer E, Troidl H. The gastrointestinal Quality of Life index. A clinical index for measuring patient status in gastroenterologic surgery. Chirurg 1993;64:264–274.

9. Drummond MF, Stoddart GL, Torrance GW. Methods for Economic Evaluation of Health Care Programmes. Oxford Medical, 1986.

Commentary

If you find this chapter challenging reading, you are probably not alone. The writing is clear, but the subject material involves complexities layered one upon the other. Where data are not readily available, assumptions must be made. Dr. Kievit's mathematical orientation leads him to a numerical answer at the conclusion of an analysis. Many of the calculations are based on probability theory, with more or less complete information comprising the elements of the formulation. It is difficult to fully comprehend all of the variables that are resolved by a defined set of parameters that ultimately constitute the calculation elements.

Dr. Kievit's approach can help us appreciate the quantitative, measurable endpoints referred to in other sections of the text, and their increased utility for mathematical analysis when compared with "softer" qualitative data. Cost-benefit, cost effectiveness, and other analytic tools in this class have a definable statistical probability of accurately representing reality, and each contributes to the scatter within the mathematical solutions developed for problems at this level of complexity.

A.S.W.

CHAPTER 59

Technology Assessment

M.F. McKneally, A.F. Pierre, and H. Troidl

Truth emerges more readily from error than from confusion.

—Francis Bacon

Introduction

Technology is the domain of knowledge that includes devices, instruments, the industrial arts, and engineering. The term is sometimes expanded to include the organization of resources or systems by which social groups provide themselves with the material objects of their civilization.

The technology of health care includes drugs and devices, and systems for the delivery of care, such as operating rooms and intensive care units. Technology assessment is the examination of new or old technologies to determine their value to society with respect to feasibility, safety, benefit, effectiveness, cost, and ethics.[1]

The timeline of technology development in medicine shows recent logarithmic acceleration that will continue. The evolution of technology seems relentless and nearly unalterable. How should we think about this dominant force?

In *Technopoly*, Neil Postman describes a technology-dominated society in which technophobes who are unable to participate proficiently in technology become an underprivileged class.[2] We need to be aware that technology is not the so-lution to all of society's problems. Surgeons are inclined to be technophiles and are less likely to be left behind by the dominating force of technology. However, we should not use new technological developments simply because we can.[3] Wisdom must guide our utilization of new technology. Surgeons will be expected to provide leadership in assessing the benefits, burdens, and costs of surgical technology and must be involved in developing policies for the proper implementation of those innovations.

The Bright Side

All knowledge, including technology, is morally neutral; its application can be beneficial or harmful. There are obvious benefits to technology; it has already helped society and medicine in many ways. Advances in communications technology make instantaneous consultation available around the globe. The environment in the operating room and in our homes is conditioned and controlled electronically. Diseased tissue is biopsied or ablated by stereotactic triangulation within the brain without craniotomy, and lasers weld detached retinas or seal anastamoses. Technophiles claim that surgeons soon will be able to operate robotically in space or on battlefields from control stations far from the patient's side.

Robotic tools will operate with remarkable precision, without biorhythms, emotions, or moments of sadness or distraction leading to inattention to detail. They have a steady arm and hand and may keep the surgeon safely distanced from bullets or lethal viruses. Advanced technology will soon allow realistic rehearsal of the necessary steps of surgery before it is performed. Algorithms of treatment can be tested and perfected in simulations before their application in a real situation. Personnel can be trained in their individual and collaborative tasks using simulators, without risk to them or to patients.

The Dark Side

Since humans are not assembled robotically on a production line like automobiles, their anatomy and biology show significant variations. Adaptation to variation is an important component of the art of surgery, and surgery as we now perform it is a blend of technology and art. Robotic precision without individualization carries significant dangers. Although some functions, such as biochemical analysis of blood samples, lend themselves to automated mechanized analysis, effectiveness deteriorates when individual tissues, normally assessed by the pathologist for their variation from normal, are subjected to similar robotic interpretation.

Safety and efficacy are the first levels of analysis of the feasibility of a new technology. But what of the human cost? Adaptation to variations in human anatomy and pathology is one challenge; adaptation to the human mind and spirit is more difficult to assess. Will humans accept robotic caregivers? The very term is an oxymoron. Will engineers become the nurses and doctors of the future? Will they hold the digitized output from robotic sensors instead of the patient's hand? The public accepts and almost worships medical technology in the abstract, even when it is inappropriate. This fascination is reinforced by politicians who enhance their political standing by endorsing and identifying themselves with popular technological imperatives. Sending an American astronaut to the moon, or rushing a prehospital trauma care team of German doctors to the scene of a motor vehicle accident is supported because the voters are thrilled by the concepts, even when the cost is not balanced by the benefit. Journalists and consumers accelerate the demand for new and expensive surgical technology from the moment it is introduced, often long before accurate conclusions can be drawn from conventional modes of assessment.

The cost of complex technology is daunting. Analyses based on the large capital investments in robotics made in the auto and aircraft industries show that some expensive technology can be highly cost-effective. The automated clinical biochemistry analytic systems are an example of expensive but cost-effective technology. Biochemical analyses of blood samples, once performed at a far greater cost by skilled laboratory technicians, are now universally automated. Which advances in surgical technology will give a comparable return on investment? Currently, research aimed at developing robotic surgical interventions is so expensive that only the U.S. Department of Defense can fund it. The expense to individual hospitals for laser angioplasty equipment for the treatment of peripheral vascular disease in the 1980s is a memorable and important example of inadequate technology assessment combined with an uncontrolled enthusiasm for the promise of technology.[4] Why did this harmful misapplication of technology continue so long, until disastrous results forced its discontinuation?

Technology Assessment

Since so many contributions of technology to civilization have been beneficial, we tend to adopt technological innovations uncritically. But new is not always better, and unexamined integration of new technology cannot continue. How should we approach this problem? Specifically, how should we evaluate each new component of surgical technology as it is brought to us for application in our patients and in different communities around the world? We are under severe time pressure as the burden of disease continues to increase. The urgency for particular innovations may be increased by the incidence or prevalence of certain diseases, war, or natural disasters. This is now and will continue to be one of the most important fields for research by surgeons. Our methodology is not well developed in this area but is represented by the term *technology assessment*.

Technology assessment is the utilization of available scientific knowledge and methodologies to analyze a new or established technology.[5] Technology can be tested using the endpoints of feasibility, safety, benefit, effectiveness, cost analysis, ease of application by the surgeon, and ethical considerations.[1,6] The grades of evidence for these assessments are summarized in Table 59-1.[1,5] Methods of assessment include randomized trials, epidemiologic studies, consensus conferences, failure analysis, mathematical modeling, and so forth. Which of these methods are used alone or in combination to analyze a technology will depend on the question asked about that technology (e.g., "Is this implantable defibrillator safer than drug treatment?") and the nature of the technology or application itself (e.g., "Are intensive care units overutilized during terminal illness?").

Contemporary methods for testing less complex treatments will still be applicable to many advanced technological interventions; for example, randomized controlled clinical trials will still be useful for comparing some technologically complex innovations with standard treatments. However, new and expensive technology must be tested for safety before its first application in such a clinical trial. The methods might include laboratory experiments in animals, and nonexperimental case-controlled studies of safety and efficacy in human patients. Observational studies are still the most commonly used evidence in support of new technology, as typified by endoscopic surgery. The confidential inquiry approach of the United Kingdom, and the audit are other useful contemporary methods.

The University of Chicago method for introducing ethically troublesome innovations is a carefully constructed, rule-based observational approach that merits wider use.[7] This method involves research ethics consultation, public discussion, and protocol publication before the introduction of the innovation. A published commitment to a second follow-up report on the results obtained in a prespecified number of cases insures that the assessment will be maximally beneficial to the society, and may be helpful to the study subjects. This approach was used with exemplary success in the introduction of living donor liver transplantation.[8]

Table 59-1. Methods of technology assessment.[a]

Method	Comment
Randomized clinical trial	Avoids bias and allows comparison with control group
Cohort studies, case-control studies, cross-sectional studies	Helpful in studying risk factors and cost-effectiveness when randomized trials may be impractical or unethical
Quantitative synthesis methods (e.g., meta-analysis)	Combines information from multiple sources in order to summarize effectiveness of therapies
Group judgment methods (e.g., Delphi method, consensus conferences)	Usually do not produce new evidence of safety, efficacy, or cost-effectiveness; subject to bias
Case series	Lack explicit study design and randomization; subject to bias; may generate new hypotheses
Failure analysis	Analysis of a problem aimed at prevention of future similar problems
Registers and databases	When associated with additional information may generate new hypotheses
Mathematical modeling	Difficult to obtain appropriate models
Decision analysis	Special form of mathematical modeling
Examination of social and ethical issues (e.g., University of Chicago method)	To consider the impact of procedures and treatments on society in general; consider fairness of the technology

[a] This summary is our adaptation of a detailed table developed by Mosteller and Frazier;[5] see this reference for a more extensive presentation.

Consensus conferences (see chapter 23) provide another method of technology assessment with specific rules that provide tentative conclusions from a panel of experts, patients, and the public. This approach provides information more rapidly than observational studies summarized, reviewed by peers, and published after customary delays in surgical journals. The National Institutes of Health (NIH) method for consensus conferences is a broad, sweeping assessment, best applied to validate a general approach. The method is somewhat cumbersome and does not provide the detail required for application of technology in daily practice. The Cologne method[9] is oriented more to the particular needs of the practitioner and focuses more narrowly on important details (e.g., the incision, the suture, or the type of mesh used in endoscopic inguinal hernia repair). Consensus conferences provide rapid feedback from a large number of centers, and can be managed in such a way that information is available in summary form for cautious general consumption early in the experience with a new technique or device.

There are two major weaknesses in the consensus conference method. First, the bias of participants is not controlled. Some participants may also feel intimidated by peer pressure. Second, the nature of a consensus conference is such that ideas are reduced to a common denominator that may suppress or neglect important concepts, alternatives, or dissent.

Failure analysis is another approach to the assessment of technology.[10] It is rapid, less expensive, and generally more applicable to surgical problems than many of the previously mentioned methods. It is widely used in industry, but has been given little attention in clinical practice.[11] The essential elements of failure analysis are addressed by four questions and are aimed at the prevention of future problems:

1. What was the clinical situation in which the failure happened?
2. What happened in that clinical situation?
3. How did it happen?
4. How can it be avoided in the future?

Failure analysis may be likened to the analysis of an aircraft disaster. One goes through the process of discovering what happened, why it happened, and, especially, how to prevent it from happening again. Sir Karl Popper felt that the adoption of failure analysis is potentially the most important advance modern medicine can make. It will require a significant revision in our approach to problems; doctors are trained to emphasize repair and reconstruction rather than prevention. In contrast, the emphasis in industry is on prevention, where technical failures in the aircraft or train cannot be repaired or corrected with a salvage operation or remedial intervention.

A significant disadvantage of failure analysis is that it is retrospective. Lessons from the analysis should be coupled with ongoing tests of the quality of the instruments, technique, and judgment, and their applications before the development of failure. This is an important area for future research in surgery.

The specter of litigation is common to both consensus conferences and the failure analysis method. We open ourselves up to attack by publicly addressing our failures and uncertainties, but it is through such dialog that we are most likely to produce the greatest good and prevent the most harm to our patients in the future. A tort-based legal system is inimical to this goal.

The models for technology assessment that are currently available for analysis include the pharmaceutical model, which is a well-developed and extensive system of agencies, procedures, and guidelines typified inter alia by the Food and Drug Act in Canada, and the Food and Drug Administration in the United States. High "launch prices" for drugs and new devices are blamed on the cost of regulation imposed by these agencies. Equipment and device regulation is being assumed by the subsets of the pharmaceutical regulatory agencies, and a suggestion has been made that a separate federal technology agency be formed. Currently, the Office of Technology Assessment, the Device Regulation Branch of the Food and Drug Administration, the Technology Assessment Committee of Blue Cross/Blue Shield, and several other ad hoc organizations varying in competence, authority, and motive form a dysfunctional array of agencies in the United States.[12] As these groups compete to fulfill this function, without notable success, industry and academic science work to produce new and expensive technology at a constantly accelerating rate.[12]

Who should pay the costs of development and testing? Who should stand responsibly at the in-

Table 59-2.   Relative impact of technology assessment in eight countries.[a]

Impact of TA[b]	CABG	CT/MRI	LC	ESRD	NICU	Breast cancer
Highest	Sweden	Sweden	Sweden	Sweden Canada	Canada	UK Sweden
	Canada	UK Canada	Australia Netherlands France UK Canada US Germany		Netherlands	
	UK			France	UK France Sweden Australia	Canada Netherlands
	France	Netherlands France Australia		Netherlands		
	Netherlands Australia			Australia UK		US Australia France
Lowest	US Germany	US Germany		US Germany	US Germany	Germany

[a]Breast cancer, screening programs for breast cancer; CABG, coronary artery bypass grafting; CT/MRI, computerized tomography and magnetic resonance imaging; ESRD, treatment for end-stage renal disease; LC, laparoscopic cholecystectomy techniques; NICU, neonatal intensive care units and ECMO; TA, technology assessment.

[b]Relative impact of technology assessment on technology adoption and diffusion (case study technologies).

Reprinted with the kind permission of the authors and Elsevier Scientific Ireland Ltd., from Battista RN, et al., Lesson from the eight countries. Health Policy 1994;30:397–421.

terface of surgical technology and society, overseeing the assessment, initial introduction, and subsequent diffusion of innovations into practice? There is encouraging activity in the development of an international forum for the exchange of information about technology assessment,[13] and a favorable disposition of governments and insurers to fund it.

Surgeons should participate in these assessments, and their education should insure that they have the skills and knowledge to contribute wisely and responsibly to the process. If we abdicate this responsibility we may lose not only control of our clinical practice but also our research interests, and the very nature of the personal relationship between doctor and patient will be altered for the worse. The assessment of medical technology cannot reasonably take place without physician input; we must participate in this decision-making process.

Finally, the diffusion of new technology into widespread practice before it is satisfactorily assessed or proven remains a significant problem. New medical technology affects not only health care, but also has social and ethical ramifications. It is driven by public enthusiasm for technology, and the enthusiasm of hospitals and caregivers for using exciting new tools. Table 58-2 shows the relative impact of technology assessment in various countries, with respect to some familiar medical innovations.[14] Nations with a centralized government–controlled health care system utilize technology assessment more than nations who do not have such a system (e.g., United States and Germany). The retarding effect of cost has been insufficient to prevent excessive application prior to adequate assessment. The American College of Surgeons Committee on Emerging Surgical Technology has taken an active role in developing randomized trials and fostering the development of models for testing new innovations. The onrush of industrial development, and the wealth of the technology-driven companies creates a tension that is exciting and potentially extremely beneficial if the proper balance can be struck among innovation, assessment, and regulation.

References

1. Troidl H. Endoscopic surgery—A fascinating idea requires responsibility in evaluation and handling. In: Szabo Z, Kerstein MD, Lewis JE, eds. Surgical Technology International III. International Developments in Surgery and Surgical Research. San Francisco: Universal Medical, 1994, pp. 111–117.
2. Postman, N. Technopoly: The Surrender of Culture to Technology. New York: Knopf, 1992.
3. Lorenz, K. "Die Rückselte des Spiegels" Versuch einer Naturgeschichte menschlichen Erkennens. Zürich: Piper-Verlag, 1973.
4. White RA, Cavaye DM. Endovascular surgery: history, current status and future perspective. Int Angiol 1993;12(3):197–205.
5. Mosteller F, Frazier HS. Evaluating medical technologies. In: HS Frazier, F Mosteller, eds. Medicine Worth Paying For: Assessing Medical Innovations. Cambridge: Harvard University, 1995, p. 9–35.
6. Jennett B. High Technology Medicine—Benefits and Burdens. Oxford: Oxford Medical Publications, 1986.
7. Singer PA, Siegler M, Lantos JD, Emond JC, Whitington PF, Thistlethwaite JR, Broelsch CE. The ethical assessment of innovative therapies: liver transplantation using living donors. Theor Med 1990;11:87–94.
8. Singer PA, Siegler M, Whitington PF, Lantos JD, Emond JC, Thistlethwaite JR, Broelsch CE. Ethics of liver transplantation with living donors. New Engl J Med 1989;321(9):620–622.
9. Neugebauer E, Troidl H, Kum CK, Eypasch E, Miserez M, Paul A. The E.A.E.S. consensus development conferences on laparoscopic cholecystectomy, appendectomy, and hernia repair. Consensus Statements—September 1994. Surg Endosc 1995;9:550–563.
10. Troidl H, Backer B, Langer B, Winkler-Wilfurth A. Fehleranalyse—Evaluierung und Verhütung Von Komplikationen; ihre juristische Implikation. Langenbecks Arch Chir Suppl (Kongreßbericht) 1993, p. 59–72.
11. Cooper JB, Newbower RS, Kitz RJ. An analysis of major errors and equipment failures in anesthesis management: considerations for prevention and detection. Anesthesiology. 1984;60:34–42.
12. McKneally MF. Can surgical innovation survive? Bull Am Coll Surg 1996;81(4):8–21.
13. Battista RN. Innovation and diffusion of health-related technologies—a conceptual framework. Int J Technol Assess Health Care 1989;5:227–248.
14. Battista RN, Banta HD, Jonnson E, Hodge M, Gelband H. Lessons from the eight countries. Health Policy 1994;30:397–421.

Additional Reading

Postman N. Technopoly: The Surrender of Culture to Technology. New York: Knopf, 1992.
Cardwell D. The Fontana History of Technology. London: Fontana, 1994.

Commentary

This chapter on technology assessment is thorough and thought provoking. There is a need for clinicians to assess new technology very carefully before introducing it into the cost-contained system we work in. Every system throughout the world is at present trying to cope with escalating cost, much of it related to technological innovations. We need a system to evaluate these costs before new practices are introduced in health care. Too often new technologies have been introduced before their costs and benefits have been fully evaluated. Incrementalism about introducing new technology is common, particularly in surgery. The explosion in laparoscopic surgery has been followed by a subsequent implosion when it was realized that laparoscopic surgery couldn't do all it was claimed to do, and that it was far too costly to be generalizable throughout the health care world. What is needed is some early warning system that triggers an evaluation of technology before it is introduced. Evaluation in a randomized trial is the design of choice for assessing expensive new technology against standard treatments.

Surgeons must work to overcome the obstacles in setting up randomized trials of new technology.

Two obstacles immediately strike a practicing surgeon. First there is the problem of the long learning curve with new technologies; the benefits of the technology are often not completely realized until the learning curve is over. Second, there is the problem of resistance to randomization as new techniques are introduced. Researchers and clinicians need to work together to devise pragmatic trials that will be acceptable to surgeons and to the public despite their fascination with the new treatment. In assessing technology, there is a need to assess all the benefits and all the costs. Those that are too remote may need some alternative strategy to identify and link them. Often the costs are logarithmic and extend far beyond what is easily identifiable in the clinical situation. The same is true of benefits that may be realized by employers and workers far removed from the usual boundaries of cost benefit analyses of surgical treatments. Results of technology assessment need to be generalizable; the results should be "rolled out" to show their impact on the whole system. This is a problem with case series, when one particular group has developed a very good technique locally but hasn't the access or facilities to measure its societal impact.

Notwithstanding all the difficulties in the area, the approaches that McKneally, Pierre, and Troidl present in this very thoughtful and cogent essay must be encouraged and adopted in the surgical community.

H.B. Devlin

SECTION VIII

Ethical Issues

CHAPTER 60

Ethical Principles in Research

D.J. Roy, P.McL. Black, B. McPeek, and M.F. McKneally

I start with the premise that medicine is a moral endeavor, and within it, surgery, by virtue of its intrinsic violence, has magnified visibility.[1]

—Alexander Walt

Research ethics is as integral a part of scientific judgment as clinical ethics is of clinical judgment.[2] Many ethical issues in research arise from a failure to think as rigorously about the conditions for ethical consistency as about those for scientific validity. The ethical principles governing all surgical, clinical, and biomedical research with human subjects are fundamentally the same. They have been listed and discussed in numerous documents and countless publications over the past 40 years.[3–10]

Although due regard must be maintained for the utility and necessity of institutional review boards, ethics committees, and public participation in the ethical evaluation of the protocols for research with human subjects, it is a mistake to view ethics as an external, authoritarian imposition of regulations or possibly arbitrary constraints on the process of clinical research. The design and the practice of research ethics should be primarily, though not exclusively, a matter of self-consistency and self-governance within clinical investigation.

Ethics and Research

Research ethics and scientific research pursue a common cognitive goal; to distinguish mere appearances from reality. Scientific research, using measurement as its cardinal procedure, seeks to ascertain the actual relationships between phenomena. Uncritical reliance on initial observations, potentially distorted by bias, can lead to a systematic divergence from the truth.[11] Rigorous research methods are devised precisely to counter the tendency to mistake a mere semblance of correlation for a judgment of fact.

Research ethics, a process of critical reflection and interdisciplinary collaboration, acts against the tendency to diverge systematically from what is right. As initial observations may fail to reveal true correlations, spontaneous desires or compulsions may not correspond with what we ought to do. What appears to be good in a limited perspective may contradict a greater and more commanding value. True values, like real correlations between phenomena, are not always immediately obvious. A spontaneous apparent good acquires the moral force of a value only after passing through a process of critical reflection in which proposed courses of action and possible objects of choice are subjected to a series of questions that result in value judgment. Value judgments, like judgments of fact and of truth, are governed by assent to sufficient evidence, not by submission to custom, convention, authority, brilliance, or emotion.

Working out the ethics of research requires the exercise of critical intelligence and judgment by a community of humans engaged in attentive and mutually corrective discourse, rather than isolated monologues. Combining interdisciplinary dialogue with the study of specific cases, whether of clinical practice or clinical research, counteracts moral atomism, rampant relativism, and what Stephen Toulmin has called the tyranny of principles.[12] Principles, guidelines, and codes, alone, do not decide concrete cases. Principles will fail to reveal their meaning—what they command, permit, and prohibit—until they are interpreted in the light of specific research situations. This approach to ethics provides a basis for institutional review boards (IRBs) or research ethics committees without, necessarily, justifying their specific modes of operation. It must be emphasized, however, that ethical judgment is an integral component of clinical and scientific intelligence; clinical investigators are expected and entitled to perform as integrated humans and professionals.

Controlled Clinical Research: An Ethical Imperative

A physician's moral obligation to offer each patient the best available treatment cannot be separated from clinical imperatives to base any choice of treatment on the best accessible evidence. The tension between the interdependent responsibilities of giving care that is personal and compassionate, and treatment that is scientifically sound and validated, is intrinsic to the practice of medicine.[13] This tension, which arises prior to and as a moral reality distinct from any conflict of interests, is a structural part of the medical profession's covenant with the human community, not merely the expression of an individual physician-investigator's disordered intentions.

Controlled clinical trials—randomized and multiply blinded (when these are feasible), ethically achievable, and scientifically appropriate—are an integral part of the ethical imperative that physicians and surgeons know what they are doing when they intervene into the bodies, psyches, and lives of vulnerable, suffering humans. The ethical requirement of precise and validated knowledge gathers force with the likelihood that clinical interventions will have decisive and irreversible impacts on patients' futures and on future patients. Future patients have faces; they cannot be lumped together as part of society and set in opposition to patients occupying hospital beds today.

The standards of good medicine, determined by professional consensus based on reliable methods of achieving validated knowledge, enter into the inner structure of the doctor-patient relationship. "What doctor and patient choose is not the untrammelled expression of the knowledge and values of each. It is limited by the professional norms that constrain the doctor's judgment and constrain it in the name of good medicine generally."[14] Something more, though, is required. If the achievement of good medicine is an ethical imperative, it must exert not only the *protective force* of a constraint on potential misguided judgment and choice, but also the *constructive force* of an invocation to comprehending and voluntary collaboration in constantly redesigning the standards of good medicine. Professionally validated knowledge, without the collaboration of individual physicians and patients, would remain a utopian dream.

When there is uncertainty or definite doubt about the safety or efficacy of an innovative or established treatment, this position supports the strong view that there *is*, not simply *may be*, "a higher moral obligation to test it critically than to prescribe it year-in, year-out with the support of custom or wishful thinking."[15] When large numbers of innovative treatments are being continuously introduced into clinical practice, rigorous testing is ethically mandatory for the protection of individual patients and the just use of limited resources. This holds true with even greater force in the light of evidence that many innovations show no advantage over existing treatments when they are subjected to properly controlled study.[16] They may even be less effective or harmful.[17]

In order to conduct a trial, three conditions must be met:[18] (1) A *genuine uncertainty, or equipoise, must exist* within the medical community regarding the comparative merits of the treatment arms of the trial. (2) The trial must be designed so that its successful conclusion will disturb equipoise; that is, the trial should be continued until the difference is *convincing* enough to resolve the dispute among clinicians.[19] (3) Finally, the *rights of the patients* to protection and the pursuit of their best interests must be safeguarded.

Benjamin Freedman at McGill University in Montreal has clarified our thinking through his definition of *clinical equipoise*:

> ### Clinical Equipoise
>
> A conflict in the opinions of members of the expert clinical community over which treatment is preferred; each side recognizes that there is evidence to support the opposing view.

It is *not* a precise balance of evidence and intuition supporting each treatment, which could be disturbed by a few patients who seem to be benefited by one particular treatment; this unrealistic and fragile balance he terms *theoretical equipoise. Clinical equipoise,* on the other hand, means only that there is a *difference of opinion among respected members of the expert clinical community* over treatments. Some may favor lumpectomy while some may favor mastectomy. Or some may favor postoperative treatment with radiation or chemotherapy after cancer resection, and others may disagree, recommending radical surgery alone. Each side recognizes that there is evidence to support the opposing view. This is all that is required for initiation and continuation of a randomized controlled clinical trial.

The trial is begun because there are differences of opinion in the expert clinical community. This does not prevent the participation of doctors who hold one of those opinions and have a *treatment preference.* Entering patients into a comparative trial when your preference is to treat them with your modality, such as surgery in a trial of surgery versus radiation, requires intellectual humility, but it does not require you to abandon your responsibility to provide the best available treatment. In fact, when a doctor concludes that one treatment is clearly best for one particular patient, for example, a patient who will not or cannot tolerate the side effects of one of the treatments, that patient should be excluded from entering the trial, or should withdraw from the arm to which he or she was assigned. When strong evidence develops in the trial that would create *consensus throughout the medical community,* it is time to stop the trial. The technical details on stopping rules are a fascinating subject beyond the scope of this chapter. Stopping a randomized trial of a treatment prematurely deprives patients and society of the benefits of the trial. Unanticipated and unacceptable *toxicity,* overwhelmingly *convincing evidence*

of a beneficial treatment effect, the *completion* of a preassigned, predetermined number of treatments predicted to give a reliable assessment of the treatment, or the development of a new and clearly *more effective treatment* that was not available at the time of initiation of the trial constitute legitimate guidelines for stopping a trial.

Conditions for the Ethical Conduct of Clinical Research

Conditional Ethics

If the practice of medicine is both morally mandatory and inherently experimental,[20] controlled clinical trials cannot be inherently unethical. Clinical trials, whatever the tactics used to control for bias, will be unethical only to the extent that they fail to meet a set of necessary and interrelated conditions. "Ethical justifiability" means consistency with the ethos and morality of the human community. Human communities vary from one culture and society to another, not only in their customs and art, but also in their governing perceptions and values regarding the body, health, disease, suffering, death, and a host of other realities affecting the practice of medicine. The conditions for ethically justifiable research with human subjects arise from the requirements for consistency along each of these dimensions.

These conditions are structured. They range from fundamental principles of science, medicine, and philosophy, across more specific norms, procedures, and regulations, to encompass the tailored ethical judgments required for the unique characteristics and designs of individual clinical trials. The ethics of clinical research is open-ended, cumulative, and unfinished. A continual process of feedback is at work between tailored ethical judgments on specific trials, and the principles, norms, procedures, and regulations requisite for the ethical conduct of clinical research. Our knowledge of right and wrong is as subject to the process of evolution and cumulative growth as our knowledge of fact and truth in science.

The concept of conditional ethics, so understood, implies that ethical justifiability is a graded, not a binary, characteristic of clinical trials. The rheostat rather than the on-off switch suggests an appropriate image.

Research Ethics and Cultural Diversity

Though science is largely transcultural, the human community has not yet developed a completely corresponding body of transcultural ethics. Differing views about what is normative in person-person, doctor-patient, and investigator-subject relationships may create the need for ethical compromise or accommodation in some multicenter trials, particularly when the collaborating centers are situated in different nations.

A Japanese physician-investigator may find it difficult to honor North American insistence on detailed disclosure to patients about the randomization process used to select treatment in a clinical trial for breast cancer or cancer of the prostate. In a culture that places great emphasis on trust in the physician as an integral part of the healing process, both physicians and patients may find an open admission of physician ignorance or uncertainty therapeutically damaging or even absurd.

North American culture emphasizes the value of individual autonomy; some Asian cultures, the value of the family and the community. The approaches to informed, comprehending, and voluntary consent may be quite different in these two cultures. In China the family and the community play a central role in resolving disputes and in obtaining a patient's consent in difficult situations.

> First, community social pressure is the first and usually very effective mode of obtaining agreement. Second, the family plays an important role in securing patient consent, even with adult patients. However, others, such as fellow-workers, are also involved.[21]

Sensitivity to the dominant values of other cultures should be an ethical requisite of international collaboration in multicenter trials. Accommodating cultural differences, even in ethnic groups within the pluralistic society of Western nations, will usually require a flexibility in procedures rather than the compromise of fundamental principles.

Equitable Selection of Participants

The equitable selection of human subjects for participation in clinical trials is one of the criteria for institutional review board (IRB) approval according to the Code of Federal Regulations of the United States.[22] Until recently, the prime ethical concern was to protect vulnerable people against exploitation in research, against being forced to carry a disproportionate share of the burdens of research. The leading contemporary perspective is that women, the economically disadvantaged, the socially marginalized, and people belonging to ethnic and minority groups often suffer discrimination and injustice by their exclusion from, or under representation in, clinical trials of promising new treatments.

The history of clinical and surgical research, and of the development of research ethics, leading up to this change of perspective and to the contemporary emphasis on equitable access to the benefits of participation in clinical trials is complex. A series of ethically most dubious, if not tragic, events stretching over nearly a century formed the perception that medical and surgical research was dangerous, of little or no benefit to participants, and that vulnerable people and minority groups were used as guinea pigs for the advancement of scientific knowledge.[23] Vikenty Veressayev, whose *Memoirs of a Physician* were published in English in 1916, chastised his colleagues as "those zealots of science who have ceased to distinguish between their brothers and guinea pigs."[24] He was writing about the use of vulnerable and helpless people in gonorrhea and syphilis research conducted during the latter half of the 1800s in Germany, France, Russia, Ireland, and the United States. The use, and we would now say the exploitation, of subjugate populations, was the trend in medical and surgical research in the nineteenth and early part of the twentieth centuries.[25] These subjugate populations included American slave women in nineteenth-century surgical research,[26,27] and prisoners and institutional persons in the early part of the twentieth century.[28,29] Exclusively helpless people were involved in the medical experiments conducted by the Nazi doctors condemned in the Nuremberg trial of 1947. Twenty years later, Dr.

Henry K. Beecher documented the unethical use of vulnerable people in research conducted in the United States.[30] There were also the reports of the Tuskegee Syphilis Study with black men,[31] and the Willowbrook Studies of Infectious Hepatitis conducted on mentally handicapped children in a New York State institution.[32,33] After the thalidomide tragedy, women of childbearing age and pregnant women came to be quite generally excluded from clinical trials that could affect the fetus.[23,25]

The recent emphasis on assuring women, ethnic and minority groups, and economically disadvantaged people fair access to clinical trials stems in part from a recognition that people often receive better treatment within a clinical trial than in ordinary practice. Moreover, the HIV epidemic has also highlighted the awareness that participation in university hospital–based or community-based clinical trials is often the only way to obtain access to promising new treatments. There is also the concern about the generalizability of clinical trial results if the trial participants are not representative of the disease population for which a treatment under study is intended.

These and other considerations have prompted recent changes in the Food and Drug Administration (FDA) and the National Institutes of Health (NIH) policies concerning equitable selection of women and ethnic and minority groups in clinical trials.[34,35] However, this concern for equity, long overdue, has to be balanced against what is scientifically meaningful and feasible,[36–38] and will be constrained by what is socially difficult.[39–41]

Scientific Adequacy

The Nuremberg Code and the Declaration of Helsinki state that research with human subjects must, as a general condition of ethical justifiability, conform to the canons of scientific methodology.[42,43] Both documents insist on respect for accepted scientific principles, knowledge of the natural history of the disease or problem under study, adequate preliminary laboratory and animal experimentation, and proper scientific and medical qualification of investigators. This emphasis, though covering the basic preconditions for a valid and credible clinical trial, may sound like a quaint overemphasis of the obvious. However, the attempt in the early 1980s to treat two β-thalassemic patients by modifying bone marrow with human β-globulin gene implants was widely criticized as premature and unethical, chiefly on two grounds. The treatment was tried without adequate preliminary experimentation with animal models of β-thalassemia, or a solid foundation of adequate basic knowledge about the regulation of gene expression.[44–48]

David D. Rutstein's maxim—"A poorly or improperly designed study involving human subjects . . . is by definition unethical"[49]—directs attention to the general rule of proportionality ethics. Inviting human beings to submit themselves to a possibly heightened risk of discomfort, inconvenience, harm, or death; consuming scarce precious resources; and raising hopes, particularly when hope is about all that patients have left, demand the balancing weight of a clinical trial that exhibits a high probability of achieving the three objectives identified by David L. Sackett. They are: "validity (the results are true), generalizability (the results are widely applicable), and efficiency (the trial is affordable and resources are left over for patient care and other health research)."[50]

Only reliable clinical knowledge merits widespread clinical application. The generalization of invalid clinical knowledge is inherently unethical, and the extensive application of nonvalidated procedures is, at best, ethically dubious. In this context, randomization has gained wide recognition as one of the most effective tactics to control for selection bias—a major form of bias that leads to false conclusions about the safety, efficacy, or superiority of a given treatment.

Although the emphasis on randomization in scientific ethical discussions of controlled clinical trials with human subjects has not been misplaced, a major shift of ethical attention is long overdue. The ethical difficulties raised by the randomization process may be less significant than the methodological confusion and deficiencies it contributes to the generation of randomized clinical trials that are humanly costly and resource intensive and whose results are clinically implemented only in very limited ways. The problem is not limited to the admitted need to translate the results of clinical trials into practice more effectively,[51] nor can it be solved by technique alone or by more intensive and restricted focus on the careful blueprinting of randomization designs.[52] Randomization, whatever its power, glorious achievements, limitations, or ethical challenges, is not the root of the basic problem of scientific adequacy as a condition for ethically justifiable clinical research with human subjects.

The problem is rooted in the current limitations of basic biomedical science. Meeting the demands of scientific adequacy as a condition for the ethical justifiability of clinical research with human subjects requires the development of what Alvan R. Feinstein has called "the basic science of clinical practice." This requirement, as yet unfulfilled, is based on the fact that "the experiments of the laboratory and the bedside have major differences in scientific orientation, motivation, hypotheses, and values."[53]

A continuing failure to implement the consequences of the differences will exacerbate the ethical problems of clinical research, however much greater the increases in the number of publications and conferences on the meaning of respect for human dignity and the specifications of informed consent. Feinstein's suggested additional basic science of clinical practice would aim to bring cogent human information, derived directly from the patient, back within the boundaries of science. The goal of this science would be to give physicians and patients power over medical science and technology "by expanding it to include human data, by aiming it at human goals, and by making it respond to human aspirations."[54]

Clinical Research: A Human Relationship

Research with human subjects is ethically unjustifiable to the extent that it fails to honor four fundamental characteristics of an authentically human relationship. Charles Fried[14] has identified these as humanity, autonomy, lucidity, and fidelity. These characteristics are essential qualifications of how physicians, clinical investigators, patients, and subjects should behave toward each other. Our attention, in this discussion, is understandably focused on the behavior of physicians and clinical investigators.

In a human relationship, a person is not treated simply as one of a class. The characteristic *humanity* stresses that each person is a unique individual with a correspondingly unique biology and individualized needs, weaknesses, strengths, and life plans. *Humanity* means attention to and respect for this "full human particularity."[14] Autonomy or self-determination implies the need and the capacity to deliberate about personal goals and the liberty to act accordingly. A relationship that fosters autonomy is notable for the absence of fraud, force, and the tendency to use another human being as a disposable resource.

Lucidity qualifies communication as honest, candid, and open to imparting all known information that is material to another's self-determination, deliberation, and choice of alternatives to realize individual life plans. This means sensitivity to another person's total life interests and capacities for comprehension. Lucidity is ill served if clinical investigators look on "obtaining informed consent" as some kind of legally imposed ritual. Clinical investigators sometimes speak as though consent is something they need for their research. They fail to grasp the reality that adequate information is primarily a need of the patient and a moral requirement of integrity in a human relationship.[55]

Fidelity means faithfulness in responding to justified expectations that are integral components of a relationship. These expectations will vary from one kind of relationship to another. Patients enter into relationships with doctors justifiably expecting, however implicitly, that their doctors are suitably qualified, up-to-date with current standards of good medicine and skillful surgery, and committed to restoring their patients to good health.

Informed, Comprehending, and Voluntary Consent

Physicians and clinical investigators have a primordial obligation to assure that their patients and volunteer subjects are adequately informed to be able to consent comprehendingly, and without coercion, to the research procedures and interventions they are being invited to undergo. This condition for ethically justifiable research with human subjects, clearly established in the Nuremberg Code,[42] has been subjected to relentless and detailed scrutiny over the past 30 years in more than 4,000 publications.[56]

The ethical norm of informed, comprehending, and voluntary consent has its origin in the four characteristics of an authentic human relationship discussed earlier. Though each shapes the process of consent, humanity is the most difficult to respect. It is, nevertheless, singularly important in gauging the scope of disclosure of information in clinical practice and clinical research.

The particularity of the patient's situation was a central issue in the Canadian Supreme Court case of *Reibl v. Hughes.* The court's decision clarifies that, of three possible standards for determining the kinds of information that must be disclosed (i.e., the professional, subjective patient, and objective patient standards) the latter is to be followed. If the professional standard would allow doctors and clinical investigators to set the threshold of disclosure "at a lower level than would serve the public interest and protection," the subjective patient standard would place physicians "at the mercy of the patient's bitter hindsight."[57]

The court clarified that the objective, or reasonable, patient standard implies the need to match information to a patient's reasonably based particular concerns and preferences.[58] This legally and ethically important case illustrates the essential moral difference between "obtaining" informed consent as a ritual kind of act performed primarily to get treatment or research moving, and "educating" a patient or subject in an open, searching conversation, carried out primarily to assure that the patient knows and understands everything required to make a free and reasonable decision.

The Canadian case also emphasizes that "informed consent" is part of a two-way transaction.[57] The doctor also needs information if the patient is to be adequately informed. How can a physician or clinical investigator serve the life plans of a patient or subject if nothing is said about them in conversations about the treatment or research? Doctors and clinical investigators are as much in need of knowing every essential of the life plans, concerns, and bodily situation of patients and subjects as the latter are in need of knowing every essential of the preferred treatments and proposed research procedures.[59,60]

Viewed by the patient as medically irrelevant, some contextual features of the patient's life may have potent consequences, as illustrated in the case of *Reibl v. Hughes.* Reibl's pension, unknown to his surgeon, became unobtainable when the patient developed postoperative hemiplegia after carotid artery surgery. This elective operation was performed before he had worked long enough to be vested in his company's pension plan, and his permanent disability prevented a return to work, leaving him destitute. The court ruled, and the ruling was upheld on appeal, that the surgeon's ignorance of this nuance of the patient's particular circumstances constituted negligence.[61] Since there is no systematic review comprehensive enough to elicit details like this one, it is useful at the time consent for a trial or treatment is obtained to ask the patient, "Are there any special circumstances in your own life that we both should take into consideration as we make this decision?"

Physicians and clinical investigators bear primary responsibility for organizing consent conversations and making certain that this mutually informing process really takes place. Insecure and vulnerable patients and subjects may easily be cowed into silence, or even acquiescence, by the awesome environment of the hospital and the authority-laden image of the doctor.[62] The hospital is the doctor's daily domain and home territory, which the patient enters as a frightened stranger. In these circumstances, voluntary consent doesn't come naturally. Sensitive perception and dedicated commitment are necessary if physicians and clinical investigators are to serve the needs and goals of those who come to them for care and cure.

Confidentiality

Protection of privacy and confidentiality, a professional obligation arising from the fiduciary character of the relationship between patient and physician, is a necessary condition for the ethical conduct of surgical and clinical research with human subjects. The therapeutic relationship requires sick people to reveal to physicians, and allows physicians to acquire, kinds of information about body and biography that the patients would rarely, if ever, be willing to share with anyone else. That sharing of personal secrets can only occur if patients can trust that physicians will honor the confidentiality demands of professional fidelity. When intimate information is divulged without a patient's knowledge and consent, and, worse still, when explicit promises of confidentiality have been broken, the integrity of sick people is harmed, as is also the integrity of clinical practice and clinical research.

Participants in research may be harmed psychologically, socially, or even financially, if their privacy is invaded or if information about them, including the fact of their participation in certain kinds of research, is not kept confidential. There is now heightened sensitivity to the critical importance of safeguards for privacy and confidentiality, particularly in surveillance studies and in epidemiological and social research on conditions that are socially stigmatizing and likely to render people susceptible to various kinds of discrimination.[63–65] The HIV epidemic, for instance, has occasioned the development of detailed guidelines and ingenious coding methods for electronic data storage to protect privacy and confidentiality in the research setting.[66,67]

Information sheets accompanying consent forms for participants in clinical research routinely state, or should so state, that rights to privacy and confidentiality of information will be respected in clinical trials. The World Medical Association Declaration of Helsinki states that every precaution should be taken to respect the privacy of research subjects.[68] The Code of Federal Regulations of the United States requires, for IRB approval of research with human subjects, that there are adequate provisions to protect the privacy of subjects and to maintain the confidentiality of data.[69]

The requirements for adequate protection of privacy and confidentiality will vary in keeping with the nature of the research, the disease or condition under study, and the laws of each country. Some countries provide legal shields to protect the confidentiality of research data against civil, criminal, administrative, or other proceedings to compel disclosure.[70] Where such shields do not exist in law,

researchers may be restricted with regard to the extent of protection of confidentiality they can guarantee research subjects. When stigmatizing conditions are under study, special coding procedures may be necessary to assure that sensitive data cannot be linked to individuals via personal identifiers. Clinical studies involving follow-up of patients after close-out of the study require that particular attention be given to protection of privacy. Research subjects should be alerted to the possibility of future contact, and they should give free and informed consent to any follow-up plan.[71] In surgical research, confidentiality could be inadvertently broken if the uniqueness of the surgical operation combined with the relative rarity of patient characteristics could lead some to deduce the personal identity of the patient or patients presented in case discussions or publications.

Clinical Research: A Therapeutic Relationship

Henry K. Beecher's statement, "Ordinary patients will not knowingly risk their health or their life for the sake of science,"[72] is as true today as it was in 1966. Sick people come to doctors for care, relief, and cure. Though cure cannot be guaranteed, and every intervention into the body carries its risk of harm, care encompasses the granting by patients, and the appropriating by doctors, "of some power over another so that the other will benefit."[73]

The expectation that doctors will help, and not harm, is the basis of the patient-doctor relationship, the primary content of the medical profession's societal mandate, and the guiding norm of one of medicine's most ancient ethical maxims.[73] Fidelity to this expectation is an essential condition for ethically acceptable clinical research.

Claude Bernard gave precision to the meaning of this fidelity in his statement of a principle of medical and surgical morality:

> It is our duty and our right to perform an experiment on man whenever it can save his life, cure him, or gain him some personal benefit. The principle of medical and surgical morality, therefore, consists in never performing an experiment

which might be harmful to him to any extent, even though the result might be highly advantageous to science, that is, to the health of others."[20]

This principle sets a basic right of patients, and a corresponding fundamental duty of doctors, that takes precedence over any utilitarian calculus that would tolerate a sacrifice of the health or lives of individuals today for the putatively greater good of society or the patients of tomorrow.

This "Bernard" principle, though clearly essential for the ethical justifiability of clinical research with human subjects, is too pure and absolute in its original wording to be realistic. Medicine is inherently experimental. It is clearly impossible, either in uncontrolled clinical practice or in controlled clinical trials, to abstain totally from interventions that might be harmful "to any extent." The factors of uncertainty and risk of harm, attendant upon any clinical intervention into the body, must be taken into account in this principle of the primacy of the therapeutic obligation.

The therapeutic obligation in clinical practice, regardless of whether physician and patient are participants in a controlled clinical trial, has to be governed by proportionality ethics. Risks of harm or detriment have to be balanced by a probability of benefit for the patient that is weighty enough to compensate for any loss or injury that might occur. This principle complements the Nuremberg and Helsinki emphasis on the proportion to be maintained between the risks undertaken by subjects in clinical research and the scientific and humanitarian importance of the research objectives.[42,43]

Harms and benefits are not totally susceptible to objective, generalizable measurement. They comprise both "hard" and "soft" data. The ethical implication is that it is impossible to determine that a proportion between harms and benefits holds for particular patients, without giving due attention and weight to their personal interpretations of the total impact of a clinical intervention on their lives. This is the target of Feinstein's justified criticism of attempts to balance harms and benefits, or to judge a treatment's efficacy, on the basis of a dehumanized array of data. Such attempts fall short of their objective because they fail to assess the "total spectrum of a treatment's impact."[74]

The Therapeutic Relationship in Randomized Clinical Trials

One of the strongest recurrent ethical criticisms of randomized clinical trials is that they sin against the therapeutic relationship.[75–79] Physician-investigators participating in such studies, so the critique runs, abandon fully individualized care of their patients and even subject some patients, via the randomization process, to inferior treatment. One assumption behind this criticism is that equipoise regarding safety and efficacy rarely exists between alternative treatments at the initiation of a controlled trial.[18,80–82] There is usually some indication that one treatment is better than another, even if the indication falls short of a statistically rigorous demonstration. Even if equipoise does seem to hold at the initiation of a trial, secrecy about interim results when these favor one treatment over another means that some randomized patients, including both early and newly entered patients, will receive inferior treatment.

How can randomizing patients to inferior treatment or maintaining them on inferior treatment until the trial reaches a certain minimum probability of error be squared with the demands of the therapeutic relationship? This bottom-line question gathers force when patients die or suffer serious deterioration of health as a consequence of the inferior treatment.

The foregoing criticism of randomized clinical trials does not reflect sufficient appreciation of the proliferation of innovations and the attendant pervasiveness of uncertainty in medicine, the associated danger of using invalidated procedures in clinical practice, and the intersection of goals in clinical therapy and interventional trials.

Surgical trials with human subjects are, with few exceptions, interventional rather than explicatory. Feinstein has identified the ethical significance of the differences between these two kinds of trial.[83] In an *interventional* trial, the goal of the treatments employed is to change a patient's clinical course, not in a passing way to study some physiological variable, but in an enduring way, and to enhance health and postpone death.

The goal of the therapeutic relationship—to care, relieve, and cure a suffering patient—is identical to the goal pursued by the physician-investigators in an interventional trial. The goal of the trial is to determine, reliably, whether the effects observed to follow upon a clinical intervention are due to treatment, or whether one treatment is safer or more effective than its alternatives.

When there is no uncertainty about the safety, efficacy, or comparative worth of treatments, there is no need for an interventional trial. To the extent that such uncertainty does hold sway, it is impertinent to ask whether physician-investigators in an interventional trial are withholding known effective treatments from patients or are consigning patients to inferior treatment. That is precisely what is unknown and can be reliably determined only by a properly designed trial. An interventional trial, assuming the fulfillment of essential scientific and ethical conditions, is more consistent with fidelity to the therapeutic relationship than unquestioning recommendation of one of several invalidated treatments whose comparative worth is in dispute.

This position does not reject the principle of conscience. A physician, convinced of the superiority of a given treatment on the basis of available evidence, would be acting against his or her personal and professional conscience in participating in a randomization of patients to an alternative treatment that causes higher mortality or morbidity in the physician's opinion. It must be realized, however, that evidence sufficiently strong to constitute ethical ground for an individual physician's refusal to participate in a randomized clinical trial may fall far short of a decisive argument against the ethical justifiability of the trial itself.

Clinical Trials and Surgical Research: Ethical Issues

To fit the reality of particular clinical trials, ethical decisions need two synchronized cutting edges: an upper blade of general ethical principles, and a continually reshaped lower blade of definite answers to specific questions.

The Ethical Use of Animals in Surgical Research

It is generally and correctly assumed that the ethical justifiability of research with human subjects depends on adequate prior experimentation with animals. This does not mean that the use of animals in research requires no further justification. However, a comprehensive response to the question about whether we are morally justified "in imposing suffering on or taking the lives of other species solely for our own benefit"[84] would require an analysis of the expanding and unfinished debate on these issues.[85-88] Since such an analysis would exceed the boundaries of this chapter, two major points have been selected for discussion.

First, differences between species do have moral significance. Ethical constraints on what we may impose on other animals to satisfy our own good and our own needs increase as the capacities and needs of the animals approach those of human beings. Second, the critical question is not whether, but under what conditions we may use animals in research.

Effective measures to assure the humane treatment of animals in research and to protect animals against wanton disregard of their needs and welfare are essential requirements of civilized scientific behavior. Fulfilling these requirements does not necessitate acceptance of any of the following positions.

Humans have no right to treat animals any differently from how they would treat any member of their own species.[89]

Animals should be used in research projects only when the results will directly benefit the animals themselves.[89]

There should be an immediate replacement of all animals used in experiments by alternative systems.[87]

Sensitivity to the needs of animals and to their differential capacities for suffering from pain, constriction, and deprivation does necessitate careful attention to Lane-Petter's five basic questions.

Is the animal the best experimental system for the problem?

Must the animal be conscious at any time during the experiment?

Can the pain and discomfort associated with the experiment be lessened or eliminated?

Can the number of animals involved be reduced?

Is the problem under study worth solving?[90,91]

Necessity of experiment, humaneness of design, and a standard of pre-and postoperative care at least as good as that required for acceptable clinical veterinary practice[92] summarize the conditions for the ethical justifiability of using animals in research.

Standards in Surgical Research

There is no controversy about the desirability of high standards of evidence in surgical research. The well-known division of opinion is about the kinds of design that are practicable and effective in producing such evidence.[93–100] The rule governing such discussions should be to avoid fervent answers to global questions. Variations in the nature of the procedures under study, the clinical conditions to be treated, and different surgical specialties require differentiated judgments about the research design most appropriate for each research project.

The principle of differentiated judgment modifies and is not a substitute for the more general ethical rule: employ every possible tactic at the most opportune moment in the development of innovative surgical procedures to reduce the devastating effects of bias. Demanding that the standards of surgical research match the highest currently attainable in clinical investigation is not the same thing as insisting on identity of research design in surgical and medical trials. Methodological sophistication may indicate the need for research designs uniquely tailored for some surgical specialties.[95,100–102]

Ethics and the Design of Surgical Research

The methodologically rigorous design of surgical trials poses several distinct and widely recognized difficulties,[103–104] which have ethical implications.

First, it is generally impossible to achieve full blinding in surgical research. The extent of blinding achievable will vary according to the purpose of the trial, that is, whether an operation is being compared with nonsurgical treatment or with the comparative safety and efficacy of two operations. Though sham operations are ethically unjustifia-

ble and would not be considered today, a measure of blinding may be possible when the physicians evaluating the patients' progress have not been involved in the trials.[94,104–106]

Second, surgery has a powerful placebo effect that may exist independently of an operation's genuine efficacy. This fact, for which internal mammary artery ligation for the relief of angina offers some evidence, underscores the importance of blinding as a tactic in a methodologically rigorous trial. It is difficult to ethically justify the continued use of surgical operations having little more than placebo efficacy.[104]

Third, Francis D. Moore has observed that "the most remarkable and effective extensions of surgery have often not required elaborate statistical analysis for their establishment."[107] Though "often" is not equal to "regularly" or "generally," this observation invites a flexible attitude toward what H.A.F. Dudley has called the central dogma, namely, "the concept of overriding need to prosecute controlled clinical trials as the only way of ensuring reliable knowledge."[108]

Fourth, there are situations in which randomized clinical trials may be both impractical and ethically dubious. The advisability of a trial is open to serious questions when "thousands of patients must be treated to establish statistically significant, but very small, differences."[107]

Fifth, randomized clinical trials may be impossible when the course of treatment for a given condition is in a state of rapid evolution. For example, the arrival of coronary artery bypass grafting led to the abandonment of a randomized clinical trial of the Vineburg surgical procedure.[101] Randomized clinical trials are perilous and dubious undertakings when innovations are likely to be rapidly replaced by even better new procedures.

Sixth, the controversy over radial keratotomy, a surgical procedure to correct myopia, has emphasized once again how difficult it is to launch controlled studies of surgical innovations after they have become popular. The standard ethical objection to randomized trials in this situation is: How can one justify withholding a widely acclaimed procedure from a control group? The radial keratotomy controversy has added another objection: How can one justify withholding business from surgeons by concentrating use of the operation to those surgeons participating in a randomized clinical trial? The lawsuit launched in the United States against George O. Waring, an associate professor of ophthalmology, and against others involved in the Prospective Evaluation of Radial Keratotomy (PERK) trial, has intensified and hardened divisions of opinion about how surgical innovations should be brought into the health care system.[109]

Although a judgment on the justification of this particular lawsuit must be withheld, the wisdom of charging clinical researchers with conspiracy to monopolize an operation and with violation of antitrust laws when they undertake the evaluation of a new operation for safety and efficacy must be vigorously questioned. The good conscience of individual surgeons will never be an adequate substitute for methodologically rigorous evaluations of surgical innovations. The PERK study indicates that this surgical operation tends to have unpredictable outcomes. The risks have to be balanced against the small gains.[110,111]

The goal of controlled clinical trials should not be confused with any set of methodological strategies or tactics. The goal is reliable knowledge. H.A.F. Dudley has emphasized that "there is a continuous rather than a discontinuous scale of reliability, not a quantum leap from none to near-total reliability."[108] The role of randomized clinical trials should be gauged against that scale and in the light of the varying constraints of different clinical situations. We are coming to a more precise identification of the circumstances in which evaluations of efficacy cannot be made with randomized prospective studies.[95,101,112] However, the recent results of the extracranial-intracranial bypass study should exercise a braking restraint on any latent enthusiasm for liberation from the rigors of controlled clinical trials.[113]

Prerandomization Learning and Early Randomization

Thomas C. Chalmers has advanced methodological and ethical reasons for early randomization, indeed for the randomization of the first patient, in the evaluation of new medical treatments and surgical procedures.[94,114] Succinctly, his position is that "randomization from the beginning, with truly informed consent, is the only ethical way to begin the exploration of new therapies."[94]

Attention should be given to two methodological considerations, one supportive, the other critical of early randomization, before analyzing the ethical issue raised in the Chalmers position.

Pilot studies and prerandomization learning periods, followed by positive observations reports, increase the likelihood that methodologically rigorous evaluations of new surgical procedures will be postponed unduly or never initiated. It becomes ethically difficult to randomize patients when one of the procedures under study has already won an enthusiastic constituency, however illusory the evidence for this enthusiasm may be.[115,116] Early randomization, if practicable and successful, counters this tendency.

Early randomization may, however, be impossible or methodologically dubious in some surgical trials. Experience, technical skill, and masterful craftsmanship have to be acquired through practice. They cannot be taught and learned before an operation is actually performed. A new operation has little chance of being judged on its own merits before the surgeons performing it in a trial have acquired sufficient mastery of the procedures to permit a sufficient degree of standardization. Short of this, the same operation in the hands of different surgeons possessing quite variable levels of skill may well have quite divergent results.[117] In such circumstances, a trial would more likely measure variances in surgical craftsmanship rather than the safety and effectiveness of the new operation. Indeed, with wide variations in surgical skill, the operation under study may not be the same. Moreover, potential promising new operations for which "it takes years to reach optimum low risk and clinical benefit"[97] could be rejected, not on the basis of their real therapeutic merit, but because of initial high mortality rates due to surgeons' inexperience.

Chalmers recognizes the force of the methodological objection to very early randomization of patients in the evaluation of surgical innovations, particularly of technically difficult new operations. He has stated that "from the scientific standpoint alone, the technique should be fully developed before the randomized trial is begun."[94] Consonant with this observation, William Van der Linden has proposed a prerandomization practice period that "should last until the participants are fully conversant with every single detail of the new technique. It is not until then that a fair trial can be run."[106]

The Chalmers position holds that running a fair trial can be in conflict with running an ethical trial. Though prerandomization practice periods would set the stage for a more reliable comparison of a new against an established operation. Chalmers observes that patients honestly informed about the potentially higher initial mortality or morbidity rates, to be expected during this period, would likely refuse to enter this surgical novitiate and demand the established operation.[94] He argues that randomization from the beginning, with truly informed consent, is the only ethical way to evaluate new operations because patients are more likely to accept randomization if they are convinced that there is "an equal chance that the new operation might be better than the old from the beginning."[94]

The Chalmers exclusive position on the ethical superiority of very early randomization is not convincing. The fact that a new operation has a good chance of being superior to an older established surgical treatment must be modified by the word "eventually." The potential intrinsic merits of a new operation, once mastered, are not an antidote to the risks of potentially higher mortality or morbidity resulting from surgeons' underdeveloped skills in performing the new procedures. Lawrence Bonchek's observation and counter-question are in order: "Randomization does not alter operative risk; it simply dictates that chance, not the patient, will determine exposure to the risk. Is such an arrangement more ethical?"[93] The real ethical issue is whether patients know about and freely assume the risks of new operations.

Informing Patients about Randomization: Conflicting Views

Do the ethical principles requiring informed, comprehending, and voluntary consent necessitate telling patients how their treatments are selected in randomized clinical trials?

The ethical justifiability of randomization does not hinge only on physician "indifference" to the treatments. Equipoise of outcome of different treatments, whether apparent only at the beginning of a trial or increasingly evident as the trial progresses, does not justify the inference that patients will be or ought to be "indifferent" about the treatment they will receive.[118] Physician-investigator uncertainty about the relative merits of alternative treatments does not mean that patient preference for one treatment over another is necessarily or even generally "capricious."[119] The treatments in a trial may exert significantly different impacts on patients' quality of life and life plans, whatever the initial state of knowledge or the eventual statistical results of the trial may be.

The management of breast cancer and cancer of the prostate are two clinical trial situations for which the following conclusion is entirely appropriate: "It is not enough for the physician to have no reason to prefer one treatment over the other, in addition, there must be no reason for the patient to prefer one treatment."[120]

The harm-benefit ratio is a result of balancing multiple factors that must include effects that patients consider personally important. Reducing the ratio to the "hard" variables the trial is designed to measure can easily amount to a disregard of a patient's particular situation. Physician-investigators are not ethically justified in perceiving and treating patients exclusively as representatives of a given disease category. It is methodologically and ethically important that surgeon-investigators pay close attention to patient-subjects' unique personal differences. Good ethics and good science demand precisely that everybody not be treated alike in consent negotiations.[121,122]

Lack of candor about randomization, and the associated additional concealments of information this would often entail, can constitute an act that bars patients from what they need to know to make the choices they consider to be the most important for their lives. This is ethically unjustifiable in a trial that would otherwise be ethically acceptable. As a rule, patients should be informed about randomization. Justifiable exceptions will have to be justified. A generalization of such exceptions could arise when the differential impact on patients' lives are perceived, by patients and surgeons alike, as being just as important as the treatments' initial putative equality of outcome. In such situations, surgeons may be no less deterred from enrolling otherwise eligible candidates into a trial than the patients themselves are from participating.

The National Surgical Adjuvant Project for Breast and Bowel Cancer (NSABP) trial to compare the relative effectiveness of total and segmental mastectomy, with and without radiation, presents a challenging illustration of these difficulties[123] (see chapter 27).

Harmonizing a surgeon's responsibilities as physician, with his or her duties as clinical investigator may be easier in word and in theory than it frequently is in act and practice. The U.K. Cancer Research Campaign Working Party in Breast Conservation has noted: "It is one thing to admit doubt among one's colleagues, quite another to have to admit it to a patient."[62] The need to confess to patients that chance, not their surgeon, is in charge of selecting their treatment is at least as difficult as admitting uncertainty or ignorance. These admissions do require "mental gymnastics beyond the abilities of many,"[124,125] surgeons as well as patients. Admittedly, this is not the way surgeons traditionally behave toward their patients in normal practice. Whether behavior in normal practice should be the norm for clinical research or vice versa is a question meriting its own discussion.

Enrolling patients into randomized surgical trials without their knowledge and consent is not an answer to these and other difficulties surgeons experience with the process of randomization. Randomizing patients to treatment groups before initiating consent negotiations seems to alleviate the difficulty surgeons have when asking patients to participate in a trial without being able to tell them what treatment they will receive. Prerandomization designs are less problematic ethically when all patient candidates, those assigned by chance to standard therapy and those similarly assigned to innovative therapy, are involved in consent negotiations. It is unethical to conduct a trial when some of the patient-subjects are totally unaware of the research process in which they have been enrolled and quite unaware of the alternative treatments they might have preferred.

Involving all patient-subjects in consent negotiations does not, however, directly guarantee that prerandomization designs are ethically innocuous. Even if patients are told that their treatment has been selected by chance—and they should be told,

the way in which the advantages and drawbacks of the alternative treatments are presented can amount to tender but real coercion.[126] The voluntary, if not the informed, character of consent may be jeopardized by a linguistic tailoring of information that manipulates the patient's will without blinding the patient's intellect.

It should be emphasized that this danger is not peculiar to randomized clinical trials, whatever the randomization tactic may be. The danger is equal or greater when a surgeon who is not participating in a trial convincingly presents one of several alternative treatments under study in a trial, elsewhere, as the best "in my judgment." This situation is the target of the U.K. Working Party's fifth practical proposal:

> Those doctors who treat patients with cancer but do not participate in randomized clinical trials should realize that they too have an obligation to discuss alternative forms of treatment with their patients. In our view the fact that they are not formally randomizing their patients does not reduce their obligation in this respect.[62]

This proposal suggests a return to the point mentioned earlier about norms of surgeon behavior toward patients in routine practice as contrasted with randomized surgical trials. Some respondents to the investigation of surgeons' reasons for not enrolling patients into the NSABP trial of treatments for breast cancer "believed that participating in a clinical trial would necessitate a major change in the traditional physician-patient interaction."[123] Some changes in that relationship, motivated or necessitated by participation in randomized surgical trials, may be highly desirable, meriting introduction into routine surgical practice. Dropping the guise of sapiential authority, when the state of clinical knowledge offers no warrant for such an assumption of power, may advance the education of patient expectations, bolster patient autonomy, and, paradoxically, strengthen the trust of patients in their physicians.

Conflicts of Interest

Confucius is reputed to have said, "If language is not correct, then what is said is not what is meant; if what is said is not what is meant, then what ought to be done remains undone." Confucius could have added another consequence of the mismatch between words and meaning: what ought not to be done may be continued as the natural and normal way to behave.

Our primary concern here is with what ought to be done about conflicts of interest. If solutions and preventive measures are to fit the problems, definitions and distinctions of problems are inescapable. We first consider what is meant by conflicts of interest and then discuss what can be done about them.

Meaning

The literature about conflict of interest seems to mirror Augustine's embarrassment when he considered answering the question about the meaning of time: "If no one asks me, I know; if I want to explain it to someone who does ask me, I do not know."[127] The meaning of the word *interest*[128] includes a diversity of relationships of persons to goods, and that diversity complicates the definitions of conflicts of interest that can be found in the recent literature.

In this chapter we consider an *interest* to be whatever is to the good, benefit, profit, or advantage of anyone.[128] These advantages are in conflict when one or several cannot be obtained or maintained without sacrificing others. A *conflict of interest,* according to a definition adopted by two Councils of the American Medical Association (AMA), is a conflict "between private interests and official responsibilities of a person in a position of trust."[129] In an excellent explanatory discussion of this subject, Thompson defines the conflict as being between *primary* and *secondary* interests. Primary interests, such as the health of patients, the integrity of research, and the education of students, relate to the professional responsibilities of a physician, researcher, or teacher. Secondary interests relate to desirable personal goods such as financial gain, prestige, career advancement, or advantages for those to whom a professional has personal and private allegiance.[130]

A conflict of interest is a situation or a constellation of circumstances in which professional judgment or institutional mission regarding primary interests, such as clinical, scientific, or academic integrity, "tend to be unduly influenced by

a secondary interest."[130] This definition is open to the AMA Councils' distinction between *potential* and *actual* conflicts of interest.[129] A *potential conflict of interest* is a situation in which a professional's primary and secondary interests *might* come into conflict. An *actual conflict of interest* is a situation in which a professional cannot honor one interest without impairing others.

The scope for potential and actual conflicts of interest is extensive, encompassing medical practice,[131–138] research,[139–142] peer review,[143] medical and scientific publishing,[144–147] and education.[148] Institutions and organizations, as well as individual professionals, can be in a conflict of interest.[149]

A conflict of interest should be distinguished from scientific misconduct, which typically consists of plagiarism, deception, or falsification or fabrication of data.[129] A conflict of interest is a situation or set of circumstances, not an act or a behavior. However, unprofessional or professionally unethical behaviors can result from conflicts of interest. For example, a scientist consciously or unconsciously might review a competing colleague's research proposal unfairly, or the authors of a review article might give exaggerated prominence to studies of treatments manufactured by companies that have funded the authors.[145]

The risk of professionally unethical conduct related to conflicts of interest can be reduced if physician-investigators do the following:

- Attend to the conflict and do something about it.
- Transparently disclose their competing interests.
- Offer reasonable cause for holding secondary interests when these might be viewed as incompatible with professional and scientific responsibilities.
- Choose between primary and secondary interests when they are irreconcilably in conflict.

Management

The sources of conflict of interest may be personal, political, academic, scientific, or philosophical, and not only financial.[139,145] Yet, special attention should be given to conflicts between the pursuit of financial gain and the exercise of professional and scientific judgment. Although collaboration between industry and academia is both essential and desirable, the expansion of these collaborative connections are cause for concern, and they merit vigilance.[142] It is not objectionable in principle that researchers and their institutions share in the financial rewards of scientific discovery and innovation, but the growing dependence of biomedical research on industrial support, and the potential magnitude of the financial rewards deriving from this collaboration, could imperil, or give the appearance of imperiling, scientific integrity.[129,142] An AMA Council has reasonably emphasized that the mere appearance or perception of conflict of interest may be sufficient to cast doubt on an otherwise exemplary research program.[129] Accordingly, there has been at least one proposal that apparent conflicts of interest should be no less seriously evaluated and managed than actual conflicts.[141]

Precisely what should be done about conflicts of interest will vary with the severity of the conflict and the seriousness of the harm such conflicts can produce.[130] Severity of conflict is proportional to the likelihood that financial interests will imperil the objectivity of professional and scientific judgment or will detour an institution from the pursuit of its primary missions. The values endangered by conflicts of interest measure the harm such conflicts can cause. The harm includes the threat to the health and even the lives of sick people;[132] weakening of trust between physician-investigators and between physician-investigators, patients, and students;[141] and loss of public confidence in a profession or an institution.

While conflicts of interest may threaten the objective and trustworthy conduct, evaluation, and reporting of research,[141] they may also exercise subtle but powerful influence on the directions of research that will be pursued or neglected, perhaps to the detriment of the common good.[130]

The approaches proposed to manage conflicts of interest include disclosure, mediation, modification of research plan, monitoring of research, abstention, divestiture, and prohibition.[130,140,142,147,150] Disclosure has been called the bedrock of any sensible scheme for managing conflicts of interest.[142] Although not sufficient, disclosure is a necessary starting point in the management of conflicts of interest. It favors the maintenance of trust by ending the possible deception "of permitting one's

judgment to appear more reliable than it really is."[141] Physicians' and scientists' disclosure of their financial interests also gives to people the information required to gauge how much trust they should place in medical recommendations and scientific results. It is reasonable to expect and require that scientists' disclosure of their financial ties to companies be made to medical institutions where the research is carried out, to funding agencies, and to journals in which the research will be published.[129]

Although disclosure alerts people to the existence of a conflict of interest, it does not of itself resolve them and may even create additional problems.[130,151] The judicious use of more severe conflict of interest control measures, such as prohibiting independent researchers from serving on the boards of directors of companies that could profit from the researcher's scientific work, or prohibiting researchers from holding equity ownership or stock options in such companies,[142] will require careful evaluation of each conflict of interest situation. These conflicts are not all of one kind or of the same degree of severity, as may be seen in the Harvard University Faculty of Medicine three-category classification of conflicts of interest–related activities. Some such activities are allowable with oversight, but only after disclosure, review, and approval by a committee; other activities, ordinarily allowable following disclosure, may require oversight; the third category is of activities that are routinely allowable.[152]

The judicious regulation of conflicts of interest serves the high Confucian purpose of assuring that what ought to be done does not remain undone. What ought to be done, and expeditiously, is methodologically sound research uncontaminated by the multiple biases, including the bias of conflicting interests, that restrict both the validity of research and the common trust research needs in order to thrive.

Human Studies Permission: Some Practical Points

Perhaps the most important practical point for the potential surgical investigator is to take human studies permission seriously. The present climate and the requirements for appropriate treatment of other human beings make it mandatory that human studies forms be filled out honestly and accurately. For purposes of this discussion, the human studies form of the Brigham and Women's Hospital in Boston will be used as a guideline. At this hospital, all protocols involving human tissue or subjects are reviewed by a research committee that meets twice a month. Four categories of information are required:

1. General information, including the name of the investigator and the department, the date of beginning and ending the study, and the coinvestigators
2. Funding information, specifically whether there are costs not covered by outside research funds or third-party payers
3. Patient-subject information, including the total number of subjects, the facilities required (inpatient, outpatient, or clinical research center), potential use of special groups (children, newborns, fetuses, medical students, the mentally handicapped, pregnant women, prisoners, or adolescents), duration of study for individual subjects, remuneration, and the use of drugs, radioactive materials, medical devices, nursing services, or dietetic services
4. A description of the research and training project

The fourth category probably has the greatest import because it essentially justifies the project for human studies. It begins with a statement of the general purpose of the research and the specific hypothesis to be tested. It moves then to the proposed experimental procedures, including background information, number of subjects to be involved in the study, procedures and methodologies to be used, names and details of medications, and the use of data to test the proposed hypotheses. The next section documents stresses or aggravation of a "chemical, physical, biological, psychological, and other nature," and the investigators' experience in this kind of research. There follows a listing of possible benefits or advantages to the individual patient or society, and potential discomfort or risks. (A risk is defined here as exposure to "the possibility of any harm, physical, psychological, sociological or other as a conse-

quence of any activity which goes beyond the application of those established and accepted methods necessary to meet the patient's needs.")

The application must describe the manner in which patients will be recruited and informed consent will be obtained, appropriate alternative procedures, provisions made to answer patient inquiries, measures taken to ensure that involved subjects will be free to omit specific procedures, and changes in experimental design that might be necessary to complete the formal information portion.

The informed consent form lies at the heart of the study. The consent form should have the following elements in it: the purpose of the study, procedures to be used, risks and discomfort, benefits, alternative procedures, standard release form, confidentiality of information, a compensational clause, and option to withdraw.

The study's goals should be clearly stated at the beginning. The section on procedures should include a description of how the proposed procedures differ from standard care, the duration of the subject's participation, the details of the procedure to be used, and any compensation for participation.

Risks, discomforts, and benefits should include direct benefits to the patient and any risks he or she might run. Alternative procedures should be discussed, and the availability of the physician in charge to answer inquiries should be emphasized. Assurance should be given that information will be kept confidential. It should be stated that the subject will not be compensated for injuries occurring and that he or she is free to withdraw at any time. Finally, there should be a statement that the procedure has been explained.

The range of potential investigative procedures is rather wide. Blood drawing for purposes of doing blood testing; chart reviews; use of nursing services, women, prisoners, or adolescents; duration of study; and the use of discarded material are all part of human experimentation and must be proposed and justified. Special information is required for drug data, isotopes, and nursing services. Short forms, to expedite processing, are available for human discarded material and for record reviews.

These requirements may seem onerous, but they ensure that the patient is not abused.

Teaching and Learning Research Ethics

Riis (chapter 61) and Lock[153] describe examples of fraud and misconduct in research that led the National Institutes of Health to require specific training in research ethics as a mandatory component of National Research Service Award Training Grants in the United States. This initiative and the decision by the Royal College of Physicians and Surgeons of Canada to require teaching of bioethics (including research ethics) in all postgraduate residency programs reflect increasing recognition of the need for discussion of values, guidelines, and ethical problems confronting the researcher. Programs of this kind are necessarily compact and incomplete, but formally recognizing the topic as part of the learning agenda opens explicit discussion between trainees and their mentors about ethical issues and the pressures that lead to unethical research practices.

The introduction of the bioethics curriculum as a mandatory component of Canada's surgical residencies will provide a broader opportunity to discuss and clarify the values and principles they use as coordinates for ethical decision making. Guidance in this important area has come only implicitly from the example of surgical mentors in the past. Pelligrino's insightful discussion provides useful answers to questions raised about the appropriateness and effectiveness of teaching medical ethics.[154] He defines stable and gradable objectives such as teaching analytic skills, raising sensitivity to enhance recognition of ethical issues, and identification of ethical assumptions underlying decisions. The educational research literature analyzing the impact of teaching programs in ethics is sparse because assessment of the impact of such programs is so difficult. However, outcome data are lacking on the impact of most educational interventions including teaching anatomy or biochemistry to medical students.[154]

Sulemasy found that a series of facilitated discussions of bioethics issues increased the confidence of residents in analyzing problems in clinical ethics; translation into daily practice was evident in the frequency and clarity of orders not to resuscitate terminal patients.[155] Pollock reported that a 6-hour research ethics course using a case-based "quandary ethics" approach provided an "ethical compass" that proved helpful to surgical research trainees.[156] Residents who participated in the course felt better prepared to deal with problems related to discarding results, gratuitous authorship, data storage, and problems with mentors. One hundred percent of surgical research trainees who completed the course were prepared to seek third-party input into an ethical dilemma involving their own work, in contrast to 37% of otherwise comparable trainees without this intervention. A list of readings for this course may be obtained from the course organizer, Dr. Raphael E. Pollock, Department of Surgical Oncology, M.D. Anderson Cancer Center, 1515 Holcombe Boulevard, Houston, TX 77030, USA.

Sachs and Siegler[157] describe a two-year "scientific integrity" program of lectures and seminars developed at the University of Chicago to provide a continuous opportunity for learning and discussing issues, values, and ethical norms in the practice of good science. A booklet on scientific integrity for researchers is available from the U.S. National Academy of Sciences (National Academy Press, 2101 Constitution Avenue NW, Washington, DC 20418, USA).[158] *Teaching the Responsible Conduct of Research Through a Case Study Approach* is a thorough case-based teaching manual with extensive annotated references, provided by the Association of American Medical Colleges.[159]

With Dr. Alexander Walt, we believe that "our immersion during residency training has the most enduring influence on the way we practice surgery over the next 35 years. This seminal experience encodes our attitudes toward our responsibilities, learning habits, new techniques, and adaptability to medico-societal changes."[1] We endorse his articulation of the constructive suggestion that ethical problems should be addressed and thoroughly discussed in surgical rounds and conferences as a fundamental part of surgical residency education. Research ethics should be a fundamental component of training for surgical research, just as formal and informal exposure to statistical methods has become an expected part of the researcher's education.

Conclusion

The opening quotation was a surgeon's reminder of the need for ethical reflection in the practice of surgery. A number of matters to which surgeon-investigators should give primary attention in planning and conducting clinical trials have been discussed, but there are many other issues that are just as important.

The most prominent of these issues might be the just distribution of burdens and benefits in the selection of patients as candidates for clinical trials; compensation for subjects injured in clinical trials; the requirements of clinical investigators' collaboration with institutional review boards or research ethics committees; the ethical conditions for terminating a controlled study; and the ethical dilemma of releasing interim results during the course of a randomized clinical trial. The discussion of these matters requires far more than the space that can be reasonably allocated to this chapter. The principle adopted was to offer in-depth discussion of the questions distinctively important for surgical trials rather than to attempt a more superficial treatment of many issues, however germane they may be to all clinical trials.

References

1. Walt AJ. Presidential address: the uniqueness of American surgical education and its preservation. ACS Bull 1994;79:8–20.
2. Pellegrino ED. The anatomy of clinical judgments; some notes on right reason and right action. In: Engelhardt HT Jr, Spicker SF, Towers B, eds. Clinical Judgment: A Critical Appraisal. Dordrecht-London-Boston: Reidel, 1979, pp. 169–195.
3. Bankowski Z, Howard-Jones N. Human Experimentation and Medical Ethics. Geneva: CIOMS, 1982.
4. Beecher HK. Research and the Individual. Boston: Little, Brown, 1970.
5. Freund PA, ed. Experimentation with Human Subjects. New York: Braziller, 1970.
6. Gray BH. Human Subjects in Medical Experimentation. New York: Wiley, 1975.
7. Katz J. Experimentation with Human Beings. New York: Russell Sage Foundation, 1972.
8. Levine R. Ethics and Regulation of Clinical Research. Baltimore-Munich: Urban & Schwarzenberg, 1981.
9. Shapiro SH, Louis TA, eds. Clinical Trials. New York: Dekker, 1983.
10. WHO and CIOMS. Proposed International Guidelines for Biomedical Research Involving Human Subjects. Geneva: CIOMS, 1982.
11. Sackett DL. Bias in analytic research. J Chronic Dis 1979;32–60.
12. Toulmin S. How medicine saved the life of ethics. Perspect Biol Med 1982;25:736–750.
13. Levine RJ. Clinical trials and physicians as double agents. Yale J Biol Med 1992;65:65–74.
14. Fried C. Medical Experimentation: Personal Integity and Social Policy. Amsterdam: North Holland, 1974, p. 151.
15. Green FHK. Quoted by Jackson DM. Moral responsibility in clinical research. Lancet, 1958;1: 903. This reference comes from Feinstein AR. Clinical biostatistics: XXVI. Medical ethics and the architecture of clinical research. Clin Pharmacol Ther 1974;15:320.
16. Gilbert JP, McPeek B. Mosteller F. Statistics and ethics in surgery and anesthesia. Science 1977; 198:684–689.
17. Silverman WA. The lesson of retrolental fibroplasia. Sci Am 1977;236:100–107.
18. Freedman B. Equipoise and the ethics of clinical research. New Engl J Med 1987;317:141–145.
19. Gail MH. Monitoring and stopping clinical trials. In: Mike V, Stanley KE, eds. Statistics in Medical Research. New York: Wiley, 1982, p. 455.
20. Bernard C. An Introduction to the Study of Experimental Medicine. Greene HC, transl. New York: Henry Schuman, 1949, pp. 101–261.
21. Engelhardt HT Jr. Bioethics in the People's Republic of China. Hastings Cen Rep 1980;10:8.
22. Department of Health and Human Services Rules and Regulations. 45 CFR 46 (Title 45: Code of Federal Regulations; Part 46), 46.111, (a) (3), here cited from: Levine RJ. Ethics and Regulation of Clinical Research. Baltimore-Munich: Urban & Schwarzenberg, 1981, appendix 1, p. 264.
23. McCarthy CR. Historical background of clinical trials involving women and minorities. Acad Med 1994;69(9):695–698.

24. Veressayev V. The Memoirs of a Physician. Linden S, trans.(Russian) New York: Knopf, 1916, here quoted from: Katz J, ed. Experimentation with Human Beings. New York: Russell Sage Foundation, 1972, pp. 291.

25. Merkatz RB, White Junod, S. Historical background of changes in FDA policy on the study and evaluation of drugs in women. Acad Med 1994;69(9):703–707.

26. Savitt TL. Medicine and Slavery: The Diseases and Health Care of Blacks in Antebellum Virginia. Urbana, IL: University of Illinois, 1978, pp. 297–298.

27. Pernick MS. The calculus of suffering in 19th century surgery. In: Leavitt JW, Numbers RL, eds. Sickness and Health in America. Madison, WI: University of Wisconsin, 1985, p. 100.

28. Ethridge E. Pellagra: an unappreciated reminder of southern distinctiveness. In: Savitt TL, Young JH, eds. Disease and Distinctiveness in the American South. Knoxville, TN: University of Tennessee, 1988, pp. 110–119.

29. Mitford J. Cheaper than chimpanzees. In: Mitford J, ed. Kind and Usual Punishment. The Prison Business. New York: Vintage Books, 1974, pp. 151–184.

30. Beecher HK. Ethics and clinical research. New Engl J Med 1966;274:1354–1366.

31. Brandt AM. Racism and research: the case of the Tuskegee Syphilis Study. Hastings Cent Rep 1978;8(6):21–29.

32. Ward R, Krugman S, Giles JP, Jacobs AM, Bodansky O. Infectious hepatitis: studies of its natural history and prevention. New Engl J Med 1958; 258:407–416.

33. Katz J. Experimentation with Human Beings. New York: Russell Sage Foundation, 1972, pp. 1007–1010.

34. Merkatz RB, Temple R, Subel S, Feiden K, Kessler DA. Women in clinical trials of new drugs. A change in Food and Drug Administration policy. New Engl J Med 1993;329:292–296.

35. U.S. Congress Public Law 103-43. National Institutes of Health Revitalization Amendment. Washington, DC, June 10, 1993.

36. Bennett JC. Inclusion of women in clinical trials—policies for population subgroups. New Engl J Med 1993;329:288–292.

37. Marshall E. New law brings affirmative action to clinical research. Science 1994;263:602.

38. Piantadosi S, Wittes J. Politically correct clinical trials. Control Clin Trials 1993;14:562–567. Letter.

39. Freeman HP. The impact of clinical trial protocols on patient care systems in a large city hospital. Cancer 1993;72:2834–2838.

40. El-Sadr W, Capps L. The challenge of minority recruitment in clinical trials for AIDS. JAMA 1992;267:954–957.

41. Brown LS. Enrollment of drug abusers in HIV clinical trials: a public health imperative for communities of color. J Psychoactive Drugs 1993; 25(1):45–52.

42. The Nuremberg Code. Trials of war criminals before the Nuremberg military tribunals under control council law, no. 10, vol 2. Washington, DC: Government Printing Office, 1949, pp. 181–182. Reprinted as Appendix 3 in Ethics and Regulation of Clinical Research.[8]

43. World Medical Association Declaration of Helsinki: Recommendations guiding medical doctors in biomedical research involving human subjects. Reprinted as Appendix 4 in Ethics and Regulation of Clinical Research.[8]

44. Anderston WF, Fletcher JC. Gene therapy in human beings: when is it ethical to begin? New Engl J Med 1980;303:1293–1297.

45. Cline MJ, Mercola KE. The potential of inserting new genetic information. New Engl J Med 1980; 303:1297–1300.

46. Gene therapy: how ripe the time? Lancet 1981;1:196–197. Editorial.

47. Grobstein C, Flower M. Gene therapy: proceed with caution. Hastings Cent Rep 1984;14:13–17.

48. Wade N. UCLA. Gene therapy racked by friendly fire. Science 1980;210:509–511.

49. Rutstein DD. The ethical design of human experiments. In: Experimentation with human subjects, Freund A, ed. New York: Braziller, 1970: 383–401.

50. Sackett DL. The competing objectives of randomized trials. New Engl J Med 1980;303:1059–1060.

51. Frederickson DS. Welcoming remarks, national conferences in clinical trials methodology. Clin Pharmacol Ther 1979;25:630–631.

52. Zelen M. A new design for randomized clinical trials. New Engl J Med 1979;300:1242–1245.

53. Feinstein AR. An additional basic science for clinical medicine. I. The constraining fundamen-

tal paradigms. Ann Intern Med 1983;99:393–397.

54. Feinstein AR. An additional basic science for clinical medicine. IV. The development of clinimetrics. Ann Intern Med 1983;99:843–848.

55. Katz J. "Ethics and clinical research" revisited. A tribute to Henry K. Beecher. Hastings Cent Rep 1993:23(5);31–39.

56. Woodward FP. Informed consent of volunteers: a direct measurement of comprehension and retention of information. Clin Res 1979;27:248–252.

57. Dickens BM. The modern law on informed consent. Mod Med Can 1982;37:706–710.

58. Reibl v. Hughes. 1980;2 S.C.R. 882.

59. Thornton H. Clinical trials—A brave new partnership? J Med Ethics 1994;20:19–22.

60. Baum M. Clinical trials—A brave new partnership: a response to Mrs. Thornton. J Med Ethics 1994;20:23–25.

61. Kluge E-HW. Informed consent and the competent patient. In: Kluge E-HW, ed. Readings in Biomedical Ethics, A Canadian Focus. Scarborough, Ontario: Prentice-Hall Canada, 1993, pp. 129–152.

62. Cancer Research Campaign Working Party on Breast Conservation. Informed consent: ethical, legal, and medical implications for doctors and patients who participate in randomized clinical trials. Br Med J 1983;286:1117–1121.

63. Fayerweather WE, Higginson J, Beauchamp TL, eds. Ethics in epidemiology. J Clin Epidemiol 1991;44(suppl I):1S–170S.

64. CIOMS. International guidelines for ethical review of epidemiological studies. Law Med Health Care 1991;19(3–4)(appendix I):247–258.

65. Tancredi L, ed. Ethical Issues in Epidemiological Research. New Brunswick, NJ: Rutgers University, 1986.

66. Bayer R, Levine C, Murray TH. Guidelines for confidentiality in research on AIDS. IRB 1984; 6(6):1–9.

67. Boe E. Pseudo-identities in health registers? Information technology as a vehicle for privacy protection. Int Privacy Bull 1994;2(3):8–13.

68. World Medical Association Declaration of Helsinki. Recommendations guiding medical doctors in biomedical research involving human subjects, here cited from: Levine RJ. Ethics and Regulation of Clinical Research. Baltimore-Munich: Urban & Schwarzenberg, 1981, appendix 4, p. 288.

69. Department of Health and Human Services Rules and Regulations. 45 CFR 46 (Title 45: Code of Federal Regulations; Part 46), 46.111, (a) (7), here cited from: Levine RJ. Ethics and Regulation of Clinical Research. Baltimore-Munich: Urban & Schwarzenberg, 1981, appendix 1, p. 264.

70. McCarthy CR, Porter J. Confidentiality: the protection of personal data in epidemiological and clinical research trials. Law Med Health Care 1991;19(3–4):240.

71. Meinert CL, Tonascia S. Clinical Trials. Design, Conduct, and Analysis. New York, Oxford: Oxford University, 1986, p. 164.

72. Beecher HK. Ethics and clinical research. New Engl J Med 1966;274:1354–1360.

73. Jonsen AR. Do no harm. Ann Intern Med 1978; 88:827–832.

74. Feinstein AR. Clinical biostatics. XLI. Hard science, soft data, and the challenges of choosing clinical variables in research. Clin Pharmacol Ther 1977;22:485–498.

75. Schafer RA. Ethics of the randomized controlled trial. New Engl J Med 1982;307:717–724.

76. Marquis D. Leaving therapy to chance. Hastings Cent Rep 1983;13(4):40–47.

77. Gifford F. The conflict between randomized clinical trials and the therapeutic obligation. J Med Philos 1986;11:347–366.

78. Hellman S., Hellman DS. Of mice but not men. Problems of the randomized clinical trial. New Engl J Med 1991;324:1585–1589.

79. Passamani E. Clinical trials—are they ethical? New Engl J Med 1991;324:1589–1592.

80. Johnson N, Lilford RJ, Brazier W. At what level of collective equipoise does a clinical trial become ethical? J Med Ethics 1991;17:30–34.

81. Botros S. Equipoise, consent, and the ethics of randomized clinical trials. In: Byrne P, ed. Ethics and Law in Health Care and Research. Chichester: John Wiley & Sons, 1990, pp. 9–24.

82. Gifford F. Community—equipoise and the ethics of randomized clinical trials. Bioethics 1995;9: 125–148.

83. Feinstein AR. Clinical biostatistics. XXVI, Medical ethics and the architecture of clinical research. Clin Pharmacol Ther 1974;15:316–334.

84. Dresser R. Book reviews: In: Dodds WJ, Barbara F, Orlans, eds. Scientific Perspectives on Animal Welfare. New York: Academic, 1982. Also in J Med Philos 1984;9:423–425.

85. Naverson J. Animal rights. Can J Phil 1977;vii: 161–178.

86. Regan T, Singer P. Animal Rights and Human Obligations. Englewood Cliffs, NJ: Prentice Hall, 1976.

87. Rowan AN, Rollin BE. Animal research—for and against: a philosophical, social, and historical perspective. Perspect Biol Med 1983;27:1–17.

88. Singer P. Animal Liberation. New York: Random House, 1975.

89. McIntosh A. Animal rights and medical research. Future Health, 1985;Winter:10–11.

90. Editorial. Animal experiments. Br Med J 1982; 284:368–369.

91. Lane-Petter W. The place and importance of the experimental animal in research. Proc R Soc Med 1972;65:343–344.

92. Russell JC, Secord DC. Holy dogs and the laboratory; some Canadian experiences with animal research. Perspect Biol Med 1985;28:374–381.

93. Bonchek LI. Are randomized trials appropriate for evaluation new operations? New Engl J Med 1979;301:44–45.

94. Chalmers TC. Randomized clinical trials in surgery. In: Varco RL, Delaney JP, eds. Controversy in Surgery. Philadelphia: Saunders, 1976, pp. 3–11.

95. Feinstein AR. The scientific and clinical tribulations of randomized clinical trials. Clin Res 1978; 26:241–244.

96. Haines SJ. Randomized clinical trials in the evaluation of surgical innovation. J Neurosurg 1979; 51:5–11.

97. Loop FD. A surgeon's view of randomized prospective studies. J Thorac Cardiovasc Surg 1979; 78:161–165.

98. Spodick DH. Randomized controlled clinical trials. The behavioral case. JAMA 1982;247:2258–2260.

99. Spodick DH, Aronow W, Barber B, Blackburn H, Boyd D, Conti CR, LoGerfo JP, Lown B, Mathur VS, McIntosh HD, Preston TA, Selzer A, Takaro T. Standards for surgical trials. Ann Thorac Surg 1979;27:284.

100. Van der Linden W. On the generalization of surgical trials results. Acta Chir Scand 1980;146: 229–234.

101. Feinstein AR. An additional basic science for clinical medicine. II. The limitations of randomized trials. Ann Intern Med 1983;99:544–550.

102. Feinstein AR. An additional basic science for clinical medicine. III. The challenges of comparison and measurements. Ann Intern Med 1983; 99:705–712.

103. Fisher LD, Kennedy JW. Randomized surgical clinical trials for treatment of coronary artery disease. Controlled Clin Trials 1982;3:235–258.

104. Merlo G. Surgical trial: possibilities and objections. Eur Surg Res 1984; 16:1–4.

105. Blindness in surgical trials. Lancet 1980;i:1229–1230. Editorial.

106. Van der Linden W. Pitfalls in randomized surgical trials. Surgery 1980;87:258–262.

107. Moore FD. Perspectives, surgery. Perspect Biol Med 1982;25:698–720.

108. Dudley HAF. The controlled clinical trial and the advance of reliable knowledge: an outsider looks in. Br Med J 1983;237:957–960.

109. Norman C. Clinical trial stirs legal battles. Science 1985;227:1316–1318.

110. Waring GO, Lynn MJ, Fielding B, Asbell PA, Balyeat HD, Cohen EA, Culbertson W, Doughman DJ, Fecko P, McDonald MB, et al. Results of the Prospective Evaluation of Radial Keratotomy (PERK) Study 4 years after surgery for myopia. JAMA 1990;263:1083–1091.

111. Radial keratotomy. Lancet 1990;335:1131–1132. Editorial.

112. Fyfe IM. The randomized clinical trial: panacea or placebo? Can Med Assoc J 1984;131:1336–1339.

113. EC/IC Bypass Study Group. Failure of extracranial-intracranial arterial bypass to reduce the risk of ischemic stroke: results of an international randomized trial. New Engl J Med 1985;313:1191–1200.

114. Spodick DH. Randomize the first patient: scientific, ethical, and behavioral bases. Am J Cardiol 1983;51:916–917.

115. Managing severe head injury—doing more and faring worse? Lancet 1980;i:1229. Editorial.

116. McKinlay JB. From promising report to standard procedure: seven stages in the career of a medical innovation. Milbank Mem 1981;59:374–411.

117. Fielding LP, Stewart-Brown S, Dudley HA. Surgeon-related variables and the clinical trial. Lancet 1978;ii:778–779.

118. Hill Sir Austin Bradford. Medical ethics and controlled trials. Br Med J 1963;I:1043–1049.

119. Esenberg L. The social imperatives of medical research. Science 1977;198:1105–1110.

120. Angell M. Patients' preference in randomized clinical trials. New Engl J Med 1984;310:1385–1387.

121. Brewin TB. Consent to randomized treatment. Lancet 1982;ii:919–921.

122. Sade RM, Miller III, Clinton M. Letter. New Engl J Med 1983;308:344.

123. Taylor K, Margolese RG, Soskolne CL. Physicians' reasons for not entering eligible patients in a randomized clinical trial of adjuvant surgery for breast cancer. New Engl J Med 1984;310:1363–1367.

124. Dudley HAF. Informed consent in surgical trials. Br Med J 1984;289:937–938.

125. Consent: how informed? Lancet 1984;i:1445–1447. Editorial.

126. Ellenberg SS. Randomization designs in comparative clinical trials. New Engl J Med 1984;310:1404–1408.

127. St. Augustine. The Confessions, book II. Ryan JK, trans. New York: Image Books, Doubleday, 1960, p. 287.

128. The Compact Edition of the Oxford English Dictionary. New York, 1971:1462.

129. Council on Scientific Affairs and Council on Ethical and Judicial Affairs. Conflicts of interest in medical center/industry research relationships. JAMA 1990;263:2790–2793. The Councils here use the definition of conflict of interest given in Webster's Third New International Dictionary.

130. Thompson DF. Understanding financial conflicts of interest. New Engl J Med 1993;329:573–576.

131. Rodwin MA. Medicine, Money, and Morals: Physician's Conflict of Interest. New York: Oxford University, 1993.

132. Perry CB. Conflicts of interest and the physician's duty to inform. Am J Med 1994;96:375–382.

133. Terry PB, Strauss M. The price of trust: conflicts of interest in medicine. Ann Allergy Asthma Immunol 1995;74:115–117.

134. Council on Ethical and Judicial Affairs, American Medical Association. Conflicts of interest. Physician ownership of medical facilities. JAMA 1992;267:2366–2369.

135. Council on Ethical and Judicial Affairs, American Medical Association. Guidelines on gifts to physicians from industry: an update. Food Drug Law J 1992;47:445–458.

136. Iglehart JK. Efforts to address the problem of physician self-referral. New Engl J Med 1991;325:1820–1824.

137. Relman AS. "Self-referral"—what's at stake? New Engl J Med 1992;327:1522–1524.

138. Wilkinson P. "Self-referral": a potential conflict of interest. The GMC should produce tighter guidelines. Br Med J 1993;306:1083–1084.

139. Elks ML. Conflict of interest and the physician-researcher. J Lab Clin Med 1995;126:19–23.

140. Kassirer JP, Angell M. Financial conflicts of interest in biomedical research. New Engl J Med 1993;329:570–571.

141. Frankel MS. Ethics in research: current issues for dental researchers and their professional society. J Dent Res 1994;73(11);1759–1765.

142. Gostin LO, Witt MD. Conflict of interest dilemmas in biomedical research. JAMA 1994;271:547–551.

143. Ellis SJ. Peer review and conflicts of interest. J Intern Med 1995;237:219–220.

144. Pitkin RM. Conflict of interest revisited. Obstet Gynecol 1995;86:293.

145. Smith R. Conflict of interest and the BMJ. Time to take it more seriously. Br Med J 1994;308:4–5.

146. Angell M, Kassirer JP. The Inglefinger rule revisited. New Engl J Med 1991;325:1371–1373.

147. Freestone DS, Miller R, Woodgush G, Pearl S, Pinching AJ, Sleight P, Partridge N, Richmond C, Goodwin P, Smith R. Supplemental Issue on Conflict of Interest. J R Soc Med 1995;88(suppl. 24):1–33.

148. Goldrick BA, Larson E, Lyons D. Conflict of interest in academia. Image J Nurs Sch 1995;27(1):65–69.

149. Emanuel EJ, Steiner D. Institutional conflict of interest. New Engl J Med 1995;332:262–267.

150. The PHS Regulation on Objectivity in Research. Federal Register. 11 July, 1995. Cited and summarized in: Mervis J. Conflict of interest. Final rules put universities in charge. Science 1995;269:294.

151. Rodwin MA. Physicians' conflicts of interest: the limitations of disclosure. New Engl J Med 1989;321:1405–1408.

152. Harvard University Faculty of Medicine. Policy on Conflicts of Interest and Commitment. Cambridge, Mass.: Harvard Univeristy, March 22, 1990.

153. Lock S. Research misconduct: a résumé of recent events. In: Lock S, Wells F. (ed.) Fraud and Misconduct in Medical Research. London: BJM Publishing Group, 1993, pp. 5–24.

154. Pellegrino ED. Teaching medical ethics: some persistent questions and some responses. Acad

Med 1989;December:701–703.

155. Sulmasy D, Terry P, Faden R, Levine D. Long-term effects of ethics education on the quality of care for patients who have do-not-resuscitate orders. J Gen Intern Med 1994;9:622–626.

156. Pollock RE, Curley SA, Lotzova E. Ethics of research training for NIH T32 surgical investigators. J Surg Res 1995;58:247–251.

157. Sachs GA, Siegler M. Teaching scientific integrity and the responsible conduct of research. Acad Med 1993;68(12):871–875.

158. U.S. National Academy of Sciences, Committee on Science, Engineering and Public Policy. On Being a Scientist: Responsible Conduct in Research. Washington, DC: National Academy, 1995.

159. Korenman SG, Shipp AC. Teaching the Responsible Conduct of Research Through a Case Study Approach: A Handbook for Instructors. Washington, DC: Association of American Medical Colleges, 1994.

Additional Reading

IRB. A Review of Human Subjects Research. This journal, edited by Robert J. Levine, was first published in 1979 and is now into its eighteenth volume. This journal tracks new and emerging ethical issues in the domains of research (clinical, behavioral, epidemiological, etc.) involving human beings.

Korenman SG, Shipp AC. Teaching the Responsible Conduct of Research through a Case Study Approach: A Handbook for Instructors. Washington, DC: Association of American Medical Colleges, 1994. The cases and annotated references in this handbook for instructors provide an excellent foundation for a course in research ethics.

Levine RJ. Ethics and Regulation of Clinical Research. 2nd edn. Baltimore-Munich: Urban & Schwarzenberg, 1986. This highly readable book covers all the major and recurring ethical issues encountered in the design and conduct of clinical trials. This book has become a standard reference work.

Lock S, Wells F, eds. Fraud and Misconduct in Medical Research. London: BMJ Publishing Group, 1993. This is a short, very well written survey, emphasizing examples in the pharmaceutical industry. Excellent general chapters on fraud and the editor, legal aspects, and a resumé of landmark cases of scientific misconduct make this book particularly interesting reading.

Thompson DF. Understanding financial conflicts of interest. New Engl J Med 1993;329:573-576. The clear thinking and language of this essay have made it a standard reference for discussion of this topic.

Commentary

Marc Siegler, America's foremost clinical ethicist, gives surgeons high marks for their ability to confront and resolve ethical quandaries on a daily basis. This chapter is not intended to address the broad range of issues in clinical ethics; it is narrowly focused on *research ethics*. An excellent source book for further reading in the general field of biomedical ethics is Beauchamp T.L. and Childress J. F. *Principles of Biomedical Ethics,* Oxford University Press, 1994.

M.F.M.

Commentary

Science once enjoyed an almost sacred status in Western culture. Like a secular religion, it was devoted to truth-seeking and universal communication of new findings to advance the common body of knowledge derived through the scientific method. This public perception of science was forever changed by Hiroshima, Nuremberg, and Tuskegee. It has been further damaged by misconduct related to conflicts of interest. Formal teaching of the values and principles of research ethics helps to strengthen the habits of mind and conduct that have always earned the best scientists an honored position in society.

H.T.
M.F.M.

CHAPTER 61

Scientific Integrity: Dealing with Scientific Fraud

P. Riis

Dramatic advances in informatics, imaging, and analytic techniques are dominating contemporary science. It is natural that attention is focused around what can be measured, described in numeric terms, reproduced, and analyzed. In this setting, science has deemphasized its foundational, cultural, and moral values.

At a time when tools for measuring, calculating, and transferring have never been so many and so efficient in medical research, it becomes more and more evident that fundamental values such as honesty, reliability, and social responsibility are *conditiones sine qua non* for all biomedical research. The eye-opening moral transgressions in science[1] have dramatized the need for a revival of ethical norms, analytical principles, and control *systems*, including education and review processes.

Definitions

Ethics can be defined in many ways. Here a pragmatic definition is used: the overall principles behind the pluralism of moral judgments in a given society.

Research is here defined as an endeavor to bring unrelated masses of information together, in order to answer a question related to the potentials of such an original combination. One of the masses can be known already, another created by the ap-

plication of a new method. The original question and the potential answer are linked by what is called *scientific methodology*, that is, the art of planning, carrying through, interpreting and publishing the results.

Research ethics within the health sciences is a *toto pro parte* expression, usually meaning ethics related to the security and respect afforded subjects involved in research, either as trial patients or healthy volunteers. Taken for its full meaning it ought to include also the ethics of the scientists, namely, the ethical norms involved in the research process as such, independent of any involvement of research subjects.

Scientific integrity is a widespread euphemism that covers good scientific standards in a moral, not technical sense. Outside such moral standards of science lie a variety of transgressions ranging from minor ones to fraud in the form of fabrication and plagiarism.

The Scope of Scientific Dishonesty

The term *scientific dishonesty* covers "all consciously fraudulent actions in the course of the application-research-publication process, and all instances of negligence so gross that they must be expected to form a corresponding strain on scientific credibility. In the last mentioned cases, it may also be difficult to disprove intent. In legal terminology, the above delimitation corresponds to the concepts of intent and gross negligence."[2]

The wide scope of scientific dishonesty is characterized by

> forgery or distortion of the scientific message or a false claim of the contribution of researchers. This includes deliberate:
>
> - Fabrication of data
> - Selective and undisclosed rejection of undesired results
> - Substitutions with fictitious data
> - Erroneous use of statistical methods with the aim of drawing other conclusions than those warranted by the available data
> - Distorted interpretation of results or distortion of conclusions
> - Plagiarism of the results or entire articles of other researchers
> - Distorted representation of the results of other researchers
> - Wrongful or inappropriate attribution of authorship
> - Misleading grant or job applications

Other types of dishonesty concern the scientific message itself only to a small degree, but rather concern the attempts of researchers to distort the perceptions in the surrounding world of themselves and their relations with other scientists through exaggerations or omissions:

- Covert duplicate publication and other exaggeration of the personal publication list
- Presentation of results to the public, thus bypassing a critical professional forum in the form of journals or scientific associations
- Omission of recognition of original observations made by other scientists
- Exclusion of persons from the group of authors despite their contributions to the paper in question[2]

Dealing with Suspected Scientific Dishonesty

Someone has to react to a suspicion, to blow the whistle, informing the scientific society that something might be wrong. This puts the *whistleblower*

in the center of an inquiry process. The whistle-blower could be a laboratory technician, a chief of a department, a colleague in the same department or laboratory, or sometimes a member of a competitive research group who has tried in vain to reproduce a set of postulated original results.

The closer the alleged transgressor and the lower the whistleblowers are placed in the local hierarchy, the more vulnerable they will be. The same rule applies if whistleblowers have to address themselves to the institution itself, and not to an independent national system. Experience has shown that whistle-blowers often suffer strongly from having acted with much moral courage. Instead of being appreciated for having done their moral duty, they are often stigmatized as traitors and condemned by the research community. This vulnerability is the reason for the decision of the Danish Committee on Scientific Dishonesty to accept anonymous allegations for serious scientific dishonesty, at least until the inquiry phase is ended. Agreement on this approach was reached reluctantly and only after consultation with legal experts. The negative side of anonymous denunciations is all too well known, but must be balanced against potential whistleblowers not acting due to fear. There is sometimes a paradoxical benefit. Bringing false accusations into the open enables an allegedly fraudulent scientist to be totally acquitted, bringing clarification that might otherwise be impossible in a jungle of rumors and gossip.

Once scientific dishonesty has been alleged, someone has to carry it through the *inquiry phase.* This could be an independent national system (a final solution foreseeable in all developed countries in the years to come) or an institution such as a university, another research institution, or a hospital. In very severe cases it can even be the nation's judicial authorities, if patients' lives have been put at risk by falsified statements about the treatment of life-threatening illness. A whistleblower would rarely take this longer step to civil or criminal proceedings, and police authorities and courts are not prepared to deal with such cases.

If the institution elects to deal with a case of alleged scientific misconduct, the following rules will help to avoid the consequences of the volatile and all too well known mixture of self-defense, guilt, and wounded vanity. The first person to be addressed by a whistleblower ought not to be the department chair alone, but a combination of the chair and a representative of the institutional president or a member of the board of trustees. Such dual arrangement will help to prevent "sweeping the problem under the rug"—a common reflex response to allegations of scientific fraud. The inquiry phase consists of correspondence with the accused and with all others involved, asking for their reactions and comments. Based on this material, the responsible authority decides if the case contains sufficient substance to necessitate a formal investigation.

The *investigation phase* should be run by an independent ad hoc group of competent persons whose impartial judgment the accused, the accusing, and the institution will accept. The material to be meticulously scrutinized by the ad hoc committee consists of raw data, research protocols, published articles, and other appropriate documents. The ad hoc group may perform control experiments or ask someone to do them. The ad hoc group ends its work by writing a report that is presented to the involved parties for comments. The commented report is then left to a national independent body for conclusion of the whole case, if such a body exists. Otherwise, the report goes directly to the responsible research institution for appropriate action. This might be complete acquittal of the accused person, probably accompanied by the issue of a public statement or press release stating the conclusion. Transgressions beyond reasonable doubt may result in real reprisals. These will vary according to the severity of the fraudulent behavior but might include the following:

- Warning or reprimand from the researcher's institution
- Transferral to other work or to another place of work
- Deprivation of public research funds, possibly for a specific period of time, and in more serious cases total or partial repayment of funding received
- Divestiture of the right to conduct university teaching *(jus docendi)*
- Divestiture of academic degrees in cases where scientific dishonesty directly affects the publications used as the basis for the award of the degrees
- Discharge or expulsion

Sanctions can be graduated as follows:

- Measures aimed at regulating conduct in cases which concern the borderline areas of dishonesty. Such sanctions must often be made conditional.
- Sanctions in effect for a period of time. Such sanctions should be employed in cases where the dishonesty evidenced is of a less serious nature which has not damaged the credibility of research nor had negative effects on patients.
- Serious and permanent sanctions which should be employed in cases that have had detrimental consequences for patients or groups of patients, or which have involved serious strains on society or seriously damaged research[2]

The Prevention of Scientific Dishonesty

As in other fields, prevention is better than punishment. All institutions involved in biomedical research ought to include courses in good scientific practice and research ethics as a part of the formal training of all young scientists. In this way excuses about not knowing can be eradicated.

Prevalence and Types of Real Cases

Based on a national system's experience, the prevalence of scientific dishonesty cases raised can be calculated to be approximately 1–3 per million inhabitants. All types of allegations appear. At the most serious end of the spectrum are allegations of fabrication of data or severe distortion in data calculations. Severe cases of plagiarism include word-by-word translations from a foreign language of a published scientific manuscript published locally, with a whole new set of authors' names, only discovered by chance by the original authors; or ghost-authorship represented by a ready-made manuscript without an author's name, sent to a reputable scientist asking him to be the author.[3]

At the other end of the spectrum one finds quarrels about priorities, sequence of authors' names in publications, and allegations of scientific dishonesty raised by pressure groups who do not like the results of published controlled trials that have cast doubt about a certain therapy. Attempts to misuse a national system to resolve petty or inappropriate issues must be resisted.

In the middle of the spectrum one finds cases of alleged unrightful authorship, disclosing this problem as a major one in the health sciences around the world. "The word *author* comes from Latin, *au(c)tor*, which means originator. If only the application of this term were in keeping with etymology, there would be no problems."[3] But there are problems.

> The increasing, now almost dominating, occurrence of group authorship which especially characterizes the health sciences has further contributed to inflate the scientific authorship so that a clearly dishonest use sometimes occurs. In many cases it only gives an illusion of the presence of a named originator.
>
> Why has it come to this? It started out all right and is based on a truth which still (beneath the sediments of substandard publications) is valid: professions which renew themselves through scientific methods must apply documentation of scientific originality and experience as an evaluation for appointments. But instead of being a qualitative criterion, it has become a monetary standard on the basis that if something is good, it must be even better to possess more. This development has also lead to a deterioration of the evaluation itself. If eight applicants are to be evaluated for an appointment, and several of them claim authorship to 150–300 articles, it is almost impossible to carry out a critical, in-depth evaluation.
>
> It is one thing to face the curse of quantity, but why does the risk of dishonesty occur? The answer is that in all known systems created by man, in which the competition is large and the unit of measurement is depersonalized or made anonymous, man is tempted to get more possessions by various short-circuiting manoeuvres. Therefore, in situations of strong competition within the health sciences—sometimes even real battles—for positions, grants and scientific pri-

orities, it is obvious that the general inflatory tendency not only increases and becomes more visible but that some people are tempted to obtain power through authorship even if the activity moves from the grey area of "bad scientific practice" into actual dishonesty.[3]

The International Group of Medical Journal Editors has tried to bring order, and consequently to reduce dishonesty, by defining *authorship* as the term is applied within the health sciences.

> All persons designated as authors should qualify for authorship. The order of authorship should be a joint decision of the coauthors. Each author should have participated sufficiently in the work to take public responsibility for the content. Authorship credit should be based only on substantial contributions to (a) conception and design, or analysis and interpretation of data; and to (b) drafting the article or revising it critically for important intellectual content; and on (c) final approval of the version to be published. Conditions (a), (b), and (c) must all be met. Participation solely in the acquisition of funding or the collection of data does not justify authorship. General supervision of the research group is not sufficient for authorship. Any part of an article critical to its main conclusions must be the responsibility of at least one author. Editors may require authors to justify the assignment of authorship. Increasingly, multicenter trials are attributed to a corporate author. All members of the group who are named as authors, either in the authorship position below the title or in a footnote, should fully meet the criteria for authorship as defined in the Uniform Requirements. Group members who do not meet these criteria should be listed, with their permission, under acknowledgements or in an appendix.[4]

Scientific Fraud in a Wider Societal Perspective

Fraudulent behavior is not confined to the health sciences or to our time. It has been identified throughout history in geology, physics, polar exploration, chemistry, and many other research disciplines and has commonly occurred outside the research sector. Norms within society interact with the norms of science. Young scientists bring their norms from school and home years with them into their scientific careers. If ethical transgressions are common in school, at home, and among friends, fraudulent behavior can be expected to be seen more often than if scientists are recruited from a society with strong moral norms. The underlying norms of honesty, reliability, and responsibility are prevalent ideals in society as a whole, and insure that most research is conducted and reported with very high standards. Only a minority deviate from these standards.

Advice to Young Biomedical Scientists

1. Beware of the very serious consequences that scientific dishonesty can have for patients, your institution, and especially for yourself.
2. Store all raw data meticulously according to the guidelines in Appendices 61-1 and 61-2.
3. If suspicion of scientific dishonesty arises in your laboratory or department, start by discussing the case with a good friend and colleague. Then go on to a national independent body if it exists, or to a superior distant from the institution, for instance, a scientific society. Bring your colleague and friend as an assessor. Unions and lawyers can come afterward.
4. Do what you can to restore authorship to its original dignity.

Advice to Leaders of Scientific Institutions

1. Include lectures and discussions on good scientific practice and research ethics in the formal training of the institution's young scientists.
2. See that all raw data are meticulously stored according to the guidelines in Appendices 61-1 and 61-2.
3. If suspicion of scientific dishonesty arises in your laboratory or department, start by dis-

cussing the case with the accused person. Then go on either to a national independent system if it exists, or to a colleague. After this bring the case in verbal form to the president or rector of the institution. Bring a colleague as an objective assessor.
4. Do what you can to restore authorship to its original dignity.

References

1. Lock S. Research misconduct: a résumé of recent events. In: Lock S, Wells F, eds. Fraud and Misconduct in Medical Research. London: BMJ, 1993, pp. 5–24.
2. Anderson D, Attrup L, Axelsen N, Riis P. Scientific Dishonesty and Good Scientific Practice. Copenhagen: The Danish Medical Research Council, 1992.
3. The Danish Committee on Scientific Dishonesty. Annual Report 1994. Copenhagen: The Danish Research Council, 1995.
4. International Committee of Medical Journal Editors. Uniform Requirements for Manuscripts Submitted to Biomedical Journals. JAMA 1993;269: 2282–2286.

Appendix 61-1.   Guidelines for the presentation of experimental records, research reports, data documentation, and data storage in basic research in the health sciences.

1. Experimental records must include date of entry, experimental classification number, and the identity of the person(s) responsible for the adequate storage of records and annexes in a way that all participants have direct access for a period of at least 10 years. The index to the record must be kept up to date. The person(s) responsible for the project are to be permitted to keep copies of the data after the termination of their employment.
2. Research records must be comprehensible and unambiguous for all involved, not only for those that plan and implement the experiments, but also for those who may later assess the results. Use standardized formats for the project's title, material, methodology, time schedule, basic documentation, and the calculations involved.
3. The general project description in the research record should be drafted prior to the implementation of the experiments so that there is sufficient time for

the preparatory work. The experimental report should be completed as soon as possible after the termination of the experiments and should include information on methods of calculation, any corrections, and the premises for such corrections, to the extent that is necessary for interpretation of the results obtained.

4. Experimental reports should be formulated in such a way that the experimental conditions can be reproduced even several years later and in other laboratories. It is therefore necessary to describe any new research objects, apparatus, chemicals, isotopes, and so forth when they are used for the first time.

5. Experimental reports must contain information on any mistakes or deviations from the work program planned and for the materials used. Such information can be decisive for assessing which data are to be excluded from the calculations. In addition, such changes in experimental circumstances can illuminate new aspects and, hence, be of scientific value. Any corrections made to the records must be carried out in such a way that the original data are legible.

6. The research reports' data must, as far as possible, contain the raw data in a form that is easily read, for example, as printouts of computer data, printouts of adhesive labels, plotters, automatic balances, meters, automatic analyzers, and calculators. Copies of key computer data should be entered in a joint database in the institution involved as soon as possible. The participant researchers can keep their own copies.

7. Annexes to the records should contain information on quality controls of crucial methods and data in the investigation and, where available, statistical assessments and results of pilot studies.

8. The experimental annexes must enable an assessment of whether the results can be reproduced and of statistical variations, both within each experiment and between different experiments. It must be possible to identify the original observations from the published data, for example, by record number.

9. It is the responsibility of the management of the research institute concerned, and of project supervisors, to ensure that the above guidelines are known to the parties involved. It is also a precondition of the implementation of projects that the researchers, supervisors, and other participants must inform each other as to the original experimental results and their processing and interpretation.

Appendix 61-2. Guidelines for the presentation of research plans, data documentation, and data storage in clinical and clinical-epidemiological research.

---

1. Research plans, questionnaires, case report forms, and other annexes must be comprehensible and unambiguous for all parties involved, not just for those who plan and carry out the research, but also for those who may later assess the results. Use a typewriter or word processor and a standardized presentation of the title of the investigation, the objective, methodology, procedures, raw data, and calculations for every investigatory plan.

2. Research plans should be presented sufficiently early to give time to test the practical utility of the case report forms, and to get necessary scientific and ethical approval.

3. Get the necessary approval of the scientific-ethical committee system, the appropriate data registration authority, radiation protection laboratory, health authorities, and other involved bodies. In addition, consent forms from the persons involved in the investigation may be followed up; this is also true of interview reports, questionnaires, and case report forms. All such documentation should be archived separately, not in case records. Anonymous codes must also be preserved to the degree that legislation so permits.

4. Research plans and annexes must contain sufficient information so that it is possible to assess whether a random sample is representative of the population in question. There should, therefore, be precise inclusion criteria for the persons investigated and conditions for entry, for example, whether it was planned to conduct the research consecutively. Conditions for drop outs should also be mentioned.

5. Data related to individuals in clinical-scientific research must be clearly identified, signed, and dated. Boxes that are not filled in should be crossed out.

6. The data in the case report forms must, as far as possible, contain the raw data in a form that is easily read, for example, as printouts of computer data, printouts of adhesive labels, plotters, automatic balances, counters, automatic analyzers, and calculators. Copies of key computer data should be kept in a joint database in the institution involved as soon as possible. The participant researchers can keep their own copies.

7. Annexes should contain the calculations carried out, including calculations of observation periods, corrections, and their premises, as documentation and to facilitate comprehension of the results achieved.

8. Information as to quality control of key data should be given and also which statistical methods and computer programs were used.

9. It should be possible to identify the original observations that are included in published tables and figures from the research annexes and the questionnaires.

10. It is the responsibility of the management of the research institute concerned, and of project supervisors to ensure that the above guidelines are known to the parties involved. It is also a precondition of the implementation of projects that the researchers and other participants must inform each other as to the original experimental results and their processing and interpretation.

Commentary

The National Surgical Adjuvant Breast and Bowel Project (NSABP) was featured in the second edition of this textbook (*Principles and Practice of Research: Strategies for Surgical Investigators*, 2nd edn. Springer-Verlag, New York, 1991) in chapter 29 on "Multicenter Collaborative Clinical Trials." Because the details are still being reviewed in court, we have elected not to attempt to analyze the prominent contemporary case of Roger Poisson at this time. We will return to the complex questions raised by "the Poisson affair" in a future edition.

M.F.M.

Commentary

Fifteen—certainly twenty—years ago nobody could have conceived of having a chapter and a commentary on this subject in such a book as this. To be sure, in history there had been alleged candidates for fraudsters, Newton, Pasteur, Mendel, and Cyril Burt among them, let alone the inspired archeological jape of Piltdown Man.[1] Yet the series of frauds emerging since 1975, when William Summerlin was found to have faked a graft of black skin in a white mouse simply by coloring a white skin transplant with a black felt-tip pen, has plunged academics into confusion, with politicians and the media forcing action on them in many countries. And, while mechanisms have been devised to deal with possible miscreants (though these are still being tinkered with as I write), there has usually been a tendency to neglect the far more important aspect of prevention, in particular, by emphasizing that the head of the department has to set standards (and especially eschew gift authorship).

Characteristically, such action has had to occur in the absence of one piece of crucial knowledge:

the prevalence of fraud. Cases in the public domain certainly number in the low hundreds, but most of us suspect that these are the tip of a deeper-than-usual iceberg. What we do know is that fraud (or misconduct, or dishonesty—all synonyms, given that the international community has still no agreed nomenclature for the phenomenon) has been reported in all countries undertaking major medical research. Surveys of scientists show anything between 10 and over 50% knowing of unaddressed suspected instances; audits of results in multicenter clinical trials disclose 0.25–0.5% that are crooked; and, despite a high profile, fresh cases continue to occur often in major departments in major academic centers (an average of six or seven cases coming to closure in every quarterly report issued by the U.S. Office of Research Integrity alone, for example).

To anatomize such cases further is to overturn some established shibboleths: we now know that forgery of data is far commoner than plagiarism, that the latter is often associated with abuse of a grant or editorial referee's access to confidential information, and that whistle blowers are still heavily penalized for their public-spirited approach to what is in reality a crime. I am still staggered by the amount of gift authorship disclosed by the investigation of papers that turn out to be based on fraudulent work; in particular, many heads of departments still assume a *droit-de-seigneur* in having their names put on papers reporting research they have had nothing to do with—indeed, couldn't have had, given that the work has never been carried out. One wag has likened this to claiming coauthorship of *Hamlet* because he happened to be around when Shakespeare wanted to borrow a pencil.

No country has done more to address this problem than the United States, though the Nordic countries with their statutory committees on scientific dishonesty run a close second. In particular, I warm to their recent distinction between crooks and jerks, because management so clearly has to be different. The crooks need a three-stage process of receipt, inquiry, and investigation, all carried out with due process (fairness to whistle blower and accused, total confidentiality, and speed), and preferably with some sort of extreme sanction for those found guilty (such as removal of the license to practice, as happens with the

---

[1]The fact that scientific fraud had also featured as a major theme in several works of fiction (Dorothy Sayers' *Gaudy Night*, Angus Wilson's *Anglo-Saxon Attitudes*, and CP Snow's *The Affair*) suggested that a little economy with the truth had always been a feature of academia.

General Medical Council in Britain). The jerks tend to operate in the middle of the spectrum between, at the one end, mistakes in good faith that all of us make (wrong observations, or wrong interpretation, for example) and, at the other end, undoubted crookery: clear-cut forgery, plagiarism, and piracy (the stealing of ideas). Jerks smooth curves, trim data, accept or confer gift authorship, publish the same article more than once in different journals without disclosing this, and split reports of a single good piece of research into several different subsets ("salami science"). So they need supervision of their research together with education in good research practice, in particular on the keeping and storage of data, authorship policies, and publication practices, and they need regular audit of their work.

The Nobel laureate Sir Peter Medawar considered that there were at least six causes of research fraud: the need to publish, for grants, tenure, or promotion; greed; vanity; mental illness; crookery; and the "Messianic complex," in which the scientist becomes so convinced of his solar-plexus ideas that he invents results to prove them right. As always, Medawar spoke wisely. As an editor, I have been amazed by the consistent link in one way or another between publication and episodes of fraud. Would, I wonder, there have been so many cases if the community had not chosen to evaluate its scientists by the *quantity* of what they publish rather than its quality? How can a profession go on excusing its well-loved and senior members (the "there but for the Grace of God go I" syndrome) who have strayed "merely" by putting their names on a report of research with which they have had nothing to do. To my mind, this is academic prostitution, deserving our obloquy and not our sympathy. Even though, at this *fin-de-siecle,* all Western societies are in a state of sleaze, with other professions such as the law and accountancy reporting similar practices to those going on in academic scientific research, is it too naive to call for a return to the concept of virtue in research? Povl Riis's paper points to the way to this Arcadia, and the Danish Central Research-Ethics Committee, in whose formation he had such a crucial role, is an exemplar of what can be achieved.

S. Lock

SECTION IX

Perspectives

CHAPTER 62

Pentathlete: The Many Roles of an Academic Surgeon

C.M. Balch, M.F. McKneally, B. McPeek, D.S. Mulder, W.O. Spitzer, H. Troidl, and A.S. Wechsler

The art and practice of academic surgery are mastered by defining and learning the pertinent basic principles and skills, and by practicing them under an experienced mentor. This requires a delineation of the personal qualities and professional skills needed to integrate surgical practice and investigation, and their attainment through an appropriately structured training program. This chapter discusses these qualities and skills, and the unique aspects of training that must be addressed by the academic surgical trainee in collaboration with his or her surgical program director.

The academic surgeon must exhibit the following:

1. Be an excellent clinical surgeon
2. Be willing to initiate and test clinically relevant ideas
3. Be a good communicator who willingly passes knowledge to others in an understandable way
4. Be highly organized and able to maintain an appropriate balance among professional and personal objectives
5. Have excellent interactive skills to facilitate research collaboration and fulfillment of administrative duties

Many have discussed the dilemmas faced by a surgeon in the university setting who attempts to acquire all these traits and master all these skills. In the words of William P. Longmire, "developing and maintaining the technical skills that will iden-tify an individual as a well-trained surgeon and at the same time qualify him or her as a scientist poses a greater challenge to surgery than to any other field of medicine."[1]

The diversity and multiplicity of challenges confronting the academic surgeon have become so great that the editors consider the pentathlete an illustrative analogy.

The Pentathlon Analogy

The modern pentathlon, an Olympic event, requires an individual athlete to be outstanding in five diverse athletic events: swimming, fencing, shooting, running, and riding—based on the skills required to qualify as a battlefield messenger in Napoleon's army. The critical characteristics of the pentathlete are personal strength, stamina, and commitment to excellence. The pentathlete is competitive in multiple areas but is not a record holder in events that are the single focus of other athletes.

Most successful pentathletes begin with a strong background in swimming and develop other athletic skills around that. In a similar way, academic surgeons build their careers around clinical skills. To achieve the level of excellence attained by someone who has chosen to focus on clinical surgery or laboratory research, the academic surgeon must be willing to spend extra time in training, and additional working hours as a faculty surgeon.

Athletes competing in the pentathlon have unique individual combinations of relative strengths, but their training and prowess must encompass all five arenas of competition. Their real field of competition lies in their versatility and ability to build a combination of strengths to a competitive level of performance in multiple areas.

The analogy is that each aspiring academic surgeon must follow a training program specifically designed to expand his or her unique combination of talents, interests, and developed skills. The effort and dedication required of each individual presupposes an honest self-assessment of relative personal strengths and weaknesses, and a willingness to develop a diverse set of skills with a high degree of initiative and self-determination. There is no stereotyped or uniform approach to becoming an effective and productive academic surgeon.

The pentathlon analogy is not perfect. Only a few can win the pentathlon, but most academic surgeons can be effective and productive in a personally rewarding way, if they prepare themselves well for the challenges and take full advantage of the opportunities around them. Those who train well and meet the challenges are all winners.

As discussed in the remainder of this chapter, several areas of professional and personal skill must be developed, perfected, and maintained to have a successful and rewarding career in academic surgery.

The Academic Surgeon as a Clinical Surgeon

Academic surgeons must, first and foremost, be excellent clinical surgeons, even though they cannot devote their time solely to clinical surgery. Because they are role models for surgical residents and medical students, they must not only display superb operative skills and techniques, they must also be compassionate and respectful in their interactions with other people.

Although excellence in clinical surgery is an essential prerequisite for success as an effective academic surgeon, we will not dwell on the training

of a clinical surgeon, since the purpose of this chapter is to describe the special features of training in other areas.

Willingness to Initiate and Test New Ideas

Ability to generate new knowledge relevant to surgical science and patient care is one of the most distinctive traits of an academic surgeon. It may be expressed through laboratory or clinical research, or a combination of the two.

Many surgical training programs emphasize scholarly acquisition of knowledge and skills, but surgical investigative trainees must also learn to be "constructive skeptics" about current scientific knowledge and standard surgical practice if they are to identify where opportunities for improvements and advances lie. They must be able to think "nontraditionally" and to channel ideas with clinical relevance into a series of formal investigations that will test them in a quantitative, analytical, and deductive manner.

Training to Be an Investigator

Because scientific methodology is the basis of evaluation and the medium of exchange of new ideas, it should be the centerpiece in the training of surgical investigators. The training program should focus on developing the ability to channel ideas into a formal, systematic scientific inquiry based on a hypothesis, a set of scientific objectives, and accepted and effective methodology for achieving the study's objectives.

What should trainees for academic surgical careers do to prepare themselves specifically for the unique challenges of their chosen careers?

A variety of pathways can lead to successful preparation for a career in academic surgery; many interesting options will suit some trainees better than others. Several programs proposed by the American College of Surgeons Conjoint Council on Surgical Research are outlined in Table 62-1.

A few core curricular requirements or fundamental courses essential to a scientific career should be incorporated in the formal/informal pe-

Table 62-1. Examples of proposed programs for training in surgical research (Conjoint Council on Surgical Research).

I	II	III	IV	V
PG1[a]	PG1	PG1	PG1	PG1
PG2	PG2	PG2	PG2	PG2
Research 1	PG3	Research 1	Research 1	Research 1/PG3
Research 2	PG4	Research 2	Research 2/PG3	PG4
PG3	PG5	PG3	PG4	PG5
PG4	Research 1	PG4	PG5	Research 2
PG5	Research 2	PG5	PG5	Research 2
Research 3	Clinical research	Research 3	Research 3	Research 3
Research 4		Research 4	Research 4	
Clinical research				

Post graduate year (PG)	Status
0	M.D. degree
1	Internship
2	Surgical resident
3	Surgical resident
4	Research
5	Research[a]
6	Surgical resident
7	Surgical resident (chief)
8	Basic/clinical research fellowship
9	Basic/clinical research fellowship
10	Basic/clinical research fellowship

[a]Board requirements met at end of PG5 year.

riod of training in scientific methodology; biostatistics and computer methodology are two of them, as indicated in the following list.

1. Statistics
2. Scientific writing
3. A basic science, such as molecular biology, immunology, and so on
4. Laboratory methodology
5. Use of computers
6. Research seminars
7. Public speaking as applied to scientific presentations
8. Grant writing
9. Scientific instrumentation
10. Teaching methods

For surgical scientists whose primary language is not English, developing a command of the English language is highly desirable for international exchange. For English-speaking scientists, development of one or more additional languages will facilitate and enrich their scientific communication skills. An adequate understanding of the language of computers and statistics is an absolute requirement for success in surgical science.

When should the trainee learn scientific methodology? Ideally, an aspiring academic surgeon should embark on learning the experimental method as an undergraduate or medical student and expand this work during residency training. For those who have not had an earlier opportunity to gain experience in research in a scientific setting, the period of research immersion should occur, ideally, upon completion of the first two or three years of surgical training. It is important to know whether an individual can perform proficiently in the clinical surgeon's role before committing resources, time, and energy to his or her training as a surgical investigator.

At the end of the second or third year of surgical training, the trainee is sufficiently flexible to derive maximum benefit from new experiences; subsequent surgical training will be enriched by the principles learned and the habits and attitudes developed in the laboratory. While flexibility and diversity are to be encouraged, deferring the period of scientific training until the end of surgical residency is not as desirable, particularly if the laboratory experience is to be divorced from hands-on surgical experience.

Where should training in scientific methodology be obtained? The most significant requirement is that the period of training in scientific methodology be an immersion in a milieu so organized that the scientific method is the dominant cultural and educational experience. The academic discipline and setting should be appropriate to the trainee's interests—a strictly surgical laboratory or such other departments as biostatistics, epidemiology, anesthesiology, immunology, anatomy, biochemistry, physiology, economics, or social science. Provided the standards of observation, hypothesis formulation and testing, analysis, critical review, and communication are high, the discipline is best chosen according to the interest and needs of the investigative trainee and the objective advice of his or her department chief or mentor.

Exposure to investigators who have different opinions and different approaches to solving problems in a given area of scientific inquiry is an important component of the surgical research training experience. *Visiting other institutions and laboratories, and meeting with visiting professors to discuss their distinctive perspectives on a problem of common interest are broadening experiences.* You will be surprised to learn how many different ways a given problem can be tackled.

Should the academic surgical trainee pursue a Ph.D. degree in basic science? Some trainees will find a Ph.D. program a sensible, enjoyable way to develop fundamental skills in scientific method. If you are facile at course work, enjoy examinations, are not deterred by thesis writing, and have an enthusiastic interest in the research and course work required for a doctorate in a given science, a Ph.D. program is an excellent route to developing a sound knowledge of scientific methodology. On the other hand, many highly successful surgical scientists and major contributors to fundamental science know that time at the laboratory bench, under the influence of an excellent scientist, can provide equal or possibly more appropriate preparation.

How do I support myself while I am learning scientific methodology? A variety of scholarships and research training fellowships are available through the National Institutes of Health in the United States, the Medical Research Council of Canada, and a variety of surgical organizations. They provide stipends to cover the trainee's living expenses and usually provide a small supplemental sum to the department for the support of the surgical research. They are generally available through such surgical organizations as the American College of Surgeons, the American Surgical Association, and others listed in chapters 42, 43, and 46. If the surgical scholar seeks out a department that fosters training in scientific methodology, departmental funds are often available to support appropriate candidates during prolonged periods of training in science.

The Academic Surgeon as a Communicator

The mere acquisition of knowledge is not sufficient; the knowledge must be communicated to the surgical and scientific community in an understandable way. Doing this requires oral and written skills, especially in English, which is now the primary scientific language.

The effective surgical investigator must know how to communicate with specific audiences in such varied settings as scientific and surgical meetings, seminars, and rounds. The role of educator requires the ability to communicate enthusiasm as well as knowledge. The dedicated surgical educator tries to arouse an interest in surgery in every student and then chooses those best suited to become surgeons.

Because the ability to assimilate meaningful information is an essential component of being a good communicator, the academic surgeon must have well-developed reading skills and be able to extract important conclusions from a wide array of frequently contradictory reports. The academic surgeon's skill in interpreting data and resolving major issues must be sufficiently sophisticated to allow the development of soundly based convictions and their courageous defense against opposition from any source.

Training to Be a Communicator

Writing and public speaking skills may come more easily to some than to others, but for most people they are the result of considerable effort. The rewards of such efforts are significant and will be garnered at scientific meetings and through published reports in the form of lucid, interesting, and effective communication with other surgical investigators. To develop skill in talking about scientific topics, start by speaking to small groups, informally; master the content and delivery of your talk before speaking to larger groups. Most of the authors of this chapter regard enthusiastic critiquing by their colleagues and mentors, in small groups, as the best preparation they ever had for the academic surgical life.

To learn scientific writing, begin with a relatively simple, straightforward clinical or scientific paper before attempting to write a complex scientific manuscript. In addition to language and writing skills, trainees must learn to use the formats required for abstracts and for scientific manuscripts destined for publication; the successful surgical investigator communicates effectively through surgical and other scientific journals. Whether you are choosing a journal or a meeting, think about the audience you wish to address. Select the audience that is not only the largest with an interest in your report but also the most creditable and respectable forum to which you can convey your new finding.

We recommend participation in courses in scientific writing and public speaking. Some surgical trainees have found that Toastmasters International, an organization that meets in most major cities throughout the world for the purpose of enhancing effective public speaking, provides a good learning experience.

The Academic Surgeon Must Be Highly Organized

Academic surgeons must be highly organized to fulfill their responsibilities for multiple simultaneous professional activities. Maintaining an appropriate balance among competing priorities requires emotional maturity and stability, and the ability to keep a clear set of goals and objectives in focus. To master the juggler's art of "keeping all the balls in the air," you must become and remain adept at setting priorities and delegating responsibilities.

A perspective derived from the frequent review of responsibilities and objectives must be the basis for setting and balancing priorities. You must weigh and take account of clinical versus scientific, institutional versus national, and professional versus personal responsibilities. Development of the ability to use time effectively and wisely and to sort the urgent from the important and prevent the former preempting the latter, is essential.

The following points will help you to learn how to be organized.

1. Look for role models. Analyze how busy, effective people organize their time.
2. Know your own strengths, weaknesses, and limitations. Have realistic expectations of yourself and others.
3. Have long- and short-range plans for all aspects of your professional activities.
4. Make your time meaningful by (a) identifying areas of wasted time, through time-motion studies if necessary, (b) developing the ability to dictate your thoughts clearly, (c) attending speed reading courses, and so on.
5. Write things down. Most of us keep a "do list" in our pocket or briefcase, on an index card, a sheet of paper, or on a tape in a pocket-size dictating machine. One of these should never be far away, day or night, so that thoughts can be captured as they come and before they evaporate.
6. Think constantly about priorities and delegations.
7. Maintain an appropriate balance between professional and personal life. Family and personal commitments are critically important. Develop areas and times for relaxation, such as hobbies, sports, and cultural and community activities.
8. Consider professional training in organizational and management skills.

We believe that family and personal commitments, including at least one relationship or friendship that is close and trusting enough to allow unburdening and sharing of very personal anxieties and aspirations, rank first among the important values to be maintained. "Burnout" is a not uncommon tragedy when rapidly rising successful young academic surgeons fail to maintain a balance in their personal lives, leading to turbulent periods of emotional instability or family disruption that undermine an individual's effectiveness in all areas.

The Academic Surgeon Must Have Interactive Skills

Multiple part-time responsibilities to collaborate in various clinical and scholarly activities demand significant interactive skills on the part of the academic surgeon. Success depends on maturity, humility, and the ability to delegate effectively. Learning to delegate is a form of training. You should arrive at an early appreciation of how to be an effective part-time, but wholehearted, coworker and learn how to establish effective, mutually beneficial partnerships in various areas of your professional life. In research, this usually means collaborating with full-time investigators within their departments or in basic science departments.

Think about the impact your activity will have on the discretionary time of the investigator and about the cost, to others, of the requests you make. Inspiring people to want to work with you requires a "give and take" personality. The successful academic surgeon strives to create "win–win" situations for all collaborators.

Learn to frame suggestions and delegations tactfully, positively, and constructively; cutting comments entail a cost! You must also learn how to challenge and criticize at the right time, in the right place, with the right approach. Insensitivity to the needs and feelings of others, or destructive public criticism, is especially counterproductive. Productive interaction presupposes a well-developed capacity for self-criticism and acceptance of constructive criticism by others. Learning interactive skills is a lifetime task in self-development.

Many of the topics just discussed are the subject matter of various books on managerial and leadership skills, but careful observation and consideration of how others work with and manage

people, either well or badly, will make major contributions to your acquisition of their most desirable characteristics. Try to see yourself as others do and listen to criticism given to or by others.

Character Traits of the Academic Surgeon

We are convinced that the skills of the academic surgeon must be developed in candidates who have basic character traits appropriate to this choice of career. *The effective academic surgeon must be intellectually honest, with deep personal integrity, as well as generosity in the art of helping others.*

1. Commitment to excellence—be willing to put forth extra effort. This requires extra stamina and dedication to follow through and complete all responsibilities, even at the end of a long day.
2. Determination and initiative. These qualities may be more important than intellectual brilliance.
3. Integrity and honesty.
4. Judgment and intuition.
5. Creativity (i.e., nontraditional and innovative thinking).
6. Analytical, quantitative, deductive thinking.
7. Curiosity.
8. Humility and grace, particularly in giving credit to others.
9. Emotional stability and maturity.
10. A compulsive attitude toward getting things done right, coupled with flexibility about the methods of implementation.
11. Patience and tolerance toward the imperfections and shortcomings of others and yourself.
12. Willingness to make financial sacrifices in exchange for intellectual and personal rewards.
13. Consistency.
14. Courage.

Conclusion

To achieve a unique composite of special skills, the pentathlete lives with the frustration of not being the best in any one athletic field. Becoming and remaining competitive as a pentathlete demands dedication to working on areas of least skill to achieve overall excellence. Most pentathletes find their athletic careers amply rewarding.

Those who have chosen academic surgery as a lifetime career are similarly content. The breadth of the experience and the diversity of the challenges combine to create an exciting, stimulating, and rewarding professional and personal life.

References

1. Longmire WP—Conjoint Council on Surgical Research. Reports of the Committees of Special Interest, 1986. Chicago: American College of Surgeons, 1986.

Commentary

The editors wrote this synthesis of our views of the life of the academic surgeon in 1990, while preparing the second edition. We agree with the values, principles, and spirit it expresses today, though we are sensitive to the increasing pressure for surgeons to devote more and more time to their clinical and administrative responsibilities. These pressures are making pentathlete academic surgeons as unusual as their athletic equivalents. The increasing complexity and depth of knowledge in cognate fields of basic science also requires more time for study and consecutive thinking. In deference to this change, Dr. Ori Rotstein has developed a new chapter (chapter 63) on the surgeon who maintains a basic science laboratory, and explains the program of training for surgical scientists at the University of Toronto.

When the "pentathlete" skills required of academic surgeons become so complex that combining them in a single individual may compromise each skill too much, a reasonable substitute is awareness and appreciation for the manner in which each of those skills contributes to the whole. The pentathlete has been largely replaced by a relay team.

M.F.M.
A.S.W.

CHAPTER 63

The Clinician with a Basic Science Laboratory

O.D. Rotstein

Introduction

In previous generations, the academic surgeon was the consummate clinician to whom the most difficult of surgical cases were referred for consultation on problems ranging from cardiovascular to gastrointestinal to endocrine systems. These individuals were invariably virtuosos of the scalpel and innovators of surgical technique, characteristics required to deal with the complexities of their surgical practices. In addition to their superior clinical abilities, academic surgeons were defined by their ability as teachers, researchers, and administrators.

The best of these academic surgeons combined their breadth of surgical knowledge with the ability to challenge the thought processes of their students. They were considered to be most effective teachers, and generally developed substantial schools of surgery that provided future leaders to the profession. The apprenticeship system of surgical training and the complexity of their surgical practices ensured that such individuals were given frequent exposure to students and more junior colleagues. The research laboratory was a natural extension of the surgeon's clinical practice. The pathophysiology of common clinical problems would be taken to the animal laboratory and unraveled using a combination of physiological and anatomical models. This new knowledge could

then be refined and readily translated back to the clinical situation, presumably resulting in improved outcome. The ability of academic surgeons to use their surgical skills to clarify pathophysiological principles in the animal laboratory and then carry them back to the clinical setting made research a natural extension of academic surgical practice. As leaders in their profession, these individuals participated vigorously in various organizational aspects of hospital and university activities.

In summary, academic surgeons of previous generations were the complete surgeons. They were the clinician-teacher-researcher-administrators whose combined skills allowed them to address all of the most difficult of surgical problems and provide definitive answers to many of them.

The Changing Environment

The mandate for academic surgeons of today is unchanged. To fulfill the requirements, they must be skilled clinicians, provocative teachers, innovative researchers, and accomplished administrators. In all areas, however, the playing field has enlarged substantially. In the clinical arena, surgical practice has evolved into a matrix of intense specialization. Even within a specialty area such as general surgery, it is now virtually impossible to be an expert in all aspects of surgical practice.

Similarly, the scope of biomedical research has undergone rapid expansion, particularly over the past two decades. To a significant extent, the shift has been away from physiology and toward the areas of cellular and molecular biology. Research methodology has become more technical and labor intensive. Competition for research funding and laboratory space has increased markedly. Most significantly, the concept of peer review has changed. Our peer group, no longer comprising surgeons alone, now includes the most fundamental of scientists. The complexities of being a surgeon-administrator have similarly increased in the present environment of fiscal restraint and managed care. This role is addressed in chapter 64, "The Academic Surgeon as Administrator."

The net result of this changing environment is the perception that most academic surgeons can no longer straddle clinical practice, research activities, teaching, and administration. Among these pillars of academic medicine, continued research productivity seems most threatened. The changes in the research environment have made it less natural for the physiological bent of the surgeon. Both the technical and intellectual aspects of the surgeon's abilities in the laboratory are stressed. The translation of clinical problems from the bedside to the fundamental study of cellular and molecular mechanisms of disease in the laboratory, and then translation back to the clinical setting, is a greater challenge than that presented to our predecessors, whose physiological research was a natural intellectual extension of their clinical activities. The technical aspects of research are less familiar and more demanding. Surgeons have a natural aptitude for the performance of surgical procedures in the laboratory, and the measurement of physiological parameters. By contrast, pursuing biochemical, molecular, or electrophysiological questions requires a skill set for which the surgeon is not trained. Further, the acquisition and maintenance of such skills combined with the need to remain up-to-date on current literature mandates commitment of a significant amount of time to research activities. While no precise data exist, this commitment seems to require more of academic surgeons today than was expected of previous generations, who might achieve outstanding success in all events of the "academic pentathlon" described in the previous chapter.

Managing the Changed Environment

Through redefinition of one's job description, the academic surgeons of today may be able to fulfill the mandate of the complete surgeon as defined by their ability to be clinicians, scientists, teachers, and administrators simultaneously. This is best accomplished through focusing of activities. Academic surgeons should strictly define their general area of expertise in the clinical realm and link it to an appropriate domain of basic science. For example, the colorectal surgeon with an interest in rectal cancer and its molecular biology should attempt to confine his or her practice to this area. This concentrated experience will develop intellectual and technical expertise in the field synergistically.

Academic surgeons can excel as surgical teachers without a change of context. They will serve as the local content experts in their specific area while maintaining a broad knowledge base in which their expertise is located. Focused interest and expertise will help to attract students, particularly at the fellowship level, to work with them. With their focus on investigation, surgeon-scientists are well equipped to serve as role models for future generations of surgeons. Their ability to pose new questions challenges students' thinking and propagates the stimulating concept that advances in clinical care are best achieved through challenging present dogma.

Maintaining an active research program in the face of responsibilities as a clinician and a teacher is the most significant challenge to an academic surgeon in the initial years on faculty. A multitude of definitions have been used to define the surgical investigator. At one extreme, there are individuals who devote the majority of time to research to the exclusion of clinical activities. At the other extreme, there are individuals who participate on the margins of research through occasional visits to a basic laboratory, or peripheral involvement in clinical trials. The actual definition of the surgeon-investigator rests significantly upon the local circumstances as defined by the expectations of the surgical chair and the institution.

The opportunities for surgeons as investigators in the present era are multiple. With the development of the science of clinical epidemiology over the past decade, clinical investigation has become far more rigorous. The role of the surgeon as a clinical investigator as well as an investigator in the area of health services and outcomes research is addressed elsewhere in this text. This discussion will focus primarily on the role of the surgeon as a fundamental biomedical scientist.

The competition for resources for basic science has increased significantly, challenging the ability of surgeons to establish themselves in this realm of research. In my opinion, surgeons can and must continue to do fundamental research. They are best qualified to define clinical questions, test them in the laboratory, and bring answers back to the clinical setting. Walter Ballinger suggested that "basic" research did not exist in surgery.[1] Whether this is true depends in part on one's definition of "basic." Surgeon-scientists are unlikely to be involved in studies that elucidate the fundamental mechanisms underlying DNA replication or regulation of ion flux. This does not preclude our use of such information and novel technologies to investigate clinically relevant problems in these domains, such as regulation of cellular proliferation in tumors or determination of intracellular acidosis during myocardial preservation. The surgical investigator uses fundamental tools to answer questions related to basic pathophysiological mechanisms of disease. This practice does not differ significantly from that carried out by our surgical predecessors, except for the fact that the tools and techniques of cellular and molecular biology are not as natural to the contemporary surgeon as those of anatomy and physiology were to surgeon-investigators of previous generations.

Training the Surgeon-Scientist

Several different models have been proposed for the optimal training of the surgeon-scientist. Important, largely unanswered questions include whether research training should be obtained during or after the residency period, whether obtaining a graduate level degree is beneficial, and whether optimal training should be sought in the laboratory of a clinician-scientist or a full-time scientist. The answers depend on the particular needs of the trainees and the university setting within which they are training. Regardless of the specific training route, it is clear that sufficient duration of training in the appropriate environment is an absolute requirement for success as an independent clinician-investigator. In his presidential address to the American Society for Clinical Investigation,[2] Dr. Joseph Goldstein coined the formula for success as a clinician-investigator: "fundamental discovery = clinical stimulus × basic scientific training." The daily problems facing the surgeon certainly provide sufficient stimuli for scientific inquiry. I will answer the question of what is the best mechanism for providing basic scientific training, based on the experience of our department.

At the University of Toronto, a formal surgeon-scientist training program has been in place for 10 years. Its goal is to provide excellent research training for surgical residents who wish to pursue a career in academic surgery. Residents who wish to participate in this program are excused from the clinical stream at the end of two or more years of core training in order to pursue research work. The research training period is formalized by the requirement to enroll in the graduate school of the university toward a degree at the M.Sc. or Ph.D. level. Supervisors may come from the Department of Surgery or other departments, and allocation of surgical residents to specific laboratories is based on the interests and long-term career plans of the individual trainee. Research programs may be pursued in the general areas of basic and clinical research, clinical epidemiology, or medical education. During the period of research training in the surgeon-scientist program, the surgical residents do not have regular clinical responsibilities. It is considered optimal for each individual to maintain contact with clinical activities by attendance at divisional, departmental, and hospital rounds as well as at formal teaching sessions. Trainees are also permitted to attend specialty clinics with direct relevance to their areas of research. Entry in the surgical scientist program is not mandatory for residents in the training program. However, the percentage of the resident pool enrolled is gradually increasing because of the attraction of the training program to individuals interested in pursuing a career in academic surgery, and an increasing number who elect to pursue a Ph.D.

Since its inception in 1984, 100 individuals have enrolled in this program. At the time of the most recent review, 20 residents completed their research and clinical training and were eligible for university faculty appointments. Eighteen (90%) had appointments at academic institutions; of these, 55% are independent investigators with external peer-reviewed funding. Eleven of these individuals have assumed faculty positions at our own institution.

These preliminary results of training in the formalized setting of a surgeon-scientist program provide evidence that this is an effective means of training individuals for a career as an academic surgeon. The high retention rate of these individuals within our own institution suggests that this approach represents an excellent means of faculty renewal. Further follow-up of these individuals and future graduates from the program is needed to verify this initial positive experience.

In addition to developing individuals who may be successful clinician investigators, the surgeon-scientist program has had a significant impact on the academic profile of the Department of Surgery in our institution. We have been able to recruit well-trained young faculty who have a profound commitment to research activities. The fact that most of the resident trainees do their research training in the laboratories of our surgical faculty has augmented the productivity of these laboratories. The definition of the program has raised the level of awareness of the role of the surgeon-scientist in the department. Other benefits include the fact that this program has attracted highly qualified applicants to the residency training program, and the productivity of the surgical trainees during their research training has improved their competitiveness for positions, either research or clinical, following the completion of the residency program.

The duration of research training correlates well with the ability of individuals to successfully compete for peer-reviewed funding. Levey et al.[3] suggested that 2 years of formal research training appeared to be a prerequisite for success in this process. However, the endpoint of an "active researcher" in this study was defined as someone who spent 20% of his or her time in research endeav-

ors, had one original publication in the previous 2 years, and had some external funding. Given the changes in the peer-review system in the 8 years since this paper was published, this number probably underestimates the required duration of training by at least 50%. In the context of the surgeon-scientist program at the University of Toronto, this would suggest that individuals completing the M.Sc. program would require additional training in research at the end of their clinical residency. The duration of this additional fellowship training would be 1 to 2 years. This relatively short period would presumably serve to focus the individual's activities in a specific area and to bring that individual up to speed with a view to establishing an independent research program. Those who obtain a Ph.D. degree, a process usually requiring 3.5 years, might choose to use the fellowship period for further research training or for specialized clinical training. Individuals who advocate delaying research training until completion of the residency program view this split in training as a major disadvantage, arguing that a concentrated and prolonged research program immediately prior to assuming a faculty position is the best preparation for success as an independent investigator. I believe that both approaches are workable, and the local situation may dictate what is preferable at a specific institution.

The initial 3 years on the faculty should also be considered as part of the training period for a successful career as a surgeon-scientist. During this reentry period, many young investigators have personal salary and research support that will sustain a research effort directed toward obtaining independent funding and establishing a productive laboratory program. The duration of this support should be a minimum of 2 years.[3] During this period, the young investigator must also learn to manage a laboratory. This includes hiring and managing new personnel, assessing and ordering new equipment, and simultaneously dealing with the rigors of translating new ideas into experimental protocols. All of this takes place in a new environment where the stresses of being a clinician and a surgical teacher are simultaneously present. This development clearly cannot be successfully achieved in isolation. Placement of new investigators within existing laboratory programs allows them to learn from the activities of others.

This approach reduces the stress associated with the complexities of establishing a research program, while providing an environment within which initial independent research activities may flourish. As the individual develops an active research program and is able to obtain peer-reviewed funding and independent publications, allocation of independent space might be appropriate. This approach also encourages the development of collaborative efforts with established investigators, a process vital to the success of surgical investigators.

At our institution, all new faculty sign a Memorandum of Agreement, a contract that clearly defines the commitment of the university to the individual, as well as the expectations for this individual during the first 3 years of appointment. For new recruits with a major commitment to research activities, we have developed a highly structured memorandum that defines protected time for research, time for clinical activities including operating room time, as well as the resource package such as laboratory space, startup funds, and salary support. The expectations with respect to research program development are outlined. This contract is reviewed on a yearly basis to ensure that all parties in the agreement are fulfilling their commitments. A formal university review of the new faculty member takes place at 3 years to determine whether the objectives outlined in the initial memorandum have been achieved. If so, the individual is granted a continuing appointment at the university. This is the equivalent of university tenure, as our Faculty of Medicine has no tenure stream. Two items mentioned in the memorandum should be highlighted. First, all new faculty are assigned a mentor, an individual who is named in the agreement. The mentor is expected to meet regularly with the new faculty member, act as an advocate and ombudsman, ensuring that all aspects of the memorandum are fulfilled in a timely fashion. The mentor attends yearly departmental reviews of progress and contributes to the evaluation and promotion process. Second, the memorandum contains a clear statement regarding the fact that all grant proposals by the new faculty are to be reviewed internally within the university prior to their submission. This requirement is based on the demonstration within our own institution that internally re-viewed grants have a higher probability of success at competitive peer-review funding agencies. To ensure compliance with this policy, participation in the process of internal review has been tied to the allocation of resources and is also a consideration at the yearly review of the individual's progress. A clearly constructed Memorandum of Agreement, by reducing hopes and expectations to written commitments, provides the contractual basis for the successful transition from promising new faculty recruit to established investigator.

The Challenge of Time Management for the Surgeon-Scientist

Owen H. Wangensteen crystallized the greatest challenge for the academic surgeon:

> One of the most important questions every Surgical Academician has to resolve is how best to divide his time among his many heavy and important responsibilities, of teaching, research, and patient care. Does he aspire to become known primarily as a talented operating surgeon or an effective teacher of undergraduate and graduate students, or innovative scientific investigator?[4]

Stephen Covey describes a steady evolution in the approaches to achieving optimal time management in business.[5] His "planning, prioritizing and controlling" formula is perfectly applicable to the needs of the academic surgeon. Through dogged determination, precise organization, and intense focus, today's surgeon is able to juggle the commitments to clinical, teaching, and research work required to achieve success as an academic surgeon.

Practice

Concentration of effort in a confined area of specialty to achieve excellence in clinical activities is best accomplished by participating in a group practice. Specific cases can be steered toward individuals with interest and expertise in that area.

Surgeons within this type of practice must agree to limit the scope of their activities to facilitate the function of the group. The precise amount of operating time required to achieve a high level of technical expertise has not been the subject of objective study. Several factors warrant consideration in this regard, including the innate abilities of the surgeon, the surgical specialty, and the types of cases performed by the individual. An informal poll of senior surgeons in our department indicated that 1–1.5 days per week of operating time is probably sufficient to maintain technical skills. Block scheduling of operating time on a weekly basis is mandatory to minimize wasted time. Some departments have utilized 3 consecutive days every 2 weeks as an alternative approach. During the early years on faculty, young surgeons should be encouraged to operate with more senior faculty on difficult cases to gain experience, enhance technical expertise, and minimize the pressures that may distract them from their research mission.

Time attending patients outside of the operating room must be regularly and strictly scheduled. One should attempt to see referred patients during a regularly scheduled day each week, and rounds on inpatients should be made at a defined time each day for a defined period of time. Extensions outside of these time slots should be minimized. Academic surgeons must also carve out scheduled time to attend multidisciplinary rounds in the area of their clinical specialty. This is vital for establishing referral lines that will promote specialized practice development.

While regimentation of clinical time will help to protect committed research responsibilities, it poses a difficult dilemma for the academic surgeon. How does one compete for clinical practice, while limiting the time spent attending to patients? The magnitude of this problem is heightened in the present era where pressures to generate clinical earnings are increased. Academic surgeons with job descriptions that include a significant commitment to research must have an institutional guarantee of personal salary support. In addition, they must be part of a practice plan wherein there is sharing of clinically generated earnings and clinical cases. Anxiety about financial security is not compatible with success as a surgeon-investigator, particularly for young faculty. However, the practice plan does not remove the requirement for practice development by an individual. The surgeon-investigators must simultaneously protect their research time, yet be accessible to referring physicians. Organization of clinical activities is essential. For elective outpatient consultations, patients should be seen during the same week, even if this means crowding or extending office hours. For urgent consultations, the academic surgeon must be immediately available to referring physicians to arrange the optimal time for the patient visit. Practice sharing with individuals with common interests in the same financial group helps to alleviate some of these problems. The importance of a capable clinical secretary in these situations cannot be overstated. This individual must be able to triage patients to the complete satisfaction of the referring physician's needs. Clearly enunciated guidelines for dealing with various situations are invaluable to the secretary.

Teaching

The surgeon-investigators have some clear advantages in terms of natural teaching skills. They are practiced in hypothesis-driven consideration of problems. This is an effective means of encouraging students to consider clinical problems in terms of what information is available, what is the likeliest diagnosis (i.e., generating the hypothesis), and what investigations are needed to prove the diagnosis (i.e., to test the hypothesis). This approach provides students with a well-defined template for the consideration of future problems. In a defined area of specialty, the surgeon-scientist can add a breadth and depth of knowledge for particularly challenging clinical problems and can pose insightful challenges to existing dogma where answers are unclear.

The actual amount of time spent teaching may limit an individual's contributions in this area. Clinician-scientists are frequently not perceived as excellent teachers by clinical residents because their time of exposure is limited. Several strategies may be used to overcome this problem. The surgeon-scientist should take advantage of time clearly committed to clinical activities. This includes time in the operating room as well as scheduled clinic time. Use the time exclusively and emphatically for teaching clinical skills. Do not bring a grant or a paper to the operating room to work on between cases. Use this time to communicate clinically with the residents, nurses, and other staff. In addition, the surgeon-scientist should aim to schedule a weekly session with the resident staff on the service. This committed time period can be used to discuss highly specialized but clinically interesting issues related to the investigator's particular area of expertise. The academic surgeon should encourage clinical projects among resident staff and medical students. This will provide an opportunity for the surgeon-scientist to teach the techniques of literature review, database management, evaluation of data, and the writing of abstracts and manuscripts. Combined together, these strategies will permit teaching commitments to be encompassed within the context of clinical activities, thereby optimizing time utilization, particularly with respect to commitments to research activities. Within our own surgical department, we have recently begun to evaluate teaching activities that take place within the context of laboratory work. The laboratory is an ideal setting for the surgeon-scientist to teach surgical residents research methodology and thinking.

The Laboratory

Having organized your clinical activities with a view to protecting research time, you are left with the multifaceted and broad-ranging challenge of running a productive and competitive laboratory. In addition to performing the research, you must manage the personnel, manage the budget, raise funds, troubleshoot equipment problems, and maintain excellent public relations. Similar to clinical activities, time in the laboratory must be used efficiently. A secretary or a laboratory manager will help offload some of the managerial aspects of being a principal investigator, but ultimate decision making must always rest with you. In the initial years in the laboratory, the surgeon-investigator should spend a significant amount of time at the bench performing studies. This work should be primarily focused on the development of new techniques, or ensuring quality control by the technical staff. As the laboratory grows and the staff becomes more established, surgeon-

scientists should relinquish much of this technical activity and use their protected time to read, write, teach, and think. Attendance at the journal club seminar series in your area of interest should have high priority. Time allocated for writing should be used for the completion of original manuscripts for submission to peer-reviewed journals. While writing chapters may help formulate your thinking, this practice should be considered a lesser priority. Authoring chapters will help to develop writing skills, to update one's knowledge in a given field, and may enhance practice development. However, their value in terms of enhancing one's scientific credentials is limited. The surgeon-scientist should limit chapter writing to high-impact publications, preferably state-of-the-art textbooks with wide circulation. Similarly, there is a temptation for young faculty members to join the speaker's circuit to promote their research and clinical activities. This practice distracts from the more important activities of developing your research program and should be minimized.

The Family

I have deferred discussion of time management related to the mechanisms whereby individuals involved in the rigors of academic surgery are able to devote adequate time to their own family life because I do not profess to have personally mastered this challenge. One comment clearly relevant to the issue of the academic surgeon and family time is used as the title of the first chapter of the book *First Things First* by Covey and colleagues[5]: "How many people on their deathbed wish they'd spent more time at the office?" Although the answer to this question is self-evident, we rarely remind ourselves to ask it. The strategies to achieve balance between home and work are nowhere clearly enunciated and not discussed enough in our conferences and conversations. Rather than address this issue directly, I will recommend Covey's book for definition of some of the principles for doing so. One important aspect of this challenge is the incorporation of maternity or parental leave into the modern surgical department. A clear policy statement regarding this issue should be integrated into the mission statement of surgical departments. Within our own institution, the policy states: "The Department of Surgery supports maternity leave for faculty members. Female surgeons must be permitted to take time off for childbearing (or adoption), without compromising their academic careers in the Department of Surgery." With this premise established, issues relating to job protection, income support, practice preservation, and academic promotion can be resolved along lines that protect the important role of the family in the life of the surgeon.

Essentials for the Surgeon-Scientist with a Laboratory

1. Train thoroughly in a well-developed program.
2. Reenter the scientific domain after senior residency with well-protected time.
3. Have a clearly written agreement specifying the obligations of the hospital and the department, to ensure adequate time, space, and support for the success of your laboratory effort.
4. Strictly define your clinical domain.
5. Clarify the linkage in this domain to laboratory research and maintain it.
6. Have a mentor in academic and in clinical work during the early years of practice.
7. Manage your time and control your schedule.
8. Do elective surgery in block time, not a random schedule.
9. Share your practice with like-minded surgeons.
10. Do not bring a grant or paper to the operating room. Use the time to teach and learn more about clinical surgery.
11. Protect time for your family life.

Conclusion

The challenges facing the academic surgeon have evolved over the years but still permit simultaneous contributions as a clinician, scientist, teacher, and administrator. Focusing clinical and research activities, combined with strict adherence to time management principles, is critical for achieving this goal. An institutional commitment to aca-

demic excellence enhances the probability that a surgeon be able to advance our understanding of disease, improve patient care and stimulate our students' thinking. Increasing numbers of women in the field of surgery, job sharing plans, and departmental programs designed to strengthen family life will encourage a more balanced and humanistic view of an academic career.

References

1. Ballinger WF II. Surgical research as a discipline. In: Ballinger WF II, ed. Research Methods in Surgery. Boston: Little, Brown, 1964, p. 3.
2. Goldstein JL. On the origin and prevention of PAIDS (Paralyzed Academic Investigator's Disease Syndrome). J Clin Invest 1986;78:848–854.
3. Levey GS, Sherman CR, Gentile NO, Hough LJ, Dial TH, Jolly P. Postdoctoral research training of full-time faculty in academic Departments of Medicine. Ann Int Med 1988;109:414–418.
4. Wangensteen OH. University selection criteria for future surgical leaders. Ann Surg 1978;188:114–119.
5. Covey SR. How many people on their deathbed wish they'd spent more time at the office? In: Covey SR, Merrill AR, and Merrill RR, eds. First Things First. New York: Simon and Schuster, 1994, pp. 17–31.

Commentary

Dr. Rotstein personifies the success of the surgical-scientist program at the University of Toronto. He lives by the recommendations in this chapter and manages a laboratory that is popular with surgical residents seeking an academic career.

The resolution of time management problems for academic surgeons is not taught well in residency. Like most academic residencies, the surgical-scientist program follows the tradition of total immersion of surgical residents in the laboratory-science phase of their training without any opportunity for continued contact and follow-up with laboratory colleagues during senior residency. Surgeons who emerge from the laboratory lose currency in their scientific field and must reestablish their linkages several years later at a time when they are establishing their clinical practices. Ideally, we would teach surgeon-scientists how to manage their time and fulfill both roles during the protected period of senior and chief residency so that the transition to postresidency life would be less arduous. To my knowledge no program has attempted this daunting task. If residents could return to the laboratory for only 3 hours per week, they would be able to maintain their mental linkages with the field they know so well when they leave it. Protected time for this purpose is an unrealized ideal at the University of Toronto and elsewhere throughout the world. It is not unrealistic, but it requires a shift in the thinking of all concerned with the responsibilities of the clinical years of residency.

M.F.M.

Commentary

The early years on a faculty for a surgeon who wishes to establish a fundamental research laboratory require all the elements discussed in Dr. Rotstein's chapter. These requirements for insuring success represent utilization of valuable resources. Institutions have the responsibility to limit resources to ventures with a high probability of success, and surgical investigators must be pre-pared to complete the research mission that they undertake. This almost certainly means specialized training prior to the time of faculty entry so that the higher institution "gets what it pays for." During the "start-up" years, administrative tasks should be shunned. Opportunities to enlarge your bibliography by writing reviews and chapters should be declined unless there is a clear-cut educational advantage that will be specifically helpful in the near term. The classic triad of clinical work, teaching, and research should be reduced to the two elements of research and practice. The immediate gratification of practice should be limited during the early years to allow investment of energy in establishing a research program, which generally brings almost no immediate gratification. It is critical that time for consecutive thinking and program development be invested in the early faculty years in order to achieve extramural funding. The academic surgeon's overall efficiency can be greatly enhanced by a supportive environment that includes an investment in physician extenders who can learn and maintain stable routines. Residents require and deserve teaching time and rotation to different clinical services. Because both of these requirements increase time demands on the young faculty member, residents are not ideal extenders for the academic surgeon during the developmental phase.

A.S.W.
M.F.M.

CHAPTER 64

The Academic Surgeon as Administrator

P.M. Walker and D.J. Anastakis

Academic surgeons have always been expected to excel as clinicians, educators, and researchers. The role of surgical administrator has been undervalued, and development of skills and experience in this domain of academic surgery has not kept pace with the growing need for effective surgical administrators.

Global changes in the delivery of health care now demand that some academic surgeons become as skilled in administration as they are in operative surgery. Most academic departments face radical changes related to continuing decline in available funding and increased pressure for fiscal accountability. Surgeons who become instruments of change and take leadership roles in the management process can ensure continued high-quality surgical care, education, and research. These surgeons can bring their highly developed attention to detail and reliable decision-making skills to the larger interface between the institution and society, defining priorities and taking responsibility for resource management. To succeed in this new and changing environment, surgical administrators must be proactive, creative, and well grounded in their knowledge of administrative methods.

The demands of an administrative position may conflict with the other academic responsibilities, trapping the surgeon in a cycle of increasing administrative activity and decreasing academic productivity. In this section, the principles and strategies that have been helpful in the administration of a large surgical department in a major university-affiliated teaching hospital will be provided. We will emphasize the skills and techniques that facilitate a successful blend of administration with other academic responsibilities.

Be Prepared

Formal training in hospital or business administration for all surgical administrators is absolutely necessary. This training should provide the surgeon with the fundamental knowledge and skills required for success in administration. Workshops or programs specifically geared toward clinician administrators are a more common and more feasible alternative to a full course of formal training. The principles of management and the development of problem-solving skills when faced with potential situational crises should be highlighted. In summary, the most important first step is being prepared, knowledgeable, and equipped to face the responsibilities of an administrative position.

Timing

When should an academic surgeon accept an administrative position? This is an important consideration for young academic surgeons focused on developing their clinical practice and research. An administrative role accepted too early on in one's career may adversely affect academic growth and development. We recommend focusing your initial efforts on the development of your clinical practice and research program. It is most important that you establish yourself as an expert in your chosen clinical and research domain. The skills developed from experience in clinical practice and in being productive in the research environment are invaluable to the surgeon-administrator. An established and respected surgeon is a good candidate for leadership, but accepting a major administrative post too late in one's career may be problematic. In today's environment, most positions now require new thought processes and endless energy.

Expertise

Establishing yourself as an expert in your chosen clinical and research domain is an important credential for a surgical administrator. The respect of the academic community is essential in order to be an effective leader and administrator. Your colleagues need to respect you as a clinician and researcher before they will follow your lead as an administrator.

Strategic Planning

As an administrator, you must have a vision of the overall direction your department should take. To effect change, a strategic plan is crucial, including outlining your goals and objectives along with the necessary actions required to attain them. Identify immediate, short- and long-term objectives and actions. Each action should have measurable outcomes associated with it. In measuring these outcomes, you will be able to monitor the effectiveness of your plan and act on problems that may develop.

A very important concept in the development of any strategic plan is "buy in" by all stakeholders. This can be accomplished by encouraging all parties to partake in the plan's development. In doing so, everyone feels ownership in the plan, and this facilitates the implementation of change.

Job Description

Before assuming any administrative position, secure a clear description of what is expected of you in your new role. Ask for a written description of what it is you are to do or accomplish. This is an important strategy. It will not only guide your actions but will be used to assess your effectiveness as an administrator.

Communication Skills

Open and effective communication skills are the hallmark of a good administrator. Clear communication prevents misconceptions from developing. A good communicator not only conveys information but is also a good listener. Listening to all the staff and colleagues you represent is vital to your success as an administrator. Effective communication is also essential in the clinical and research domains, allowing you to maintain vital links to all those involved in your clinical practice and research laboratory.

Strategy for Task Completion

As an administrator there will be numerous tasks for you to complete. Given the demands of clinical practice, research, and teaching, you will not be able to complete every one of these tasks personally. An overall approach that is productive and helpful for task completion is illustrated in Figure 64-1.

The first step in this strategy is to define the outcome that you desire as the administrator. The outcome you desire should be clear, precise, measurable, and in most cases a part of the strategic plan you have prepared.

The next step involves delegating the responsibility to an individual. Delegating a task represents more than just clearing your desk of work and responsibility. The individual(s) you choose to carry out the task have to be carefully selected.

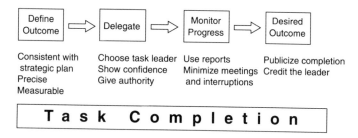

Figure 64-1   Strategy for task completion.

They represent you and carry responsibility for your success. They should possess the skills and knowledge you feel are required to complete the task. Express your confidence in their abilities, and respect for their authority. They also need to be empowered by you to complete the task without interference.

After assigning a task, you need to make it clear that you are available to provide additional information, help solve problems, and troubleshoot. The individuals working on the task need to know that you are responsive to their needs should any arise. Interruptions and endless meetings to check on progress are signs of ineffective management. Nevertheless, you do need to be abreast of all that is happening. Periodic progress reports allow the most effective use of your time. Completion of the task must be publicized with appropriate credit to the task leader.

Conclusion

As academic surgery continues to change, surgeons will assume very demanding administrative roles. This responsibility added to an already busy academic practice can be difficult to manage. This summary for the academic surgeon as administrator is very brief and does not purport to be a thorough overview of administration. We have provided a few of the most useful tips that can be helpful to any administrator in surgery, including those who continue to participate actively in clinical and laboratory research.

Additional Reading

Burrows M, Dyson R, Jackson P, Saxton H. Management for Hospital Doctors. London: Butterworth Heinemann, 1994. This is one of the few books that gives perspectives of both management and clinicians. At the end of most chapters, there is a section that tries to demonstrate the impact of management programs on the practice of medicine. This book is specifically related to a situation in England, which makes it somewhat less useful for North American readers.

Anthony RN, Young DW. Management Control in Nonprofit Organizations, 5th edn. Burr Ridge, IL: Irwin, 1994. This book outlines in great detail the financial management and control systems in place in hospitals. It provides all the information necessary for clinicians to understand the accounting processes within most hospitals, and should be read by all individuals interested in assuming a role in medical administration.

Commentary

The administrative position may allow you to develop your research with broader scope ("The eagle view of the pond, not the frog view" [Troidl]) and may even enhance the resources available for your studies. Be sure the terms for such an expansion are clearly and widely understood before you assume the leadership position, to avoid conflict of interest or resentment in the department. For most surgical researchers, graduating to an administrative position attenuates and modifies the research component of a surgical career to the role of team leader or coach. This transition is beneficial to younger researchers; the chief should not be in competition with fledgling investigators.

M.F.M.

CHAPTER 65

Surgical Research around the World

W. Lorenz, M. McKneally, and H. Troidl, with J.K. Banerjee, J. Benbassat,
C. Dziri, P.-L. Fagniez, J.M. Little, J. Wong, and H.R. Wulff

A Clearing Conference on Surgical Research from around the World

This chapter was written as a formalized inter-action of a group of surgeons and basic scientists from various countries to address some contemporary issues in surgical research. It was conducted as a conference through written questions. When we talk about consensus, we frequently, and paradoxically, mean totally different things.[1] H. Wulff proposed that we avoid this term altogether. We did not seek or achieve formal consensus; there was general agreement and clear disagreement on several issues.

Consensus conferences constitute a formalized process to seek advice about a complex decision problem (how to treat prostatic cancer, when and how to use blood and blood substitutes, etc.). The process of seeking and getting advice is organized by rules that are derived from a scientific, social psychological background[2] and intends to produce in a short time (usually a few days) as much agreement as possible between people of common sense and/or expertise about the complex decision problem. H.R. Wulff (personal communication) has criticized consensus conferences as artificial and of doubtful validity as far as real and long-lasting consensus is concerned. He acknowledges the potential benefits of formalized processes of putting

information, statements, and judgments together in order to present the problem in a clearer light, state the present positions of various people, define the deficits in agreement, and indicate where further research is needed. *Clearing the issues* at a given point of time is therefore considered a more useful term for such a process of seeking advice than *consensus*, and we think of the exchanges of ideas recorded here as a clearing conference.

Our objective was a survey on surgical research around the world: its aims, methods, content, and the group dynamics among academic surgeons and basic researchers. A questionnaire was developed after discussion by a steering committee comprising the first three authors. It was sent to a selected group of participants in January 1996. Some of the questions and answers were transformed into tables (Tables 65-1 through 65-4) from which the structure of the questionnaire can be understood. Letters explained some answers, revealing more details, judgements, and reflective consideration.

Twelve participants of the conference were selected by the steering committee. H. Troidl remained as an independent referee. M. McKneally—in addition to his steering functions—served for North America (USA and Canada), and W. Lorenz for Germany. Most commonly, surgeons were surveyed, one from each country. In addition, sociologists, surgical methodologists (theoretical surgeons[3]), methodologists in internal medicine (clinical theory), and philosophers were questioned. Three members who elected not to fill out the questionnaire were excluded from the analysis. All members of the conference were asked to consider first what would be the "typical" response of a person from their country, society, or culture to each of the questions, and thereafter present their own opinion. These two opinions sometimes differed.

Our approach to the problem of "surgical research around the world" is not perfectly representative and is certainly incomplete, but in the spirit of Popper or Reichenbach,[4] it may be considered as a hypothesis that we believe to be valuable for refutation.

Statement of the Clearing Conference on Surgical Research: How Much Is Heterogeneity Based on Cross-Cultural Differences?

Aims of Surgical Research (Table 65-1)

Primary Aims. All respondents counted "curing and caring through surgical management and techniques" as a primary aim of surgical research. The hierarchy of longevity > good health > quality of life persists in most countries surveyed. A balance between prolongation of life with good quality was described for Denmark. There seems to be increasing emphasis on quality of life in other countries. We were surprised that life prolongation was so highly valued in India despite

the widespread belief in reincarnation and renunciation. J.K. Banerjee explains, "Since renunciation is a voluntary effort, the person doing it does not feel miserable at all. Longevity is not linked to an achievement. The word that has been used is 'immortality,' which means continuing to live in the form of 'soul' after death without a physical body, as a part of the Supreme Being." Research on pain was viewed as a primary aim of surgical research by only four respondents: India, Tunisia, Australia, and Germany, suggesting underestimation of this problem by surgeons elsewhere[5] or its delegation to anesthetists.

J.K. Banerjee discussed the three stages of surgical research: (1) discovery of an idea, (2) development of the idea in the laboratory and hospital, and (3) delivery of the result to the people who need curing and caring. He criticized the Western world for not taking the third stage sufficiently into account. In India, a few institutions such as the Association of Rural Surgeons of India conduct research on new discoveries to manage surgical situations associated with India's socioeconomic restraint and cultural setting. If surgical research is to be meaningful around the world, then the benefits of research should be delivered not just to the 650 million people of the Western world, but to the 6 billion who make up the total global population. Bannerjee emphasized that *simplifying and innovating the means of delivery* should be viewed as a central aim of effective surgical research.

J. Benbassat of Israel suggests three aims: (1) The development of methods to evaluate how patients regard their future quality of life. These should be clear enough to be routinely applicable for individual patients.[6] Evaluation of quality of

Table 65-1. Aims of surgical research.[a]

Aims of surgical research	1 Ind	2 Isr	3 Tun	4 Fra	5 Aus	6 Ger	7 NAm	8 HK	9 Den
Curing and caring by surgical management techniques	+	+	+	+	+	+	+	+	+
Hierarchy: longevity > good health > good quality of life	+	+	+	0	+	0	+	+	0[b]
Good health defined by objective well-being criteria	+	+	+	0	+	+	0	+	
Quality of life defined by subjective criteria	+	+	+	0	+	+	+	+	
Role of pain in surgery	+	0	+	0	+	+	0	0	

[a] +, yes; 0, no.

[b] A balance between long life and a good quality of life.

life necessitates interpersonal skills and an involvement of the patient in clinical decision making. Medical decisions require an understanding of how patients view alternative treatment outcomes in order to insure their participation in the choice between management options.[7] (2) Use of *failure analysis* as a method of quality control focused on *why* the error happened, rather than *who* committed an error. Such methods correct system faults rather than eliminate poor performers. They identify problem-prone clinical processes and suggest interventions with a view toward making the health care system as "error-proof" as possible.[8] This primary aim has been strongly advocated by H. Troidl[9] and by Leape.[10] (3) Appropriate clinical guidelines should be generated. These should not be counterintuitive, formulaic rules that take the art out of clinical medicine, but effective means to reduce the disturbingly high rates of medical errors and health care costs.[11]

M. Little recommended attention to a more fundamental level: "There is far too little research being done on the *value-base* which justifies medicine and surgery and rationalizes assessments of quality-of-life and outcomes."[12]

Secondary aims. Secondary aims of surgical research might include advancement, fame, grants, wealth, or greater personal efficiency. M. Little expressed the unanimous opinion of our authors: "Research prowess does not translate into high income." The demonstration of efficiency (e.g., performing good studies, writing papers for high-impact journals) and garnering more financial support of research were viewed as significant secondary aims in most countries. Efficiency is becoming increasingly linked to the other secondary benefits, particularly in North America because of the industrial revolution overtaking health care. The pathway to advancement may be smoother for the proficient surgeon-manager than the productive surgeon-scientist in this setting. Outcome research and research documenting efficiency link the skills of the scientist and the manager.

Complexity. The service impact on society was identified by J.K. Banerjee as the specific aim of surgical research: "Health insurance and social security have failed to meet the surgical cost of nearly 5 billion of the world population. The specific aim of surgical research in any area is to develop surgical services for this category of people

by their contribution and the surgeons' innovation." This point is strongly supported by H. Gibbs.[13] We regard this, and all research that incorporates the interactive social, governmental, and cultural forces, as research in complex systems, requiring a departure from the deterministic or stochastic reductionism that has characterized much of surgical research.

Studying complexity was not identified as a specific aim of surgical research for the United States, Israel, Australia, or Germany. The trend toward simplification and linear thinking was summarized by M. Little: "The question about complexity as a specific aim is an interesting one. I think that one of the problems with surgical research in this country arises from a devotion to reductionism. We are very much in the thrall of the British and American empiricists, and I think that we have suffered from this by denying the importance of holism with all its attendant complexity."

Only J. Wong (Hong Kong) considered complexity as a specific aim for surgical research. Perhaps this is a cross-cultural difference. In their *Illustrated Guide to Chaos Theory*, Briggs and Peat[14] state that the first culture to investigate the interaction of order and chaos was China.

The dawning realization that complex systems can and should be analyzed by surgeons requires an important change in methodology, and a shift in our thinking away from linear thinking about unique molecules such as tumor necrosis factor or nitric oxide. A more holistic look at all interacting reactions will bring us closer to understanding the complex systems interacting in cells, organisms, and whole societies. The reductionist linear and stochastic models learned in the surgical laboratory may constrict the viewpoint of surgical leaders trying to solve large-scale problems in surgical services research and national health policy. This problem will be discussed further in the Commentary section.

Methods in Surgical Research (Tables 65-2 and 65-3)

There was no single research methodology that all participants unanimously agreed upon. The heterogeneity of views was greater than in any of

Table 65-2.   Methods in surgical research.[a]

Methods in surgical research		1 Ind	2 Isr	3 Tun	4 Fra	5 Aus	6 Ger	7 NAm	8 HK	9 Den
Scientific criteria	• Measurability	+	0	+	+	+	+	+	+	+
	• Repeatability	+	0	+	+	+	+	+	+	+
	• Avoidance of bias	+	+ +	+	+	+	0	+	+	+
	• Ethical soundness	+	+	+	0	+ +	+	+ +	0	+
Research disciplines	• Biomedical (e.g., molecular biological)	+	0	0	0	+	+	+	+	+
	• Clinimetric (scores, decision making)	+	+	+	+	+	+	(+)	+	+
	• Information science (networks)	+	+	+	+	+	+	0	+	
Approach to problem solving	• Laboratory (cells, animals)	+	0	0	0	+	+	+	+	+
	• Clinical trial	+	+	+	+	+	(+)	+	+	+
	• Thorough analysis	+	+	+	0	+	+	+	+	+[b]
	• Intuitive (surgery as art)	+	0	0	0	0[c]	+	+	+	0
Concepts of analysis	• Deterministic (one cause, one effect)	+	0	0	+	+	+	+	+	0
	• Stochastic (some probability)	+	+	+		+	0	+	+	+
	• Fractal (chaos related)	+		0		0	0	0	+	0
	• Intuitive	+	0	0		0	+	0	+	0

[a] + +, very important; +, important; (+), less important; 0, no.

[b] The first 3 are equally important.

[c] Australia is in contrast to the author, who very much appreciates intuitive (reflective) research.

the other parts of the survey, especially when the preferences for a methodology to solve a clinical research problem were asked for (Table 65-3). However, there was general agreement about the importance of such scientific criteria as objectivity, measurability, repeatability, avoidance of bias, and ethical soundness, reflecting the currency of determinstic and probabilistic analysis. Clinical problem solving in surgery included laboratory analysis (biochemistry, molecular biology) in all countries except Israel, Tunisia, and France.

Formal surgical decision analysis. Clinimetric methodology, including formal mathematical scoring and decision analysis, was accepted in all responding countries, but given different levels of importance. In Germany this approach is now considered equally important to all forms of biomedical research within the German Surgical Society; in the United States, clinimetric approaches are far less prevalent in surgery. The abstracts of the Society for Medical Decision Making from the United States are predominantly from internal medicine; only one group in surgery regularly participates (J.R. Clarke, Philadelphia). In Germany, surgical units dominate the contributions to the European Society of Medical Decision Making, just the opposite to the United States. This difference was documented in 1996 in the two country profiles for clinical research in *The Lancet*.[15,16]

The preference among surgical researchers for biomedical versus clinimetric methods in surgical research varied considerably between the countries (Table 65-3). J. Benbassat: "an emphasis on clinimetrics, decision sciences, clinical guidelines, observational analysis detects institutional failures that cause medical errors. Biomedical methods have secondary importance. The basic science of clinical practise is clinical epidemiology."[17]

M. Little saw a balance between biomedical and clinimetric data sorting. M. McKneally stated, "Biomedical methods still seem to predominate over clinimetrics and information science in the United States." The situation in Germany is similar to that in Australia.[15]

Controlled clinical trials. Clinical trials were al-

Table 65-3. How are research problems approached in your country?[a]

Country	Nomination and ranking
India	1. Invitation of surgical specialists for discussion 2. Invention of simpler techniques than those with high costs
Israel	1. Laboratory analysis 2. Thorough logic analysis
Tunisia	Controlled clinical trials
Australia	Controlled clinical trials
Germany	1. Laboratory analysis 2. Thorough logic analysis (Cartesian type) 3. Intuitive, expert analysis and controlled clinical trials on equal level
North America	1. Controlled clinical trials 2. Laboratory analysis
China (Hong Kong)	Controlled clinical trials
Denmark	Laboratory analysis, thorough logic analysis and controlled clinical trials on equal level

[a]Items of problem solving taken from Table 65-2. Preference expressed by ranking; no ranking means preference for only one approach.

most universally accepted (Table 65-2), but preferences differed (Table 65-3). In Germany, there is continued resistance.[15,18] Can the wide support described for controlled clinical trials be a reflection of personal bias, rather than the scientific conformity of all the countries including the Middle and Far East with the Western world? Or may it also reflect medical education that is strongly oriented to the Western world? These questions about the heterogeneity of "surgical research around the world" require research beyond this survey.

J. Benbassat denoted the avoidance of bias as the main methodological issue. The most frequent bias in surgical clinical research is the placebo effect of surgery, and selection bias—an argument stressed by H. Troidl.[9] Avoidance of these biases is fraught with methodological difficulties and ethical uncertainties for which methodologists have no ready solutions. M. Little emphasized the influence of strong teachers on Australian surgery:

> We have been obsessed by a statistical correctness in this country for many years, and a number of influential people, including Hugh Dudley, John Lubrook, and John Hall, have written extensively on good statistics in surgical research. The search for objectivity, numbers, and ways of treating numbers is therefore paramount in our clinical research. So is the design of trials.

Experience-based intuitive judgment. We found considerable cross-cultural difference of opinion about intuition.[19] In the German tradition, intuition was judged to be much more reliable ("the experienced clinician is usually right") than in the Western community ("intuition is distorted by misjudgment of probabilities").[19,20]

J. Benbassat: I am biased against the intuitive approach that regards medicine in general and surgery in particular as an art. This claim is only too often used as an excuse for an inability to explain to others "how I did it."

M. Little: We are still somewhat overconnected to determinism, but the national interest in statistics has made all researchers aware that most biological outcomes are stochastic rather than purely deterministic. The devotion to reductionism, however, still keeps people looking in a deterministic fashion, particularly in their laboratory investigations. I am aware of a few projects using fractal theory but neither fractals nor chaos have penetrated our surgical thinking much. I might detect a slight cultural problem with the word *intuitive*. In common parlance in Australia it means something like "inspired guess work." I think it has other philosophical meanings that are much richer. Many of my surgical colleagues are now starting to see that there is a real value in reflective research of the philosophical kind, as they meet problems that are not met by conventional models of ethics nor by the conventional reductionist approaches.

J.K. Banerjee: Intuition was highly valued by philosophers and their students both in China, India, Greece, and Egypt. And this was the basis of the entire philosophical and mathematical development in the earlier part of human civilization.

An individual analysis[19] and a group discussion forum[21] drew attention to a related difference between cultures: the German public and its clinicians very much dislike the term and concept of uncertainty,[22] whereas great parts of the Western culture revere *"the art and science of uncertainty."*[23] They understand uncertainty not as a threat, but as a status that one can comfortably live with. "Clinical equipoise,"[24,25] or a balance of conflicting opinions within the expert community, is the ethical prerequisite for a randomized trial.[15,22] The attitude to randomized trials differs between cultures, strongly influenced by different approaches to problem solving and concepts of analysis.[18]

Ethical correctness. The dominant influence of *research ethics review* was not reported from France and China. It was heavily emphasized in Australia and the United States, for different reasons.

> M. Little: The ethical movement in Australia is strong. We have been particularly influenced by Peter Singer from Melbourne and by numerous bioethical institutes that have sprung up in every major city. I am concerned, however, that much of the ethical deliberation is somewhat mechanistic. Nevertheless, there has been a welcome upsurge of interest in all levels in the last few years. The Royal Australasian College of Surgeons, for example, is turning its main plenary session at the next scientific meeting into a series of workshops on major ethical topics.[1]

> M. McKneally: Ethical correctness and occasionally excessive political correctness have become clear-cut concerns; for example, the National Institutes of Health requires that clinical studies be designed so that treatment effects can be evaluated among female patients and minority group members. This is a reaction, or perhaps an overreaction, to the exclusion of women in the childbearing years because of feared consequences to the fetus.

Ethical issues are also of concern in India.

> J.K. Banerjee: Ethics is a variable factor depending on a society's values at any given point of time. In the next National Conference of Rural Surgery here in India we are holding a sympo-

sium on ethical and legal issues in rural surgical practice in India. While our law forbids anesthesia being given without a qualified anaesthetist, a large number of rural surgeons are operating on emergencies by giving anesthesia themselves, out of the need to save lives of those who would otherwise die due to lack of transportation facilities. So what is ethical in a given situation in our world today is greatly dependent on available resources and human judgement.

Results of Surgical Research

Respondents were presented with a table listing the content (items) of surgical research and an array of fields of study such as oncology, infection, and perioperative risk to help formulate their thinking. Items listed were (1) techniques and technical aspects, (2) increase of knowledge about patients, (3) improvement of outcomes ("biological" equates with hard data), (4) improvement of outcomes ("clinimetric" equates with soft data, e.g., on quality of life, patient's expectations and satisfaction), (5) others (in order to stimulate new, innovative items).

The responses of the participants were remarkably uniform. The importance of outcome-related research was emphasized in all comments—and this is a dramatic change over the last 10 years. The importance of outcomes measured with clinimetric methods, of health status, quality of life, of outcomes expressed by patient's introspection and subjective judgment (data obtained by the qualitative, hermeneutic approach) was also emphasized in all comments—and this is again a dramatic change over the last 10 years! The three following comments illustrate this:

> J. Benbassat: The central importance of outcome research has been emphasized. I do not see any difference between so-called hard and soft measures. The main technique to be developed is the interpersonal skill whereby surgeons can elicit patients' preferences regarding quality of life. Perioperative risk research is my preference. Essentially, surgery is expected to be safe and effective. During the last decade, safety has improved dramatically. Anesthesia is an example of a clinical subspecialty that succeeded in reducing errors through continuous quality improvement,[8]

namely, through an analysis of errors and improved monitoring. The escalating frequency of negligence claims will be an additional motivation for the focus of surgical research on reducing perioperative risk and postoperative complications such as infections. I believe that the orientation to safety is foremost in importance.

M. Little: Australians still spend quite a bit of time investigating and reporting technical aspects of surgery. Their clinical research is very much aimed at practical outcomes and increased knowledge of patients and their diseases. What outcome research is being done depends both on biometric and clinimetric data. I am somewhat unhappy calling clinimetric data soft data, because it performs rather well in comparison to what is generally called hard data. I am personally very much devoted to concepts of further understanding societal values, by which we may better judge the outcomes of our surgical procedure.

M. McKneally: Techniques and technical aspects were once the dominant area of North American surgical research. Outcome evaluation is gaining precedence. There is less in-depth research about the real impact of interventions in patients lives and some confusion in the outcome variables measured; for example "return to work" is a complex endpoint, where motivation confounds the analysis. When serious illness such as cancer or heart disease results in a surgical intervention, the operation may frighten the patient away from further work or validate his claim that his illness is serious enough to stop working. I am currently looking at qualitative research techniques[26] to clarify the questions and answers on outcome from surgical interventions. This approach involves the use of focus groups and interviews emphasizing open questions. It provides a complementary source of information to quantitative studies. (See chapter 29 on "Qualitative Research.")

Group Dynamics in Surgical Research (Table 65-4)

Publication and language bias. "Political correctness" requires that certain questions not be asked in public. We thought that it was necessary to propose a few of them, because sometimes those questions were asked by journalists,[13] and because we consider them as interrelated with the aims and content of surgical research. We would neglect important influences if we were too polite. In the introduction to the questionnaire we defined a general policy, that we should not be so polite that we would not be able to find new hypotheses and refutations of current beliefs.

M. McKneally: There is a strong trend toward more publication of research from international sources in the surgical scientific literature of the United States, particularly in journals enjoying a large international circulation.

Imitation of the powerful leadership of the United States is present in the English-speaking countries, in Israel, and—in particular—Germany,[15] but quite typically not in France and the francophone society of Tunisia or in the very individualistic Scandinavian societies.

M. McKneally: Language problems have a definite impact in Quebec, where francophones do not have a suitable scientific journal as an outlet for their surgical research contributions in their own country. The French-speaking departments publish occasionally in the *Annales de Chirurgie* in Paris, but in general tend to publish in English for a wider readership in their own province and country. (A. Duranceau, personal communication)

The same issue, namely, that clinicians want to read clinical research in their own language, also influences publication strategies in Germany.[15]

Publication bias was not considered a problem by France and some other countries, but it was described in India, Germany, and China (Table 65-4). For example,

J.K. Banerjee: The rural surgeon is a victim of publication bias in our country and abroad. We feel this is because the delivery dimension of surgical research is ignored by surgeons of the developed world and their counterpart, the professorial surgeons of the developing world, with a few important exceptions.

M. Little: I think that we are the victims of a rather curious publication bias. Australians pub-

Table 65-4. Group dynamics in surgical research[a]

Group dynamics	1 Ind	2 Isr	3 Tun	4 Fra	5 Aus	6 Ger	7 NAm	8 HK	9 Den
Do language problems affect surgical research?									
• In reading	+	+	0	0	0	0	+	+	0
• In publishing	+	+	+	0	0	+	+	+	0
Do you feel you or others in your area are victims of publication bias?									
• In your country	+	0	0	0	+	+	0	0	0
• World wide	+	0	0	0	0	+	0	+	0
Do research teams create problems?									
• Loss of power by delegation?	0	0	0	+	0	0	+	0	0
• Should younger people work in lab, older in clinical trials?	0	0	0	+	0	+	0	+	0
Are international teams built in your area?	0	0	+	+	+	+	+	+	+

[a] +, Yes; 0, no.

lish very widely in the English language surgical journals around the world. Our output of publication is high. Our problem arises from the weighting assigned to surgical journals when research outputs are being assessed. Medical journals, such as *The Lancet* or the *New England Journal of Medicine* are weighted far more highly than any equivalent surgical journal. (See chapter 14 "Where Should You Publish Your Paper?") This means that a physician with the same or even a smaller number of publications will have higher publication weightings than his surgical colleague. This probably tells you that Australians are very prone to use formulae to measure outputs of this kind. I think that this is a real problem for surgical workers.

These comments have important implications: (1) Surgical researchers in countries or regions that do not belong to the English-speaking Western world adapt very much to the latter as a dominant culture, and do not find adequate means to express their own needs and feelings. (2) Surgical research is generally undervalued, a problem very much recognized in Germany.[9,15]

Participation in Trials. This section was developed from leading questions, for example, "Are there problems in creating research teams, such as losing power by delegation? Should younger surgeons work in the research laboratory, and older ones in clinical trials?" The latter question was stimulated by Vandenbroucke's provocative suggestion that

> progress in medicine is dependent upon young creative researchers who approach the problems with an abundance of novel ideas, while the final demonstration of the effectiveness of some therapy by randomised trials might be left to their burnt-out superiors who are only good for administration and organisation.[27]

Vandenbroucke was deliberately impolite, but he said what many basic scientists in the biomedical field think, and what many academic clinicians parrot, because of their inferiority complex toward "very basic research." H.R. Wulff refuted Vandenbroucke's challenge:

> The planning of randomised trials presents a *great intellectual challenge* and I disagree strongly with Vandenbroucke's remark. Young doctors should engage themselves in that type of research all over the world. I actually find it a scandal that surgeons introduced endoscopic surgery in the absence of evidence from properly conducted trials. . . . [Alleged] advances in medicine are no substitute for the accumulation of simple empirical evidence.

Respondents from France, Germany, and North America favored an individualistic approach, expressed in the comment of M. McKneally:

Large trial groups create authorship problems. These are poorly resolved by publication of very long lists of participants. Younger people tend to want to distinguish themselves through work in the laboratory following an old tradition, but in recent years more of them are seeking training in epidemiology and trying to gain leadership roles in clinical trials early in their careers.

The view is quite different in Australia.

M. Little: In this country, we do not really lose power by delegation, and I do not see that as a major problem. Each person has his own insecurities, and there are certainly some who decline to delegate. Nevertheless, I do not see those who delegate as losing power. I think this in part reflects the egalitarianism of this country. I would not necessarily assign just the younger people to the laboratory and the older to clinical trials. Some of our best laboratories have been run by very active researchers in their 60s.

It should be emphasized that almost all countries have a positive attitude toward international teams.[15]

Two answers to the question, "Is scientific terminology related to your culture?" should complete this section.

M. Little: There is no question that terminology is a problem between cultures. My comments on the word *intuitive* reflect this. European education stresses philosophy and the philosophy of science far more than ours does. In the United Kingdom, there is a reasonable strand of philosophy in school education, but there is practically none in Australia. For this reason discussion of conceptual matters can pose problems. Your (W. Lorenz's) mention of the word *theoretical* emphasizes this point. British empiricism dominates, and words like *dialectic* and *hermeneutic*[15,28] are almost unknown among surgical researchers in this country.

M. McKneally: Scientific or medical terminology does have cultural impact and specificity. The term *theoretical surgeon,* though well established in Germany since the time of Semelweiss, seems an oxymoron in English because of the strong emphasis on empiricism and practical applications in the conduct of surgery. Some other

words have excessive emotional overtones. The use of the word *client* to designate a patient enrages surgeons because of its connotation of market transactions that degrade the patient-physician relationship. *Rationing* inflames and confuses discussions of resource allocation despite its appropriate place in studies of expensive, innovative technologies.

Closing

The clearing conference on Surgical Research around the World was intended as a formalized procedure to exchange views among participants from different societies, countries, and cultures. The selection of topics and the structure of the questionnaire was clearly subjective and dominated by the steering committee, although the participants had many chances to escape its restrictions.

H.R. Wulff addressed three missing issues of the clearing conference:

There is a great need for classical randomized clinical trials in surgery and for meta-analyses of such trials. I know that there are still many who disagree with this point of view, but also many who agree, and I miss a detailed discussion of this issue. . . . I also miss critical discussions of technology assessment and quality assurance. I think that these are the main issues that must be faced by the international surgical community in order to harness the introduction of new technology.

In his preface to *Invitation to Social Psychology,*[2] Philipchalk drew attention to cultural influences on behavior.

This emphasis reflects a growing awareness among social psychologists that culture affects virtually everything we do. As modern communication and mass migration increasingly brings diverse cultures into contact, and multicultural societies struggle to cope with their diversity, the potential for cultural clashes is enormous. At the end of the twentieth century, understanding culture's impact is a very practical necessity.

The part that social psychology plays in medicine in general and in surgery in particular is not only social cognition, which deals with diagnostic and therapeutic decision making, but also prosocial behavior: helping others. Why and how doctors help the patients is a subject of great interest to social scientists.[2] Two interesting cross-cultural perspectives on this issue have been published;[29,30] L. Payer's[30] lively account is focused on surgery (bypass operations and hysterectomy) in four countries of the Western world. Cross-cultural and cross-national issues in clinical trials, especially in relation to quality of life and to pharmacoeconomics, are extensively covered in Spilker's second edition.[31] However, most of the articles refer to technical and methodological aspects and do not relate to clinical issues.

It is incumbent on surgeons to become familiar with these approaches, and to provide realistic appraisals based on their unique insights. As we have learned in assembling this chapter, there is a rich variety of viewpoints and values that can strengthen surgical research and practice.

Commentary: Reflections on Surgical Research around the World

Over the past 10 years, there have been three quite different editions of *Principles and Practice of Research*. The changes reflect the positive impact of research on the larger practice community and innovative developments in the conduct of research. In previous editions, there has been a strong suggestion that there are quite different forces that influence surgical research within different countries and cultures. This commentary is a reflective consideration of some of these forces.

1. *Globalized information.* Information about human beings has been globalized within a small frame of simultaneity, giving the impression that we have nearly achieved global unity through information.

- One of the consequences is an increased pressure to establish emotional equality among all human beings. Clinicians, for example, who visit colleagues all over the world, develop great personal sympathy for them. Thereafter when they watch disasters on television in areas they

are now familiar with, for example, in India, Philippines, China, or South America, they feel compassion toward these regions, not on a national level but on the level of the individual.

- A second consequence of international contacts is increased pressure to establish fairness in medical care and clinical research. This pressure probably arises from the painful fact made obvious by the information superhighway—that the presentation of discoveries and newly established knowledge at present is unbalanced because of domination by an elite group of First World countries.[13]

- A third consequence of the globalizing of information is awareness of the different ways in which people in the various societies, regions, countries, and cultures value and conceptualize health and scientific research.[19,32,33] The paradigms[34] of illness, risk, quality of life, and the theoretical and intuitive approaches to medical problem solving differ greatly, even in terms of etymology.[28] International partners in research from different communities sometimes despair that they will ever establish a common vocabulary, much less come to some form of research consensus. This issue prompted some of the language and conceptual probes we included in the questionnaire.

2. *Rise of molecular biology.* The explosive advances in molecular biology and particularly molecular genetics over the past 10 years has created a powerful influence over surgical research, promising solutions to some general problems of mankind, such as lethal sepsis, tumor development and progression, hypertension, autoimmunity—even physiological and pathological aging. As this new discipline attempts to explain its findings, it also creates its own highly specialized language and terminology, paradoxically isolating clinicians and inhibiting communication.

More importantly, it can lead to unrestricted reductionism[15] based on a purely mechanistic model of illness.[28] The dangers become obvious when preemptive surgery is recommended for genomic abnormalities, for example, prophylactic mastectomy in patients with *BRCA1* and *BRCA2* inherited susceptibility mutations, because they carry an increased risk for mammary cancer.[36] Exaggerated optimism based on belief in the benefits of technology shocks critical clinicians (Wulff et al.[28]). Technology can diminish compassion and awareness of the ethical requirement to "do no harm." It does not engender respect for the importance of the relationship between the patient and the doctor. These problems fall within the domain of social psychology;[2] we suspect that they will be handled differently in various countries.

3. *Outcome movement.* The outcome movement[37] is a more recent cause of paradigmatic shift urgently demanding changes in surgical research. There are two major factors responsible for this movement: the economic crisis of health care[37] and the demand and capability for performance of quality-of-life research.[38,39] Quality of life is now an important endpoint of studies in diseases with high mortality, such as cancer, and low mortality, such as gallstone disease. Outcome research also includes the analysis of individual choices between endpoints. The leading scientific methodologies used to carry this out are utility analysis[40] and cost-effectiveness analysis.[41] The values given to different outcomes of treatment vary in different human societies. As in the case of India, reported by Banerjee in this chapter, choices made under economical restraints have considerable influence on surgical research.

4. *Concept of complexity.* In contrast to the first three major sources of influence, it is less obvious how the "new" methodology of handling complexity forces us to alter and to broaden surgical research.

We are at the beginning of a scientific revolution, in the terminology of Kuhn;[34] some of its highlights have gained publicity and carry an emotional charge: *chaos* as a turbulent mirror of biology,[14] *complexity* as a new science at the edge of order and chaos,[42] *self-organizing systems,*[43] and, finally, *the science of wholeness.*[14] Despite this unfamiliar and somewhat poetic terminology, these new models and methodological systems offer us solutions for important unsolved clinical problems such as the management of sepsis,[44–47] the measurement of wound healing,[48,49] and assessment of the increased perioperative risk in senescence.[50]

Terminology. In order to understand the analysis of complexity, we have constructed a glossary of definitions that do not follow mathematics or formal logic (chapter 55). Popperian definitions are descriptive denotations of the term, with as

many specific attributes as possible. (See chapter 1, "Toward a Definition of Surgical Research").

- *Stochastic.* This attribute in a model of the real world implies the presence of at least one random variable (i.e., a variable with uncertainty). It describes concepts derived from statistics or from probability theory. The Greek root, *stochazesthai,* means to aim at a target; people dealing with stochastic processes tend to forecast future events, with the aim to be true, but to accept some calculated uncertainty or scatter. Much contemporary science relies on stochastic or statistical inquiries and analyses.

- *Deterministic.* This attribute in a model of reality implies that no random elements, only fixed elements, are included. Hence the future course of the system, as a prediction, is determined precisely by natural laws and the exact state of its components at some fixed time point. Deterministic systems are rigid, but usually more simple than stochastic ones. Determinists deny the existence of chance and emphasize the influence of laws and explicit causes.

- *Chaotic.* Chaotic processes are no longer considered to be expressions of irrationality. They follow rules that can be formulated by special nonlinear equations (e.g., $g(z) = z^2 + c$, from Mandelbrot[51]). The attributes for such processes (and therefore also predictions for an outcome in the future) are not one-dimensional, two-dimensional, and so forth. Parts between one and two or between two and three are called fractals obtained from repeated iterations of the nonlinear equations.[52] Chaotic processes do not accept the classical differentiation between stochastic and deterministic events (predictable with some uncertainty or with an absolute necessity), but combine them. Chaos is stochastic behavior occurring in a deterministic system. Chaos predicts that *very small causes* may elicit—by iterative processes—very severe effects (the poetic but not fanciful example often quoted is that the wing stroke of a butterfly in China might be the cause of a hurricane in the United States a few weeks later[14]). The analysis of chaotic processes provides a new way to approach the understanding of complex systems[53] and new models for the transition between regular and irregular behavior in physiological or pathophysiological systems such as ventricular fibrillation or septic shock.

- *Fractal.* Fractal models can be described as complex shapes (e.g., in wound healing[48,49]) that cannot be described by classical geometry with one (line), two (surface) or three (space) dimensions. Fractal analysis is derived from chaos theory; it uses the nonlinear equations mentioned previously. A fractal line has a dimension between a line and a surface, and a fractal surface has a dimension between a surface and a volume or space.[49] Other attributes of fractals include self-similarity, a very important attribute in chaos theory: at smaller and smaller scales similar forms (sets of variables) are repeated within the same shape.[49] Thus retention of complexity is guaranteed, whether on the molecular, cellular, whole animal, or clinical level.

- *Complex.* The simplest way to describe a complex system is that it is a great many independent variables (agents, effectors, mediators) interacting with each other in a great many ways.[42] This definition does not predict the model of handling the many variables, which might be stochastic, deterministic, chaotic, or fractal or something else. (See L.J. Cohen[54] for an excellent discussion of this point). The system in the real world (the patient in his clinical situation) is modeled (by the doctor, the nurses, the health managers) using particular items and the relations between the items. If the items and their relationship are affected by or change over time, the term *dynamic* instead of *static* systems is used.[55] This is usually the case in clinical situations. The more items and relations a system demonstrates, the greater is its complexity. Intricacy is an expression of the inhomogeneity of the items. In clinical practice, the complexity can be measured by clinical algorithms structure analysis (CASA).[56,57] Using the same clinical situation (e.g., anastomotic leakage after resection for colorectal cancer), the CASA values for managing the patient (case-related clinical practice guidelines) may vary from 19 to 168 units (Table 65-5). Com-

plexity and intricacy are important analytic concepts in our routine clinical world.

- *Intuitive.* Attributes of intuitive reasoning for diagnostic and therapeutic processes consist of multistage inferences with partly unproven steps.[19] Experience is essential for making intuitive decisions correctly; this was very nicely defined by leading information scientists, in the Dreyfus scale of clinical expertise[58] (Table 65-6). One attribute of complex systems, self-organization, fits very well with intuition: "In every case the very richness of these interactions allows the system as a whole to undergo spontaneous self-organization."[42] This statement supports experience-based intuition as a valid strategy of surgical decision making (see R.M. Hamm[59] for a contrasting view). This has important implications for cross-cultural attitudes to clinical practice guidelines[60] because it no longer places the experience-based intuitive judgment of the experienced surgeon at the bottom of the cognitive continuum for solving clinical inquiries and clinical research problems.[59]

Application of methodology. How can we use these models in finding treatments and predicting outcomes in complex clinical situations?[61] Let us look at sepsis, a frustrating problem. In contrast to optimistic predictions derived from reductionistic experiments of basic scientists,[62] the clinical reality in sepsis remains dismal. One randomized trial after another has failed to demonstrate reduction in mortality or morbidity.[63] Our classical reductionistic approach using deterministic cell and animal models (Koch-Dale criteria[52]) could not solve this problem. The jump to the next level of complexity, integrating diagnosis, scoring, operations, antibiotics, and intensive care in large, multicenter clinical trials applies the same deterministic, reductionistic thinking. We look for a single "magic bullet" such as a cytokine, antibody, or drug; but when we find one in the laboratory and test it in a clinical trial, we always fail to show effectiveness.[63]

An example. The example of adverse cardiovascular effects of antimicrobial agents in a clinical trial will help to clarify the complex interaction of stochastic and deterministic events. Two of us (W.L. and H.T.) were engaged in a randomized

Table 65-5. Measurement of clinical guidelines (algorithms) complexity.

a) *Seed algorithm:* Patient with colorectal cancer and postoperative leakage of anastomosis

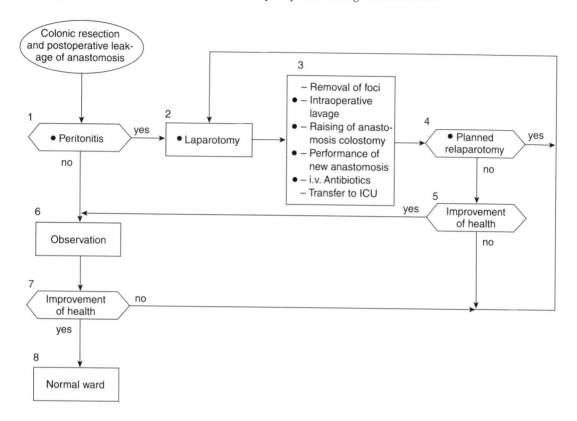

b) CASA Scores for case-based algorithms of individual centers on anastomotic leakage

Center (surgical clinic)		CASA score
Columbes-Paris	(France)	19
Cologne	(Germany)	20
Siegburg	(Germany)	20
Altötting	(Germany)	22
Frankfurt	(Germany)	29
Delmenhorst	(Germany)	29
Eindhoven	(Netherlands)	31
Bristol	(UK)	80
Brooklyn	(USA)	81
Hamburg	(Germany)	168
Seed algorithm (see above)		53

CASA (scores) $= 2\,D_x + D_0 + \sum_{i=1}^{n} L_i$, when D_x = number of decision box ($<\ >$), D_0 = number of all action and state boxes ($\boxed{}$), L_i = weighted sum of all boxes between loop origin and reentry, and n = number of loops. The seed algorithm was proposed from all individual centers for a consensus process in Marburg, January 7–9, 1997.

Table 65-6.   The Dreyfus Scale of Expertise (from Hilden[59]).

Stage	Characterization
Novice	The novice uses rules to pick out elements of a task and make simple decisions. When the car reaches a speed of 20 mph, it must be shifted into third gear. To interpret an ECG, first try to identify P waves and check their regularity.
Advanced beginner	The advanced beginner starts perceiving clusters of situational elements as a whole (the sound of the car engine or in the stethoscope), but must still rely on rules for making simple decisions.
Competent	The competent clinician has internalized most of these functions, but for high-level planning of diagnosis and treatment he or she must still rely on cookbook reasoning.
Proficient	The proficient individual handles tasks without hesitation or apparent effort. He does more than just drive the car: he simply goes where he wants to. She has acquired a flair for the important features of her task, while irrelevant ones recede into the background. (Flair may thus be acquired.) Even strategic ideas or hypotheses suggest themselves without conscious use of specific rules or heuristics, but major decisions are still analytical in many situations.
Expert	The true expert has internalized all aspects of the decision process. He or she sees the problem, sees the solution, and acts accordingly.

controlled trial[64] that included the measurement of histamine release in the perioperative period. A catastrophic event, cardiovascular collapse, was observed at unpredictable intervals. The clinical situation was complex, including an activated network of cytokines and an uncontrolled array of up to ten different drugs. Any of these factors might be contributory, but hypotension occurred unpredictably 10% of the time after prophylactic administration of cefuroxime with metronidizole.

We followed the classical approach of Descartes, who is not only one of the fathers of reductionism[65] but also of the analysis of complexity; "[I resolved] to direct my thoughts in an orderly manner, by beginning with the simplest and most easily known objects in order to ascend little by little, step by step, to knowledge of the most complex, and by supposing some order even among objects that have no natural order of precedence."[66] (See also chapter 1, "Toward a Definition of Surgical Research.")

We analyzed our clinical problem by modeling,[61] using animals, in vitro studies, and the intuition of experienced clinicians, to perform a Cartesian decomposition of the swirling mass of variables associated with sepsis and its treatment. Surely, within this complex array of treatments, effects, intentions, complications, expertise, and misfortune, there had to be deterministic, causal

components as well as random events. There was an intelligible summation of causes, but it did not lend itself to the usual reductionistic pharmacological analysis. Complex interactions of antibiotics and endotoxin, not simple direct effects, were detectable using isolated vascular tissue from the guinea pig aorta (Figure 65-1). The more the experimental model captured the conditions of the complex clinical scenario, the more predictable were the complications, even though we could not entirely explicate the causal network. Different antibiotics behaved differently. They elicited or modulated histamine-related and histamine-unrelated cardiovascular instability only in the complex experiment in piglets that modeled components of an anterior resection of the colon. Hypotension did not occur in the simpler experiment of intravenous anesthesia followed by intravenous antibiotics, a model more typical of pharmacologic reductionism, but not typical of the complex clinical situation in which hypotension was occurring unpredictably in our trial.

The lessons we derived from this experience included the following:

• A realization of the accuracy of Nobel prize winner J.W. Black's insight: "It must be axiomatic that all biochemical events are occurring

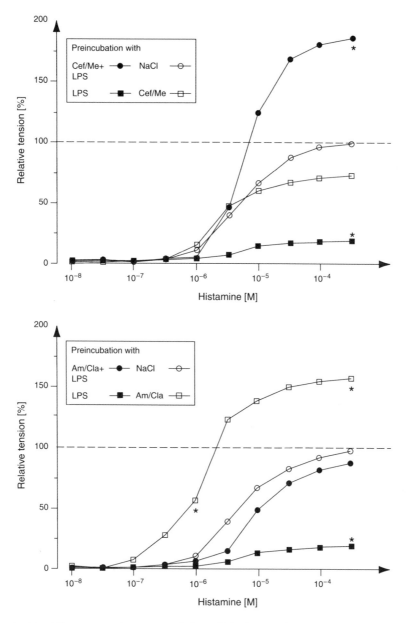

Figure 65-1. Isolated tissue experiments modeling clinical complexity. Concentration-effect curves of histamine concentration in the organ bath fluid and contraction of guinea pig aortic rings. Mean values from 8–12 experiments fro each of the doses used in the experiments. (a) Influence of cefuroxime-metronidazole on vascular contraction is shown, but works only in combination with LPS. (b) Influence of amoxicillin/clavulanic acid on vascular contraction is shown but does not work in combination with LPS. *$p < 0.05$, t-test. From Künneke et al.[61]

instantaneously, in parallel, so that, potentially, every chemical event could be influenced, however remotely, by every other event."[67]

- Recognition that seemingly random events within a controlled, logically predictable system reflect a chaotic order we do not fully understand, but can eventually explicate. Like the example of the seemingly random contours of a coastline, ultimately explained in chaos theory as a summation of multiple predictable causal factors, our incomprehensibly complex clinical situation began to yield a logic we could begin to comprehend.

- Greater understanding and respect for the role of the clinician in the basic science laboratory, as a guide to relevant issues and components of complex unsolved clinical problems, not simply a primitive user of reductionistic biomedical methods.

Sepsis, cancer, trauma, cardiovascular disease, and the myriad clinical problems facing surgical researchers around the world will not yield to randomized trials, nor to Bayesian approaches, Markov processes, or reductionistic searches to isolate single molecular causes.[52] The paradigm of surgical research is shifting toward a more holistic analysis, seeking to understand a multitude of contributory factors, including societal and cultural influences, that we are just beginning to take into consideration in our studies.

Acknowledgments. Supported in part by a grant from Deutsche Forschungsgemeinschaft Ba 1560/2-2 and the Lucerne Study Group on Sepsis.

References

1. Lorenz W, Troidl H, Fingerhut A, Rothmund M. Introduction—the different ways to reach consensus. Eur J Surg 1996;576(suppl):5–8.

2. Philipchalk RP. Invitation to Social Psychology. Fort Worth, Philadelphia, San Diego: Harcourt Brace College Publishers, 1995.

3. Lorenz W, Rothmund M. Theoretical surgery: a new specialty in operative medicine. World J Surg 1989;13:292–299.

4. Reichenbach H. The Rise of Scientific Philosophy. Berkeley, Los Angeles: University of California, 1951.

5. Neugebauer E, Troidl H. Meran conference on pain after surgery and trauma. A consensus conference on various clinical disciplines and basic research. Theor Surg 1989;3:220–224.

6. Tsevat J, Weeks J, Guadagnoli E, Tosteson AN, Mangione CM, Pliskin JS, Weinstein MC, Cleary PD. Using health related quality of life information: clinical encounters, clinical trials and healthy policy. J Gen Intern Med 1994;9:576–582.

7. Kassirer JP. Incorporating patients' preferences into medical decisions. New Engl J Med 1994;330:1895–1896.

8. Berwick DM. Continuous improvement as an ideal in health care. New Engl J Med 1989;320:53–56.

9. Troidl H. Surgical research. Lancet 1996;348:1637–1638.

10. Leape LL. Error in medicine. JAMA 1994;272(23):1851–1857.

11. Gottlieb LK, Margolis CZ, Schoenboum SC. Clinical practice guidelines at an HMO: development and implementation in a quality improvement model. Qual Rev Bull 1990;16:80–86.

12. Little M. Humane Medicine. Cambridge: University, 1995.

13. Gibbs WW. Mißachtete Forschung der Dritten Welt. Spektrum der Wissenschaft 1996;82–90.

14. Briggs J, Peat FD. Turbulent Mirror. An Illustrated Guide to Chaos Theory and the Science of Wholeness. New York: Harper & Row, 1989.

15. Lorenz W. Worse or just different. Lancet 1996;348:1638–1639.

16. Brook RH. Practice guidelines: to be or not to be. Lancet 1996;348:1005–1006.

17. Sackett DL, Haynes RB, Tugwell P. Clinical Epidemiology: A Basic Science for Clinical Medicine, 2nd edn. Boston: Little Brown, 1991.

18. Lorenz W. Attitudes to controlled clinical trials. Lancet 1982;i:1460–1461.

19. Gross R, Lorenz W. Intuition in surgery as a strategy of medical decision making: its potency and limitations. Theor Surg 1990;5:54–59.

20. Abernathy CM, Hamm RM. Surgical Intuition. Philadelphia: Hanley & Belfus, 1995.

21. Lorenz W, Hobsley M, Dudley HAF, Pollock AV, McPeek B, Habermann E, Healy MJR, Hilden J, Elstein AS, Cohen LJ, McPeek D, Janich P, Fox R, Gross R, Rothmund M. Discussion forum on intuition in surgery as a strategy of medical decision making: its potency and limitations. Theor Surg 1991;6:74–109.

22. Lorenz W, Ohmann C, Immich H, Schreiber HL,

Scheibe O, Herfarth C, Feifel G, Deutsch E, Beger HG. Patientenzuteilung bei kontrollierten klinischen Studien. Chirurg 1982;53:514–519.

23. Hamm RM. Clinical intuition and clinical analysis: expertise and the cognitive continuum. In: Dowie J, Elstein A, eds. Professional Judgment. Cambridge: Cambridge University, 1988.

24. Lindenschmidt T-O, Beger HG, Lorenz W. Kontrollierte klinische Studien: Ja oder Nein? Aufgaben und Grenzen kontrollierter klinischer Studien (KS) aus der Sicht des Chirurgen. Chirurg 1981; 52:281–288.

25. Freedman B. Equipoise and the ethics of clinical research. New Engl J Med 1987;317:141–145.

26. Denzin NK, Lincoln YS. Handbook of Qualitative Research. Thousand Oaks: Sage, 1994.

27. Vandenbroucke JP. Is there a hierarchy of methods in clinical research? Klin Wochenschr 1989;67: 515–517.

28. Wulff HR, Pedersen SA, Rosenberg R. Philosophy of Medicine. Oxford, London, Edinburgh: Blackwell Scientific, 1986.

29. Gergen KJ, Morse SJ, Gergen MM. Behavior exchange in cross-cultural perspective. In: Triandis HC, Brislin RW, eds. Handbook of Cross-Cultural Psychology, vol 5. Boston: Allyn & Bacon, 1980, pp. 121–153.

30. Payer L. Medicine and Culture. New York: Henry Holt, 1988.

31. Spilker B. Quality of Life and Pharmacoeconomics in Clinical Trials, 2nd edn. (Cross-Cultural and Cross-National Issues, vol. 7) Philadelphia, New York: Lippincott Raven, 1996, pp. 575–585.

32. ARC, Hay J-M, Fingerhut A, Michot F. French vocabulary terms of sensitivity expressed as percentages. Theor Surg 1993;8:181–193.

33. Hilden J, Hilden M. Comment on French vocabulary terms of sensitivity expressed as percentages. Theor Surg 1993;8:187–192.

34. Kuhn TS. The Structure of Scientific Revolutions, 2nd edn. Chicago: University of Chicago, 1970.

35. Lewontin RC. Biology as Ideology. The Doctrine of DNA. Concord: Harper Perennial, 1991.

36. Holtzman NA. Testing for genetic susceptibility to common cancers: clinical and ethical issues. Adv Oncol 1997;13:9–15.

37. Relman S. Assessment and accountability. The third revolution in medical care. New Engl J Med 1988;319:1220–1222.

38. Troidl H, Menge K-H, Lorenz W, Vestweber K-H, Barth H, Hamelmann H. Quality of life and stomach replacement. In: Herfarth C, Schlag PN, eds. Gastric Cancer. Berlin, Heidelberg: Springer Verlag, 1979, pp. 312–317.

39. Eypasch E, Troidl H, Wood-Dauphinee S, Williams JI, Reincke K, Ure B, Neugebauer E. Quality of life and gastrointestinal surgery—a clinimetric approach to developing an instrument for its measurement. Theor Surg 1990;5:3–10.

40. Clarke JR. A scientific approach to surgical reasoning. Theor Surg 1991;6:166–176.

41. Sox HC, Blatt MA, Higgins MC, Marton KI. Medical Decision Making. Boston, London, Durban: Butterworths, 1988.

42. Waldrop MM. Complexity. The Emerging Science at the Edge of Order and Chaos. New York, London, Toronto: Simon & Schuster, 1992.

43. Yates FE. Self-organizing systems. In: Boyd CAR, Noble D, eds. The Logic of Life. Oxford, New York, Tokyo: Oxford University, 1993, pp. 189–218.

44. Bone RC. Let's agree on terminology: definitions of sepsis. Crit Care Med 1991;19:973–976.

45. Pilz G, Fateh-Moghadam S, Viell B, Bujdoso O, Döring G, Marget W, Neumann R, Werdan K. Supplemental immunoglobulin therapy in sepsis and septic shock—comparison of mortality under treatment with polyvalent i.v. immunoglobulin versus placebo. Theor Surg 1993;8:61–83.

46. Solomkin J. Sepsis as a descriptor, not a disease. Theor Surg 1994;9:12–13.

47. Glauser MP, Heumann D, Baumgartner JD, Cohen J. Pathogenesis and potential strategies for prevention and treatment of septic shock: an update. Clin Infect Dis 1994;18(suppl 2):205–216.

48. Velanovich V. The box-counting method of fractal analysis for complex biological shapes, illustrated with reference to wound healing. Theor Surg 1994; 9:68–71.

49. Walsh MS, Goode AW. The measurement of open wounds: order out of chaos. Theor Surg 1994;9: 108–110.

50. Lipsitz LA, Goldberger AL. Loss of complexity and aging: potential applications of fractals and chaos theory to senescence. JAMA 1992;267: 1806–1809.

51. Mandelbrot BB. The fractal geometry of nature. New York: Freiman, 1982.

52. Sitter H, Lorenz W, Klotter HJ, Lill H. Models for causality assessment. In: Neugebauer E, Hola-

day JW, eds. Handbook of Mediators in Septic Shock. Boca Raton; CRC, 1993, pp. 499–522.

53. Holaday JW, Neugebauer E, Carr DB. Meta²—an analysis of meta-analyses of mediators in septic shock. In: Neugebauer EA, Holaday JW, eds. Handbook of Mediators in Septic Shock. Boca Raton, Ann Arbor, London, Tokyo: CRC, 1993, pp. 523–534.

54. Cohen LJ. Can human irrationality be experimentally demonstrated? Behav Brain 1981;4:317–330.

55. Mittelstraß J. Komplex. In: Enzyklopädie Philosophie und Wissenchaftstheorie, Bd 2 H-O. Mannheim Wien Zürich: BI-Wissenschaftsverlag, 1984, 427–428.

56. Pearson SD, Margolis CZ, Davis S, Schreier LK, Gottlieb LK. The clinical algorithm nosology: a method for comparing algorithmic guidelines. Med Decis Making 1992;12:123–131.

57. Sitter H. Prünte H, Lorenz W, Christensen JP, Scherrer JR, McNair P. A new version of the programme ALGO for clinical algorithms. In: Brender J, ed. Medical Informatics Europe '96. IOS, 1996, pp. 654–657.

58. Hilden J. Intuition and other soft modes of thought in surgery. Theor Surg 1991;6:89–94.

59. Hamm RM. Clinical intuition and clinical analysis: expertise and the cognitive continuum. In: Dowie J, Elstein A, eds. Professional Judgment. A Reader in Clinical Decision Making. Cambridge: Cambridge University, 1988, pp. 78–105.

60. Lorenz W. Leitlinien in der Chirurgie: Aus der Sicht der klinischen Forschung. Langenbecks Arch Chir (in press).

61. Künneke M, Stinner B, Celik I, Lorenz W. Cardiovascular adverse effects of antimicrobials in complex surgical cases. Eur J Surg 1996;576 (suppl):24–28.

62. Dinarello CA, Thompson RC. Blocking IL-1: interleukin 1 receptor antagonist in vivo and in vitro. Immunol Today 1991;12:404–410.

63. Bone RC. Why sepsis trials fail. JAMA 1996; 276:565–566.

64. Lorenz W, Duda D, Dick W, Sitter H, Doenicke A, Black A, Weber D, Menke H, Stinner B, Junginger T, et al. Incidence and clinical importance of perioperative histamine release: Randomised study of volume loading and antihistamines after induction of anaesthesia. Lancet 1994;343:933–940.

65. Descartes R. oder Der Metaphysiker hält Diät. In: Fischer EP, ed. Aristoteles, Einstein & Co. München Zürich: Piper, 1995, pp. 138–153.

66. Descartes R. Selected Philosophical Writings. Cottingham J, Stoothoff R, Murdoch D, trans. Cambridge, England: Cambridge University, 1988, p. 29.

67. Black J. Foreword. In: Boyd CAR, Noble D, eds. The Logic of Life. Oxford New York Tokyo: Oxford University, 1993, pp. v–viii.

CHAPTER 66

International Exchange for Surgical Education

L. Köhler, C.K. Kum, M. Miserez, D. Rixen, and S. Saad

Let our young [doctors], particularly those who aspire to teaching positions, go abroad. They can find at home laboratories and hospitals as well equipped as any in the world, but they may find abroad more than they knew they sought—widened sympathies, heightened ideals and something perhaps of a Welt-cultur *which will remain through life as the best protection against the vice of nationalism.*
—Sir William Osler, Philosophical Essays, "Chauvinism in Medicine," 1902

International exchange for surgical education has a long and rich tradition. William Halsted, for example, took his postgraduate training in Europe from 1878 to 1880. During this period abroad, Halsted gained experience in surgical techniques unknown to many North American surgeons. He formed close relationships with a number of clinical and laboratory professionals. When he became chief of surgery at the Johns Hopkins Hospital, he adopted a training program for residents similar to what he had observed in Europe. The knowledge and experience he gained was not only a personal benefit, but it also contributed substantially to the development of North American surgical training programs.

This chapter will provide some guidelines for surgeons who would like to study abroad. The ideas expressed are based on the personal experience of the authors. Two of the authors (C.K. and M.M.) visited Cologne, Germany, for a 1-year period. Two others (L.K. and D.R.) trained in the United States for 1 and 2 years, respectively, and one author visited Japan for 2 years (S.S.).

Why Go Abroad?

We are convinced that the training of an academic surgeon should include at least 1 year abroad in another academic institution. There are several good reasons to do so. You will see and learn different techniques of surgery, investigative methods, and experimental approaches to unsolved problems. This will expand your repertoire as a surgeon-investigator and stimulate new ideas. You may have the opportunity to learn a specific technique from a master in that field. When working together for a prolonged period, scientists tend to influence each other's thinking. You will learn alternatives for solving problems, and new concepts, ideas, and methodologies that you will be able to bring back to your own clinic. You will be able to compare standards of other institutions with those of your own institution, and to judge your own position in a particular field. You will learn about differences in culture and custom, health care policies, socioeconomic structures, and political systems. This will help you to understand the reasons for differences in various diagnostic and therapeutic management protocols.

Another very important benefit is the opportunity to form new friendships. These friendships often last a lifetime, and allow further exchange of thoughts and experience. Moreover, going abroad is often an enrichment in terms of personal development, such as building skill in foreign languages.

When and Where to Go

To benefit from foreign training, prior experience in basic surgical skills is a minimal requirement; we feel it is best to go abroad toward the end of surgical training. It is also useful to have had some experience in research methodology and scientific writing. One year is short, and you should not waste it on learning fundamentals.

Foreign training may consist of exclusively clinical activities, an exclusively scientific experimental mandate, or a combination of both. The search for a suitable location for foreign training should primarily take into account the specific purposes of your visit, for example, training in laparoscopic surgery. The center you choose should be reputable. Check the literature carefully for the areas of interest of the clinic and surgeons. If the center fulfills the objectives in your area of interest, try to interview current or former residents about their experiences there.

Institutions with experience in foreign resident training are often more open to foreigners, and the facilities, such as housing and administration, are more directed toward visitors from abroad.

Preparation

Planning is crucially important; taking training abroad without adequate preparation is the biggest mistake you can make. Ideally, planning should start 2 years before the estimated date of arrival at your chosen place of study abroad. You will need to make sure that you can communicate with your future colleagues in at least one language, for example, English. If this is not the native language, you may have to learn that in addition. You should read as much as possible about the people, culture, history, and social customs of

the country you are visiting. You will want to find out what clothing is suitable, especially in the professional setting.

Financial arrangements should be made as soon as possible. The least cumbersome procedure is to be paid by the hospital or institution abroad. However, finding such a position is not easy. Many foreign resident programs may be available, but only a few of them include specific financial compensation. In most cases a scholarship is needed to finance a resident's training abroad. Scholarship applications often need to be processed more than 1 year in advance, so information on specific scholarships to support foreign training should be gathered early.

If you wish to participate in patient care, a license to practice medicine is obligatory. The administrative formalities to be fulfilled differ from country to country, for example, the German medical license is not accepted in the United States. However, all countries have one thing in common—the application procedure takes quite a long time!

After determining the site of training abroad, a formal application with curriculum vitae should be forwarded. If the answer is positive, a short visit should be organized, to provide the opportunity to get to know the hospital and to make contact with the chief of the surgical department and the residents. During this visit, ask the following questions: Is a project already planned, or are you expected to initiate it? Can you perform clinical work? What time of the year is best to come? Is there a salary? Are accommodations provided? If not, are there inexpensive, subsidized accommodations for residents who are alone or those with a family? What about medical and personal insurance? Are there special visa requirements? Is a working permit necessary?

If your scientific project has not been planned prior to acceptance into the program abroad, it is urgent to prepare a plan as soon as possible. Writing a research protocol, funding the project, and getting approval from the animal care committee and other institutional committees are time-consuming activities that must be done in advance. You want to be able to start the project right away upon your arrival, rather than losing valuable time (sometimes 3 to 6 months) finding a project, dealing with the bureaucracy, and planning experiments. On the other hand, it is the responsibility of the host to help plan the stay of the resident. Accepting a foreign resident without a clear and practical plan for what the resident will do is unfair.

If you travel with your family, preparation takes longer and is more intense. It may be wise for you to arrive first and have your family follow you in a few weeks—after you have settled in, found an appropriate place to live, and overcome the initial culture shock.

What to Do When You Are There

Always remember that you are a guest. After your arrival, you will first have to become acclimatized to your new situation. You will now be very grateful for your earlier efforts to become acquainted with the culture, language, and social customs.

There will be an initial time of probation, when your hosts watch you carefully to learn about your personality, knowledge, and experience. It is advisable to have one responsible staff person as your mentor; this is often the director of the department. You should meet with your mentor on a regular basis, perhaps every 2 weeks, to discuss progress. It is important not to let unresolved problems accumulate until your departure. An open conversation in which all experiences, problems, ideas, and initiatives can be freely discussed is very worthwhile for the success of your stay.

If the major purpose of your study abroad is development of technical surgical skills, it is advisable to have a detailed list of operations in which you would like to participate. Constructive discussion with the local residents concerning this topic is mandatory. Using your privileged situation of being a foreign resident to perform only

the nice jobs is not fair; you should become a cooperative member of the surgical team and participate in all aspects of everyday practice. If, in your opinion, some techniques or procedures performed are inferior to prior methods you have learned, you should not criticize. Always be polite and tactful.

You should prepare a reasonable timetable for the year and try to keep to it. Leave a few weeks of unscheduled time at the end of the year for unexpected delays. If possible, attend courses in such areas as statistics or epidemiology. Finish writing up your project before your departure. It is much easier for your supervisors to discuss and edit your work while you are still there. If this is not possible, a return trip should be considered.

It is important to participate in festivals and cultural events and to learn as much about the country as possible. Meeting people and making friends, participating in social activities, and traveling around the country are good ways to prevent homesickness.

After completion of your foreign training, you will want to report your experiences to colleagues back at your home institution. You should document your visit, take notes, photographs, and videos, and prepare for presentation. A diary can be very helpful for putting your experiences into perspective.

Final Note

There is no question that integrating yourself into another medical care system is challenging personally and professionally. The new techniques and approaches that you learn, and the durable collaborations and friendships you create through training abroad will enrich your institution and your country as well as your own professional and personal life.

CHAPTER 67

Survival Essentials for the Surgeon-Scientist in Training

D.J. Hackam

The surgical resident who has just become comfortable in the clinical world faces a number of challenges on entering the unfamiliar world of scientific study. A supervisor must first be selected, and a research project carefully chosen. You must decide whether to enter a graduate training program, and if so, courses and a thesis committee must be selected. Once research training begins, you must make the transition to graduate student in science. This process results in significant separation anxiety from the surgical floors and operating room, as well as frustration with the pace of the research process. As the pressures of adjusting to laboratory life ease, the next challenges arise. These include the submission of abstracts to scientific meetings and attending and presenting at national and international conferences.

Planning Your Research Program

The first choice made by every resident entering the laboratory is that of a research supervisor. This will be predetermined if a particular scientist has recruited you to his or her laboratory. In most cases, the resident is interested in "learning science" and has no preselected mentor; the choice of a supervisor from the myriad of scientists at an institution can be a daunting task. The following suggestions may facilitate the process. (1) The less

research training you have, the more hands-on supervision you will require. In these circumstances, choose a lab with a variety of expert teachers in the form of postdoctoral fellows, technicians, and other students. (2) Consider the track record of your prospective supervisor. Unlike the stock market, past performance in research is a predictor of future performance and should be carefully investigated. A quick MEDLINE search can readily acquaint you with the productivity and diversity of an individual's research program. (3) Meet with the supervisor and tour the laboratory. Given the long-term investment being considered, the personal interaction between supervisor and student becomes paramount. Don't feel obligated to choose a particular supervisor because you like him or her, but be absolutely certain to avoid a supervisor that you dislike.

The next decision often centers around whether to enter a formal graduate program leading to a master's or doctoral degree. While the ultimate decision remains a personal one, remember that the time for completion is approximately 2 years and 4 years, respectively. If a degree program is entered, complete the course requirements as soon as possible. Base your course choices on practical grounds and don't be embarrassed to take easy courses with an emphasis on material previously acquired in medical school. You'll do lots of focused reading in your area of research, so the amount of time spent in peripheral areas should probably be minimized as much as possible. Choosing a thesis committee becomes extremely important. Remember that the committee must read and approve your thesis before you defend it, so select members with a reputation for efficiency and partnership.

Making the Transition from Surgeon to Scientist

As the surgical resident embarks on laboratory training, anxiety related to separation from surgery can be a major hurdle in making the adjustment to a new life. Until you get "turned on" to the research process, anxiety created by losing touch (and ground) with resident colleagues can be significant. Coping strategies at this time can include attending clinical rounds regularly and taking occasional call on surgical services, if the program permits. Remember, reading a clinical paper will generally be easier and less stressful than a pure scientific one and will keep you in touch with an important part of your life and the developing definition of yourself as a professional.

An important part of the transition that is seldom discussed is that the focus in science is so different from that in the clinical world. In simple terms, scientific training emphasizes a *process*, clinical training emphasizes an *outcome*. Understanding this difference may alleviate the extremely common anxiety associated with the apparently slow pace of scientific research. As residents, we are accustomed to knowing results within hours—whether our patient makes it to the floor or stays in the intensive care unit, the response to a saline infusion, the result of an X ray. In science, we must become accustomed to knowing results within days or weeks—the results of gel electrophoresis, the expression of a plasmid, the sequence of a protein. The sooner you realize and accept the difference in time scale, the easier it is to make the adjustment. As a rough guide, consider this timeline for the achievement of the following milestones from entry into the laboratory as fairly typical: fear, anxiety, confusion (up to 4 weeks), pure laboratory neophyte/clinical clerk equivalent (3 months), growing confidence (6 months), some independence in performing experiments (8 months), flying solo (12 months).

Laboratory Life

Life in the laboratory for surgical trainees can be as variable and as intense as clinical rotations. It depends very much on your goals, the supervisor's expectations, and the general pace of the laboratory. Most often, the hours are as long as clinical hours, to the surprise of clinical colleagues. A few simple rules will help you plan a laboratory routine. (1) Plan on everything taking approximately twice as long as you think it should. This reality won't necessarily please your supervisor, but it will assist you greatly in designing a research schedule. (2) Don't be afraid to ask widely about experimental protocols. Most things in the lab have been done before by at least one person, and scientists are generally extremely willing to share experiences and even reagents. This can save immense amounts of time and effort and can lead to useful collaborations. (3) Talk often with your supervisor, especially in your early research training, both about the planning of experiments and the results. There are many ways for an experiment to fail, and generally only one way for it to succeed. There is a good chance that your supervisor will know how to ensure the latter.

Suitcase Life: Submitting Abstracts and Attending Meetings

Submitting abstracts and attending conferences is an important part of the scientific research process that allows interaction with colleagues in the same field and provides an opportunity for communication and personal advancement. Basic science meetings tend to be less formal than clinical meetings, and graduate students generally present in poster format. This is an excellent way to meet and receive direct feedback from people specifically interested in your work and may provide important ideas for further study. Clinical meetings offer the opportunity to meet like-minded colleagues and may occasionally provide a podium for the presentation of your research to the wider community of surgeons. Both types of meetings should be attended at least once, since the experiences will be quite different. The easiest way to attend a given meeting is to submit an abstract and have it accepted. Your supervisor will be of critical importance here, both in the selection of the meeting and the design of the submission.

Once the abstract is accepted, a few golden rules will ease a great deal of stress as the meeting approaches:

1. Book flights and hotels early. Meetings are often well attended, and the number of flights may be very limited, particularly in smaller cities. Similarly, hotels near the meeting site can become occupied at a rapid rate, literally leaving a student out in the cold. Take advantage of a conference's accommodation or hotel-booking service if available.

2. Register in advance if possible. The feeling of control over one's life that one gets when walking to the front of a block-long registration line to pick up a prepared identification badge is indescribable.

3. When attending a meeting, pack lightly and call home often.

Survival Essentials

1. Choose a lab with excellent supervision and technical expertise.
2. Use MEDLINE or another search program

---

to review the publication track record of the supervisor and lab you are considering.
3. Interview your supervisor and the laboratory members to be sure you will be productive in the new setting.
4. Get your courses out of the way as soon as possible.
5. Choose your thesis committee carefully.
6. Have a defined controlled exposure to clinical work, on a regular basis.
7. Consult regularly with your supervisor, especially early in your training.
8. Register early and book flights and hotels early for meetings, especially if you are presenting.

Commentary

Chairpersons far removed from the day they entered the laboratory will be reminded of the resident's unique needs, which are well expressed by Dr. Hackam. Long before they enter the laboratory, residents should have time to read the protocols, papers, and abstracts covering material that they may investigate. This period of mutual assessment can help insure that the right resident is in the right laboratory. We look for residents who are self-starters and have good organizational skills, a record of getting things done, and proven ability to write. The attitude, skill, and values that bring success in clinical medicine generally apply with equal weight in the research laboratory.

M.F.M.

CHAPTER 68

Future Horizons in Surgical Research

F.D. Moore

. . . and a horizon is nothing save the limit of our sight.

To glimpse what lies beyond our horizon, it is wise to examine the terrain from whence we come. Since World War II, surgical research has functioned in four modes.

1. *Developing new procedures.* Examples of new procedures developed where none existed before include open-heart operations using a pump oxygenator, organ transplantation, microsurgery of the brain and middle ear, laser surgery of the detached retina, direct arterial suture and repair (including aortic aneurysm), and prosthetic replacement of major joints.
2. *Building bridges to the basic sciences.* Bringing basic science directly to the bedside has resulted in advances in our understanding of the metabolic needs of surgical patients, intravenous feeding, the biology of convalescence, the use of anticoagulants and antibiotics, and the role of immunology in surgery.
3. *Collaborating with clinical colleagues.* The blossoming of cancer surgery into a multimodality collaborative treatment, improved orthopedic management of rheumatoid arthritis, and the use of pacemakers, ultrasound, and computed axial tomography are but a few examples of the effectiveness of collaboration between surgeons and other clinical colleagues.

4. *Improving existing procedures by surgical engineering.* The improvement of surgery is often triggered by self-examination and self-criticism. This time-honored practice by surgeons is now augmented by incisive research. The evolution of surgery for breast cancer, liver resection, prostatectomy, pituitary neoplasms, and fracture stabilization illustrates how surgical care has changed and improved through repeated performance and a clearer understanding of its own shortcomings. Advances in the evaluation of new procedures and technology assessment belong in this category.

Surgical research has two basic requirements.

1. *People, institutions.* The recruitment and academic support of young people interested in surgical research require the establishment of surgical laboratories and their expansion and integration. To accomplish this, collaborative bridges must be built with basic science departments, and the support of surgical research by boards of trustees, hospital directors, university deans, and science colleagues must be won. It also requires an adequate understanding of the significance of the mission of surgical research and its accomplishments in producing some of the most remarkable biomedical advances of this century.
2. *Financial support.* When young people embark on careers as investigators, they do not have

bibliographies or research backgrounds that will command outside financial support for the pursuit of their ideas and their personal or family needs. Later, the full backing of home universities and nonsurgical faculties becomes a critical factor in successful searches for funds from large donors, foundations, and institutions, but it is, in some areas, very difficult to obtain.

Two questions have to be answered by each surgical department head about the surgical research in his or her department.

1. *What is the role of modern basic quantitative biology in surgical research?* Like their colleagues in medicine, pediatrics, psychiatry, or radiology, very few surgeons are basic biologists. As the methods of modern science become progressively more challenging, fewer expert clinicians master them. Should there be more collaborating scientists in surgical departments?
2. *Where does health policy fit in surgical research?* Health policy research includes the role of surgical care in social rehabilitation, cost-benefit analysis, surgical manpower, the organization of surgical departments, the establishment of new procedures and practice patterns, law and ethics, the burden of malpractice litigation, and the application of highly technical methods to life support in critical illness. Since all the foregoing enter into the practice of surgery, these areas cannot be neglected by research, despite their not having been considered a part of surgical research in the past. If surgical investigators overlook or avoid them, critical decisions about surgery will be made by inadequately informed sociologists and legislators.

To have impact on the care of the sick, surgical research must be done *with or by surgeons, or under their guidance. Whether the surgical investigator plays the key or a more modest role, the inspiration, driving force, and scientific and clinical insight of the surgical presence are essential for the success of surgical research.*

Now, within the same framework, we might take a quick glance—albeit not quite in focus—at the horizon.

New Procedures

In 1935 very few people would have predicted perfection of the pump oxygenator to support surgery on the open heart. Such a technological development and the transplantation of organs between unrelated individuals were termed impossible by the experts in 1952 and 1953, respectively. From the turn of the century onward, surgeons were taught that large foreign bodies in a wound were a sure recipe for disaster, to say nothing of artificial heart valves or such large plastic prostheses as new hip joints. Success in such endeavors is now the rule. These examples illustrate the possible fate of negative predictions about new surgical procedures. One must be quite presumptuous to imagine what might be on surgeons' operating lists even 10 or 15 years hence.

I would guess that transplantation will be further perfected and extended to include additional organs and tissues. Although these operations will hardly be called "new," transplantation of the pancreas and long sections of small bowel are among the many unsolved challenges.

Head injury, whether inflicted by automobile or home accidents, child abuse, or military activity, remains the commonest cause of death from trauma. Microvascular operations for intracranial bleeding or for infarction caused by head injury might become a reality. The evaluation of head injuries to discern those that might be remedied by early direct examination of the brain and its vasculature remains an important goal. New imaging modalities such as nuclear magnetic resonance and positron emission tomography may be crucial to success in this effort.

The development of artificial organs will surely continue for many decades. Such organs fall into two general categories. First are the artificial organs that are physiologically outside the body, even if implanted under the skin. Extracorporeal pump oxygenators (the first effective artificial organ), pacemakers, artificial kidneys, and artificial pancreases belong in this group, although the first two are now in such wide use that we scarcely think of them as artificial organs.

The second group comprises those artificial organs truly incorporated in situ. The artificial heart is one example, although it currently suffers from a surpassing difficulty. In animal models, the tendency to cerebral microembolism may be masked by the inadequacy of our knowledge of the subtleties of animal behavior (speech, affect), or by actual differences in the coagulability of blood. In any event, microembolism, usually to the brain but possibly to other organs as well, has been a major complication in most of the patients in whom artificial hearts have been implanted. This unfortunate complication keeps this valuable, albeit expensive, bulky, and awkward form of life support, from providing a life of acceptable quality for patients.

The recent development of an endothelium-stimulating growth substance, fibroblastic growth factor (FGF), holds great promise. It seems reasonable to expect that implantable hearts and other left ventricular assist devices will eventually have endothelial linings grown within them to make them essentially physiologic as regards coagulation induction. If this becomes possible, the use of artificial hearts will be limited only by the awkwardness of the extracorporeal power source. The work of several investigators who are attempting to develop an electrical, magnetic, or nuclear implantable power source is important, and it should occupy the time and attention of several capable collaborative groups encompassing energy conversion, engineering, medicine, and surgery.

The human heart transplant requires toxic immunosuppressive drugs, the artificial heart implant capricious anticoagulants. The tradeoff has not been as simple as it appeared.

Will there be some new form of operation applicable to many forms of cancer? It could, conceivably, be an organ implant, such as lymph nodes or spleen containing "educated" lymphocytes to assault the tumor; a microfilter; or a microfilter containing gene-engineered microorganisms that synthesize diffusible substances such as interleukin 2 or antiangiogenin. Though these might not be new operations, they would basically be the application of new immunologic and genetic knowledge to surgical care.

When mastoidectomy yielded to antibiotics, and polio reconstruction disappeared following the advent of the Salk vaccine, no surgeon objected. Indeed, all were elated. There are, however, other losses to surgical practice, such as

ultrasound-guided deep needle biopsy, angiographic embolization in hemorrhage, percutaneous angioplasty, and colonoscopic polyp removal, where a steady surgical hand and the longstanding "field familiarity" of surgeons are still needed. Although surgery (*chirurgie*) is "doing with the hand" and can be learned by others, the surgeon should insist on participation, in some cases. Other new areas will require that the surgeon "keep a hand in" by mastering new techniques and learning new concepts from other fields, as has already happened in relation to the treatment of deafness and coronary disease.

Building Bridges to the Basic Sciences

Immunology looms large with respect to building bridges between surgery and the basic sciences because molecular immunology should surely be applicable to cancer, transplantation, and surgical infection. Most immunologists who worked through the difficult decades of the 1940s, 1950s, and 1960s readily acknowledge the stimulus they received from surgery, given that the growth of tissue transplantation, the description of the HLA groups, and enhanced understanding of the events of tissue rejection were all central to the rebirth of immunology and its movement from pragmatic clinical testing to basic molecular biology. Several Nobel laureates (Burnet, Baltimore, Medawar, and Benacerraf) have worked on tissue types, immune competence, histocompatibility, and antigen genetics.

Many young surgeons are now selecting immunology as their basic science field, just as they may select physiology, metabolism, neurology, microbiology, or biomaterials. Although, when viewed in the harsh light of the 1990s, molecular immunology has not yet revolutionized anything in surgery, my own scientific faith affirms its tremendous surgical potential.

Immune therapy for cancer seems, finally, to be on the verge of widespread applicability. The work of Rosenberg and his colleagues at the National Institutes of Health has an unmistakable ring of the future about it. Using their method, the patient's lymphatic system is stimulated by interleukin 2 (IL-2), as are also the patient's lymphocytes (in some instances from tumor infiltration itself). The combined treatment is very toxic, but it has produced some remarkable effects, such as the complete disappearance of some very large metastases of certain types of tumor, such as hypernephroma, lung cancer, and melanoma.

IL-2 treatment has been criticized as having an inadequate response rate but, in cancer treatment, the attention of the biologic and medical community should be focused on the nature and quality of the response rather than the fractional response rate. Although some tumors may, for example, display a response rate as high as 75% to certain chemotherapy regimens, almost all the patients die of their tumors without the tumors ever regressing completely. The response rate is high, but the quality of the response is very poor. With IL-2 treatment, tumors have disappeared completely following immune intervention—an entirely new phenomenon in cancer therapy. The fact that some stay away while others return when the treatment is stopped raises the possibility of chronic immune therapy to maintain remission.

Immune modulation of this type will surely be applicable to other forms of cancer. By extension, some analogous form of immune treatment might become available for severe surgical sepsis and its attendant multiple organ failure.

Although our expanding knowledge of immunological processes seems to be establishing the basis for specific therapy, clinical case management has not yet altered much. It now seems clear that certain types of surgical trauma inhibit the production of immunoreactive globulins and may adversely affect the activity of specific lymphocyte subpopulations, possibly through an overload mechanism. All clinicians are familiar with the phenomenon of sequential failure of several organs and death as a consequence of sepsis following trauma or surgery with multiple treatment modalities and successively changed antibiotics. These terminal events suggest widespread immune deficiency and raise the possibility that repair of the patient's immune system, were it feasible, might be lifesaving.

The 1940–1970 era may well go down in history as one whose prime characteristic was the mishandling of antibiotics. The adverse effects included immunosuppression from overdosing with antibiotics, and the acquisition of antibiotic resistance by successive strains of organisms. Patients were converted into bacteriologically sterile but immunologically suppressed settings for the overgrowth of ordinary commensals such as fungi and the cytomegalovirus. A better knowledge of the immune sequences in such complex cases may enable the surgeon to employ new agents more intelligently.

The induction of specific immunologic tolerance for transplant antigens from one organ source, without global immunosuppression, remains elusive. Significant as the replacement of azothiaprine by cyclosporin has appeared to be for many transplanted organs, particularly liver, cyclosporin is but another nonspecific immunosuppressive drug with neoplastic by-products.

Bringing basic science to the rescue of the surgical patient, through physiologic support systems, has several inviting possibilities. New knowledge about hormone mediators that translate peripheral injury into central organ damage, nitrogen loss, conversion of energy sources to lipid oxidation, and activation of the stress response holds much promise. The possibility that treatment modalities may exist in the endocrine area is brighter than ever. If, after severe injury, catabolic activity could be modified and necessary substrates could be simultaneously released from within the body, or be introduced, a more serene clinical course might be anticipated. Recent evidence suggests that glutamine may have specific nutritional functions for the GI tract and that human growth hormone may hasten recovery.

If such methods of stress modulation become available, their misuse and overuse can be predicted. It has been observed since the beginning of surgical metabolic research that healthy young men who show a very vigorous or brisk endocrine and catabolic response do very well clinically. The plentiful release of endogenous substrates for fibroplasia, leukocyte activity, and immune globulin production appears to be an obvious though unproven explanation. When some hormone becomes available to abate this response, the appearance of the vigorous young man with his "brisk and florid" endocrine response will rapidly be "mollified" to resemble that of a weakened old man having his fifth operation, totally devoid of physiologic response. The use of such potent and dangerous hormones, if and when they become available, will require a great deal of sophistication, but the dismal antibiotic record provides little assurance that a large group of surgeons and physicians will be able to use them intelligently.

Collaborating with Clinical Colleagues

The evolution of cancer treatment in the past decade has been one of the most spectacular examples of collaboration. Formerly limited to essentially "do or die" surgical operations whose effectiveness was based largely on early diagnosis, treatment now includes other modalities and often produces very good results. Nevertheless the net effect has often been overrated by the public media because of enthusiasm about the very existence of these methods. This is particularly true vis-à-vis chemotherapy for solid tumors, and radiotherapy with supervoltage equipment.

Despite many disappointments and failures, cancer patients now have a better prospect than ever before of prolonged disease-free survival, with a good quality of life. This is due not to any single "breakthrough" but to noncompetitive collaboration in comprehensive cancer centers, where the welfare of the patient is more important than any specialty ambitions. When one visits such units, one can quickly discern whether the practitioners of the various and potentially competing treatment modalities, and the domains of sovereignty, such as surgery, radiotherapy, and chemotherapy, are truly collaborating for the welfare of the patient, or if they are actually seeking the enrollment of patients in their own "protocols" in order to get more money, more publicity, more patients, or a higher group income.

A professional is defined as a practitioner who places the welfare of the patient or client above the practitioner's own social, scientific, personal, or financial advancement. The availability of multiple cancer therapies and therapists has truly placed the professionalism of all physicians on the line. Although most multiple-modality cancer treatment centers demonstrate a high order of professionalism, it is evident that, in a few, research protocol enrollment rather than the welfare

of the patient governs the outcome. Although collaboration now prevails in many fields, the psychology of professional interaction is an important component that remains to be analyzed.

Clinical and research collaboration promises many rewards for the surgical patient. The development of ultrasound and computed axial tomography are tremendous advances in surgical care. To appreciate them, one has only to reflect on the painful and uncertain procedures of encephalography and ventriculography to diagnose hemorrhage in the skull or disorders along the spinal column, and contrast them with the specificity and anatomic precision of tomographic scanning.

Nuclear magnetic resonance (NMR) and positron emission tomography (PET) hold great promise. Although NMR seems to have almost no adverse effects, current apparatus is expensive, cumbersome, and awkward, and does not lend itself either to the scanning of extremely ill patients or to any sort of emergency procedure. PET scanning has the unique feature of demonstrating areas of functional activity within the brain. The development of this type of combined engineering and its application to neurosurgery and various mental, behavioral, and psychiatric problems open a new horizon for neurosurgery. It is possible to hope that these techniques, combined with very prompt attention, immediate and focal diagnosis, and microsurgery or CNS excision, will provide a way to save a few patients from that large group that now accounts for most of the mortality among civilian and military casualties.

Improving Existing Procedures through Surgical Engineering

While most of the quantum advances in surgery during the past century have come from university centers, gradual improvement and perfection of surgical procedures have often come via practitioners, clinical practicing groups, and community hospitals. As an applied form of biological science or human engineering, surgery improves with practice. The marked reduction in patient mortality and the tremendous increase in the fractional survival of transplanted kidneys between 1965 and 1978, when there was no qualitative improvement in immunosuppression, is but one of many examples that demonstrates perfection by gradual engineering.

The same is true of open-heart surgery, particularly coronary bypass operations. This formerly imposing and immensely complex surgery has become much safer, rather than more hazardous, with its widespread performance. The mortality over large areas of the United States is now around 1%.

The introduction of laparoscopic techniques for major surgery is a beautiful example, becoming increasingly prominent over the last 5 years, of the improvement of existing surgical procedures by engineering. The use of thorascopes for the division of pleural adhesions, of gastroscopes and esophagoscopes for biopsy, and of sigmoidoscopes for diagnosis and treatment, go back to the turn of the century or shortly thereafter. The increasing use of endoscopic procedures on the bile ducts, and of colonoscopy, became prominent approximately 25 years ago. Now, the much more extensive technical developments of laparoscopic procedures for cholycestectomy, herniorrhaphy, appendectomy, and even exterpative maneuvers in thoracic, abdominal, and arthroscopic surgery have become commonplace. A thread of technical development underlies this whole area, namely, the use of television presentations based on electronic imaging. The engineering steps have therefore involved not only the optical and electronic devices, but the presentation screen. Through the further development of these procedures we can expect a very considerable simplification of surgical procedures over the coming decades, with earlier discharge of patients and a lower morbidity and mortality. One major precaution remains. Namely, that surgeons doing this type of less invasive television-presented surgery must be themselves expert in the entire anatomy and classic surgical care of the diseases under treatment.

Very few clinicians or scientists outside the field of surgery understand its remarkable capacity for self-improvement. Many adverse views of surgical operations are based on early results before surgery's built-in learning curve becomes manifest. Liver transplantation is one of the most difficult and complex of the frontier group of surgical procedures, but its perfection and the consequent improvement in morbidity and mortality have been spectacular. Liver transplantation should be undertaken only by a master surgeon with self-confidence and specific training. Within those limitations, its repeated performance has resulted in an improvement in results beyond expectation; It is highly challenging to the neophyte individual or hospital at the beginning of the learning curve.

Every hospital, clinical unit, group practice, or academic department conducting surgical operations in any quantity should periodically review its results in terms of immediate mortality and morbidity, and late survivorship and rehabilitation. While modern computer techniques render this very simple, there must be an established program that is adequately supported at the outset and periodically evaluated. This is a matter of pressing importance at the horizon of surgical research.

Hospitals that cling to old operations, such as radical mastectomy in breast cancer or subtotal gastrectomy for duodenal ulcer, should have the research fortitude, often called "discipline" or "guts," to examine their own results in the light of recent advances. If they can, indeed, document superior results with the time-honored procedures, they should be encouraged to do so and to stand up in the court of professional opinion to defend their view. The same principle applies to such frequently performed standard operations as prostatectomy, colectomy for cancer, heart valve surgery, laminectomy for disc removal, and arterial replacement of the aorta or in the lower limb. It should be an obligation of every surgical unit, wherever located, to know its own results, compare them with those published by peer groups, and set its house to rights if its results are inadequate. The support of research to accomplish this should come from the institution itself.

The Two Basic Inputs: People and Support

We can say with perfect confidence that young surgeons devoted to a life in science will be as rare in the future as they have been in the past. The coercion of all young interns and residents to laboratory "projects" is positively unrewarding; it merely results in crowding the literature with trash. Nevertheless, the door to the laboratory should be open to all young surgeons so that, if their talents call them in that direction, they may give them a fair trial. The analogy with playing a musical instrument is too close to withhold: forcing every young person to practice 3 hours a day would produce only a large crashing of noise. And yet, one cannot learn to play by attending concerts: one must perform oneself and practice every day! The instrument—a laboratory—should be there, along with a teacher—the professor—so that each resident in an academic unit can develop his or her talent, if it exists.

The backwardness of institutions in providing space for surgical research is depressing. Surgical research is not demanding of space, although animal facilities have sometimes been difficult to establish and maintain. Antivivisectionist pressures have been a problem for surgical research for almost a century. It is an obligation of the professor of surgery to convince the dean and the hospital director of what the necessary components of surgical research are and to call to their attention that only where research thrives and inquiring minds are given scope, will the quality of clinical surgery be maintained at its optimal level and the hospital attract patients and residents.

Financial support for career development in surgery must come, increasingly, from practice income, although this has an ethical aspect that requires examination. If a practicing group such as a private group clinic of the United States model (Mayo, Lahey, Crile) sets aside professional fee income for research, the problem of fee splitting must be considered. Patients, or their insurance companies, are being charged for an activity (i.e., research) that they may be totally unaware of and unprepared to underwrite. If such fee diversion becomes extensive, it is clearly unethical. This also applies when the dean or the university taxes practice income from academic clinicians. It is, in essence, a tax on the patient's pocketbook or on the insurance company, for the conduct of a medical school, which the patient may not feel is intrinsic to the treatment of her breast cancer.

This ethical concern is counterbalanced, however, by the fact that all enterprises in a free society require the diversion of some revenue to research and development. Given a proper explanation, even the most conservative patient would willingly make a reasonable contribution to the improvement of surgical practice.

Determination of what is a "reasonable" fraction must depend on the scene and circumstances, but somewhere in the region of 10 to 15% would seem to be appropriate. Some sort of notification should be included in hospital publications or be given to the patient at admission, to make it clear that some of the professional charges incurred for his or her care will be devoted to assisting the research education of young surgeons. With that proviso, academic surgical group practices can provide fellowships and a few basic laboratory components for young people embarking on research careers. Although group practices can never supply the broadly financed support required by modern quantitative biology, they can play a critically important role by providing the seed money and the strong surgical supporting voice that the young surgeon must have to compete successfully on the national scene for continuing grant funds.

Where Does Basic Science Collaboration Fit?

Surgical research will, in the future, involve a more searching appraisal of the role of basic science than it has in the past. The young surgeon embarking on research should spend a year or two acquiring the vocabulary, skills, and concepts of some area of basic biology, molecular immunology, genetics, or bioengineering and then have a period of collaboration with scientists holding Ph.D. qualifications. To make this happen, surgical departments must willingly give appointments in surgery to Ph.D. scientists. Medicine, pediatrics, and psychiatry have already assigned such appointments to scientists from other fields, but surgery has not done so very often.

Young people with the talents required to meet the mechanical, spatial, and operative challenges of surgery may not have the mental bent appropriate to thinking in terms of molecular interactions. The same limitation is found in medicine and pediatrics: as molecular biology becomes ever more challenging, an increasing proportion of total research funding in clinical departments is held by Ph.D. scientists. Surgery must do the same, if it is to move ahead.

Health Policy

Health policy research is one of the most interesting features of the surgical research horizon.

Surgical research has three phases: discovery, development, and delivery. *Discovery* covers the revelation of some important bioscience finding related to surgical care; *development* occurs during the period of surgical bioengineering improvement already discussed. *Delivery* is concerned with providing new modes of surgical care, and with the manpower, economic, and regulatory constraints within which surgery operates in every nation.

The manpower limitation in surgery is usually misunderstood by people outside the field and sometimes even by large national surgical organizations. Because surgeons operate on specific disease entities, the requirement for surgeons is limited by the epidemiology and prevalence of those diseases. In many fields of surgery, 75% or more of the total operations performed may be devoted to a few disease entities. Thus, while the public "appetite" for family practitioners seems to be insatiable, that for surgeons is clearly limited. Failure to recognize this may lead to the training of an embarrassing and crippling excess of surgeons by postgraduate programs in the United States.

There is no point to expanding surgical training programs or recruiting additional people into surgery when the requirement for them is fixed and already met. Although many young people wish to enter surgery, boards of surgical examiners and colleges of surgeons must enforce strict and even "brutal" criteria to weed out everyone who cannot meet the highest standards. However, because it is not only uneconomic but also inhumane to cut people off at this late stage of their training, it is essential that potential incompetents be identified by in-house examinations as early as possible and be counseled accordingly.

Malpractice litigation is a major disincentive to surgical practice in the United States and accounts for 3 to 5% of the total financial cost of medical and surgical care. The problem arises from the lack of any statutes of limitation relating to the care of children, judgments, and legal fees. Lawyers' concern for the welfare of the "victims" of incompetent physicians is rarely accompanied by an equal concern about the victims receiving only a tiny fraction of the settlements awarded. Although there is a persisting need for high standards of quality assessment and constant surveillance of physicians for such damaging disorders as senility or drug and alcohol abuse, many crippling malpractice suits are launched against individuals who are delivering medical care of the highest quality. It is widely accepted in the press, with no basis in fact, that all malpractice judgments favoring the plaintiff reveal an incompetent practitioner.

The impotence of national surgical organizations in the United States in this area is largely the result of a lack of sound, relevant social research in collaboration with lawyers and judges. Other nations face or will soon face the same problem. Relief will come only from changes in public policy based on sound social research done by surgeons.

L'envoi

As we peer or peep over the horizon, we see many things promised and many challenges posed. On the basis of the past, many problems will be solved and many challenges will linger on.

It is my guess that two of the lingering challenges will be death from head injury and from widespread sepsis with multiple organ failure. In my own 50-year surgical career, to date, I have seen very little progress on either front. Such spotty advances as have been made have been overwhelmed, in some ways, by the larger number of early cases that have survived to show us the futility of existing modes of treatment.

Every professorial head of a surgical department should support an active research program that would, I hope, include health policy, the evaluation of clinical procedures used within the department and, most of all, a periodic assessment of the areas in which injured or diseased patients still die despite our best efforts.

Our future failures will be those of blindness to the power of surgical research and of lack of focus in research. We will possess both vision and research focus if the surgical profession of each nation supports its own research establishment, and the leading departments of surgery take bold new initiatives in the outstanding salients of surgical mortality. Such new ventures will be far more rewarding than the pursuit of small details down some well-trodden path and will be inspired only by surgeons who study their own patients.

Index

About the Editors

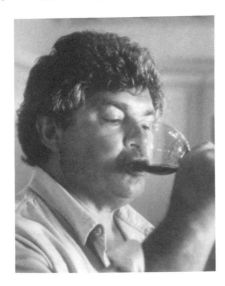

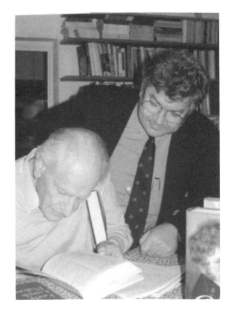

Hands Troidl with Sir Karl Popper.

Hans Troidl, Prof. Dr. med., Dr. h.c.
Professor and Chairman
II Department of Surgery
University of Cologne

Born in Bavaria in a small town, Schwarzenfeld,
July 5, 1938

Studied medicine in Munich, 1959–1964
Educated as a general surgeon in Munich by
Professor R. Zenker from 1964–1968;
in Marburg by Prof. H. Hamelmann 1969–1978;
in Kiel by Prof. H. Hamelmann from 1979–1981.

He has acted as Professor and Chairman at the
University of Cologne since 1981.

Main teachers:
    Peter Kiefhaber
    Wilfred Lorenz
    Prof. Hamelmann

    Prof. Goligher
    Sir Karl Popper
Main interests:
    Pathophysiology of duodenal ulcer
    Endoscopy
    Outcomes
    Epistemology

Awards:
Honorary Fellow of the Royal College of Sur-
    geons of England
Honorary Fellow of the Surgical Society of France
Doctor Honoris Causa, University of Bordeaux
Honorary Fellow of the Trauma Society of the
    American College of Surgeons

Married for thirty years to Ulla Troidl, with four
    children: Susanne, Christian, Stephan, and Va-
    nessa.

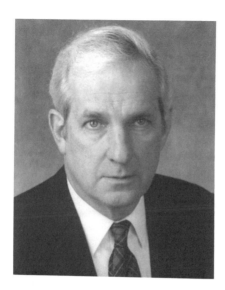

Martin F. McKneally

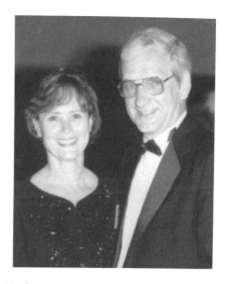

Dr. Martin McKneally with his wife, Deborah.

Martin F. McKneally received his M.D. from Cornell University Medical College. He completed general and cardiothoracic surgical training under Dr. Owen Wangensteen and Dr. Richard Varco at the University of Minnesota in 1968 and received his Ph.D. in immunology there in 1970 under Dr. Robert A. Good. He established an active academic clinical program focused on general thoracic surgery at the Albany Medical Center in Albany, New York. He was Professor of Surgery and Chief of the Division of Cardiothoracic Surgery at Albany Medical College until 1990. He was principal investigator for several NIH-sponsored laboratory and clinical studies testing the efficacy of stimulation of the immune system after surgical resection for lung cancer, the efficacy of surgery in coronary artery disease, and innovative adjuvant and surgical treatments in the Lung Cancer Study Group.

He served as Chairman of the Division of Thoracic Surgery at the University of Toronto from 1990 to 1995 and is currently Professor of Surgery at the University of Toronto, the Joint Centre for Bioethics, and The Toronto Hospital. His current research focus is on ethical issues in surgery and the education of surgeons in bioethics. He has served as a Director of the American Board of Thoracic Surgery, Secretary of the American Association for Thoracic Surgery, Co-Chairman of the AATS/STS Joint Committee on Video-Assisted Thoracic Surgery, and President of the Thoracic Surgery Directors Association. He is Vice-Chairman of the American College of Surgeons Committee on Emerging Surgical Technology, and President of the Thoracic Surgery Foundation for Research and Education.

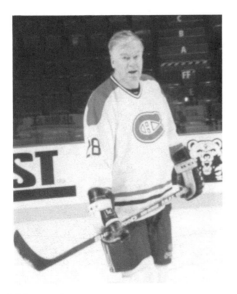

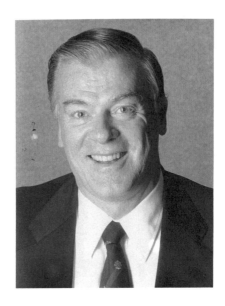

David S. Mulder

David S. Mulder was born in Eston, Saskatchewan, where he received his elementary education. He obtained an M.D. from the University of Saskatchewan in 1962. Rotating internship at the University Hospital in Saskatoon preceded a move to the Montreal General Hospital and McGill University where he did his entire general surgical training under the direction of Dr. Fraser N. Gurd. This was followed by training in cardiovascular thoracic surgery at the University of Iowa under the direction of Dr. J.L. Ehrenhaft. He then returned to the McGill University Department of Physiology where he completed a further year of research training under the supervision of Dr. David Bates. He received an M.Sc. in Experimental Surgery in 1965 for a thesis on "The Use of Percutaneous Left Heart Bypass in Hemorrhagic Shock."

Dr. Mulder was appointed to the staff of the Montreal General Hospital and McGill University on July 2, 1970. He was appointed Surgeon-in-Chief at the Montreal General Hospital on January 1, 1977, and continues to serve in this role. He was named Professor of Surgery at McGill University in 1978 and served as Chairman of the McGill Department of Surgery from 1983 to 1988, and from 1993 to the present. He has been President of the American Association for the Surgery of Trauma, the Trauma Association of Canada, and is presently Honorary President of the Pan-American Trauma Association. He is Chair of the Canadian Association of Surgical Chairmen and Vice President of the James IV Surgical Association.

Dr. Mulder's scientific interests have been in the field of cardiovascular surgery and trauma. His major research interests include basic investigations into the adult respiratory distress syndrome following hemorrhagic shock. This has more recently continued as basic investigations in the differentiation of pulmonary sepsis and acute rejection following lung transplantation. Studies in trauma have included laboratory and clinical investigations in airway trauma, peripheral vascular injury, and thoracic trauma. He has also been interested in improving the organization of trauma care in Canada and the United States and has worked actively as a member of the Committee on Trauma of the American College of Surgeons. Dr. Mulder's extracurricular activities have always included sports-related activities. He is currently on the medical team of the Montreal Canadiens and Director of the McGill Sports Medicine Centre.

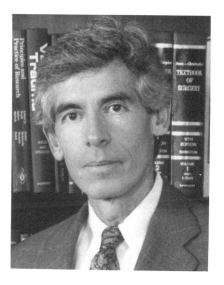

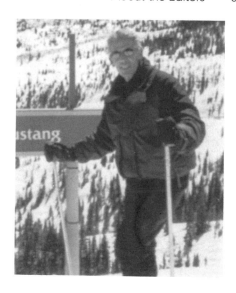

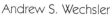

Andrew S. Wechsler

Andrew S. Wechsler, M.D., is the Stuart McGuire Professor of Surgery at the Medical College of Virginia of Virginia Commonwealth University where he serves as Chairman of the Department of Surgery. He is also Professor of Physiology and Head of the Division of Cardiothoracic Surgery. After two years of medical training at the Peter Bent Brigham Hospital in Boston, he spent two years in the laboratory of Dr. Eugene Braunwald, and subsequently received his surgical training at Duke University Medical Center. He served on the Duke faculty for 14 years. He is author or coauthor of over 300 scientific articles and has participated actively in the postdoctoral training of 19 research fellows who have worked in his laboratory. He served as Chairman of the Surgery and Bioengineering Study Section of the National Institutes of Health and is on several editorial boards including those of *Circulation,* the *Journal of Cardiac Surgery,* and the *Journal of Thoracic and Cardiovascular Surgery.* He has served on the Research Committee of the American Heart Association, as Vice-Chairman of the Forum Committee of the American College of Surgeons, and as a Director of the American Board of Thoracic Surgery. He is a member of the Research and Education Committee of the American College of Surgeons and is Treasurer of the American Association of Thoracic Surgery.

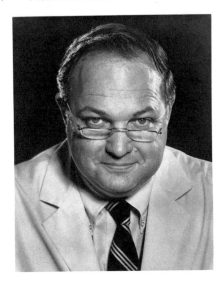

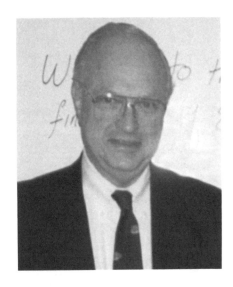

Bucknam McPeek

Bucknam McPeek, M.D., has been a student and teacher at Harvard University since 1951. He received his A.B. in 1955, his M.D. in 1959, and holds the certificate in Health Systems Management from the Harvard Graduate School of Business Administration. After a year on the Harvard Surgical Service at the Boston City Hospital, he became resident in Anesthesia at the Massachusetts General Hospital under Professor Henry Beecher. He joined the faculty in 1962 and is currently Associate Professor of Anaesthesia at Harvard University, Anesthetist to the Massachusetts General Hospital, and Director of its Acute Pain Service. For more than 20 years he has served as Deputy Director of the Harvard Anaesthesia Center and the Anaesthesia Research Training Program. He has taught in Harvard College and three of its graduate schools. His major research interests lie in population studies of risk and postoperative outcome, research on the assessment of health and medical practices, and information-gathering strategies for policymaking. He served as coeditor of the journal *Theoretical Surgery.* A previous book, *Data for Decisions,* is widely used in policy courses in graduate schools of government, business, and public health.

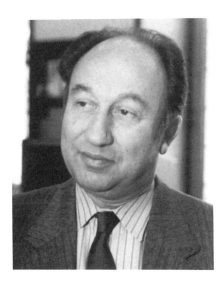

Walter O. Spitzer

Walter O. Spitzer graduated in medicine from the University of Toronto in 1962. After completing postgraduate studies in health administration at the University of Michigan and in epidemiology at Yale University, he joined the Faculty of Biostatistics at McMaster University in 1969. In 1975 he was appointed Professor of Epidemiology at McGill University, with a cross appointment in Medicine. He was at McGill until 1995, serving as Strathcona Professor and Chairman of the Department from 1984. During his tenure in Montreal, he was appointed National Health Scientist of Canada (1980) and elected to be a member of the Institute of Medicine of the National Academy of Sciences of the USA in 1985. He was editor of the *Journal of Clinical Epidemiology* from 1980 until 1995, and also founded the Canadian medical journal, *Clinical and Investigative Medicine,* in 1979. Today he serves as Professor Emeritus at McGill University and is Clinical Professor of Medicine at Stanford University, as well as Research Professor in the School of Medicine at the University of California at San Francisco (UCSF). He is Senior Epidemiologist and Director at Genentech, Inc., San Francisco.

Professor Spitzer has published 101 original, peer-reviewed articles in subject areas that include clinical epidemiology, cancer epidemiology, environmental epidemiology, health services research, the measurement of quality of life, and pharmacoepidemiology. A keen interest throughout his career in research and teaching has been the development of methods in clinical investigation and epidemiology. In recent years he has pursued his methodological interest in close collaboration with surgical and academic colleagues, focusing on measures of quality of life and other outcomes of clinical interventions.